The Science and Practice of Intramedullary Nailing

Second Edition

The Science and Practice of Intramedullary Nailing

Second Edition

Bruce D. Browner, M.D.

Gray Gossling Professor and Chairman
Department of Orthopaedic Surgery
University of Connecticut Health Center
School of Medicine
Farmington, Connecticut

Director
Department of Orthopaedic Surgery
Hartford Hospital
Hartford, Connecticut

SANS TACHE

Williams & Wilkins

BALTIMORE • PHILADELPHIA • HONG KONG
LONDON • MUNICH • SYDNEY • TOKYO

A WAVERLY COMPANY

1996

Executive Editor: Darlene B. Cooke
Managing Editor: Fran Klass
Production Coordinator: Danielle Santucci
Project Editor: Susan Sfarra

Williams & Wilkins
Rose Tree Corporate Center
1400 North Providence Road
Building II, Suite 5025
Media, PA 19063-2043 USA

Accurate indications, adverse reactions, and dosage schedules for drugs are provided in this book, but it is possible they may change. The reader is urged to review the package information data of the manufacturers of the medications mentioned.

Printed in the United States of America

First Edition 1987

Library of Congress Cataloging in Publication Data

The science and practice of intramedullary nailing / [edited by] Bruce
D. Browner. — 2nd ed.
p. cm.
Includes bibliographical references and index.
ISBN 0-683-01123-5
1. Intramedullary fracture fixation. I. Browner, Bruce D.
[DNLM: 1. Fracture Fixation, Intramedullary—methods. WE 185
S416 1995]
RD103.I53S35 1995
617.1′5—dc20
DNLM/DLC
for Library of Congress 95-14195
CIP

The Publishers have made every effort to trace the copyright holders for borrowed material. If they have inadvertently overlooked any, they will be pleased to make the necessary arrangements at the first opportunity.

96 97 98 99
1 2 3 4 5 6 7 8 9 10

Reprints of chapters may be purchased from Williams & Wilkins in quantities of 100 or more. Call Isabella Wise, Special Sales Department, (800) 358-3583.

Dedicated to Barbara

whose love and wisdom
have supported and guided
me for twenty-five years.

Preface

The first edition of this book published in 1987 was an outgrowth of a meeting entitled "Intramedullary Nailing—An Advanced Course and Symposium," which was held in Baltimore, Maryland, May 7 and 8, 1982. The faculty included surgeon developers of the most important modern nails from the United States and Europe. More than 300 orthopaedic surgeons from 42 states attended this meeting to listen to lectures and participate in workshops that were supervised by these leaders in intramedullary nailing. Although the chapters, which subsequently composed the text, paralleled the basic science and clinical topics of the lectures, manuscripts for the text were prepared as separate text book chapters not in the form of the recorded symposium. Additional clinical experience was incorporated into the chapters, which were written over the 4 years subsequent to the meeting. The final text was an accurate reflection of the state of the art of intramedullary nailing in the mid-1980s.

Almost a full decade has passed since the first edition of this book was written. Availability of the locking nails, which have broadened the indications for closed intramedullary nailing in all of the long bones, has led to the wide spread adoption of these techniques for the femur, tibia, and humerus. Many manufacturers have produced variations of the original locking nails. While some have maintained designs that closely resemble the original clover leaf cross section of Küntscher, others have produced closed-section implants which no longer bear the longitudinal slot. Some companies have changed from stainless steel to new alloys containing titanium and other metals. Certain implants that were used more extensively at the time of publication of the first edition have been used much less frequently, as surgeons have turned to the closed intramedullary nailing technique employing these newer implants. Ender nails, which were used in the early 1980s to treat fractures of the proximal femur and the shafts of the femur, tibia, and humerus, have been abandoned by all but a few surgeons in the United States. The chapters relating to these techniques have not been included in the second edition. Nails developed by Dana Street, M.D. and Robert Zickel, M.D., which were not cannulated, were inserted primarily with an open nailing technique. For this reason, they have been replaced in most hospitals by the cannulated locking nails, which can be inserted by closed nailing techniques. Original chapters covering these now less popular techniques were also not included in the second edition.

A second generation of locking femoral intramedullary nails has been developed to decrease the likelihood of implant failure and improve the fixation and rate of union of complex proximal femoral fractures. The Reconstruction Nail, developed by Thomas Russell, M.D. and Charles Taylor, M.D. is the first device in this class. Since its original introduction, a number of other manufacturers have developed similar implants. The majority of these devices contain two diagonal channels in the proximal end through which lag screws are inserted upward into the femoral neck and head. The enlarged proximal diameter and increased wall thickness of these nails is designed to resist the high forces in the subtrochanteric area. The second generation of femoral locking nails allows secure fixation of fractures that are more proximal in the femur than those which could be treated with the first generation locking nails. The deforming forces of muscle pull on subtrochanteric fractures and the subtle differences in implant geometry and instrumentation between the devices produced by different manufacturers has made the use of these second generation nails more complex and demanding than standard locked intramedullary nailing of femoral shaft fractures. When used correctly, these devices have led to excellent results in these historically problematic fractures.

Stuart Green, M.D., David Seligson, M.D., and Steven Henry, M.D. have developed a specialized locking supracondylar nail that is inserted retrograde to the distal end of the femur. This implant, which is similar in design to the Huckstep nail, permits closed intramedullary fixation of fractures more distal than those that could previously be fixed with the standard first generation locking nail. Many of these fractures were previously treated by open reduction using blade plates, distal condylar screws, or condylar buttress plates. Although these techniques have given excellent results, the supracondylar nail can be inserted with less dissection having the theoretical advantage of lower infection and higher union rates.

Since the last edition, small-diameter, locking nails have been developed to be inserted into the tibia without reaming. Following a number of successive reports concerning the use of this technique in the treatment of open tibia fractures, there has been a widespread decrease in the use of external fixation as surgeons have switched to this new technique. In retrospect, because of the great consistency in the earlier results obtained by Otto Lottes, M.D. in his extensive series of unreamed tibial nailings, which contained a large number of open fractures, the chapter that he wrote for the first edition has been retained even though the nail bearing his name is now used much less frequently.

A variety of other specialized intramedullary devices have been developed in the last 10 years including the intramedullary hip screw, locking nails for the humerus, implants for the radius and ulna, the limb-lengthening rod for the femur, and the self-guiding nail that was designed to eliminate the difficulties associated with the distal transfixion screw insertion and standard first generation locking nails. Chapters covering these techniques have been included in the second edition. The basic science section at the beginning of the book has also been revised to reflect new information on bone vascularity, biomechanics, and fat embolization.

The authors discuss the design rationale, indications, surgical technique, pitfalls and complications, and results from using each intramedullary device. Numerous manufacturers have produced locking nails for the shafts of the femur, tibia, and humerus. Although the chapters on these portions of the anatomy may include illustrations of a particular implant, the authors' comments should be interpreted to apply to an entire class of nails of which the illustrated device serves as a generic example. Although the general principle discussed may be germane, a surgeon wishing to use another similar device would have to follow the manufacturers surgical technique closely to avoid specific system related pitfalls. I believe that this text strikes an excellent balance between theoretical and practical information, and I hope that it will be of use to orthopaedic and trauma surgeons in training and in practice.

Farmington, Connecticut

Bruce D. Browner

Acknowledgments

I am grateful to the authors and their staffs for compiling the text and illustrations for their contributions. As chapter writing receives little formal academic recognition, their willingness to share their experience and present organized discussions of this subject matter represents a true commitment to teaching. I am grateful to Darlene Cooke, the Executive Editor of this project, for convincing me to produce the second edition of *The Science and Practice of Intramedullary Nailing.* Her sensitivity, patience, and professionalism have been a source of support and guidance during all phases of the construction of this second edition.

Special thanks go to Fran Klass, Managing Editor, who worked closely with Laurie Michaud of my office, communicating through countless letters, faxes and phone conversations with the authors and their assistants to keep the work on schedule and to ensure the necessary components of the manuscripts, illustrations, and permissions were submitted. I would also like to thank Susan Sfarra, the Production Editor for this book, whose skill as a copy editor resulted in stylistic and grammatical improvements in our writing while preserving its scientific content.

Contributors

Samuel G. Agnew, M.D.
Assistant Professor
Head, Section of Trauma
Department of Orthopaedic Surgery
University of Arkansas for Medical Sciences
Little Rock, Arkansas

Samir N. Azer, M.D.
Associate Professor Orthopaedic Surgery
Howard University
Chief of Orthopaedic Surgery
Greater Southeast Community Hospital
Washington, DC
Chief of Orthopaedic Surgery
Fort Washington Hospital
Fort Washington, Maryland

Joan E. Bechtold, Ph.D.
Director, Orthopaedic Biomechanics Laboratory
Midwest Orthopaedic Research Foundation
Hennepin County Medical Center
Assistant Professor, Department of Orthopaedic Surgery
University of Minnesota
Associate Professor, Department of Biomedical Engineering
University of Minnesota
Minneapolis, Minnesota

Frederick S. Bennett, M.D.
On Staff in Orthopaedic Surgery
University of Tennessee Medical Center
Knoxville, Tennessee
Courtesy Staff Privileges in Orthopaedic Surgery
Fort Sanders Regional Medical Center
Academic Faculty, University of Tennessee Medical Center at Knoxville
Clinical Instructor, Department of Surgery
Knoxville, Tennessee

Bruce D. Browner, M.D.
Gray Gossling Professor and Chairman
Department of Orthopaedic Surgery
University of Connecticut Health Center
School of Medicine
Farmington, Connecticut
Director, Department of Orthopaedics
Hartford Hospital
Hartford, Connecticut

Michael W. Chapman, M.D.
Professor and Chairman, Department of Orthopaedic Surgery
University of California, Davis
Chief, Orthopaedic Trauma Service, UCD Medical Center
Davis, California

J. Dean Cole, M.D.
Matthews Orthopaedic Clinic
Orlando, Florida

Charles M. Court-Brown, M.D., F.R.C.S.(E.D.) Orth.
Consultant Orthopaedic Surgeon
Edinburgh Orthopaedic Trauma Unit
Royal Infirmary of Edinburgh
Edinburgh, Scotland

William G. DeLong, Jr., M.D.
Associate Professor of Surgery
Robert Wood Johnson Medical School
Chief, Division of Orthopaedic Surgery
Cooper Hospital/University Medical Center
Adjunct Clinical Assistant Professor of Orthopaedic Surgery
Hospital of the University of Pennsylvania
Adjunct Clinical Assistant Professor of Orthopaedic Surgery
Thomas Jefferson Hospital
Philadelphia, Pennsylvania

William R. Dobozi, M.D.
Professor of Orthopaedic Surgery
Loyola University Medical Center
Maywood, Illinois

Victor H. Frankel, K.N.O., M.D., Ph.D.
President, Hospital for Joint Diseases
Orthopaedic Institute
Professor, Orthopaedic Surgery
New York University
New York, New York

Robert F. Hall, Jr., M.D.
Associate Professor of Orthopaedic Surgery
University of Illinois
Chairman, Department of Orthopaedic Surgery
Cook County Hospital
Chicago, Illinois

Sigvard T. Hansen, Jr., M.D.
Professor and Chairman Emeritus
Department of Orthopaedics
University of Washington and
Harborview Medical Center
Seattle, Washington

M. Bradford Henley, M.D.
Associate Professor, Orthopaedic Surgery
Harborview Medical Center
Department of Orthopaedic Surgery
University of Washington
Seattle, Washington

James F. Kellam, B.Sc., M.D., F.R.C.S.(C.), F.A.C.S.
Vice Chairman of Orthopaedic Surgery
Carolina Medical Center
Charlotte, North Carolina

Klaus Klemm, M.D.
Head of the Department of Posttraumatic Osteomyelitis
BG-Unfallklinik Frankfurt Am Main
Germany

Kenneth J. Koval, M.D.
Orthopaedic Fracture Service
Hospital for Joint Diseases
Orthopaedic Institute
New York, New York

William R. Krause, Ph.D.
Adjunct Associate Professor
Department of Mechanical Engineering
Department of Orthopaedic Surgery
University of Virginia
Charlottesville, Virginia

Frederick Kummer, Ph.D.
Associate Director, Bioengineering (HJD-OI)
Research Professor, Department of Orthopaedics
New York University Medical School
New York, New York

Richard F. Kyle, M.D.
Chairman, Department of Orthopaedic Surgery
Hennepin County Medical Center
Associate Professor, Department of Orthopaedic Surgery
University of Minnesota
Minneapolis, Minnesota

J. Otto Lottes, M.D.*
St. Louis, Missouri
*Deceased

Keith Mayo, M.D.
Department of Orthopaedics
Hutzel Hospital
Detroit, Michigan

Sven Olerud, M.D.
Professor Emeritus
Former Head of the Orthopaedic Department
University Hospital
Uppsala, Sweden

Hans Christophe Pape, M.D.
Department of Trauma Surgery
Hannover Medical School
Hannover, Germany

Stephan M. Perren, M.D.
Professor Dr. Med. Dr. Sci.(H.C.) Chirurgie FMH
Davos, Switzerland

Gerd Regel, M.D.
Department of Trauma Surgery
Hannover Medical School
Hannover, Germany

Barry L. Riemer, M.D.
Professor of Orthopaedic Surgery
Director, Division of Orthopaedic Fractures
Medical College of Pennsylvania/
Hahnemann University
Allegheny General Hospital
Pittsburgh, Pennsylvania

Thomas A. Russell, M.D.
Associate Professor of Orthopaedic Surgery
University of Tennessee Center for Health Science
Staff Surgeon, Methodist Hospital
Memphis, Tennessee

David Seligson, M.D., F.A.A.O.S., F.A.C.S.
Professor and Vice Chairman
Department of Orthopaedics
University of Louisville
Chief, Fracture Service
University of Louisville Hospital
Attending Orthopedist, Louisville Baptist Hospital, Norton's Hospital and Kosair Children's Hospital
Louisville, Kentucky

Dana M. Street, M.D.
Professor Emeritus of Orthopaedic Surgery
Loma Linda and UCLA Universities
Courtesy Staff, Orthopaedic Hospital
Los Angeles, California

Harald Tscherne, M.D.
Professor and Director
Department of Trauma Surgery
Hannover Medical School
Hannover, Germany

Robert G. Veith, M.D.
Clinical Associate Professor
University of Washington
Department of Orthopaedic Surgery
Seattle, Washington

Robert A. Winquist, M.D.
Clinical Professor of Orthopaedics
University of Washington
Seattle, Washington

Mark Wolgin, M.D.
Clinical Instructor, Adult Foot and Ankle Orthopaedic Clinic
Harbor/UCLA Medical Center
Private Practice
Torrance, California

Daniel M. Zinar, M.D.
Chief, Division of Orthopaedic Surgery
Chief, Orthopaedic Trauma Service
Harbor/UCLA Medical Center
Associate Clinical Professor
Department of Orthopaedics
UCLA School of Medicine
Los Angeles, California

Contents

Section V. The Upper Extremity

Section VI. Special Techniques

1

The Evolution of Intramedullary Nailing

Dana M. Street

Intramedullary nailing is one of this century's greatest advances in the treatment of fractures. While there was considerable development in intramedullary nailing during the first decade, there has also been much in the sixth or last decade. I have been privileged to be a first-hand observer and participant in this development.

Prior to the use of metal nails, intramedullary fixation was sporadic. The first instance was reported by the Conquistadors in the 16th century. They observed that the Incas and Aztecs used resinous wooden pegs in the medullary canal of long bones for the treatment of nonunions.[1] This report is found in a brief paragraph in the Spanish archives, but the report gives no details of technique, numbers employed, or results. No excavations to date have found bones confirming the Conquistadors' report.

Ivory pegs were used by Bircher[2] and others in 1886 and again were reported by König of Germany in 1913.[3] The ivory peg grafts apparently worked well if strict asepsis could be maintained. They did not become encapsulated like a foreign body, such as a bullet, but gradually underwent resorption over a period of years. Hoglund reported the use of bone rather than ivory pegs in 1917.[4]

Lambotte of Belgium employed grooved nails in the clavicle and also long screws inserted at the tip of the greater trochanter and extending into the medullary canal of the proximal third of the femur for intertrochanteric and subtrochanteric fractures about 1907. This was reported in his book in 1913[5] and by Soeur[6] in 1946, who also cites Joly's use of Kirschner wires in the clavicle and smaller bones and Danis' use of Kirschner wires in the forearm. Nicolaysen of Norway is credited by Watson-Jones as being the father of intramedullary nailing. He outlined the principles of intramedullary nailing in an 1897 publication,[7] emphasizing the need to span the canal with nails of maximum length. However, his work appears to be confined to the femoral neck rather than the shaft.

The first use of rods which filled the medullary canal and extended the entire length in long bones appears to be the work of Schöne of the Kiel clinic in Germany. In his report in 1913,[8] he describes his use of 3 and 4 mm square, silver rods in the radius and ulna and he details how they controlled rotation. The silver tended to control any bacterial contamination. Also included in the report was the mention of a suitable extractor. Apparently this report has been overlooked by later investigators who speak of the great difficulty in treating the forearm, particularly the radius.

Hey Groves of England used intramedullary fixation on gunshot femur fractures during World War I. He used a long cortical graft in one case. However, in three cases nails were used which closely resembled nails currently used. Hey Groves had three patterns, a perforated tube, a rod with X-shaped cross section, and a solid rod (presumably round), which he preferred because it had no crevices to harbor infection.[9] The nails filled the canal, but extended only about 3 inches into the distal fragment. All the nailings failed, the patient with the bone graft died after amputation, and he apparently abandoned the method with no further trials, as no further reports can be found.

In 1937, L.V. Rush and H.L. Rush contributed the first American description of intramedullary fixation, since the report of the Conquistadors. They used medullary Steinman pins for ulnar fractures[10] and later (1939) reported pin fixation for femoral fractures as well.[11] L.V. Rush went on to develop a flexible nail system, including four different diameters of pins for use in all parts of the body, which were described in his book published in 1956.[12] Other early reports of the use of medullary wires include those of Lambrinudi[13] (forearm and femur) in 1940, Murray[14] (clavicle) in 1940, and the American surgeon Dickson (forearm) in 1944.[15]

Successful intramedullary nailing, as we know it, began during World War II with the work of Küntscher, whose first publication appeared in 1940.[16] In the following divisions, the history and evolution of intramedullary nailing is divided into six decades that serve as a convenient time frame for the various developments.

THE FIRST DECADE (1940 TO 1949)

Küntscher's initial work with animals employed three-flanged nails similar to those used for the femoral neck. However, his first presentation of the method as used in humans described the V-shaped nail which filled the canal and was also compressible, providing a snug fit for greater stability. By the time of his first publication, the Küntscher method was already well advanced and it even included the Y nail for intertrochanteric fractures.

Although other orthopedists in Germany at first resisted the concept of intramedullary nailing and regarded it as unphysiologic,[17] the advantages were so apparent that they soon concurred and reports began to appear by Küntscher's colleagues. Under the impetus of World War II, the method quickly spread throughout Germany and Austria and later into France and Italy. By the end of 1942, there were over 38 references to intramedullary nailing in the European literature by 20 surgeons, as found in the combined lists of Böhler and Küntscher.

Noteworthy among the early reports was one by his chief, Fischer, and associate, Maatz, describing instrumentation for the method.[18] These included a windlass type of extractor, the C-shaped extractor which became standard (Fig. 1–1), and also a windlass traction apparatus. Maatz, who had a degree in engineering before studying medicine, was a gadgeteer, and according to Alvis,[19] he played a major role in the development of the sound mechanical principles of the method and design of nails and instrumentation. Among other contributors was Stör, who implemented an extractor consisting of a rod with a hook at one end that inserted into the eye of the nail and a heavy, weighted sleeve that slid along the rod, impacting against a stop at the other end.[20]

The first book on the subject by Küntscher and Maatz was written for publication in 1942, but because of the war, it was not published until late 1944.[21] The text on intramedullary nailing was a limited edition of only 1000 copies, half of which disappeared.[19] In the preface to this book by their Kiel clinic chief, Fischer, there is a clear statement of the essence of the Küntscher method.

> The essential feature of the Küntscher method is the introduction of a foreign body from a place apart from the fracture site, which differs from all other methods of operative treatment. Through the use of a specially shaped, very stable, properly constructed nail-like splint, which forges an elastic union with the inner surface of the marrow cavity, the greatest possible stability of the fracture is achieved, so that further support by plaster cast or traction apparatus is not required. By this method the disadvantage of a prolonged immobility is avoided.

The difficult part of the closed nailing procedure, that of reducing the fragments to align the canal, was initially performed using circumferential straps above and below the fracture, which were pulled transversely in opposite directions by ropes anchored to hooks in the walls of the operating room[18] (Fig. 1–2). The reduction, however, was more easily accomplished with the apparatus of Linsmayer,[22] in which lateral traction was applied by windlasses in a frame allowing freer access to the operating table (Fig. 1–3). A similar effect was achieved with the reduction apparatus of Wittmoser[23] using gear-controlled rings (Fig.

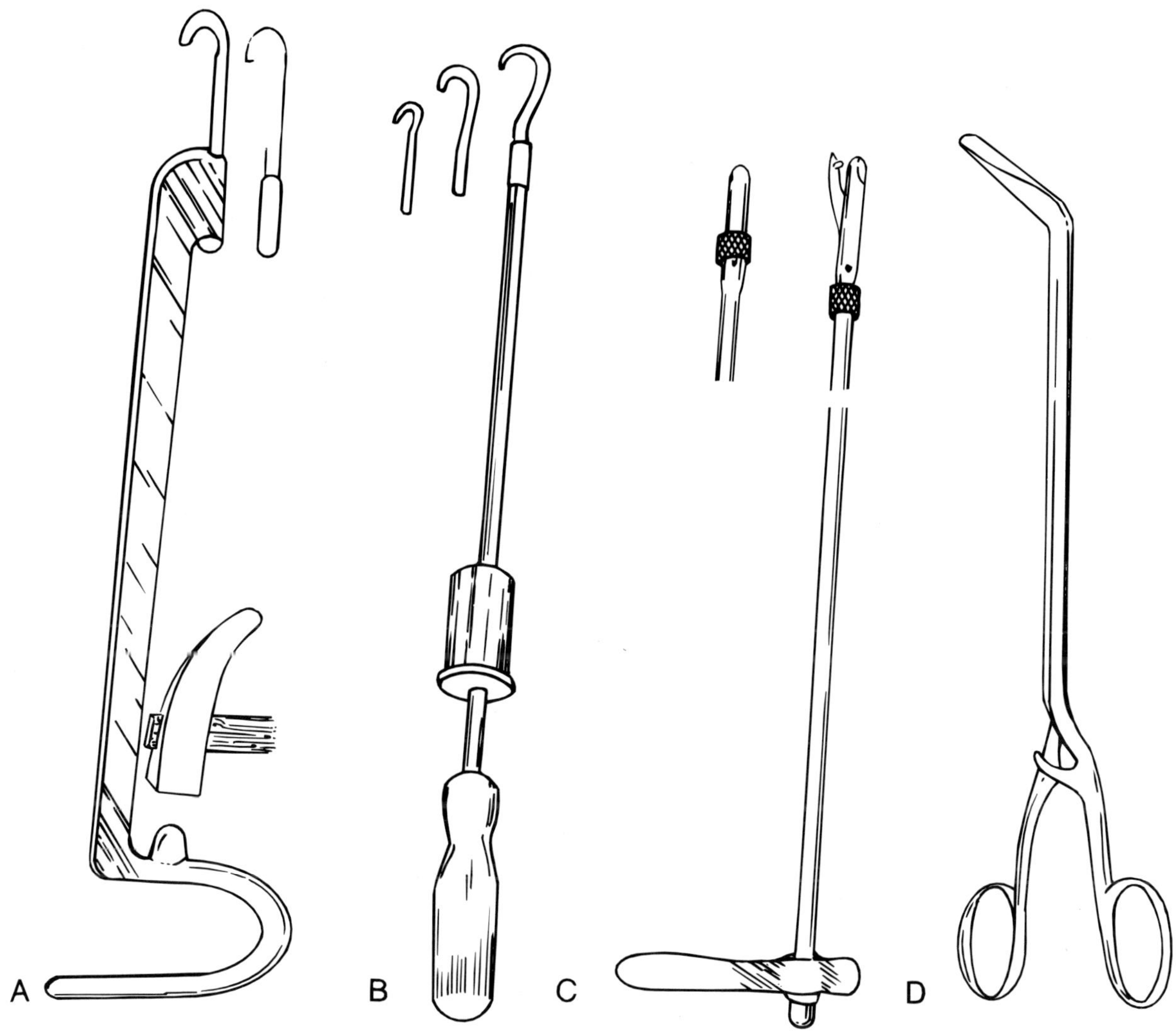

Fig. 1–1. *A,* C-shaped extractor designed by Maatz. *B,* Slide weight extractor designed by Stör. *C,* Toothed extractor designed by Westerborn. *D,* Intramedullary forceps designed by Maatz.

1–4). Unless they were well padded, the rings would appear to cause contusion of the muscles if applied over an extended period.

Küntscher later used a crutch with a strap applied near the large end (Fig. 1–5) that would control both fragments and used the crutch as a long lever arm. This appears in his book in 1962.[49] Currently, we are using two tennis rackets with the strings removed that are slipped over the extremity when it is placed in traction. The metal-framed rackets show better than the wooden ones in the image intensifier view when positioned above and below the fracture site (Fig. 1–6).

By 1943 most of the apparatus and nail patterns had been designed and included the change from the V-shaped nail to the cloverleaf nail for use in the femur. The cloverleaf nail provides greater strength and follows a guide pin better.

By the end of 1944, 60 investigators had published 150 articles on Küntscher nailing. Böhler[24] reviewed over 500 cases, including 236 from his own clinic. In 1944, he published Volume III of his book *The Technique of Fracture Treatment in Peace and War*, which was devoted entirely to the medullary nailing of Küntscher. He thought it was time to restrain enthusiasm for this new method and called attention to serious complications.

Küntscher and Maatz had developed intramedullary nailing for the femur, tibia,

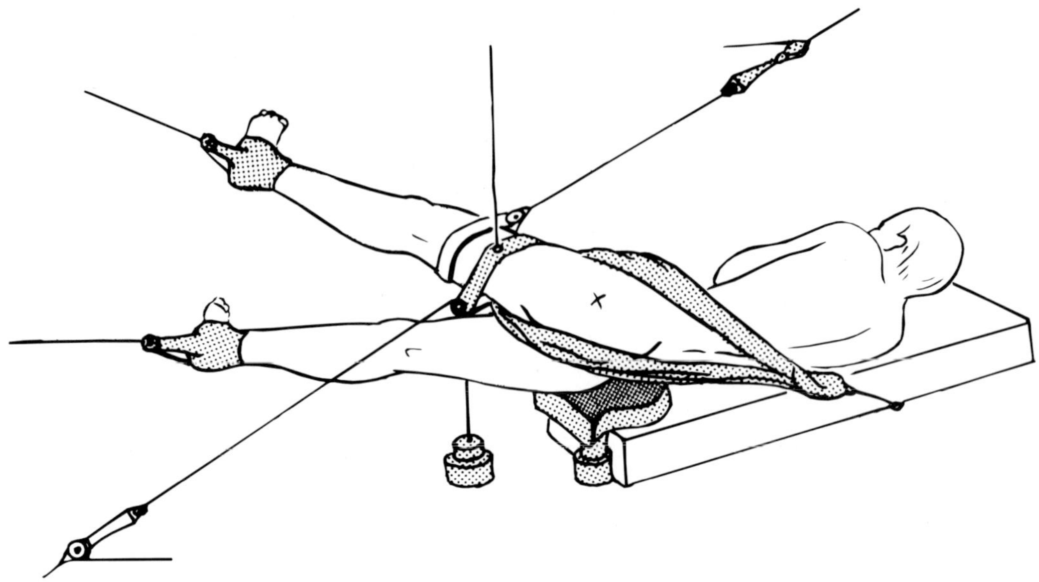

Fig. 1–2. Early closed reduction performed with the use of multiple slings.

humerus, and forearm. Although Böhler recognized the great advantages of this method for femoral fractures, he restricted its use in his clinic for all other bones.[25] The fatalities attributed to fat embolism following immediate open nailing were felt to result from the combination of fat embolism, initial shock from injury, and the trauma of extensive surgery. Therefore, he held that open nailing should not be performed in an emergency situation and advised nailing after the patient's condition was stable. Böhler felt primary closed nailing was acceptable, and he delayed nailing of open fractures until after debridement.

In summary, at the end of the first 5 years, Küntscher had established a method with highly developed instrumentation that had undergone trial in hundreds of cases in Europe, although there was little knowledge of it in North America. The method was based on two principles. First, it provided a stable fixation that allowed the patient to return immediately to normal activities. This was done by using longer nails than those of Hey Groves and larger nails

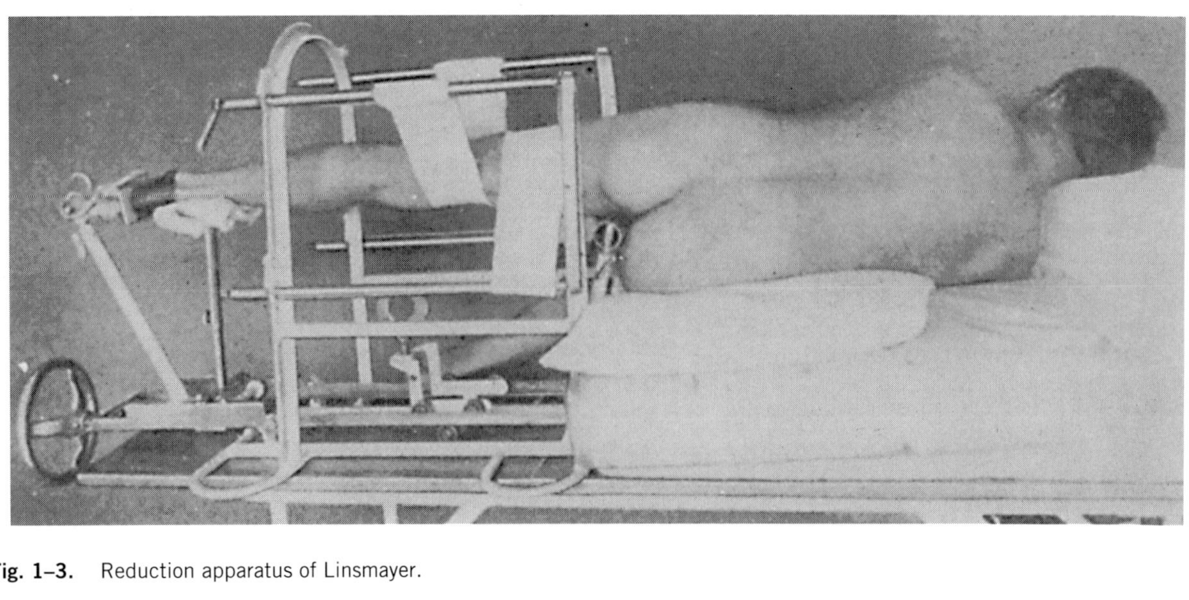

Fig. 1–3. Reduction apparatus of Linsmayer.

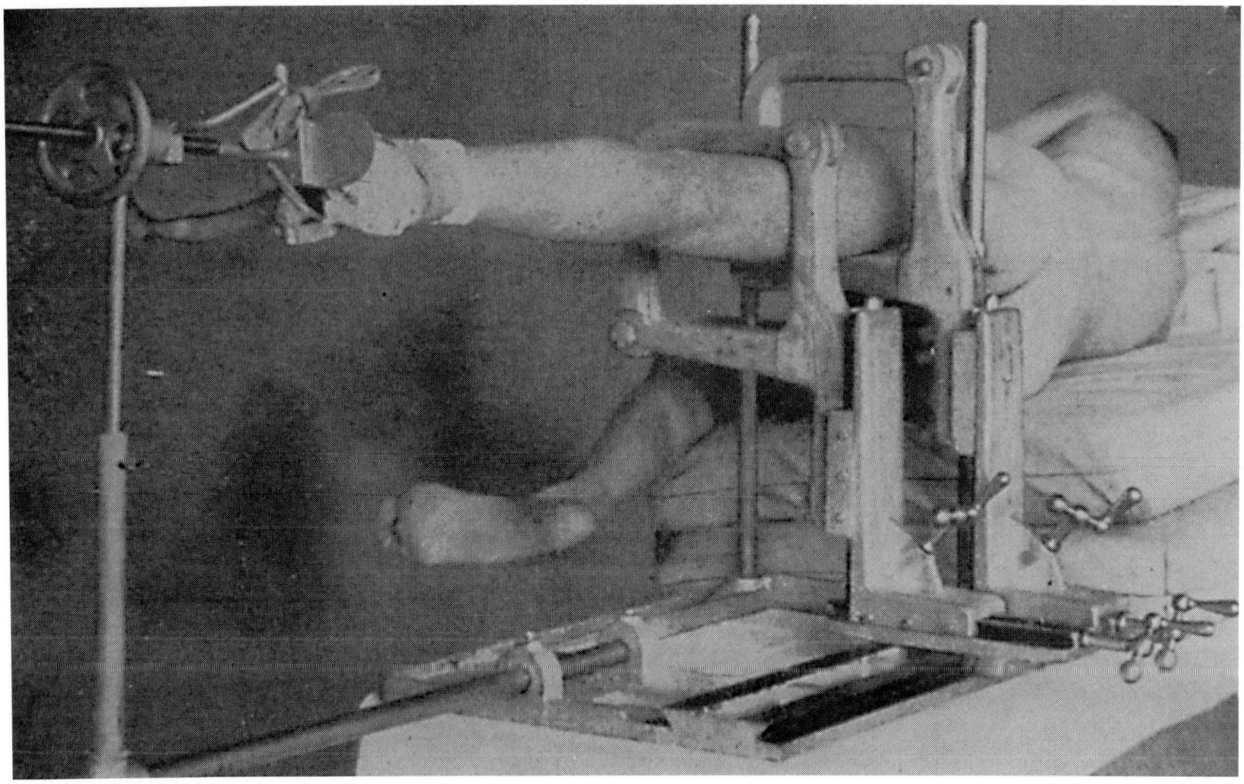

Fig. 1–4. Reduction apparatus of Wittmoser.

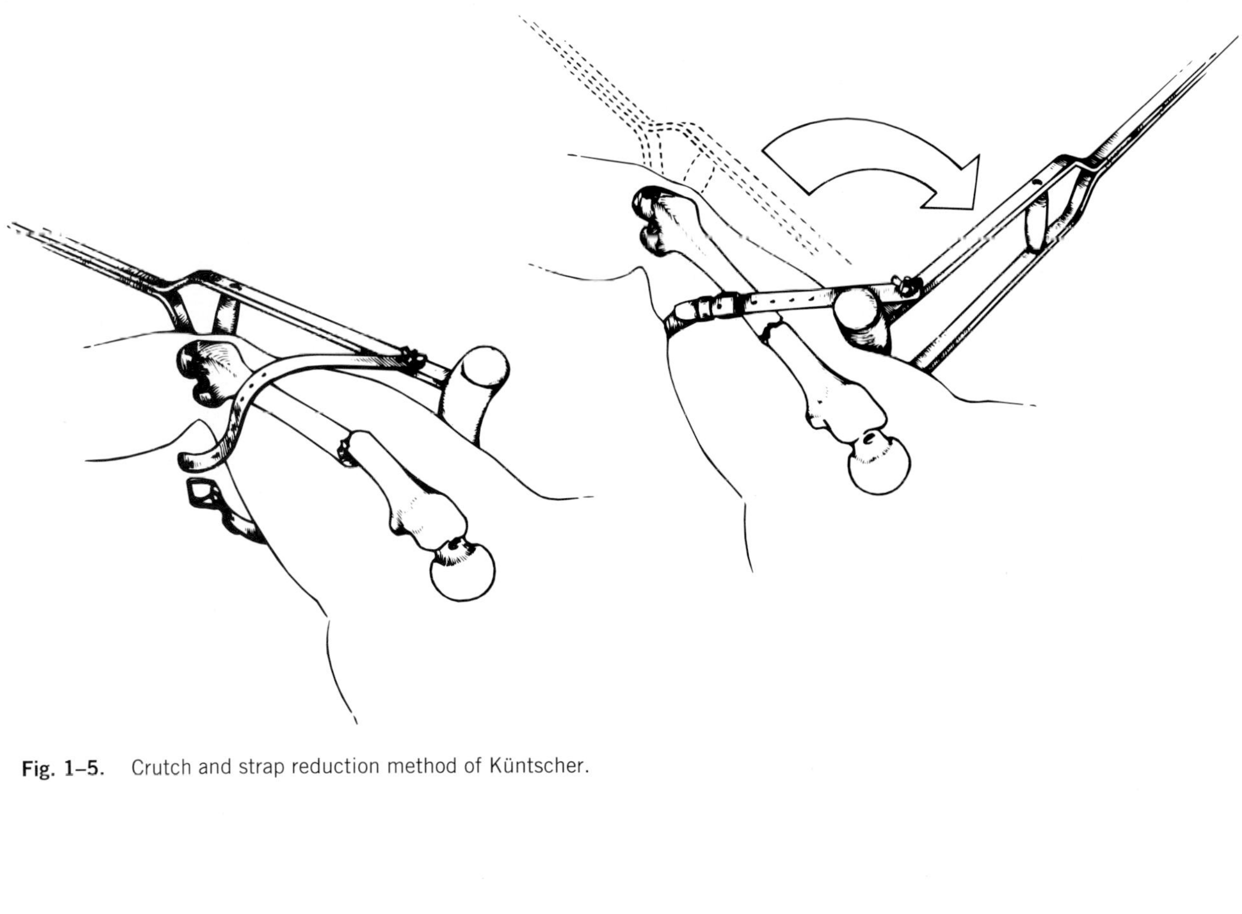

Fig. 1–5. Crutch and strap reduction method of Küntscher.

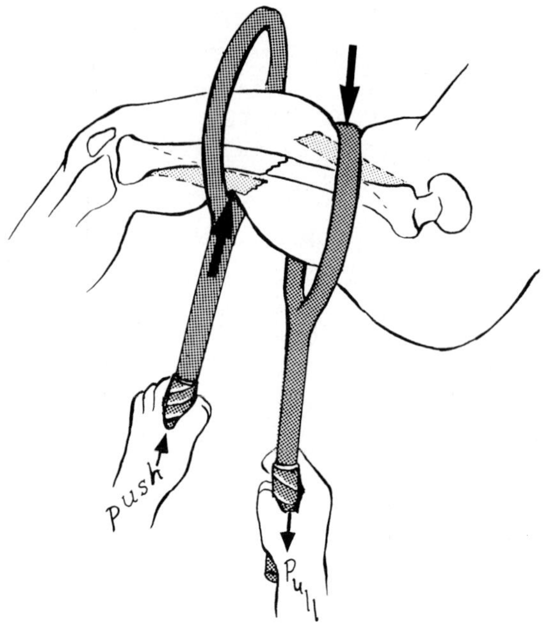

Fig. 1–6. Reduction with two tennis rackets, pushing with one and pulling with the other.

than the bolts of Müller-Meernach.[26] These nails were compressible to give a snug fit. Küntscher compared the holding power of his nail to a nail driven into wood, where the compressible wood binds the firm nail, and similarly the compressible nail binds in the firm bone (Fig. 1–7). However, this is only true when fixing isthmus fractures where the nail obtains a snug fit on both sides.

The second principle was that of closed nailing, with the point of insertion far-removed from the fracture site. Closed nailing limits the damage to parosteal soft tissues and blood supply, thereby lowering the risk of infection and nonunion. Prior to the development of the image intensifier, radiographic control of reduction and nailing required the use of the head fluoroscope (Fig. 1–8). This resulted in the surgeon's thyroid being exposed to excessive radiation.

Other similar nails developed during World War II included those of Soeur and Westerborn. Soeur's nails[27] were grooved, round V2A steel bars (essentially Küntscher U-shaped) with a sharp, oblique point on one end and an eye at the other. His nails were relatively small, less than 9 mm for the femur, but straight, thereby wedging into the irregular bowed canal. The nails were long enough to transverse the entire length of the femur (Fig. 1–9).

He used the Stör extractor and a novel driver with a sleeve containing a punch that had graduations showing the nail penetration (and also the extent of nail protrusion above the bone.) He began nailing in 1943 and by the time of his report in 1946, he had a series of 55 cases including 23 nailed femora, 10 nailed tibiae, 9 nailed humeri, and 16 nailed forearm bones.

Westerborn of Gothenburg, Sweden, also began nailing in 1943. He reported his first 28 cases in 1944,[28] but later noted that there had been little in American literature concerning "marrow nailing". He therefore published his expanded series of 100 cases in the *Annals of Surgery* in 1948.[29] He discussed the three major concerns of the earlier investigators and of the profession at large, namely, the risks of fat embolism, osteomyelitis, and possible anemia. Loss of marrow had little significance because many amputees had lost much more marrow with no ill effects. Fat embolism, though a cer-

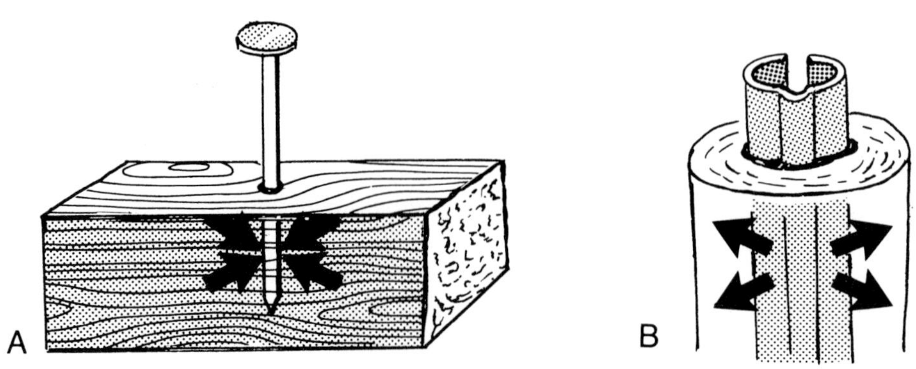

Fig. 1–7. *A,* The nail achieves fixation in the wood through the elastic compression of the wood. *B,* The cloverleaf Küntscher nail achieves fixation in the isthmus through the elastic expansion of the compressed nail.

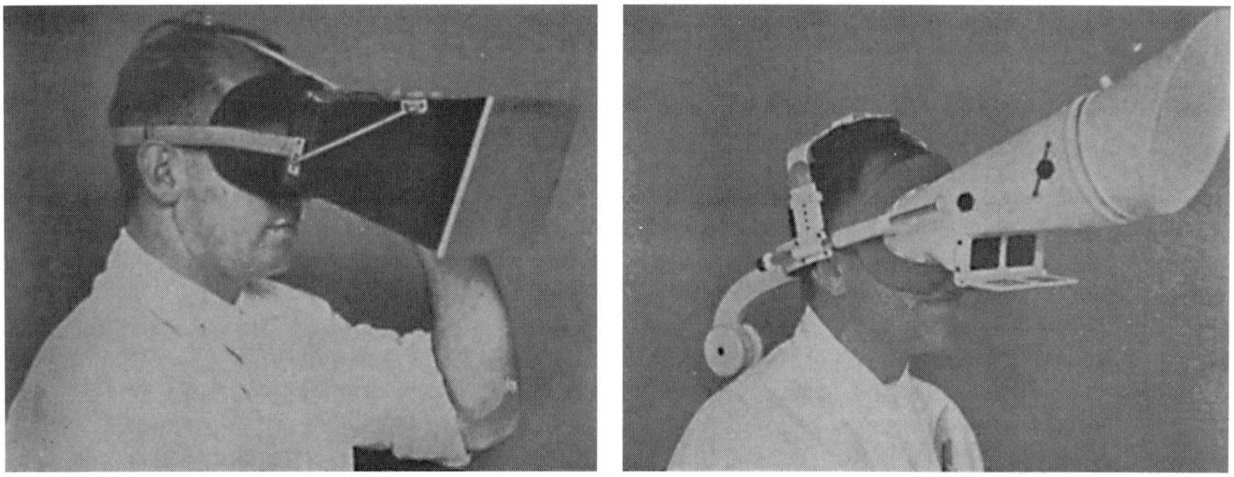

Fig. 1–8. Early headworn fluoroscopes.

tain risk, could be caused by either the fracture or by nailing. Osteomyelitis as an extensive infection was rare. Westerborn confirmed the experience of Küntscher, Fischer, Böhler, and others that when deep infection occurred it remained a local osteitis at the fracture site because pus escaped along the nail, thereby preventing rising pressure. Also noted was Küntscher's advice to drain the area but leave the stable nail in place. He reported a series of nailings including 22 femora, 32 tibiae, 31 humeri, 13 forearm bones, and 2 metacarpals.

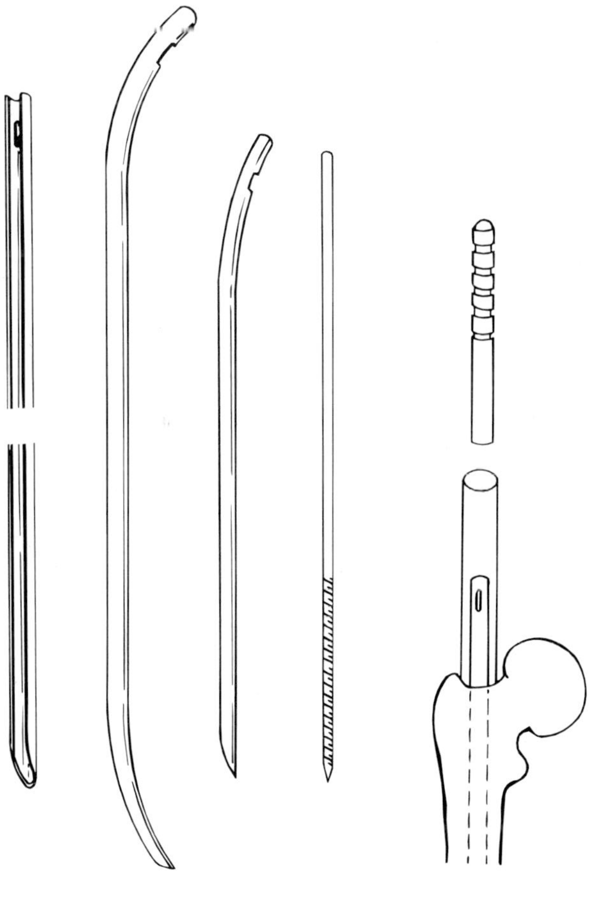

Fig. 1–9. Nails of Soeur.

Westerborn continued with the V nail for the femur as well as for other bones. Although snug fixation was considered mandatory, an advantage of the V nail was that in the event one nail was not sufficiently tight, a second could be driven in the groove of the first, particularly in the tibia and humerus. This was the basis for continued use of the V nail by others as well.[30]

Westerborn's stainless steel nails, manufactured in Gothenburg, had a series of six holes spaced in the butt end that would allow a nail to be shortened yet still retain a hole for extraction (Fig. 1–10). He had a unique extractor shaped like the jaws of a snake with a single fang that would engage the hole in the nail and would lock by a drop ring.

North American surgeons first became aware of Küntscher nailing in 1945 when prisoners of war returned from Europe carrying nails inside well-healed femora and tibiae with little or no sequelae. Their initial reactions were shock and disbelief. It was immediately branded as unphysiologic and problems such as anemia were predicted.

The first publication in American literature that dealt with the use of nails, rather than pins, in major long bones was by Tordoir and

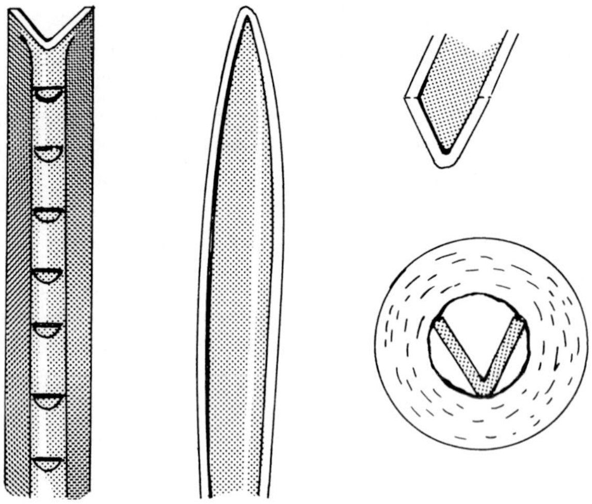

Fig. 1–10. Westerborn V nail.

Moeys[31] in July 1945. At about this time, nails designed by Hansen and Street, MacAusland, and others appeared in America.

In 1945, Harvey C. Hansen and I were working together in the Army. He had previously removed a round nail from a tibia, which had healed in 17° of external rotation. Hansen thought a diamond-shaped nail would control rotation. I had the nails made in the base shop, and together we nailed four successful cases, which were reported in 1947.[32] These nails became the Hansen-Street nail.

In 1947, my residents and I began a comparative study treating femoral fractures with skeletal traction, dual plating, open nailing, and closed nailing (Fig. 1–11). We quickly abandoned traction and plating, as they were considered inferior procedures. Despite initial good results with closed nailing, we abandoned it in favor of open nailing, because of radiation exposure for the surgeon and after observing a radiograph burn on a patient's skin.[33] Open nailing was simplified by retrograde insertion of the nail at the fracture site.

In the late 1940s in America, there was a tantalum nail developed by MacAusland[34] and C-shaped or split tubular nails reported by Wiggins.[35] These were never widely accepted because of the inherent weakness of the C nail design and the brittleness of the tantalum.

In the second half of the decade, Lottes designed three flanged femur and tibial nails. The femur nail was never widely used, but the tibial nail became the only extensively used tibial nail in America. Both nails employed a screw-on driver-extractor.[36,37]

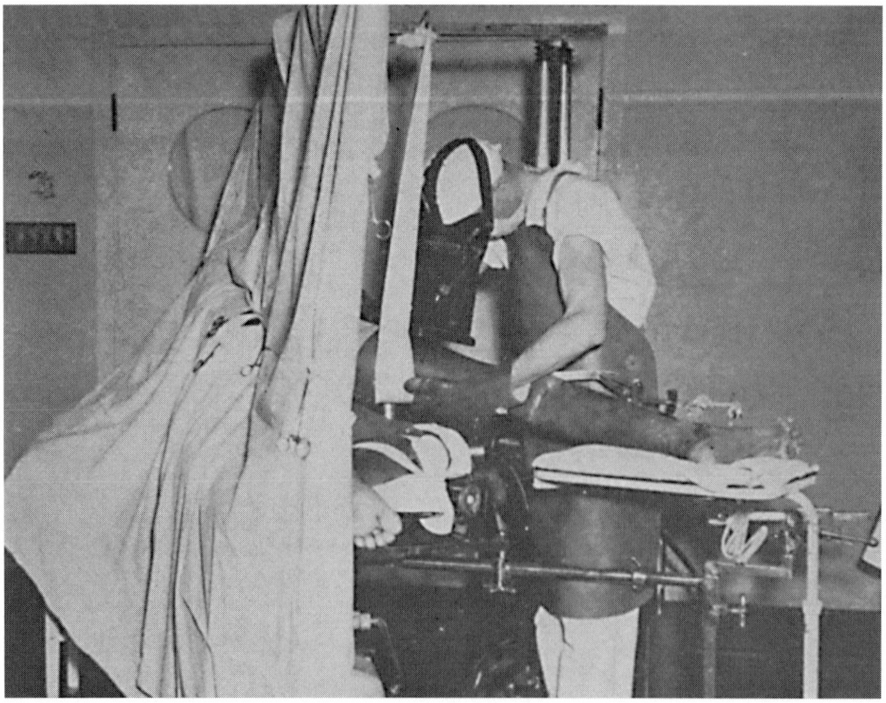

Fig. 1–11. Positioning and draping used in early closed nailing (1948). Vertical drape separates sterile operative field from unsterile manipulative field. Note author visualizing closed reduction with head-worn fluoroscope.

From 1947 to 1950 closed nailings in this country were performed chiefly in university centers. However, these centers soon abandoned closed nailing for several reasons. A foremost concern was the extensive exposure to radiation when using the small fluoroscope (see Fig. 1–8) necessary to allow manipulation of the extremity. Although closed rodding minimized infection, Americans felt more secure using penicillin, which was not available to the Germans in World War II. A third concern was the unpredictable duration of the closed nailing procedure. While a thin individual who had received adequate skeletal traction preoperatively could be nailed quickly, the stocky, muscular male with insufficient traction presented a lengthy exercise. It was these "wrestling matches" that added to the initial shock and possible fat embolism led to intraoperative deaths in some earlier cases.

At first there was concern that retrograde introduction of the nail would explode the trochanter. Initially we thought it was necessary to cut the cortex in the region of the anterior margin of the trochanteric fossa with a ¼ inch osteotome, then turn it 90° and drive it through again. In 1948, (unfamiliar with J. Otto Lottes' work), we replaced the eye in the end of the nail with a threaded stud to take a screw-on driver-extractor, eliminating the hook extractor, which had given us many problems. If the hook was too malleable it would straighten out and if hard enough not to straighten it would break. Also, it was often difficult to locate the eye at the bottom of a small exposure. Then with a sharp end on the nail we felt it no longer necessary to cut the cortex. At first we used an arrowhead point on the stud, which was unscrewed after driving the nail out through the trochanter (Fig. 1–12). Then we found that a sharp end on the stud would raise only a small chip of cortex.

By the end of the first decade, open femoral nailing had become well established in America by two main techniques, one using the cloverleaf nail and the other using the diamond nail. The single Rush pin for the femur shaft fractures never had much following, because it

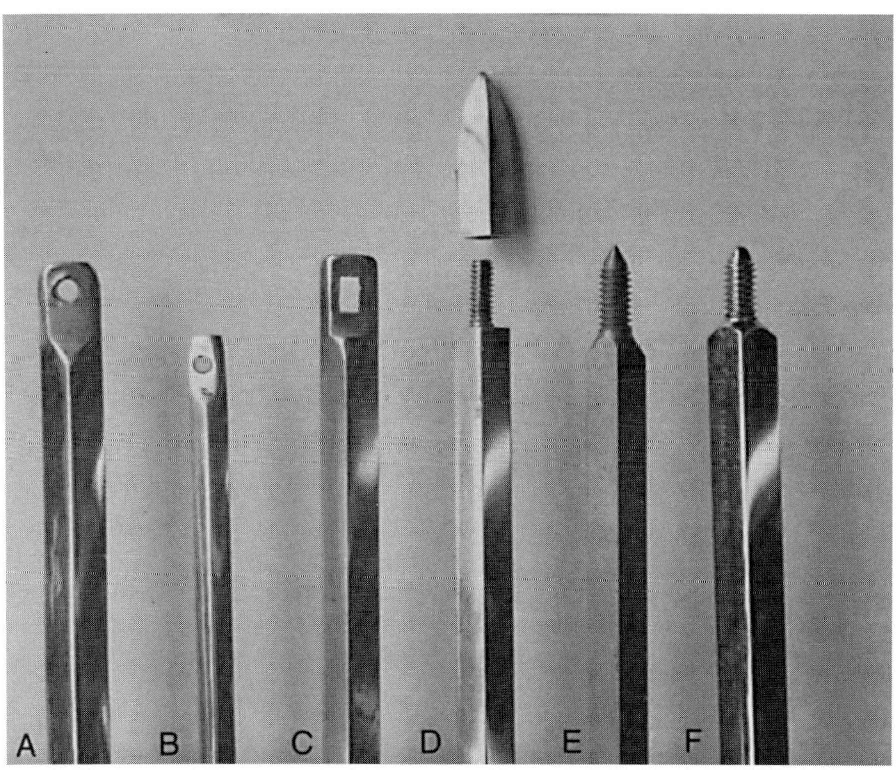

Fig. 1–12. *A,B,* Original Hansen-Street nails: 12.5 mm for femur, 7 mm for humerus, both with round holes for extraction. *C,* Later nail (1948): 11 mm nail with rectangular hole for stronger extraction hook. *D,* Arrowhead-point screwed on 3⁄16 inch threaded stud when nail is passed retrograde through the trochanter (1949). *E,* Conical point on ¼-inch stud (1951). *F,* Bullet or hemispherical point for less irritation of gluteal muscles (1954).

apparently required about 6 weeks of recumbency to allow a good start on healing before encountering the stresses of ambulation.

The Küntscher nail was promoted in America by two major projects. One was by the Navy under Captain Alvis, who spent considerable time with Küntscher and prevailed upon him to write a book of approximately 8 looseleaf volumes, each of about 200 mimeographed pages. The other was by the Army and National Research Council under Hugh Smith.

The cloverleaf nail, relying on a snug fit at the isthmus, gained good fixation in the proximal fragment but poor fixation in the distal fragment, in fractures below the isthmus. The nail, being a straight nail, extended to the upper pole of the patella to avoid possible penetration of the anterior cortex under the patella. It needed an assortment of nail diameters, reamers, and guide pins to match, and also a separate driver, nail set, and extractor. The total cost of the starter set was about $400 in 1950. Smith placed this inventory in about a dozen different universities.

By contrast, the diamond nail relied on the holding power in the cancellous bone at both ends and controlled rotation by reason of the nail pattern. This placed the emphasis on maximum length rather than snugness at the isthmus. The nails were bowed to approximate the anterior bow of the femur[38] and one size was employed (11 mm × 8 mm). A smaller 9-mm size was manufactured, but not recommended for the femur, because it was considered too weak. The 13-mm size was not made until 1957.

The surgeons performing open nailing using the Küntscher cloverleaf nail inserted a guide pin retrograde, reamed from above, removed the guide pin, reduced the fracture, and then reinserted the guide pin from above, followed by the nail. Problems sometimes arose in nailing high fractures when the retrograded guide pin hugged the medial cortex and exited the femoral neck too far medially, causing the reamer to angle laterally and ream too much lateral cortex and causing some comminution when driving the nail. Conversely, when hugging the lateral cortex, it exited the tip of the trochanter and comminution of the medial cortex occurred. (This was not seen when retrograding the diamond nail.) To avoid this, a series of nested tubes, like cork borers, was devised that could be placed in the canal of the proximal fragment.

I was never aware of the reason, until recently, why Küntscher and his European followers used the tip of the greater trochanter as the point for nail insertion. I assumed it was a matter of convenience. However, they feared disturbance of the circulation to the femoral head and possible avascular necrosis or risk of infection involving the hip joint with a more medial approach.

Having used retrograde nailing almost from the beginning of my surgical experience and seeing no avascular necrosis following the use of the more medial point of insertion (nor having heard of it in thousands of cases), I do not consider it a risk. The same applies to hip joint infection, even after superficial infection or drainage at the point of insertion or with chronic infection at the fracture site. Regarding vascularity, one encounters very little bleeding approaching the neck-trochanter junction from a point directly above.

Küntscher reserved the term "nagel" for the implant that could exert pressure against the more rigid bone, like the cloverleaf nail and might call the diamond nail a bolt. On the other hand, bone has elasticity when compared with a solid-core nail, similar to a nail in wood. The diamond nail obtains fixation in cancellous bone at both ends of a bone, which exerts pressure or friction on the nail regardless of the level of fracture. This is why it is difficult to remove the nail at 4 months but easier after bone resorption at 1 year.

THE SECOND DECADE (1950 TO 1959)

At the start of the decade, an important contribution was the broach by Stryker, as an alternative for reaming. This he suggested in 1950 and proceeded to manufacture it in both a diamond and cloverleaf pattern[39] (Fig. 1–13). We adopted it immediately for the diamond nail, because it allowed use of a nail in smaller canals in a size of adequate strength (11 mm). It provided maximum holding power to resist torque, and it also avoided reaming the entire canal circumference. The cloverleaf pattern of broach never gained acceptance, which in my opinion was a mistake, because it would have provided better control of torque than the reamed canal.

A comprehensive review of the complications of nailing in which 12 surgeons participated was published by Watson-Jones in

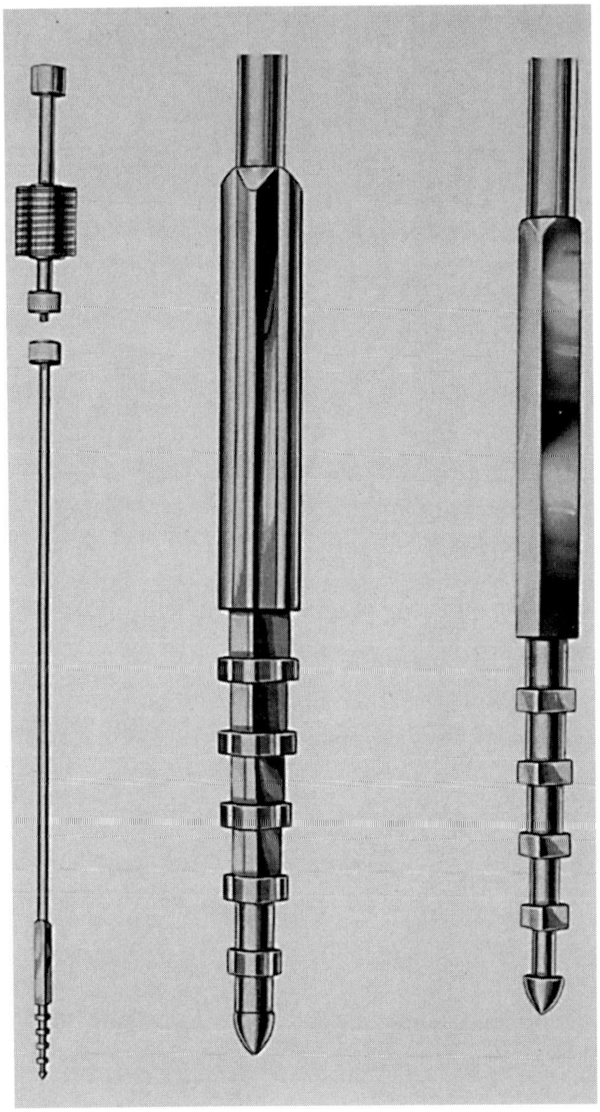

Fig. 1–13. Stryker broach.

1950.[40] This report focused on closed nailing. In addition to problems discussed earlier, the report brought attention to the complications of guide pin malposition, causing injury to the femoral artery or radial nerve, incarcerated nails and guide pins, distraction leading to delayed union, tight nails splitting the shaft, bent and broken nails caused by small diameter or malleable metal and nail migration.

In a multicenter study in 1951 involving 700 patients, Smith[41] reported the incidence of broken nails was twice as frequent in the cloverleaf nail than the diamond nail (i.e., 1.3% vs. 0.6%), whereas bent nails were 3 times more common in the diamond nail than in the cloverleaf nail. These problems were largely overcome by the use of larger nails and stronger metal. It was my privilege to analyze the data for this study with the help of F. James Funk, at that time in his residency. We used the punch card, key-sort method. Today it would no doubt be done by computer.

Several new nails appeared in the early 1950s. The Livingston bar, a short I-beam pattern pointed at both ends, had short slots for cross-pinning with screws[42] (Fig. 1–14). This was probably the first interlocking nail. It was made of Vitallium and designed to remain in the bone indefinitely. Its lack of acceptance was probably caused by the risk of infection with difficult removal. It was inserted at the fracture site into one fragment, then backed into the other until it spanned both equally. Another nail that used the same technique, but was not cross-pinned was designed about the same time by Breck for the humerus.[43] It was L-shaped and ¼ inch wide, but as made, it proved too weak. A third nail, which allowed cross-pinning but extended the full length of the canal was designed by Modny and reported in 1953.[44] This nail has an X-shaped cross section with holes throughout its length that are spaced 1 cm apart. The holes are round and located at the center of the X so that screws can be passed through them in either of two planes at 90° angles to each other. The nail showed distinct advantages for supracondylar fractures and for comminuted fractures in which supplementary screws were needed. It was also useful in holding the distraction in a lengthened femur or keeping the contact in a shortened femur.

In 1951, Schneider designed the Schneider nail (Fig. 1–15), which incorporated both double-ended stud and self-broaching features.[45] The nail was also fluted with a square cross section. Self-broaching was later incorporated in the Street square forearm pin in 1956 and provided control of torque stress not found in the then popular Rush pin.

In 1952, Schneider presented an exhibit at the AAOS meeting illustrating the use of his nail for hip fusions.[46] Here the nail was inserted into the posterior iliac spine and crossed the acetabulum into the modified head and down the neck and shaft of the femur. To avoid excess flexion and abduction, the nail must be inserted into the crest of the ilium just lateral to the posterior superior iliac spine. I have used this technique successfully with the diamond nail,

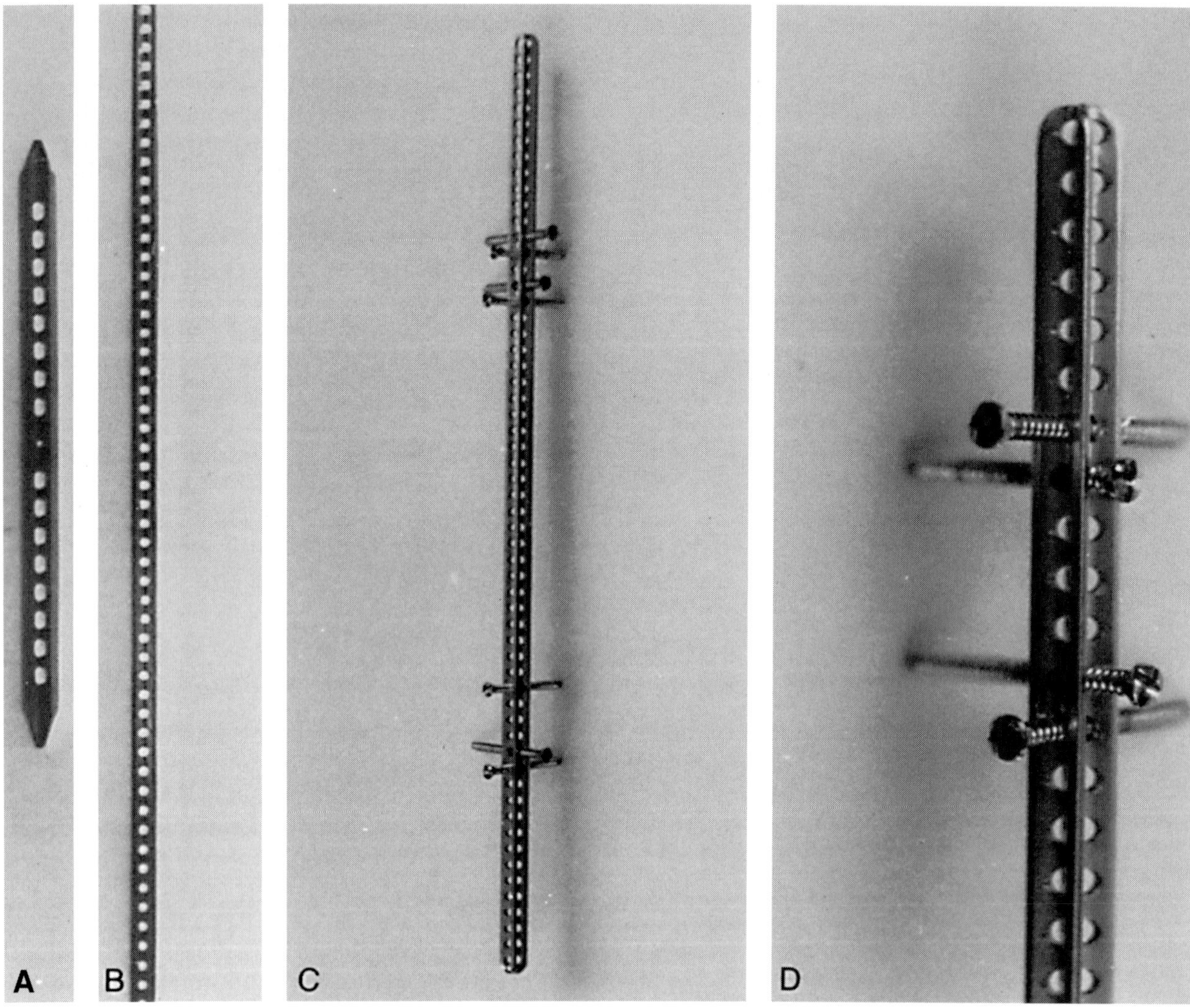

Fig. 1–14. Early nails for transfixion screws. *A*, Livingston bar. *B*, Modny nail. *C*, Modny nails with screws inserted. *D*, Close-up view of Modny nail.

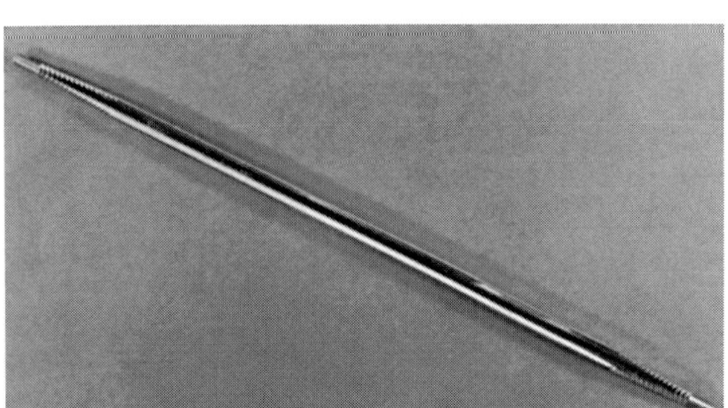

Fig. 1–15. Schneider nail.

which has some advantage here over the square nail, because the lesser of the two diameters fits better in the narrow space between the tables of the ilium.

Another device, which I learned of from McElvenney, is a key-shaped plate that engages a slot in the cortex at both sides of a fracture, is inserted over the guide pin, and is held in place by the cloverleaf nail[47] (Fig. 1–16). This resembles a key by Küntscher,[48] but which remained outside of the nail. A similar device was used for the diamond nail consisting of a sleeve of several turns of sheet metal wrapped around the nail to increase its diameter for large canals. If still too loose, the outer turn could be spread, or if too snug, part or all of a turn could be re-

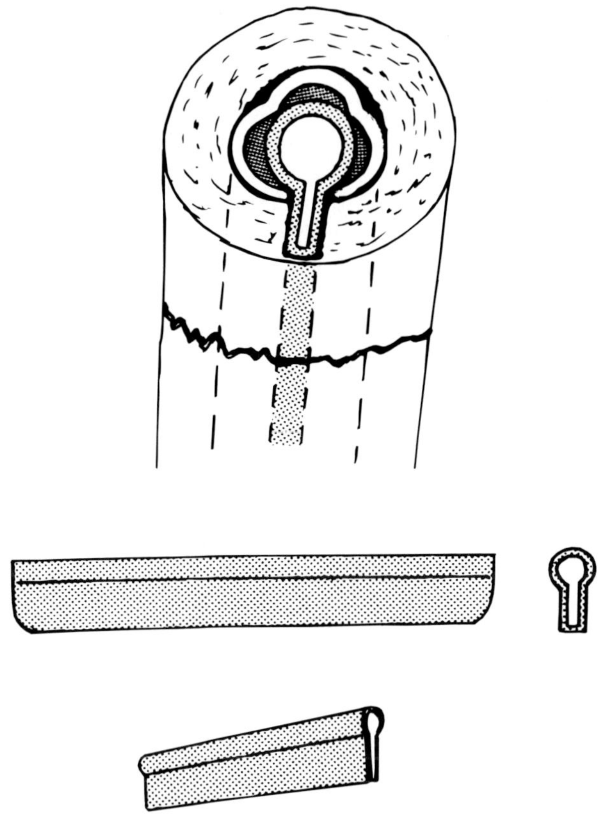

Fig. 1–16. McElvenney plate used as an adjunct to the cloverleaf nail to control rotation.

moved (Fig. 1–17). The last turn could end in a fin that engaged a slot in the cortex.

At the 1957 American Association of Orthopadeic Surgeons (AAOS) meeting, Küntscher was the guest speaker, and his speech awakened new interest in the cloverleaf nail. Küntscher illustrated flexible reamers and recommended reaming to permit use of larger nails and to obtain a larger area of nail-bone contact. He also stated that the significant reaming was well tolerated because the periosteum lays down new bone around the nail. His changes in apparatus and technique were published in his book in 1962.[49]

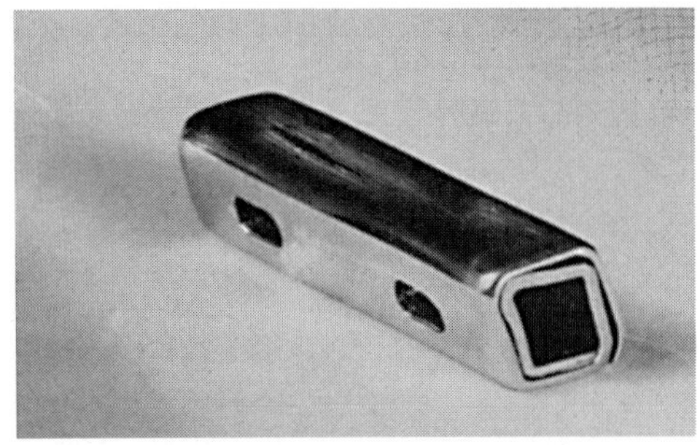

Fig. 1–17. Sleeve to fill large canal. Can spread last turn to make larger or remove with file to make smaller.

In 1958, Vesely and I, independently thought of splitting the diamond nail. I thought of splitting the midportion for the humerus and Vesely favored splitting the distal end for supracondylar femur fractures. We both went to Frank Wright to manufacture the nail and he said we had the same idea and should combine our efforts, hence the Vesely-Street nail. Together we hand-split nails with a hacksaw and tested them in cadaver femurs. We presented AAOS exhibits in 1959[50] and 1961 and a subsequent paper with 103 cases at the AAOS meeting in 1962.[2] (Fig. 1–18). Vesely later thought of the double-split nail for combined subtrochanteric

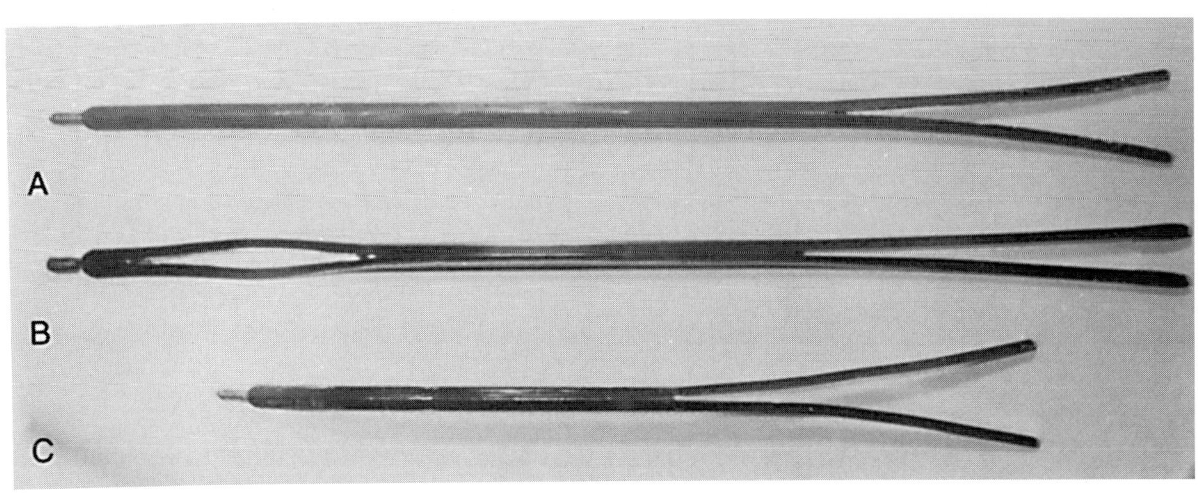

Fig. 1–18. *A*, One of the original nails hand split with hacksaw (11 mm). *B*, Double split for high and supracondylar femoral fractures (13 mm). *C*, Tibial split nail (11 mm).

and supracondylar fractures. The nail in humerus was reported by Vesely in 1965,[51] and in the femur, tibia, and humerus by Street in 1970.[52]

THE THIRD DECADE (1960 TO 1969)

The 1960s gave rise to several techniques that did not take root until the 1970s. Foremost of these new techniques was the use of the image intensifier, which became generally available about 1967. This lessened the risk of radiation exposure and permitted a return to closed nailing with its lessened physiologic insult, lower risk of infection, and better healing. I practiced this closed nailing using the diamond nail, while Clawson, Smith, and Hansen of Seattle used the cloverleaf and Schneider nail.[53]

The latter part of the 1960s, however, was a time when compression plating was sweeping the world and nailing was no longer of central interest in fracture treatment. For this reason, the contribution by Kaessman[54] of compression nailing in 1966 also attracted little interest. Kaessman employed a tie rod within the Küntscher nail (Fig. 1–19) that was anchored by cross-pinning in the distal fragment. Pressure was then maintained on the proximal end of the

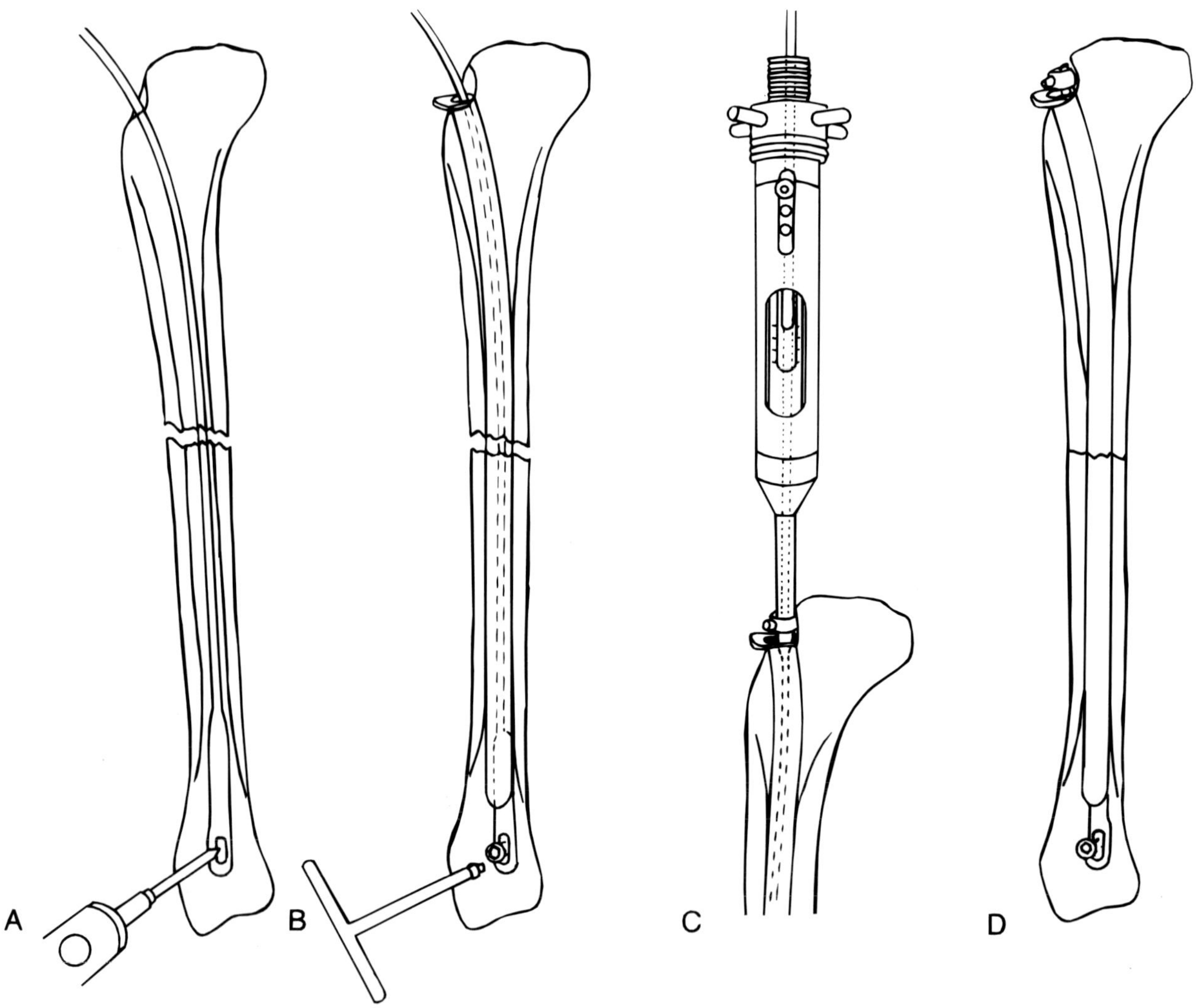

Fig. 1–19. Kaessmann compression nail. *A,* Locating the hole in the mandrel. *B,* Insertion of the transverse screw through the mandrel followed by insertion of the C-shaped nail. *C,* Compression is applied with a special calibrated compression device. The screw in the proximal locking cup is then tightened on the mandrel to hold the compression. *D,* Compressed fixed fracture with the implant in place.

nail by a collar locked with a set screw after applying pressure with a removable spring-loaded device. An American series using this nail was not reported until 1977.[55]

Compression was also independently employed by both Huckstep and me in 1967. Rather than use a separate rod, I cross-pinned the distal end of the Hansen-Street nail and compressed by screwing a cap on the threaded stud, which remained in place (Fig. 1–20). An exhibit at the AAOS in 1971 was reported later in the same year.[56] In Huckstep's method, using his own solid square nail, he cross-pinned the nail distally with one or more screws, applied compression proximally, then cross-pinned the nail proximal to the fracture. This was reported in 1972.[57] Another compression nail for the tibia was presented by Derweduven, of Belgium, in 1979.[58]

It was not until the mid-1970s that compression plating began to lose favor for the femur and nailing again became the treatment of choice. Any nail is compressed while weight bearing, provided it is not locked with cross-pins above and below the fracture. A compression nail, however, is of some advantage in the first few weeks after nailing, by providing greater stability before that of soft-tissue heal-

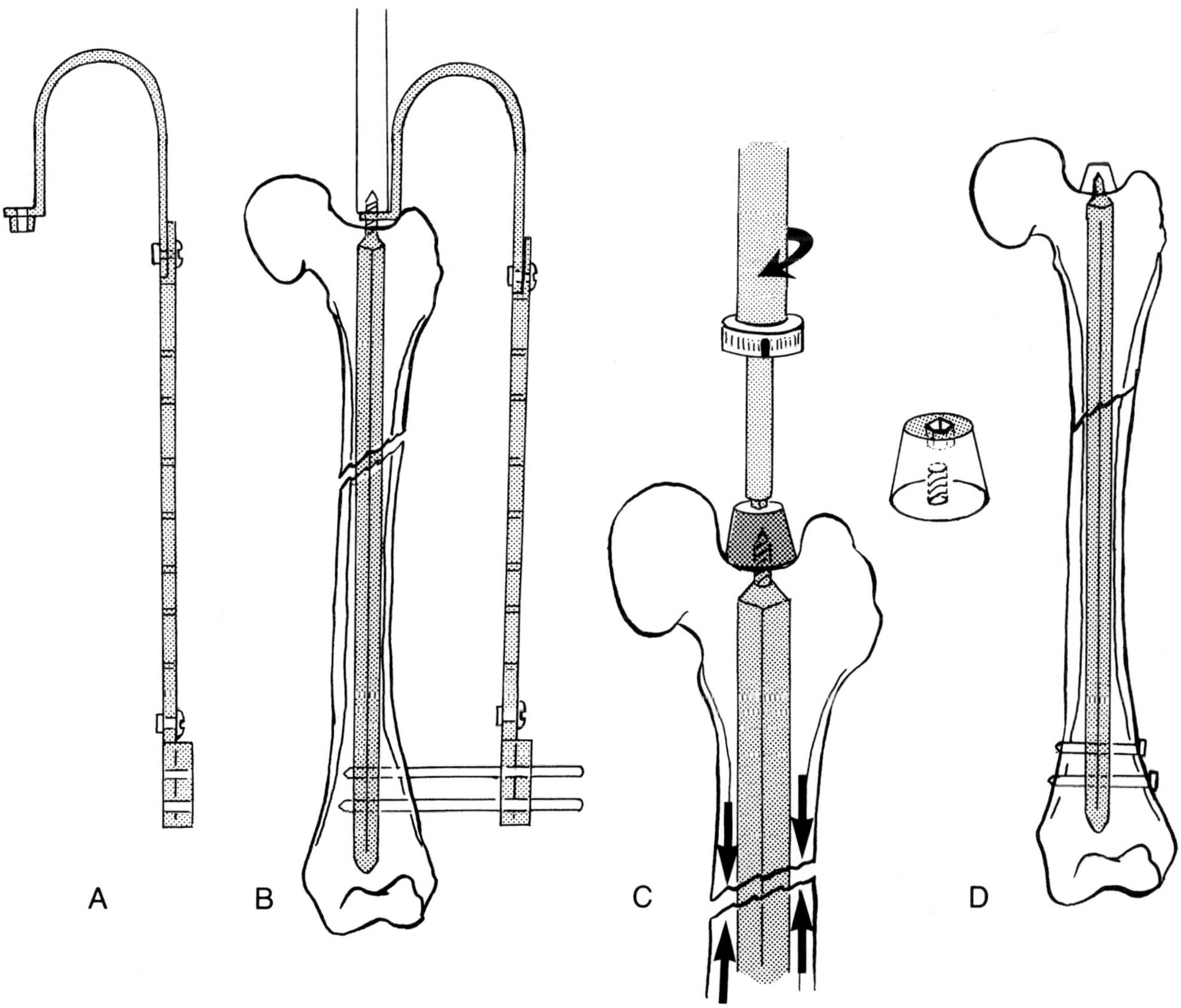

Fig. 1–20. Street compression nail. *A*, Nail mounted target device for distal transfixion screw insertion. *B*, Distal target device in use. *C*, Application of the compression cap to the threaded stud at the top of the nail produces compression at the fracture site. *D*, Fixed compressed fracture with implant in place.

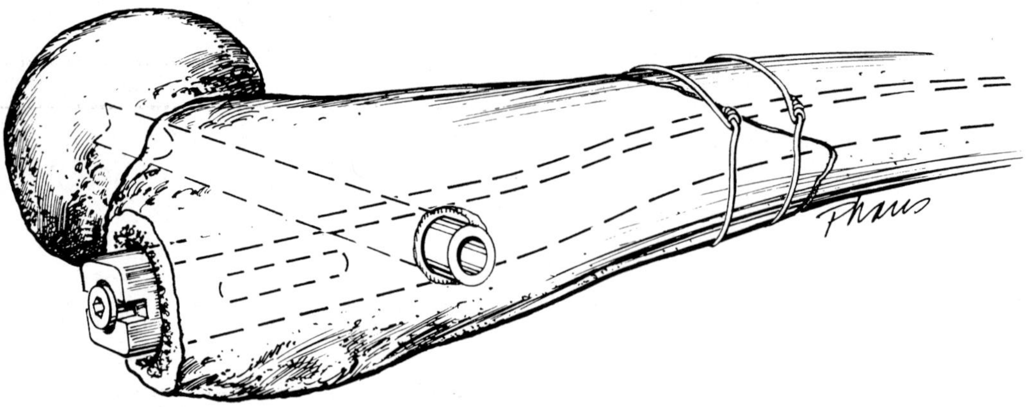

Fig. 1–21. Accessory fixation of oblique fractures with cerclage wires.

ing, and before weight bearing is begun. It is also of distinct advantage in femoral shortening where laxity of the shortened muscles allows distraction and is advantageous in controlling rotation prior to soft-tissue healing in lower third fractures.

The third technique that began in the 1960s, but did not develop until the 1970s, was condylocephalic nailing of intertrochanteric and subtrochanteric fractures. In 1950, Lezius[59] reported a technique for inserting a short nail through a window high on the medial cortex of the femur. It was not until Küntscher dropped the point of insertion to the medial condyle that the easier approach made the method practical. Küntscher reported his use of a prebowed, somewhat lighter cloverleaf nail in 1966 in German,[60] which was followed by a report in English in 1970.[61] Küntscher's technique was further reported by Collada and others in Spain in 1968 and 1973.[62,63] I began using the Hansen-Street nail as a condylocephalic nail in 1973, which led to the development of the Harris nail in 1975. Concurrent with Küntscher's development of the condylocephalic nail, J. Ender introduced the multiple, prebent flexible pin. He

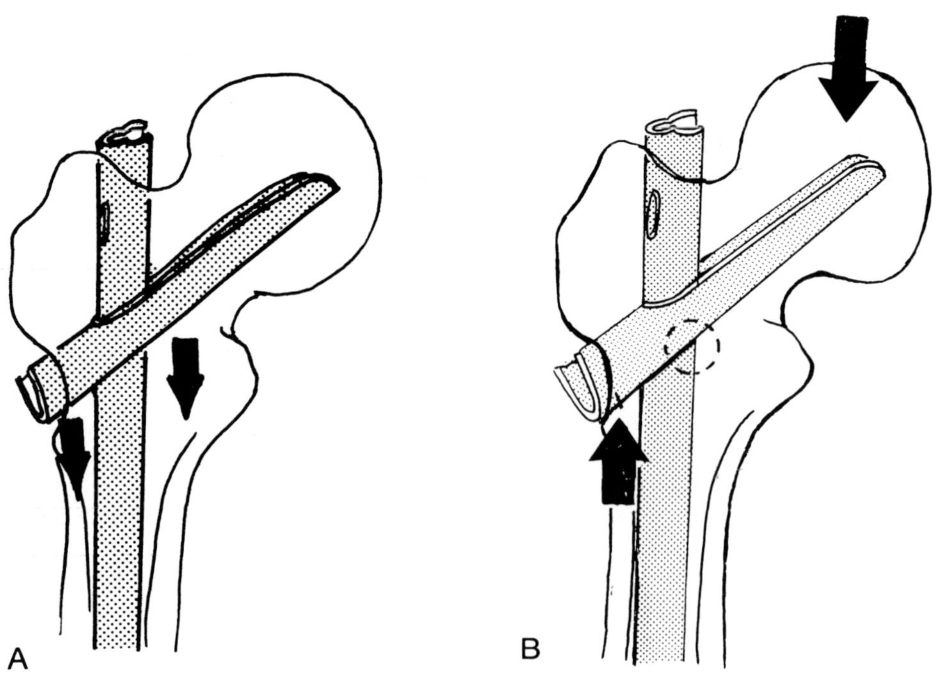

Fig. 1–22. The Y nail principle. *A,* With unloading, the head-neck nail can "walk" distally. *B,* With loading, the friction lock jams the head-neck nail on the femoral nail.

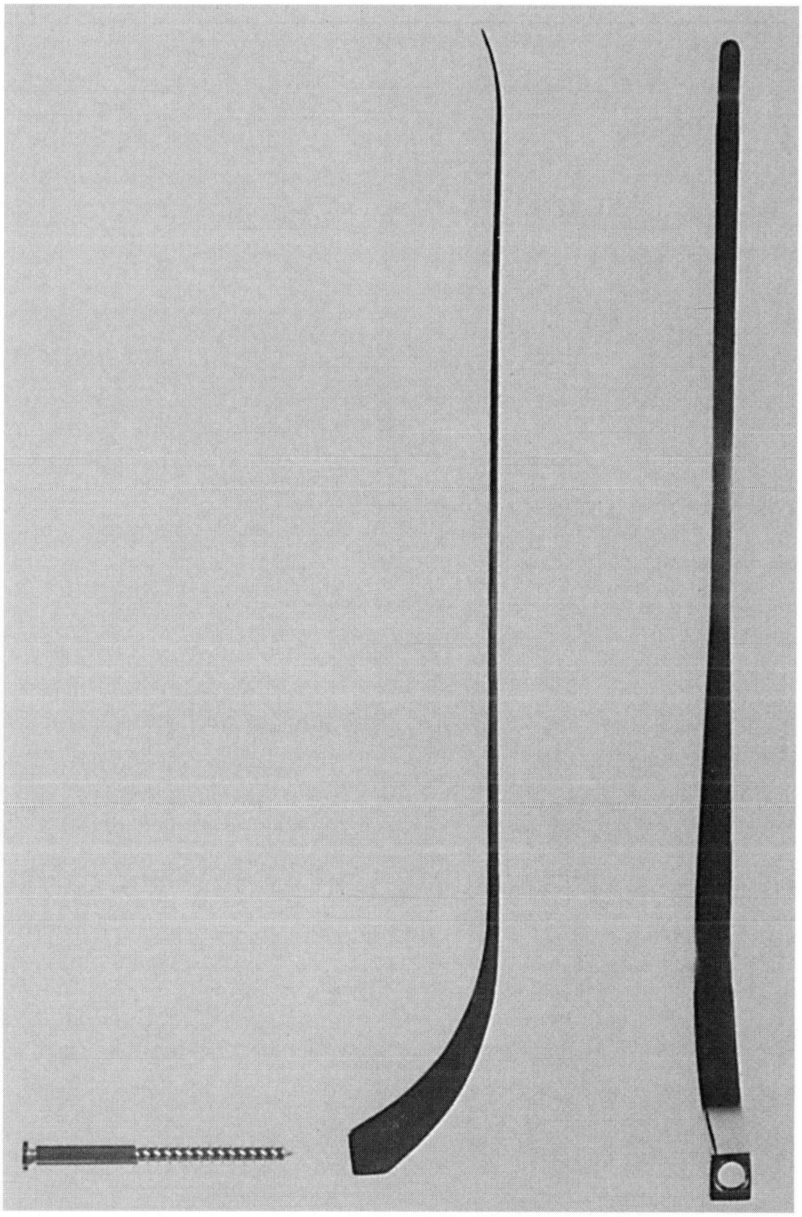

Fig. 1–23. Medium-sized supracondylar rod (two views) and compression screw.

reported this technique in 1970.[64-66] It was further developed and popularized by his son, H. G. Ender.[67,68]

In 1967, Zickel reported his nail for subtrochanteric fractures.[69] The design of this nail included an enlarged proximal end containing a tunnel through which a flanged nail extended into the femoral neck and head. It was prevented from backing out by a set screw in the end of the shaft nail (Fig. 1–21). For this type of fracture Küntscher had previously attempted introducing a small femoral neck nail through a hole in the proximal end of a cloverleaf nail, but this was abandoned because of difficulty with insertion. He subsequently developed the Y nail for proximal femoral fractures (Fig. 1–22). In this implant a cloverleaf shaft nail passes through a hole in the head and neck nail. In principle, the Zickel nail resembles the first Y nail.

The Zickel nail for supracondylar fractures appeared later (Fig. 1–23).[70] This nail is used in pairs in the manner of dual Rush pinning, and an enlarged diameter of the basal end of the nails allows a hole for a screw that further stabilizes comminuted fractures and prevents the nails from backing out. This corrects the main drawback of the dual Rush pinning, in which distal migration of the medial pin has been a major problem.

Yet another technique which had its start in the 1960s but developed in the 1970s was interlocking nails. Küntscher presented his "Detensor" nail in 1968,[71] using a single cross-pin above and below a comminuted fracture. This was also cited by Maatz,[48] who also credits Herzog with using this principle in 1949 to hold the length of a femur. Küntscher worked on the idea with Klemm before he died and they agreed on the term "interlocking".

THE FOURTH DECADE (1970 TO 1979)

This period was characterized by the decline of compression plating and firm reestablishment of medullary nailing for the femur, with the return to closed nailing. There was also the full development of condylocephalic nailing, with extensive use of Ender pins, even extending to include shaft fractures.

Klemm reported his interlocking nail series with Schellman in 1972.[72] Grosse and Kempf further developed the interlocking nail changing the angle of the proximal screw from Klemm's 60° to 45° and moving the distal screws closer to the end.[73]

Other new nails in the fourth decade include one by Halloran[74] in an I-beam pattern, which like the Modny nail and the Hansen-Street nail might allow more room for endosteal circulation than a snug-fitting Küntscher nail (Fig. 1–24). The series of short slots were said to be easier to hit when cross-pinning than round holes. It was potentially locking, like the

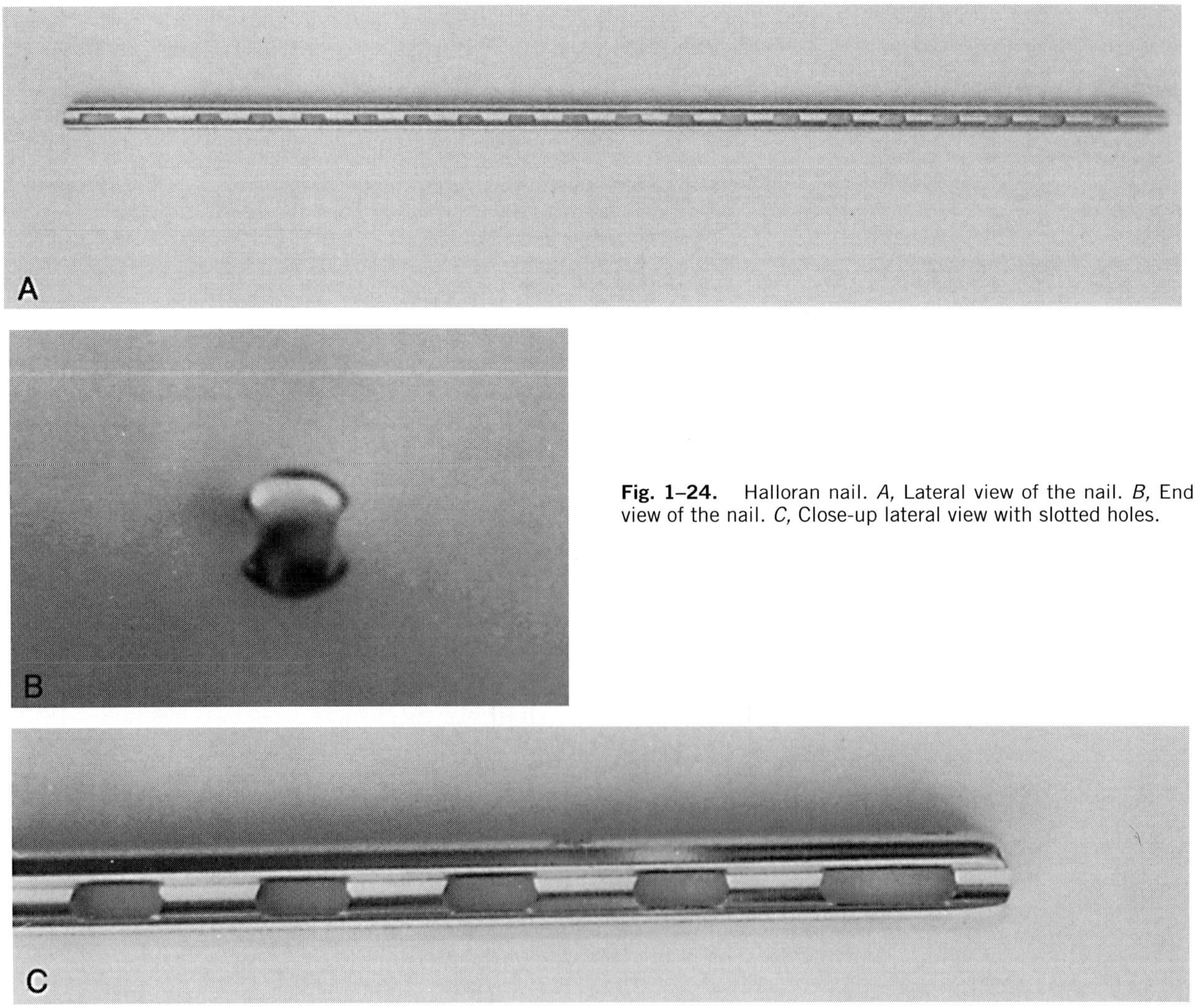

Fig. 1–24. Halloran nail. *A*, Lateral view of the nail. *B*, End view of the nail. *C*, Close-up lateral view with slotted holes.

Modny nail, but appeared before the popularity of interlocking and did not gain much following.

The Samson fluted-nail,[75] a closed circle tubular nail with eight equally spaced flutes between sharp ridges, came early in the decade. It was hailed as the strongest rod. One with enlarged diameter proximally was introduced toward the end of the decade for subtrochanteric fractures.[76]

THE FIFTH DECADE (1980 TO 1989)

In the fifth decade, I found a total of 234 nailing reports, of which 165 dealt with the femur, 50 dealt with the tibia, 15 dealt with the humerus, and 4 dealt with the forearm. Although these figures are not strictly accurate, they do show the level of interest in nailing for the respective bones.

The fifth decade was characterized by the rapid spread of the cloverleaf nail, improved by the tapered and conical point, curved to approximate the bow of the femur,[77] and cross-pinned with screws as in the Klemm-Schellman, Grosse-Kempf, and AO nails. Although Küntscher and Klemm originated the term "interlocking" and began an extensive development in nailing techniques, they were not the first to use this principle. Maatz cited Herzog's use of it in 1950,[48] Modny cross-pinned his nail in 1953,[44] and the next year Basom and I[78] used the Hansen-Street to interlock supracondylar fractures. With threaded holes in the nail and screws threaded the full length, the proximal screw in the distal fragment promptly backed out. For this reason, smooth pins were employed for the compression nail.

There were eight nonlocking femur nails, which declined or became obsolete in the 1980s. The Ender nail, as a condylocephalic nail appeared in 13 reports in the English language in the first half of the fifth decade, in 4 reports in the second half of the fifth decade, and in 1 report thus far in the sixth decade. It also declined for subtrochanter and shaft fractures, since the statically fixed nails control shortening and lack complications of migration and loss of fixation. Ender nails have been recommended only for stable intertrochanteric fractures in the elderly.[79]

The Harris condylocephalic nail apparently never gained a following, because there were only 3 reports, 2 by Harris[80,81] early in the first half of the decade and a negative report in the second half; this is surprising, since it seemed like a sound procedure. However, the technique is exacting and needs to be perfected with inserting the one diamond nail, which cannot be rotated but is very stable. Harris' excellent results in 185 cases with a 22-minute operating time indicates a learning curve, which contrasts with the third report where the procedure was abandoned after 35 attempts.[82] My experience in 55 cases, with a Hansen-Street nail bent for condylocephalic use, also indicated it is a good procedure for the high-risk patient with a stable intertrochanteric fracture,[83] (and very stable when combined with two Ender pins). The good results with experience is confirmed by Navarro-Quilis who reported good results with the Küntscher condylocephalic nail in 2660 cases in Spain.[84]

The fluted nail or Samson nail received, to my knowledge, only 5 reports in the fifth decade and 1 report in the sixth decade. Groh[85] had a large series with excellent results, but Star[86] reported breakage and difficulties removing it. Heiple[87] reported excellent results in open nailing of nonunited femurs; however removal was not routine. I have always been puzzled why the designers of the nail went to the trouble of adding an attachment to provide an eye for a hook extractor when they already had a threaded hole in the end of the nail which would have taken a screw-in driver-extractor. The screw-in type has worked well for the Hansen-Street nail for 30 years and the screw-on type has endured for 45 years. Also the Grosse-Kempf and the AO nails have a closed-circle threaded proximal end for this purpose. The nail was considered too rigid, increasing comminution. If the flutes extended the full length of the nail, the attachment omitted, and the nail made of titanium for greater flexibility, it could still be a useful nail.

The Rush nail never gained a following as a single nail for use in the shaft of the femur. It was reported for dual nailing of supracondylar femur fractures.[88] It is the most versatile nail, which has been used for every long bone in the body.

The Hansen-Street nail has been detailed in few reports, though it is still being manufactured and used in some areas. The good results reported in the one series early in the fifth decade[89] are surprising because the investigators used 9-mm nails, which my residents and I have generally considered too weak for the femur.

The Modny nail had 3 reports in the latter half of the decade,[90] one by Modny reporting 261 cases. Although used as a locking nail, it never gained much following, possibly because of the rather complicated open procedure for the nail's insertion. With a closed nailing technique it might still be useful, because the screws are rather easy to insert and can be placed in two planes.

The Zickel subtrochanteric nail, which was quite popular in the 1970s and early 1980s, declined with 4 reports in the fifth decade and 1 report in the sixth decade. Besides nonlocking, there were iatrogenic refractures during removal because of the angle at the proximal end, which was necessary because of the point of insertion at the tip of the greater trochanter.[91] Also prominence of the nail at this site caused pain while lying on the affected side. The Zickel nail for supracondylar fractures has also been replaced by locking nails.

Alternatives for the Zickel nail were the fluted nail with an enlarged proximal end, the Street sleeve with a fin in the trochanter (which was never manufactured), and a new nail, the Scherfel[92] nail (a Küntscher nail with three fins on the proximal end, used mainly in Europe). Other alternatives also included interlocking nails, the Küntscher Y nail, and, later, a Y nail by Williams.[93] Use of the Küntscher nail also gradually declined, although it continued to be used for stable femur fractures in the fifth decade, and now it has been replaced by the locking nails.

Although the locking nails took precedence over the other nails in the decade, the techniques were more exacting and time-consuming with potential difficulty inserting the distal screws. The external jigs for locating the distal holes have not worked, because the slotted nails tend to distort while being driven. They worked better for closed circle and solid nails.

The Brooker-Wills nail (Fig. 1–25) appeared in 11 reports in the fifth decade and in 2 reports in the sixth decade. It has encountered difficulty in setting the distal fins,[94] has less firm hold of length than screws with axial loading,[95] and has a reported breakage of the central rod when removing the fins.[96] Although this system would seem to have advantages of eliminating need for distal screws and somewhat arduous insertion of screws, it apparently has not

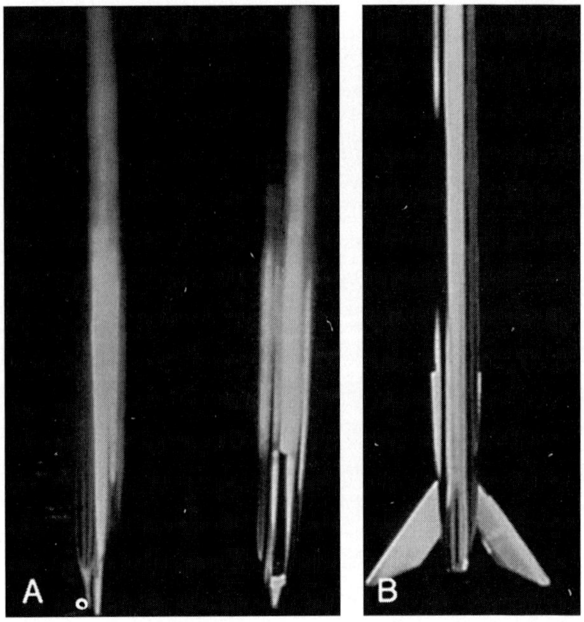

Fig. 1–25. *A,* Comparison of the distal ends of a standard Küntscher nail and the slotted Brooker-Wills nail. *B,* Distal transverse fixator deployed through distal slots.

developed widespread usage, although it is still manufactured by the Orthopedic Equipment Company.

There were late complications with the locking nails, particularly with the distal one-third fractures close to the more proximal of the distal screws. The stress riser of the proximal hole led to fatigue fracture of the nail, as reported by Buckholz in seven cases.[97] He indicated the need to delay weight bearing until evidence of union and the need to use nails larger than 12- or 13-mm or nails with smaller than 6.3-mm holes, reinforced holes, or thicker walled nails. Screw breakage has also been reported. These problems have been addressed by the new nails in the next decade.

A pitch might be made here for the less complicated compression nailing. This allows early weight bearing through increased stability in stable fractures by maintaining firm contact of meshing surfaces in all but smooth transverse osteotomies. The first compression nail, designed by Kaessmann, was again reported for the tibia by Böstman in 1984.[98] A new nail, the Derby nail, was reported by Papagiannopoulos in 1986.[99] It is a 12-mm tubular nail with a central 6-mm rod that screws down to spread wings distally and has a collar placed proximally. Huckstep, whose original report was in 1972, reported in 1980, 1983, and twice in 1986.[100] His nails for the femur, tibia, and humerus both compress and interlock. The Vicenzi compression nail[101] is a cross-pinned Küntscher nail compressed with a screw and washer proximally. Perhaps the Street nail is the simplest, with a single cross-pin in the diamond nail distally, a cap which screws on the stud for the femur, and a screw with washer which screws into a hole in the proximal end of the type II nail for the tibia and humerus. This type had the advantage that by using a threaded hole 2 cm deep, if the nail proved too long it could be shortened without removal up to about 1.5 cm and still allow enough for extraction.

For the tibia in the fifth decade, there was interest at first in flexible multiple Ender and Rush pins for acute fractures,[102] although Küntscher nailing with the Herzog angle was successful in mid one-third closed fractures.[103] It was soon evident that reaming was more serious in the tibia than the femur, because of less soft- tissue coverage and the ease with which periosteal circulation could be impaired. Because the advantages of nailing over nonoperative treatment, such as walking casts or functional bracing, were not as apparent as with the femur the development was less rapid and more with nonunion, malunion, and open fractures. However, the results in closed unstable fractures with closed reamed nailing were superior to those with other methods,[104] provided good aseptic technique could be carried out. Some even reported good results with type I and II open fractures.[105]

The contention has been more with open fractures and when open nailing is necessary. The long-term success of the unreamed Lottes nail led to interest in interlocking unreamed nails and new nails appeared toward the end of the decade.

The Chandler nail is essentially an interlocking Lottes nail that can be advantageous when cross-pining only one end in a high or low fracture and relying on the configuration of the nail to control rotation in the major fragment. A prototype for this nail was made by Neufeld in 1984, but it was brought out by Chandler in about 1987 and had a successful clinical trial in 1988.[106] The two proximal screws were in the sagittal plane and the nail has not gained a following.

The humerus was less commonly nailed, because conservative treatment is less confining than for the tibia and femur and generally satisfactory. Loss of reduction, malunion, nonunion, and nerve compromise proved the main incentives for internal fixation. Closed nailing with Ender or Rush multiple pins was successful in selected acute cases, [107] such as in elderly patients or in patients with tumors undergoing nailing for pain relief. These pins had the advantage they could be inserted quickly, also inserted off from the joint surface, avoiding disturbance of the rotator cuff.

The Hackethal pin, of somewhat smaller diameter than the Ender, was used to pack the canal of the humerus for bundle nailing used mainly in Europe.[108] Another nail for the humerus was presented by Gallagher in 1985.[109] This nail locks the proximal end with a cap, which screws onto the nail and into the cancellous bone with a larger thread, a principle used later with the True/Flex nail. Yet another nail for the humerus was the Mouradian, a modified Zickel supracondylar nail, which had a curve allowing it to be inserted at the greater tuberosity and two screws through it into the humoral head.[110]

The forearm nailing received almost no attention with only 6 reports in the fifth decade, 2 of which were my own, and 4 reports in the sixth decade.[111,112] However, I feel this will soon change, given the advantages of nailing in the forearm.

Another nail, which appeared in the late 1980s was the Inyo nail, specifically used for the distal fibula.[113] It flairs widely to span the distance between the cortices distally and tapers markedly for the narrow canal in the diaphysis. A Rush pin does a good job in this area, because the bone is cancellous in the distal fragment supporting the pin. However, the Rush pin requires a precise point of insertion for a good reduction, which may be assured by the Inyo and it can be interlocked for stability and prevent backout.

THE SIXTH DECADE (1990 TO 1995)

The sixth decade continues to show an expanding literature with over 208 reports in English, almost as many as in the fifth decade with it not yet half over. The ratio for the different bones is about the same: 132 for the femur, 55 tibia, 17 humerus, and 4 forearm at last count.

Several targeting devices have been developed for inserting the distal screws,[114] one using a laser claims 97% accuracy[115] and one using ultra sound is for hospitals lacking an image intensifier.[116] This might also have merit in eliminating risk of radiation exposure for the entire surgical team.[117] Others find freehand targeting satisfactory after enough experience.[118] I sometimes performed targeting without an image intensifier by a careful measurement, drilled the lateral hole, then felt the hole in the nail with a Kirschner wire. This can require slight adjustment in the position of the nail and is not recommended for a snug cloverleaf nail. The Self-Guiding Nail,[119] an unslotted tubular diamond-shaped nail, places the distal screws with a more efficient external jig. As yet, I know of no reported series.

With proximal shaft fractures one can use a single distal screw.[120] A single screw is sufficient proximally unless the fracture is above the isthmus. With distal fractures, the two screws are necessary to prevent rocking of the distal fragment.

A subtrochanteric nail, the gamma nail, has a lag screw extending up the neck at a 135° angle, is straight, is cross-pinned distally, and ends about mid femur. It has an angle proximally to allow it to be inserted at the tip of the trochanter. According to Stapert,[121] it has been used in over 1500 cases in the Netherlands. He discusses complications such as femur fracture at the stress riser of the distal screws and reports the long gamma nail extending to the distal femur, which being straight can also fracture the femur in driving.

In treating comminuted subtrochanteric fractures with the Grosse-Kempf nail, Wiss reversed the side for which it was used to place the proximal screw up the femoral neck, reporting two broken screws in which they were not reversed.[122] The second generation reconstruction nails are now used for fractures at this level. These and other nails are further discussed in later sections of this book.

Another nail for both the femur and tibia is the Marchetti-Vicenzi nail.[123] This nail has a tubular proximal portion, which is cross-pinned with an oblique screw similar to the Grosse-Kempf nail. More distally it divides into five flexible segments for bundle nailing in the shaft. Küntscher would call it a brush nail.

For the tibia, secondary nailing after first using external fixation became popular in treating open fractures, because infections were more common in open fractures and with open nailing after reaming,[124,125] although type I and II fractures have been successfully treated by reamed nailing.[105] Unreamed nailing is now recommended when nailing all open tibial fractures.[126] The Russell-Taylor and Delta nails had their start in the fifth decade, though they were reported in the sixth decade.[127] The AO tibial nail is solid, and basically triangular, but unlike the Chandler, has considerable rounding of the corners.

The tibial nails are not without complications. The Grosse-Kempf nail and the Chandler nail had proximal screws in the sagittal plane, which gave a potential complication of injury to the posterior tibial nerve or popliteal vessels from overdrilling or too long a proximal sagittal screw.[128] Current nails place both proximal screws transversely or also allow one or two sagittal screws. Other complications are heterotopic bone formation, which may occur proximal to the end of the nail,[129,130] and also there is breakage of nails and screws. Screws threaded only for the far cortex have been recommended for more core strength for a given diameter, allowing a smaller hole in the nail for nail strength. This is the type illustrated by Hempel.[131] Screws threaded the full length have been recommended as easier to remove and less apt to back out[132] and are currently popular in this country.

For the humerus, while the flexible pins still allow quick insertion for the poor risk or elderly person, the fixation is less secure than with interlocked nails such as Seidel's,[133] a 9-mm slotted tubular nail with three distal flanges, which are spread with a screwdriver and employ two screws proximally. Use of only the transverse proximal screw was advised to avoid injuring the radial nerve.[134] However, it does not control rotation as well as nails locked with screws distally. Some control of rotation distally was provided by the screwdriver-type point on a Hansen-Street nail as modified by Watanabi.[135] Currently a reamed interlocked nailing is advised by Ingman,[136] who uses retrograde nailing for quicker shoulder rehabilitation and places the distal screws in the sagittal plane for less risk to the radial nerve.

There has been a steady increase in use of the supine position for nailing the femur, rather than the lateral one. This has advantages for the multiply injured patient, is easier, quicker, and is more routine to set up and better for the anaesthetist and pulmonary impaired patients. However, it requires marked adduction, which may cause varus deformity of proximal fractures and may cause difficulty in locating the point of insertion, particularly in obese patients.[137] Also it crowds the whole sterile procedure of driving the nail close to the patient's trunk and head of the table. If arthritis limits adduction, the hip can be flexed.[138] Yet, with a long nail and the need for range to swing the mallet in line with the femur shaft, this would also put the procedure low with respect to the drapes. In one hospital where the supine position had become routine, it led to great difficulty with a morbidly obese patient.[139] Probably the lateral position is the better routine.

However, these difficulties are with antigrade femoral nailing. The GSH nail[140] for supracondylar fractures is inserted retrograde through the knee using the supine position. I have used this transgenicular approach seven times in unusual circumstances with no short-term untoward knee sequellae. It remains to be seen whether hemarthrosis or debris will cause problems over the long haul. There is also the question whether a tubular nail might not conduct synovial fluid to the fracture site and delay union, which Key and Conwell[141] considered one of nine causes.

The lengthy and sometimes complicated process of inserting the distal screws continues, and some surgeons are turning back to unlocked nails for stable fractures, such as the Hansen-Street nail, and supplementing with screws as necessary.[142]

There is currently interest in solid core nails,[143] one surgeon even reports a series of femur fractures treated with the AO tibial nail.[144] Also, there is a strongly positive report for the Hansen-Street nail in this decade.[145] Perhaps it should be interlocking. At this time intramedullary nailing continues to be an exciting, developing, and beneficial line of surgical procedures.

REFERENCES

1. Farill, J.: Orthopedics in Mexico. J. Bone Joint Surg. *34A*:506, 1952.
2. Bircher, H.: Eine Neue Methode unmittelbarer retention bei Fracturen der Röhrenknochen. Arch. Klin. Chir. *34*:410, 1886.
3. König, F.: Ueber die Implantation von Elfenbein zum Erzatz von Knochen und Gelenkenden. Nach experimentellen und klinischen Beobachtungen. Beitr. Klin. Chir. *85*:91, 1913.
4. Hoglund, E.J.: New intramedullary bone implant. Surg. Gynecol. Obstet. *24*:243, 1917.
5. Lambotte, A.: Chirurgie Operatoire des Fractures. Paris, Masson, et Cie, 1913.
6. Soeur, R.: Intramedullary pinning of diaphyseal fractures. J. Bone Joint Surg. *28*:309, 1946.
7. Nicolaysen, J.: Nordiskt medicinskt Ackiv. *8*:16, 1897.
8. Schöne, G.: Behandlung fur Vorderarmfrakturen mit Bolzung. Münch. Med. Wochenschr. *60*:2327, 1913.
9. Groves, E.W.H.: Ununited fractures with special reference to gunshot injuries and the use of bone grafting. Br. J. Surg. *6*:203, 1918.
10. Rush, L.V., Rush, H.L.: A reconstruction operation for comminuted fractures of the upper third of the ulna. Am. J. Surg. *38*:332, 1837.
11. Rush, L.V., Rush, H.L.: Technique for longitudinal pin fixation of certain fractures of the ulna and of the femur. J. Bone Joint Surg. *21*:619, 1939.
12. Rush, L.V.: Atlas of Rush pin techniques. Meridian, Berivon Company, 1956.
13. Lambrinudi, C.: Intramedullary Kirschner wires in the treatment of fractures. Proc. R. Soc. Med. *33*:153, 1940.
14. Murray, G.: Method of fixation of fractures of clavicle. J. Bone Joint Surg. *22*:616, 1940.
15. Dickson, J.A.: Intramedullary fixation of certain fractures of both bones of forearm: Report of two cases. Cleve. Clin. Q. 11:*62*, 1944.
16. Küntscher, G.: Die Marknagelung von Knochenbrüchen. Arch. Klin. Chir. *200*:443, 1940.
17. Nordmann, L.: (discussion of paper by Küntscher). Arch. Klin. Chir. *200*:443, 1940.
18. Fischer, A.W., Maatz R.: Weitere Erfahrungen mit der Marknagelung nach Küntscher. Arch. Klin. Chir. *203*: 531, 1942.
19. Alvis, H.J.: Project II, U.S. Fleet, U.S. Naval Forces, German Technical Section (Medical).
20. Stör, O.: Uber ein instrument zum ziehen der Knochenagel nach Küntscher. Zentralbl. Chir. *70*:754, 1943.
21. Küntscher, G., Maatz, R.: Die technic der Marknagelung, Leipzig. Thieme, 1945.
22. Linsmayer, H.: Ein Gerät für die Marknagelung nach Küntscher. Chirurg *15*:48, 1943.
23. Wittmoser, R.: Enistellgerät für die Marknagelung. Chirurg *15*:52, 1943.
24. Böhler, L.: Die Technik der Knochenbruchbehandlung im Frieden und im Kriege. Wien, Verlag Wilhelm Maudrich, 1942.
25. Böhler, L.: Medullary Nailing of Küntscher. (Translation by Hans Tretter), Baltimore, Williams & Wilkins, 1948.
26. Müller-Meernach: Bolzung der Brüche der langen Rohrenknochen. Zentralbl. Chir. *29*:1718, 1933.
27. Soeur, R.: Intramedullary pinning of diaphyseal fractures. J. Bone Joint Surg. *28*:309, 1946.
28. Westerborn, A.: Nailing in the marrow cavity in cases of recent fractures and pseudarthrosis. Report of 28 cases. Acta Chir. Scand. *90*:89, 1944.
29. Westerborn, A.: Marrow nailing of recent fractures, pseudarthrosis and bone plastic. Experiences in 100 cases. Ann. Surg. *127*:377, 1948.
30. Romney, H.: Personal communication, 1950.
31. Tordoir, B.M., Moeys, E.J.: The treatment of certain types of fractures with a V A steel nail in the medullary cavity. JAMA. *128*:792, 1945.
32. Street, D.M., Hansen, H.C., Brewer, B.J.: The medullary nail. Presentation of a new type and report of 4 cases. Arch. Surg. *35*:423, 1947.

33. Street, D.M.: Medullary nailing of the femur. JAMA. *147*:709, 1950.
34. MacAusland, W.R.: Medullary nailing of fractures of long bones. Surg. Gynecol. Obstet. *84*:85, 1947.
35. Wiggins, H.E., Lewis, G.B.: Intramedullary fixation of fractures of the femur. Naval Med. Bull. *48*:161, 1948.
36. Lottes, J.O.: Treatment of fractures of the femur with a heavy, large cored, three-flanged medullary nail. Surgery *29*:668, 1951.
37. Lottes, J.O.: Blind nailing technique for the insertion of the triflanged medullary nail. JAMA. *155*:1039, 1954.
38. Street, D.M.: Medullary nailing of the femur. In AAOS Instructional Course Lectures Vol. 10, Ann Arbor, J.W. Edwards, 1953.
39. Stryker, H.H.: A broaching tool to facilitate intramedullary nailing. J. Bone Joint Surg. *34A*:30, 1952.
40. Watson-Jones, R.: Medullary nailing of fractures after 50 years. J. Bone Joint Surg. *32B*:694, 1950.
41. Smith, H.: Symposium on medullary fixation. In AAOS Instructional Course Lectures. Vol. 8, Ann Arbor, J.W. Edwards, 1951.
42. Livingston, Austenal Co. advertisement. J. Bone Joint Surg. *34A*: 1952.
43. Breck, L.W.: Personal communication, 1954.
44. Modny, M.T., Bambora, J.: The perforated cruciate intramedullary nail: Preliminary report of its use in geriatric patients. J. Am. Geriatr. Soc. *1*:579, 1953.
45. Schneider, H.W.: Use of the 4-flanged self-cutting intramedullary nail for fixation of femoral fractures. Clin. Orthop. *60*:29, 1968.
46. Schneider, H.W.: Hip fusion using intramedullary nail fixation. J. Bone Joint Surg. *39A*:714, 1957.
47. McElvenney, R.T.: Personal communication, 1954.
48. Maatz, R., Lentz, W., Arens, W., Beck, H.: Intramedullary nailing and other intramedullary osteosyntheses. (Translated by Karl H. Mueller), Philadelphia, W. B. Saunders Co., 1986.
49. Küntscher, G.: Praxis der Marknagelung. Stuttgart, Schattauer, 1962.
50. Street, D.M., Vesely, D.C.: The split diamond nail. J. Bone Joint Surg. *41A*:1361, 1959.
51. Vesely, D.G.: The use of the split diamond nail for fractures of the humerus. Clin. Orthop. *41*:145, 1965.
52. Street, D.M.: Medullary fixation in multiple injuries. Orthop. Clin. N. Am. *1*:169, 1970.
53. Clawson, K., Smith, R.F., Hansen, S.T.: Closed intramedullary nailing of the femur. J. Bone Joint Surg. *53A*:681, 1971.
54. Kaessman, H.J.: Stabile Osteosynthese durch den Kompressionsnagel. Chirurg *37*:272, 1966.
55. Hutter, C.G., Oden, R., Kirk R.: The intramedullary compression rod. Clin Orthop. *122*:165, 1977.
56. Street, D.M.: Compression nailing (Exhibit at meeting AAOS, 1971). J. Bone Joint Surg. *53A*:1242, 1971.
57. Huckstep, R.L.: Rigid intramedullary fixation of femoral shaft fractures with compression. J. Bone Joint Surg. *54B*:204, 1972.
58. Derweduven, J.: A new intramedullary compression device for fractures and pseudarthroses of the long bones. Acta Orthop. Belg. *45*:659, 1979.
59. Lezius, A.: Intramedullary nailing of intertrochanteric and subtrochanteric fractures with curved nail. J. Int. Coll. Surg. *13*:569, 1950.
60. Küntscher, G.: Zur operativen Behandlung der pertrochanteren Fraktur. Zentralbl. Chir. *9*:281, 1966.
61. Küntscher, G.: A new method of treatment of pertrochanteric fractures. Proc. R. Soc. Med. *63*:1120, 1970.
62. Collado, H., Mijiers, G.: Anales de Medicina *55*:578, 1969.
63. Collado, F., Vila, J., Beltran, J.E.: Condylocephalic nail fixation for trochanteric fractures of the femur. J. Bone Joint Surg. *55B*:774, 1973.
64. Ender, J.: Probleme beim frischen per-und subtrochanteren Oberschenkelbruch. Hefte Unfallheilkd *106*:2, 1970.
65. Ender, J., Simon-Weidner, R.: Die fixierung der trochanterer Brüche mit runden elastischen condylennageln. Acta Chir. Austriaca *1*:40, 1870.
66. Ender, J., Simon-Weidner, R.: Die fixierung der Brüche der Trochantermassivs mit elastischen Rundnageln. Aktuel. Chir. *9*:71, 1974.
67. Ender, H.G.: Fixierung trochanterer frakturen mit elastischen Kondylennageln. Chir. Praxis *18*:81, 1974.
68. Ender, H.G., Schneider, H.: Subtrochantere Brüche des Oberschenkels: behandlung mit Federnageln. Aktuel. Chir. *9*:359, 1974.
69. Zickel, R.E.: A new fixation device for subtrochanteric fractures of the femur. Clin. Orthop. *54*:115, 1967.
70. Zickel, R.E.: A new intramedullary device for the distal third of the femur. Clin. Orthop. *122*:165, 1977.
71. Küntscher, G.: Die marknagelung des trümmerbruches. Langenbecks Arch. Klin. Chir. *322*:1063, 1968.
72. Klemm, K.M., Schellmann, W.D.: Dynamische und statische verriegelung des Marknagels. Monatschrift Unfallheilkunde *75*:568, 1972.
73. Kempf, L., Grosse, A., Lafforgned, L.: L'enclouae avec blocage de la rotation on "clou bloque" principles, technique, indications et premiers resultants. Communication a la journee d'hiver Sofcot, 1976.
74. Halloran, W.X.: The slotted femoral rod increases vascularity, thus promoting early fracture healing and faster rehabilitation. Orthop. Rev. 9:1057, 1980.
75. Allen, W.C., Heiple, K.G., Burstein, A.H.: A fluted femoral intermedullary rod. J. Bone Joint Surg. *60A*: 506, 1978.
76. Heiple, K.G., Brooks, D.B., Samson, B.L., Burstein, A.H.: A fluted intramedullary rod for subtrochanteric fractures. J. Bone Joint Surg. *61A*:730, 1979.
77. Seiler, J.O. III, et al.: A prospective evaluation of the AO/ASIF universal nail in the treatment of traumatic and reconstructive problems of the femur. J. Trauma *31*:121, 1991
78. Basom, W.C.: Personal communication, 1954
79. Levy, R.N., Siegel, M., Sedlin, E.D., Siffert, R.S.: Complications of Ender pin fixation in basicervical, intertrochanteric and subtrochanteric fractures of the hip. J. Joint Surg. *65A*:66, 1983.
80. Harris, L.J.: Condylocephalic nailing of intertrochanteric and subtrochanteric fractures of the femur. AAOS Instructional Course Lectures. Vol. 29, St. Louis, C.V. Mosby Co., 1980.
81. Harris, L.J.: Condylocephalic nailing of proximal femoral fractures. AAOS Instructional Course Lectures Vol 32, St. Louis, C.V. Mosby Co., 1983.
82. Sherk, H.H., Foster, M.D.: Hip fractures, condylocephalic rod versus compression screw. Clin. Orthop. *192*:255, 1985.
83. Street, D.M.: Condylocephalic nailing of intertrochanteric fractures. AAOS Instructional Course Lectures Vol. 29, St. Louis, C.V. Mosby Co. 1980.
84. Navarro-Quilis, A., Carrera, L.L., Pellise, F., Aguirre, M.: Condylocephalic nailing in pertrochanteric fractures. Clin. Orthop. *283*:90, 1992.
85. Groh, G.I.: Fractures of the femur treated intramedullary nailing using the fluted rod. A report of 193 consecutive cases. Clin. Orthop. *225*:223, 1992.
86. Star, A.M., et al.: Difficulties during removal of fluted intramedullary rods. J. Bone Joint Surg. *71A*:341, 1989.

87. Heiple, K.G., Figgie III, H.E., Lacey, S.H., Figgie, M.P.: Femoral shaft nonunion treated by a fluted intramedullary rod. Clin. Orthop. *194*:218, 1985.
88. Shelburn, K.D., Brueckman, F.R.: Rush pin fixation of supracondylar and intercondylar fractures of the femur. J. Bone Joint Surg. *64A*:161, 1982.
89. Hogh, J., et al.: Hansen-Street nailing of fractures of the femoral shaft. A study of 70 consecutive cases. Injury *14*:440, 1983.
90. Modny, M.T., et al.: Transfixion intramedullary nail. Orthop. Rev. *15*:83, 1986.
91. Yelton, C., Low, W.: Iatric subtrochanteric fracture: a complication of Zickel nails. J. Bone Joint Surg. *68A*: 1237, 1986.
92. Scherfel, T.: A new type of intramedullary nail for internal fixation of subtrochanteric fractures of the femur. Int. Orthop. *8*:255, 1985.
93. Henry, S.L., Werner, J., Seligson, D.: Intramedullary fixation of subtrochanteric fractures with the Williams Y nail. J. Orthop. Trauma *2*:139, 1988.
94. Browner, B.D.: Pitfalls, errors and complications in the use of locking Küntscher nails. Clin. Orthop. *212*: 192, 1986.
95. Bankston, A.B., Keating, E.M., Saha, S.: The biomechanical evaluation of intramedullary nails in distal femoral shaft fractures. Clin. Orthop. *276*:277, 1992.
96. Ebraheim, N.A., Miller, C.A., Jackson, W.T.: Complications in removal of the distal locking device of Brooker-Wills. Clin. Orthop. *290*:275, 1993.
97. Buckholz, R.W.: Fatigue fractures of the interlocking nail for the femur. J. Bone Joint Surg. *69A*:391, 1987.
98. Böstman, O., et al.: Infra-isthmal longitudinal fractures of the tibial diaphysis:results of treatment using closed intramedullary compression nailing. J. Trauma *24*:964, 1984.
99. Papageannopoulos, G., Karpinski, M.R., Nowton, G., Cargill, A.O'R.: Medullary femoral nailing of pathological fractures using the Derby nail. A report of 22 cases. Injury *17*:240, 1986.
100. Huckstep, R.L.: The Huckstep intramedullary compression nail. Indications, technique and results. Clin. Orthop. *212*:48, 1986.
101. Vicenzi, G., Graci, A., Moroni, A., Toni, A.: Intramedullary compression osteosynthesis for fractures of the femur. Ital. J. Orthop. Traumatol. *10*:61, 1984.
102. Pankovich, A.M., Tarabishy, I.E., Yelda S.: Flexible intramedullary nailing of tibial-shaft fractures. Clin Orthop. *160*:185, 1981.
103. Babin, S.R., et al.: The risk non-union following closed-focus nailing and reaming. Results in 1059 interventions using the Küntscher method. Int. Orthop. *7*:133, 1993.
104. Olerud, S., Karlstrom, C.: The spectrum of intramedullary nailing of the tibia. Clin. Orthop. *212*: 101, 1986.
105. Henley, M.B.: Intramedullary devices for tibial fracture stabilization. Clin. Orthop. *240*:87, 1989.
106. Chandler, R.W.N.: Personal communication, 1995.
107. Pritchett, J.W.: Delayed union of humeral shaft fractures treated by closed flexible intramedullary nailing. J. Bone Joint Surg. *67B*:715, 1985.
108. Durbin, R.A., Gottesman, M.J., Saunders, K.C: Hackethal stacked nailing of humeral shaft fractures. Clin. Orthop. *179*:168, 1983.
109. Gallagher, J.E., Black, R.J.: Humeral medullary nailing—a new implant. Injury *16*:374, 1985.
110. Mouradian, W.H.: Displaced proximal humeral fractures. Clin. Orthop. *212*:209, 1986.
111. Street, D.M.: Intramedullary forearm fractures. Clin. Orthop. *212*:219, 1986.
112. Zanasi, R., Franceschini, R., Rotolo, F., Romano, P., Galmarini, V., Zanasi, L.: Intramedullary osteosynthesis. 4. Kuntscher nailing in the ulna. Ital. J. Orthop. Traumatol. *16*:369, 1990.
113. McLennan, M.G., Ungersma, J.: Evaluation of the treatment of ankle fractures with the Inyo nail. J. Orthop. Trauma *2*:272, 1988.
114. Browner, B.D., Wiss, D.A.: Grosse-Kempf locking nail for the femur. The Science and Practice of Intramedullary Nailing. Philadelphia, Lea & Febiger, 1987.
115. Goulet, J.A., Londy, F., Saltzman, C.L., Matthews, L.S.: An improved method of screw placement combining image intensifier and laser light. Clin. Orthop. *281*:199, 1992.
116. Mahaisavariya, B., Laupallarakasem, W.: Ultra sound or image intensifier for closed femoral nailing. J. Bone Joint Surg. *75B*:66, 1993.
117. Miller, M.E., Davis, M.L., MacClean, Davis, J.C., Smith, B.L., Humphries, J.R.: Radiation exposure and associated risks to operating room personnel during use of fluoroscopic guidance for selected orthopaedic surgical procedures. J. Bone Joint Surg. *65A*:1, 1983.
118. Wiss, D.A., Fleming, C.H., Maria, J.M., Clark, D.: Comminuted and rotational unstable fractures of the femur treated with an interlocking nail. Clin. Orthop. *212*: 35, 1986.
119. Azer, S.N., Krause, W.R., Salman, N.N.: Self guiding interlocking nail. A new device. AAOS Exhibit, Anaheim 1991.
120. Hajek, P.D., Bicknell, H.R. Jr., Bronson, W.E., Albright, J.A., Subrata, S.: The use of one compared with two distal screws in the treatment of femoral shaft fractures with interlocking intramedullary nails. J. Bone Joint Surg. *75A*:519, 1993.
121. Stapert, J.W., Geesing, C.L., Jacobs, P.B., DeWit, R.J., Vierhout, P.A.: First experience and complications with the long gamma nail. J. Trauma *34*:394, 1993.
122. Wiss, D.A., Brien, W.A, Stetson, W.B.: Interlocking nailing for the treatment of segmental fractures of the femur. J. Bone Surg. *72A*:724, 1990.
123. Marchetti, P.G., Vicenzi, G.: Made by Zimmer UK Ltd., England.
124. Wheelwright, E.F., Court-Brown, C.M.: Primary external fixation and secondary intramedullary nailing in the treatment of tibial fractures. Injury *83*:373, 1992.
125. Wu, C.C., Shih, C.H.: Complicated open fractures of the distal tibia treated by secondary interlocking nailing. J. Trauma *34*:792, 1993.
126. Boynton, M.D., Schmeling, G.J.: Nonreamed intramedullary nailing of open tibial fractures. J. AAOS. *2*:107, 1994.
127. Wittle, A.B., Russell, T.A., Taylor, J.C., Lavelle, D.G.: Treatment of open tibial fractures with the use of intramedullary locked nails without reaming. J. Bone Joint Surg. *74A*:1162, 1992.
129. Tornetti, P., Barbera, C.: Severe heterotoptic bone formation in the knee after tibial intramedullary nailing. J. Orthop. Trauma *6*:113, 1992.
130. Gosselin, R.A., Belzer, P., Contreras, D.M.: Hetertopic ossification of the patellar tendon following intramedullary nailing of the tibia. J. Trauma *34*:161, 1993.
131. Hemple, D., Fischer, S.: Intramedullary Nailing. (Translation by Hans Koening & Thomas Koening) New York, Thieme-Stratton, 1982.
132. Winquist, R.A.: Locked femoral nailing. J.AAOS *1*:95, 1993.
133. Seidel, H.: Humeral interlocking nail: A preliminary report. Orthopedics *12*:219, 1989.

134. Riemer, B.L., Butterfield, S.R., D'Ambrosia, R., Kellam, J.: Seidel intramedullary nailing of humeral diaphyseal fractures: A preliminary report. Orthopedics *14*:239, 1991.
135. Watanabe, R.S.: Intramedullary fixation of complicated fractures of the humeral shaft. Clin. Orthop. *292*:255, 1993.
136. Ingman, A.M., Waters, D.A.: Locked intramedullary nailing of humeral shaft fractures. Implant design, surgical technique, and clinical results. J. Bone Joint Surg. *76B*:23, 1994.
137. Wiss, D.A., Matta, J.M.: Comminuted and rotational unstable fractures of the femur treated with an interlocking nail. Clin. Orthop. *212*:35, 1986.
138. Moran, C.J., Gibson, M.J., Cross, A.T.: Intramedullary locking nails for femoral shaft fractures in elderly patients. J. Bone Joint Surg. *72B*:19, 1990.
139. McKee, M.D., Waddell, J.P.: Intramedullary nailing femoral fractures in morbidly obese patients. J. Trauma *2*:208, 1994.
140. Lucas, S.E., Seligson, D., Henry, S.L.: Intramedullary supracondylar nailing of femoral of femoral fractures. A preliminary report of the GSH supracondylar nail. Clin. Orthop. *296*:200, 1993.
141. Key, Conwell: Fractures, Dislocations and Sprains. St. Louis, C.V. Mosby Co., 1937.
142. Funk, F.J., Wells, R.E., Street, D.M.: Supplementary fixation of femoral fractures. Clin. Orthop. *60*:41, 1968.
143. Sanders, R., Koval, K.J., DiPasquali, T., Nelfet, D.L., Frankle, M.: The treatment of open tibial shaft dractures using an interlocking intramedullary nail without reaming. J. Orthop. Trauma *8*:504, 1994.
144. Mahaisavariya, B., Kesprayura, S., Laupattarakasem, W., Suthiyuth, T.: Subtrochanteric fractures: Fixation using the AO tibial nail. Injury *23*:231, 1992.
145. Grimberg, B.: The use of the Hansen-Street intramedullary nail in mid shaft fractures of the femur. Bull. Hosp. Jt. Dis. *53*:45, 1993.

2

The Role of Intramedullary Nailing in Fracture Management

Michael W. Chapman

The rationale for the use of intramedullary fixation in the management of fractures is intrinsically tied to the indications for internal fixation of fractures in general.[1–5] Intramedullary nailing is by definition confined to the long bones; therefore, fixation of the femur, tibia, humerus, radius, and ulna will be discussed. Because of the inherent risk of anesthesia and the unavoidable complications of internal fixation, intramedullary nailing of long-bone fractures should be done only when the benefits of intramedullary fixation are sufficiently better than those of nonoperative treatment and when the risks are justified.[6–7] Intramedullary fixation of fractures is becoming more common, as the complication rate, especially when using closed techniques, is quite low.[8,9] Intramedullary fixation, particularly using cross-locking screws and other more stable devices, almost completely eliminates the need for external fixation or protection. Early rehabilitation with muscle strengthening and joint range-of-motion exercises is often possible. If good bone contact is achieved, early weight bearing is possible.

OPEN VERSUS CLOSED TECHNIQUE

Open nailing means that the fracture site is opened directly through the surrounding muscle envelope to achieve reduction and insertion of the nail. Closed technique means that the muscle envelope around the fracture is not opened, the fracture is reduced by external manipulation, and the nail is inserted through the end of the bone.

Opening the fracture is usually much faster than closed nailing techniques, except when one takes into account the time required to close the wound. In addition, the nailing can usually be achieved without the assistance of a fluoroscope, assuming that cross-locking using current techniques is not necessary. The disadvantages of open nailing are that blood loss is usually greater and disruption of the soft-tissue envelope and exposure of the fracture to the operating room environment increases the infection rate and decreases the blood supply to fracture, thereby increasing the rate of nonunion. Closed techniques are technically more difficult, often require special tables, and always require visualization by fluoroscopy. Closed technique is commonly not possible because the trauma patient is on an unsuitable table or in an inappropriate position. However, intramedullary nailing using closed technique has distinct advantages, including less blood loss, lower infection rate, a higher rate of union, and, in some cases, more rapid surgery.

A review of the English language literature,"Closed Intramedullary Nailing of the Femur," in the first edition of *The Science and Practice of Intramedullary Nailing* showed an accumulated experience of 1,499 nailings.[10–31] The infection rate in these reports average 0.4% and the incidence of nonunion was only 1%. The functional results reported were generally excellent. Intramedullary nailing using open techniques showed less favorable results, particularly in open fractures. In a total of 1,950 femur fractures treated by open technique, the deep infection rate averaged 3.5%, which is quadruple the rate in closed nailing.[15,32–45] The infection rate reported in immediate open nailing of open fractures averaged 17.7%. Open nailing had an average rate of nonunion of 2.1%. The overall superior results of intramedullary nailing with closed technique, when compared to open nailing, justifies the complexity and difficulty of closed nailing.[46]

On the other hand, a modified technique of open nailing, particularly for the femur, is extremely useful in patients with multiple injuries and in my experience has not had a higher complication rate than closed techniques. In the patient with multiple injuries, it is often necessary for the trauma surgeon to rush the patient to the operating room for lifesaving procedures involving the chest and abdomen. For this reason the orthopaedic surgeon frequently first encounters these patients after laparotomy and/or chest procedures in a supine position on a regular operating table that may or may not be radiolucent. Transfer of these patients to a fracture table for intramedullary nailing of the femur using closed techniques is time-consuming and occasionally hazardous, particularly if the patient has a tendency to be hemodynamically unstable. A modified open technique is ideal for these patients. Fluoroscopic control is gained by placing a C-arm across the top of the table in the inverted position. This gives an excellent anteroposterior (AP) view of the full length of the femur. Placing the leg in a frog position will provide a reasonable lateral view (Fig. 2–1).

The patient is placed into the lateral/decubitus position with the fractured femur uppermost. The entire lower extremity is prepared and draped including the buttocks, as one would use for traditional medullary nailing. The procedure is expedited if two surgeons can operate simultaneously. One surgeon opens the fracture through a short lateral incision just long enough to insert the fingers of the hand without actually exposing the fracture unless it is absolutely necessary. An average incision is 4 inches in length. Upon incising the deep fascia, a defect in the quadriceps can usually be found which represents a tear of the muscle caused by the fracture fragments. This can be split bluntly with a periosteal elevator or the fingers to expose the ends of the fracture fragments. With this technique, additional trauma caused by surgical splitting of the muscle at a different site is avoided. The exposure is extremely fast. At this point there is no need to reduce the fracture. The fracture hematoma is left in place and the fracture is not irrigated. If muscle is found to be impaled on the ends of the fracture fragments, it should be removed with a curet.

Simultaneously, the second surgeon makes a gluteal-splitting incision approximately 4 inches in length, beginning at the tip of the greater trochanter and extending proximalward. The usual entry site for the nail is made directly above the intramedullary canal at the junction of the femoral neck with the greater trochanter and somewhat on its posterior aspect. I prefer to place a 3.2-mm guide pin first and then ream over it with a cannulated 14-mm reamer. This is more accurate and easier than using an awl. Because the position can be verified on the fluoroscope prior to reaming, injury to the femoral neck is avoided. Next slide a ball-tipped reaming guide pin down to the fracture site. The surgeon at the fracture site should have a finger over the end of the open end of the proximal fragment and feel the ball-tipped guide pin as it exits the fragment. In many cases the fracture is easily reduced and then the guide pin manually passed into the distal fragment through manipulation by the surgeon at the fracture site. In transverse or short oblique fractures with overriding, reduction can be difficult. Reduction is best achieved by placing a bone hook in the end of each fragment, angulating the fracture into varus to oppose the medial corners of the fracture, and then aligning the fracture as the guide pin is pushed into the distal fragment. This is much easier in comminuted fractures. Verify appropriate position of the guide pin with the fluoroscope.

In very comminuted fractures and also in transverse fractures with overriding in which reduction is expected to be difficult, application of an AO femoral distractor greatly enhances passage of the guide pin. Occasionally, in the hands of a skilled surgeon, reduction can even be done using a closed technique. Once the guide pin has been passed, the surgeon rapidly closes the thigh wound in layers while the other surgeon proceeds with reaming of the fracture. The reaming should be done using closed techniques so that the reaming materials are contained around the fracture site as a bone graft.

If the nail is driven down to subchondral bone at the knee, surprisingly good rotation control can often be obtained. In all locking intramedullary nails on the market today, locking of the nail proximally can be achieved with a guide that eliminates the need for radiographs, except to verify proper location and length of the screw. This should always be done. In the multiply injured patient, distal cross-locking can be deferred until the patient's condition is more stable. Postoperative management with a knee immobilizer and antirotation device on the foot will suffice if the fracture is unstable. If distal cross-locking is desired, it can be achieved by flexing the hip to bring the leg off the fracture table so that access for the C-arm fluoroscope can be obtained. Having the patient on a fully radiolucent operating table is a major advantage, and many trauma centers use these routinely.

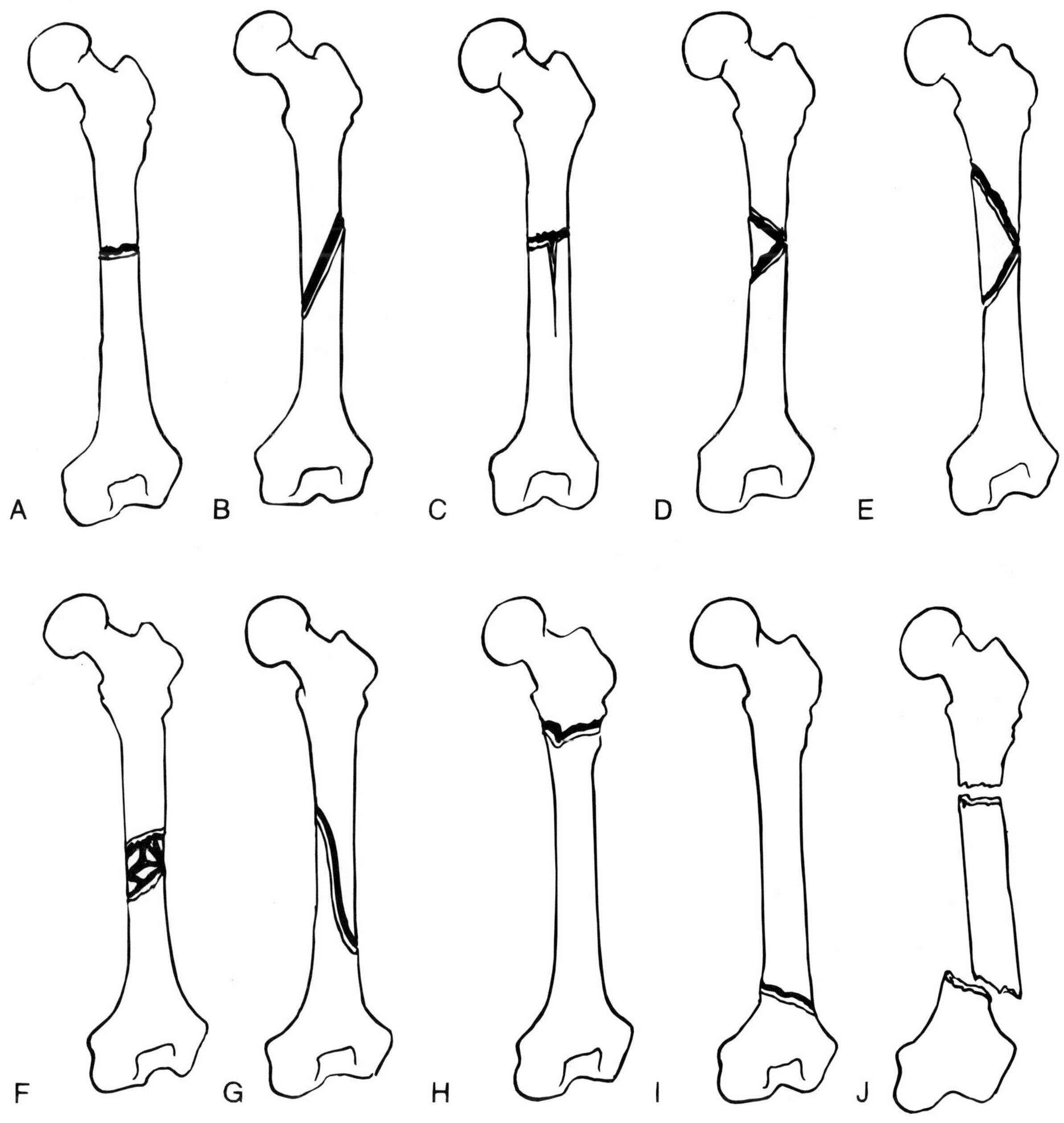

Fig. 2–1. Fracture configurations suitable for nailing.

An alternative technique that can be used under circumstances where the fluoroscope cannot be used, but cross-locking is felt to be absolutely essential, is as follows. Be certain during the drive of the nail that the distal cross-locking holes are located directly in the midline facing the lateral aspect of the femur. Take a rod of identical length and place it beside the thigh with its upper end even with the rod in the femur and mark the level of the cross-locking holes on the distal thigh. Make an incision down to the femur in this area. Using the other rod as a guide, mark on the femur the location of the cross-locking screws. Take a large drill point, at least ¼ inch in diameter, and make a hole in the lateral aspect of the femur directly over where you feel the hole in the rod is located. Then using a Kirschner wire, feel for the hole in the rod. In most cases, it is easily identified. If the initial hole is not quite in the correct location, enlarge it so that it is directly over the hole in the rod. Next, insert the appropriately sized drill point and drill the opposite cortex. The cross-locking screws can then be easily inserted. This technique has the disadvantage of sacrificing purchase in the near cortex, but in a lifesaving situation, this may be a small price to pay. Bone graft harvested from the entry site at the greater trochanter can be packed around the screw if you feel it is necessary.

ADVANTAGES OF INTRAMEDULLARY NAILING

Intramedullary nailing, particularly using closed techniques, provides good bone stability with limited soft-tissue exposure and dissection. Preservation of the muscle envelope around the fracture preserves the extraosseous blood supply to bone. This enhances revascularization of the injured bone and promotes periosteal callus formation. The lack of additional injury to muscles enhances the potential for early joint and muscle rehabilitation.

Intramedullary nailing, whether by reamed or unreamed techniques, does interfere with the endosteal blood supply to bone.[47–49] Rhinelander[50] has shown that the endosteal blood supply rapidly reconstitutes itself after intramedullary nailing with unreamed nails, such as Rush rods[51] and Street and Lottes nails.[52] Reaming obliterates the nutrient artery and endosteal blood supply, but this will reconstitute itself if the nail has channels along its length to permit revascularization. Rhinelander showed that the Küntscher nail shows the least revascularization when compared to nails with flutes. However, this advantage is short lived as the normal blood supply to bone becomes centripetal and the bone revascularizes rapidly from the periosteal surface to the marrow cavity. This phenomenon may enhance periosteal callus formation and be advantageous to bone healing.

When compared to plates and screws,[53–55] intramedullary nails have the advantage of being load-sharing devices. In fractures where the configuration of the fracture provides axial stability, early weight bearing is possible. The load is born primarily by the bone, rather than by the nail. Evidence suggests that this promotes fracture healing, prevents disuse osteoporosis, and reduces the effects of stress protection. For these reasons, breakage of intramedullary nails is uncommon when compared to plates and screws.

Removal of intramedullary nails generally involves less surgery than the removal of plates and screws. The lack of disuse osteoporosis and absence of screw holes near the fracture means that problems with refracture after intramedullary nail removal are rare.

REAMED VERSUS UNREAMED NAILING

In general, reamed intramedullary nailing provides better stability because of the increased contact between the rod and medullary canal. As larger nails can be used, the nails are generally stronger and less likely to fail because of fatigue. Unreamed nails are usually simpler to use and can be inserted more quickly, but their smaller diameter provides less solid fixation. In the femur, equally good results have been reported with reamed and unreamed nailing. Mechanical problems have been less with reamed nailing. With the advent of interlocking nailing, reamed nailing has become the treatment of choice for fractures of the diaphysis of the femur and closed fractures of the diaphysis of the tibia. Unreamed nailing in the tibia is preferred for open fractures because of the poor blood supply to the tibia and its subcutaneous location. If infection intervenes, the complications with unreamed nails are likely to be less severe. Excellent results with unreamed nails such as Lottes, Ender, and more recently, locking nails has been reported.[56–65] Because of the small size of the forearm bones, reaming is technically difficult, therefore, unreamed nails have generally been used. Unreamed nails have particular advantages in the humerus because of the problems of access at the proximal and distal ends of the bone. Reamed nails are useful for nonunions of the humerus, but problems with the rotator cuff at the entry point are more frequent.

Recent studies[66–68] have shown that there is significant embolization of marrow contents to the heart and lungs with reaming and pressurization of the intramedullary canal of the femur. Pape and colleagues[69–71] have shown that this may increase the incidence of adult respiratory distress syndrome (ARDS) in multiply injured patients who have had a pulmonary injury. For that reason, there has been a recent revival in interest in unreamed nailing of the femur. Locking nails made of titanium alloys are particularly advantageous for this application because of their increased flexibility and strength. The effectiveness of changing to nonreamed nails in the femur of the multiply injured patient at this point has not yet been proven, although the evidence is highly suggestive that this may be an important consideration.

LOCKED VERSUS NONLOCKED NAILS

Intramedullary nails that provide for cross-locking screws are now available for all of the major long bones. Because all of these can be used in a nonlocking mode, there is probably no reason to use nonlocking nails at the present time, except for their reduced cost. The exception is smooth, unreamed nails such as the Ender pins and Rush pins, which still have special indications that will be discussed later. Although locking nails provide enhanced fixation that can almost always guarantee that unexpected shortening, angulation, or malrotation will not occur, the holes in the nails do create a stress riser and therefore increase the incidence of nail breakage. Bucholz[72] has pointed out that this is a particular problem in supracondylar fractures of the femur in which failure through the more proximal screw hole in the nail can occur, particularly if an unstable fracture is subjected to early weight bearing. These problems can be minimized by using large diameter nails, filling all holes with screws, placing the screws as far away from the fracture as possible, and by delaying weight bearing. Screw failure is also a concern. Special screws which are designed for transverse cross-locking are available and are much stronger than standard, fully threaded cortical screws. Unreamed and smaller nails present a particular problem in that the transverse cross-locking screws must, by necessity, be much smaller in diameter, generally averaging between 3.5 and 4 mm in diameter. Failure rates in stainless steel screws used in the tibia have been reported as high as 30% and as high as 7% in titanium 4-mm screws. For this reason, in the tibia, I tend to pass one or two reamers gently in an effort to always place a 10-mm nail which will take full 4.5- to 5-mm standard transverse cross-locking screws.

GENERAL INDICATIONS

Intramedullary nailing must be considered when the advantages of anatomic alignment, early weight bearing, and early unrestricted joint and muscle rehabilitation are felt to be of advantage to the patient.[73–84] In patients with multiple injuries,[85,86] ARDS is best prevented if long-bone fractures are stabilized and the patient is immediately mobilized.[87–90] This optimizes cardiopulmonary care and may ameliorate the systemic inflammatory response that leads to pulmonary failure. This is particularly true for fractures of the femur and less so for fractures of the humerus.

Floating hip (fracture of the pelvis or acetabulum and femoral shaft)[91] and floating knee are other strong indications for intramedullary nailing. Combined fractures of the femur and tibia can present problems in maintaining alignment, and rehabilitation of the knee is extremely difficult with ipsilateral concomitant[92,93] fractures above and below. These are best managed by internal fixation of the femur and tibia, although nonoperative management of the tibia is possible in some cases. The same rationale applies to the floating elbow where nail fixation of the humerus and plate fixation of the forearm is advantageous.[94]

In vascular injuries requiring repair, particularly if the vascular injury was caused by the fracture, stabilization of the fracture may be indicated. To protect the vascular repair, the majority of these will be done using open technique, especially if done at the time of vascular repair.

FRACTURE CONFIGURATION

When using noninterlocking reamed and unreamed nails, particularly in weight-bearing bones, the fracture configuration must provide rotational and axial stability to be nailed without cross-locking. Only a short oblique fracture with no comminution or hidden microcracks, offer sufficient stability. Often, small cracks cannot be seen, however, and even in apparently stable fracture patterns, late extension of the fracture can occur with loss of stability. For that reason, I routinely use interlocking nails regardless of the fracture pattern. Indications for non-locking nails can be modified if the fracture is to be protected postoperatively by non-weight bearing, traction, or a cast. This is rarely practical or advisable.

Fracture configurations suitable for nailing are illustrated in Figure 2–1. When interlocking nails are used, the indications for intramedullary nailing can be extended. Interlocking nails are now available for all of the major long bones. The fracture configurations illustrated in Figure 2–1 can generally be translated to the tibia and humerus. Fractures in the proximal quarter of any of the major long bones represent extended indications for intramedullary nailing. The nailing of these fractures requires considerable experience. Angulation or inadequate fixation with cross-locking screws can be a challenging problem. When fixing fractures towards the ends of long bones, the surgeon must be certain that there are no cracks extending into the juxta-articular area that will compromise cross-screw fixation.

Extremely comminuted fractures, particularly those which represent a combination of fractures are well managed by locked intramedullary nailing; however, a large butterfly fragment may remain quite displaced, leaving a considerable defect in the midshaft of the femur, particularly when closed nailing techniques are used. It is not uncommon for the fracture to heal with a large defect in these cases. In these circumstances, closed intramedullary bone grafting is worthwhile, considering another alternative would be to open the fracture to cerclage the displaced fragment into place. The latter technique is hazardous, as considerable devascularization might occur; therefore, gentle technique is required. In spite of the comminution, these fractures usually heal.

OPEN FRACTURES

In the recent past, immediate reamed intramedullary nailing of open fractures has been felt to be contraindicated because of the increased risk of infection and the additional devascularization that is caused by destruction of the endosteal blood supply. However, clinical experience has shown that immediate reamed nailing of open fractures of the femur and humerus is possible with a minimal increase in the risk of infection.[95–99] Immediate nailing offers significant advantages in the management of the multiply injured patient and in the management of the soft-tissue injury. There is little controversy about immediate reamed nailing of Gustilo grade I to IIIa open fractures. However, some authorities still express reservations about immediate reamed nailing of grade IIIb open fractures.[96]

In the open fracture of the tibia, the risks of infection and devascularization are much higher because of the poor soft-tissue envelope over the anteromedial aspect of the tibia. Because nonreamed nails work so well in the tibia, the standard of care at the present time is to do immediate unreamed nailing, rather than reamed nailing.[100]

It goes without saying that meticulous irrigation and debridement and appropriate high-dose bactericidal intravenous antibiotics are necessary to minimize the risk of infection. Immediate intramedullary nailing of open fractures should not be performed by surgeons who are not experienced and intimately familiar with the soft-tissue care necessary to prevent infection in open fractures.

The major advantage of intramedullary nailing of open fractures is that the stability achieved is usually superior to that of external fixation, and it requires far less soft-tissue stripping than plate and screw fixation. If soft-tissue complications occur, they are usually more easily managed with an intramedullary nail in place, than with a plate or screws which may be exposed. Management of the soft-tissues is far simpler with an intramedullary nail as compared to external fixation, because the surgeon need not deal with the external fixation pins. External fixation pins have a risk of infection in and of themselves and can interfere with soft-tissue procedures such as local and free microvascularized flaps.

Delayed intramedullary nailing, particularly

with reamed nails, is advocated by some as a method for reducing the immediate risk of infection and for the treatment of potential or actual delayed unions or nonunions.[101–104] In the conversion from external fixation to intramedullary nails, care must be taken to minimize the risk of infection.[105–107] The best protocol is to convert early before the external fixation pin tracks are infected or pin loosening occurs. If the external fixation pins are loose or infected, then the risk of infection with subsequent reamed intramedullary nailing is quite high. Some feel that conversion to intramedullary reamed nailing is contraindicated. On the other hand, removal of the external fixator with curetment and treatment of any potentially infected pin sites, followed by a suitable delay and infection free interval, can minimize the risk, assuming that the advantages of conversion to an intramedullary nail are worthwhile.

From a technical viewpoint, it is wise to do the initial irrigation and debridement with one surgical setup. This should be followed by a second surgical prep and draping and the medullary nailing should be carried out with a new set of instruments. This minimizes contamination.

FEMUR

Having trained and practiced in the era of nonoperative treatment of femur fractures and after 25 years of experience with closed intramedullary nailing, I personally feel, along with the vast majority of other surgeons, that all fractures of the shaft of femur in adults should be treated with closed intramedullary locked nailing if the patient's condition warrants the procedure and the fracture pattern permits.[108–126] At the time of the first publication of this book, nonlocking nails such as the AO nail, Küntscher nail, Schneider nail, and Street nail[52] were in common use. Because none of these nails offered adequate protection against shortening and malrotation in unstable fracture patterns, complications of shortening, malrotation, and angulation clouded the otherwise excellent experience with nailing of the femur. With the development of the first truly interlocking intramedullary nails by Klemm and Schellman and Grosse and Kempf in the late 1970s, stability of nailing was vastly improved, and the complications of unexpected shortening, malrotation, and angulation nearly disappeared.[123–128] These nails were introduced to North America in the early 1980s and because of their high success rate, intramedullary nailing of the femur became the treatment of choice. The vast majority of surgeons have learned to perform intramedullary nailing using closed techniques. Locked intramedullary nails were subsequently developed that were stronger, had closed sections, and used different materials such as titanium alloys. Two distal transverse cross-locking screws has remained the standard; however, differing configurations for proximal cross-locking have developed, the most common of which at present is two transverse screws. Subsequently, a second generation of locking nails that permit fixation into the head and neck were developed. These extended the indications of intramedullary nailing to include most subtrochanteric and complex fractures involving the proximal femur, including intertrochanteric-subtrochanteric and concomitant ipsilateral fractures of the femoral neck and shaft.[129–131] With these nails, nearly every fracture pattern in the femur can now be managed by intramedullary nailing, including extremely distal supracondylar fractures. The only limitations are poor quality of bone and the absence of enough intact bone distally and proximally to allow adequate fixation for the screws of the nail.

Advances in the techniques of intramedullary fixation of the femur has greatly enhanced our ability to treat patients with multiple injuries. It has been shown by Bone and others[87–90] that immediate stabilization of fractures of the femoral shaft in patients who are multiply injured significantly reduces the incidence of pulmonary complications, treatment time in the intensive care unit, and incidence of death. No authority questions the remarkable advances that have been made in the care of multiply injured patients by the introduction of immediate medullary nailing of the femur. On the other hand, embolization of bone marrow contents caused by reaming and driving of the intramedullary nail has been well demonstrated. There is recent evidence to suggest that embolization of bone marrow contents to an injured and compromised pulmonary bed may increase the incidence of ARDS.[67–71] For that reason, there has been increased interest recently in the use of unreamed locked nails as they minimize the incidence of embolization. The difficulty with these smaller nails is that mechanical failure of the nail and nonunion is more likely. Early conversion to larger, stronger nails may be indicated. The evidence on this issue is not yet sufficiently strong to recommend unreamed over reamed nails in the multiply injured patients. My advice at present would be that in the multiply injured patients with preexisting pulmonary injury, that unreamed or minimally reamed intramedullary nails should be used. Careful follow-up with guarded weight bearing will be necessary in these patients and conversion to a larger reamed nail may be necessary after they have recovered from their pulmonary injury, assuming that the risk of failure of the nail is high.

Our thinking on dynamization of locked intramedullary nails has also changed over the past decade. It was initially feared that locked intramedullary nails would be nonunion machines because of the potential for distraction at the fracture site. For this reason, it was initially advised that in stable fracture patterns that the cross-locking screws be removed from one and/or the other of the nail to allow the fracture to compress early during the treatment of the fracture. Brumback[125] has shown that dynamization is not necessary to achieve union and that the vast majority of fractures will go on to heal well with the cross-locking screws in place. However, in spite of this experience the majority of nonunions of the shaft of the femur which I have seen have been caused by locking with distraction or defects in the fracture caused by comminution. Some recent nail designs have included slotted holes for the cross-locking screws to allow for automatic dynamization. Whether this is necessary, or even wise, is not known.

The practice at the University of California, Davis, has been to impact at the time of initial nailing all fracture patterns with enough bone contact to allow impaction immediately. This can be achieved by either using the slide hammer driver on an Alta nail or similar design, or by placing an AO femoral distractor across the fracture site and compressing the fracture prior to cross-locking. In the former case, this is done by distally cross-locking first, impacting the fracture, and then cross-locking proximally. In the later instance, a bicortical Schanz screw can be used distally in the femur and a unicortical screw proximally with the distractor to achieve compression. Where bone contact between the distal and proximal fragments with over 50% contact of the cortex is achieved, and where there is no longitudinal crack threatening the stability of the fixation, early weight bearing is possible. The majority of patients will be fully weight bearing with good quadriceps rehabilitation by 6 weeks. In unstable fracture patterns, I recommend that the nail be left statically locked until union occurs. If the fracture was open and had bone deficiency, or if there is evidence of delayed union by 12 weeks, then early bone grafting should be considered.

Contraindications to closed nailing of femur fractures are few and include those fractures involving the femoral neck and the intertrochanteric area which are too comminuted to obtain adequate fixation, particularly where the bone quality is poor, such as in senile osteoporosis. On the other hand, intramedullary reconstruction type nails may be the only device that will work in these type of fractures. Low supracondylar fractures in which two transverse cross-locking screws cannot be placed are a relative contraindication to closed intramedullary nailing. In the hands of experienced and skilled surgeons, even T-type intraarticular, supracondylar fractures of the femur are occasionally managed by intramedullary nailing. The intraarticular portion of the fracture can be fixed initially with intrafragmentary screws placed anteriorly and posteriorly to avoid impingement by the intramedullary nail. The nail can then be placed down to subchondral bone at the knee, which with some nail designs will permit at least three cortexes and sometimes four cortexes of screw fixation. Retrograde nailing is advocated by some.[132,133]

The primary contraindication to intramedullary nailing is infected skin lesions about the buttocks or other areas which would make the risk of infection too high. Active systemic infection with an organism that could infect the operative site is also a contraindication. In some conditions, femoral nailing may be unnecessary.[38,109–120] For example, fractures of the shaft of the femur in quadriplegics can often be managed by pillow splints.

TIBIA

With the introduction of locked, unreamed intramedullary nails for the tibia, the indications and use of medullary fixation for fractures of the tibia has increased substantially over the past decade, particularly for open fractures of the tibia.[62–65]

The majority of simple fractures of the diaphysis of the tibia can be managed by closed reduction and immobilization with a weight-bearing cast or cast brace.[75] In closed fractures, indications for intramedullary nailing include (1) the floating knee, with an associated fracture of the femur; (2) associated ligamentous injury of the knee, in which stability of the tibia is necessary for rehabilitation; (3) associated injuries of the foot or ankle, in which a similar philosophy applies; and (4) unstable closed fractures, in which satisfactory reduction cannot be obtained or maintained.

Patients today are less tolerant of malunion than patients in the past. Heavy laborers must perform at a high level to be competitive, and sedentary workers are frequently athletically quite active. It is always dangerous to generalize, but I would consider locked intramedullary nailing, when shortening of more than 1 cm, varus or valgus of more than 10°, and malrotation of greater than 10° cannot be controlled by nonoperative techniques. Locked intramedullary nailing is ideal for the middle third of the tibia. As fractures become more proximal and distal to the isthmus, they become more difficult to nail in anatomical condition and fixation with the cross-locking screws becomes increasingly precarious. Fractures in the proximal and distal quarters of the tibia are relative contraindications to locked intramedullary nailing. The majority of locking nails provide for two transverse distal cross-locking screws, which can control a short distal fragment if the nail is placed quite distal; however, the bone quality must be good, cracks must be absent, and the surgeon must be skilled with the technique and assure that acceptable alignment is present. Proximally the pull of the patellar tendon tends to cause the proximal fragment to loosen and angulate anteriorly at the fracture site. Cross-locking with a minimum of two solid screws, and preferably three, must be obtained to control the proximal fragment. Nailing of these fractures can be quite difficult and should be tackled only by those experienced and skilled with the technique. Some undisplaced intraarticular fractures of the distal or proximal end of the tibia can be managed by percutaneous cannulated screw fixation combined with intramedullary nailing, but this certainly represents an extension of the technique to be used only by those who are highly skilled. Be aware that unrecognized comminution may lead to failure of this type of fixation.

The indications for nonlocking, unreamed nails of the tibia such as the Lottes and Ender are quite limited because of the versatility of locking nails.[51,56,58,59] The major advantage of these nails is their low cost and simple instrumentation. Fracture patterns must be stable. External protection with a cast and limited weight bearing is usually required until healing occurs. For that reason, the majority of surgeons use locking nail systems. These can be used either as unreamed or reamed nails. Most systems can be used with either technique, depending upon the size of nail required. In closed fractures, I always ream large enough to place a nail that will permit the use of the largest transverse cross-locking screws which generally are 4.5 to 5 mm in diameter. This minimizes the risk of transverse cross-locking screw failure in the event the patient weight bears against advice or a nonunion occurs. The breakage rate in small transverse cross-locking screws (3.5 to 4 mm in diameter) in unreamed nails is significant and has been reported up to 7% in titanium and 30% in stainless steel nails.

The primary indication for unreamed, locked nails of the tibia are open fractures. Recent reports have shown results which are comparable to or better than those achieved with external fixation which has been the standard of care in the past.[62–65,100-107] The advantages of medullary fixation, compared to external fixation, are identical to those already discussed. Recent work by Swiontkowski and his associates, studying the blood flow to the sheep tibia using the laser Doppler, shows that reaming of the tibia compromises the circulation to the diaphysis in the initial post fracture period as compared to nonreamed nails.[134]

For that reason, I do not use fully reamed nails as the primary fixation in open fractures of the tibia. If possible, I use a nonreamed nail, but if necessary to obtain a 5-mm transverse cross-locking screw, I will employ minimal, gentle reaming with one or two reamers. Usually this involves increasing the medullary canal size from 9 to 10 mm. Some investigators have had satisfactory experience with primary reamed nails in open fractures of the tibia, but this has not been the general North American experience.[62] Controversy exists on whether nails should be used at all in grade IIIb fractures of the tibia. We have been nailing these routinely at the University of California, Davis, since 1988 with results comparable to external fixation, from the standpoint of infection, and superior to external fixation, from the standpoint of nonunion and malunion. Titanium nails have a particular advantage in the tibia because of the increased strength and flexibility in the smaller unreamed nails.

HUMERUS

As with the tibia, the majority of fractures of the diaphysis and metaphysis of the humerus can be managed by nonoperative means; however, if it is necessary to open the fracture, to extricate the radial nerve for example, a plate with interfragmentary screws is the usual means of internal fixation.[136] When open reduction is not required, plate fixation is less desirable in cases where the necessary large dissection for surgical exposure is contraindicated. On the other hand, intramedullary nailing of the humerus has never been popular because the fixation is frequently unstable and the entry sites into the humerus are either difficult or interfere with joint function at either end of the humerus. In spite of this, many fixation devices have been advocated for the humerus, including Rush rods,[137] Küntscher nails,[138] Steinmann pins, Supramid pins, Stack (Hackethal) nails, Ender pins, Sampson fluted nails, Street nails, and Lottes nails.

The most common indication for closed intramedullary nailing of the humerus is the inability to achieve satisfactory alignment of the fracture using closed techniques. Alignment can be a problem when the fracture is just distal to the deltoid tubercle, where the deltoid acts as a major deforming force on the proximal fragment. A similar situation can occur in surgical neck fractures in which the pull of the pectoralis major may be a problem. Other indications are fractures of the humerus in patients with multiple injuries, particularly chest trauma, where nonoperative management of the humerus fracture would interfere with pulmonary care. Likewise, nailing may be necessary for the unconscious patient who is agitated and threatens to compound a closed fracture of the humerus.

As with the other long bones, the recent introduction of locking nails for the humerus has significantly broadened the indications for nailing.[139–143] Clever methods for locking these nails without the use of distal transverse cross-locking screws (such as in the Seidel nail) have been developed. In my experience, these locking techniques have not proven to be sufficiently reliable as rotational instability frequently persists which can lead to nonunion if external immobilization is not used until fracture healing occurs. For that reason, more traditional locking nails using both proximal and distal cross-locking screws have been developed for the humerus. I prefer the Alta nail because the curvature of the nail allows it to be inserted with minimal impingement on the insertion of the rotator cuff. The disadvantages of these nails are that the stresses induced by proximal insertion can cause longitudinal fractures. I believe that unseen cracks are often present preoperatively. Distal cross-locking remains a challenge and generally must be performed open because of the danger of injury to the neurovascular structures around the elbow.

FRACTURES OF THE RADIUS AND ULNA

Displaced fractures of the radial diaphysis alone or in combination with fractures of the ulna usually require anatomic reduction and internal fixation in adults. Isolated fractures of the ulna rarely require internal fixation. Because plate fixation offers better stability, a more anatomic position, and a low failure rate, I have almost abandoned intramedullary nailing of forearm fractures. However, in situations where plate fixation is contraindicated, such as when the skin is in poor condition, intramedullary rod fixation provides an alternative.[144] Likewise, closed nailing of the forearm fractures deserves consideration when the patient's general condition will not permit the magnitude of procedures required for plate fixation.

The devices used for intramedullary nailing of the forearm are Rush rods,[145] Sage nails,[146–148] Street nails, and stacked Kirschner wires or Steinmann pins. For intramedullary nailing of the radius, the Sage rod is by far the best, as it is specifically designed for the anatomic curvatures of the radius. For the ulna, almost any intramedullary device suffices, but I have most frequently used the Rush rod. Rod fixation of both bones usually requires continued protection in a splint or cast because of rotational instability. If the rods rotate, there is a tendency for the interosseous membrane to collapse. We have abandoned the combination of plate fixation for the radius and rod fixation for the ulna because of the high incidence of nonunion in the ulna.

In the past couple of years, intramedullary nails made of titanium, which offer limited cross-locking capability, have been introduced for fractures of the radius and ulna. There is no reason not to expect these to be successful. At this point, I have no experience with these and the literature does not yet support intramedullary nail fixation of forearm fractures. The obvious advantages of being able to manage complex fractures of the forearm without having to perform an open reduction and internal fixation is obvious. Time will tell whether these devices will offer enough safety in use and enough stability to equal the superb results obtained by current methods of plate and screw fixation.[149]

PATHOLOGIC FRACTURES

Intramedullary nailing, particularly if combined with methyl-methacrylate to fill defects and obtain better bone purchase, is an excellent technique for the treatment of pathologic fractures of the diaphysis of long bones. Because the tumors from metastatic disease frequently involve multiple areas of long bones, plate fixation has the disadvantage of producing a stress riser at either end of the plate where further pathologic fracture can occur. This is particularly true in the weight-bearing long bones of the lower extremity. For this reason, intramedullary nailing is the fixation of choice where possible.

More recently, allografts have become more popular for pathologic fractures in which radical resection of the tumor is required to save the patient's life but where limb salvage is preferred. These cases that involve replacing just the diaphysis of a long bone as opposed to replacing the articular surface of the end of the bone as well tend to be more successful. The key to success with intramedullary nailing of pathologic fractures incorporating diaphyseal allografts is rigid internal fixation and bone grafting at the allograft-host junction to enhance healing and reinforce strength at this site. Revascularization of diaphyseal allografts takes place over many years and late failure is not uncommon. For that reason, the medullary nail used should be large so that the risk of fatigue failure is minimized. I use a circumferential bone graft and a small plate at the allograft-autograft junction as well to eliminate micromotion and to enhance incorporation.

INTRAMEDULLARY NAILING IN ADOLESCENTS AND CHILDREN

Fractures of the long bones in children with open physes generally are treated nonoperatively, as their capacity to heal and ability to remodel does not necessitate the more accurate reduction and stronger fixation required for good outcomes in fractures in adults. In addition, medullary nails inserted through the end of the bone can threaten the growth plate and lead to deformity. For those reasons, intramedullary nailing in the upper extremity in children with open growth centers is essentially never done. In the lower extremity, the same rationale applies to fractures of the tibia. If some type of fixation is required for the treatment of a severe open fracture, then generally external fixation is the treatment of choice.

The possible exception lays in fractures of the shaft of the femur. It is possible to insert a small-diameter unreamed or small reamed intramedullary nail into the femur from the proximal end without interfering significantly with the overall growth potential of the femur. By staying proximal to the distal/femoral physis, injury to that physis can be avoided as well. There are some indications for nailing of femur fractures in adolescents, in particular, and in some children.[150–152] Fractures of the femoral shaft occurring in males over the age of 15 and females over the age of 12 to 13 years can essentially be treated as in adults, as the remaining growth potential in the bone is minimal and the child's size makes internal fixation worthwhile in most cases. In the younger adolescent the need for medullary fixation of the femur is driven primarily by the size and maturity of the child and the associated injuries.

In children with severe multiple injuries and with severe head injuries, management of the femoral shaft fracture can be exceedingly difficult. The need for early mobilization to avoid pulmonary complications and the need to avoid malunion in the agitated head-injured child may mandate some type of fixation. The choices are plate fixation, external fixation, and intramedullary nailing. In general, intramedullary nailing works best. Timmerman and Rab[92] have demonstrated that the incidence of malunion and length of hospitalization in these patients can be significantly reduced by early medullary nailing.

REFERENCES

1. Lam, S.J.: The place of delayed internal fixation in the treatment of fractures of the long bones. J. Bone Joint Surg. *46B*:393–399, 1964.
2. Loomer, R., Meek, R., DeSommer, F.: Plating of femoral shaft fractures: The Vancouver experience. J. Trauma *20*:1039–1042, 1980.
3. Magerl, R., et al.: Plate osteosynthesis of femoral shaft fractures in adults. Clin. Orthop. *138*:62–73, 1979.
4. Roberts, J.B.: Management of fractures and fracture complications of the femoral shaft using the ASIF compression plate. J. Trauma *17*:20–28, 1977.
5. Smith, J.E.M.: The results of early and delayed internal fixation of fractures of the shaft of the femur. J. Bone Joint Surg. *46B*:28–31, 1964.
6. Brown, P.E., Preston, E.T.: Ambulatory treatment of femoral shaft fractures with a cast brace. J. Trauma *15*: 860–868, 1973.
7. Browner, B.D., Kenzora, J.E., Edwards, C.E.: The use of modified Neufeld traction in the management of femoral fractures in polytrauma. J. Trauma *21*: 779–787, 1981.
8. Bucholz, R.W., Jones A.: Fractures of the shaft of the femur. J. Bone Joint Surg. *73A*:1561–1566, 1991. (UI: 92084756)
9. Benirschke, S.K., Melder, I., Henley M.B., Routt M.L., Smith D.G., Chapman, J.R., Swiontkowski, M.F.: Closed interlocking nailing of femoral shaft fractures: Assessment of technical complications and functional outcomes by comparison of a prospective database with retrospective review. J. Orthop. Trauma, 1993, *7*: 118–122. Abstract available. (UI: 93210578)
10. Böhler, J.R.: Closed intramedullary nailing of the femur. Clin. Orthop. *60*:51–67, 1968.
11. Chapman, M.W., Blackman, R.C.: Closed intramedullary nailing of femoral shaft fractures: A comparison of two techniques. J. Bone Joint Surg. *58A*:732, 1976.
12. Christensen, N.O.: Technique, errors, and safeguards in modern Küntscher nailing. Clin. Orthop. *115*: 182–188, 1976.
13. Clawson, D.K., Smith, R.F., Hansen, S.T.: Closed intramedullary nailing of the femur. J. Bone Joint Surg. *53A*:681–682, 1971.
14. Cloke, J.H.: Closed nailing of femoral shaft fractures. J. Bone Joint Surg. *52B*:774–775, 1970.
15. Dencker, H.: Shaft fractures of the femur. A comparative study of the results of various methods of treatment in 1003 cases. Acta Chir. Scand. *130*:173–184, 1965.
16. Eriksson, E.: Ender nailing in fractures of the diaphysis of the femur. J. Bone Joint Surg. *61A*:1175–1181, 1979.
17. Fedders, O.: Femoral shaft fractures treated with closed intramedullary nailing. Acta Orthop. Scand. *50*:104, 1979.
18. Hansen, S.T., Winquist, R.A.: Closed intramedullary nailing of the femur. Clin. Orthop. *138*:56–57, 1979.
19. King, K.F., Rush, J.: Closed intramedullary nailing of femoral shaft fractures: A review of one hundred and twelve cases treated by the Küntscher technique. J. Bone Joint Surg. *63A*:1319–1322, 1981.
20. Küntscher, G.: Die Marknagelung von Knochenbruchen. Arch. Klin. Chir. *200*:443, 1940.
21. Küntscher, G.: The intramedullary nailing of fractures. Clin. Orthop. *60*:5–12, 1968.
22. McMaster, W.C.: Closed insertion technique for the prebent Sampson femoral rod. Clin. Orthop. *138*: 238–242, 1979.
23. Pankovich, A.M., Goldflies, N.L., Pearson, R.L.: Closed Ender nailing of femoral shaft fractures. J. Bone Joint Surg. *61A*:222–232, 1979.
24. Rascher, J.J., et al.: Closed nailing of femoral shaft fractures. J. Bone Joint Surg. *54A*:534–544, 1972.
25. Rothwell, A.G., Fitzpatrick, C.B.: Closed Küntscher nailing of femoral shaft fractures. J. Bone Joint Surg. *60B*:504–509, 1978.
26. Stryker, W.S., Fussell, M.E., West, H.E.: Comparison of the results of operative and nonoperative treatment of diaphyseal fractures of the femur at the Naval Hospital, San Diego, over a 5-year period. J. Bone Joint Surg. *52A*:815, 1970.
27. Weller, S., Kuner, E., Schweikert, C.H.: Medullary nailing according to Swiss study group principles. Clin. Orthop. *138*:45–55, 1979.
28. Wilber, M.C., Evans, M.D.: Fractures of the femoral shaft treated surgically. J. Bone Joint Surg. *60*: 489–491, 1978.
29. Winquist, R.A., Hansen, S.T., Jr.: Comminuted fractures of the femoral shaft treated by intramedullary nailing. Orthop. Clin. North Am. *11*:633–648, 1980.
30. Winquist, R.A., Hansen, S.T.: Segmental fractures of the femur treated by closed intramedullary nailing. J. Bone Joint Surg. *60A*:934–993, 1978.
31. Zravkovic, D., Damholt, V.: Quadriceps function following indirect nailing of femoral shaft fractures. Acta Orthop. Scand. *49*:73–77, 1978.
32. Allen, W.C., Heiple, K.C., Burstein, A.H.: A fluted femoral intramedullary rod. J. Bone Joint Surg. *60A*: 506–515, 1978.
33. Carpenter, E.G., Couk, D.E.: Complications of intramedullary nailing of the femur. J. Bone Joint Surg. *52A*:815–816, 1970.
34. Dencker, H.: Technical problems of medullary nailing. A study of 435 nailed shaft fractures of the femur. Acta Chir. Scand. *130*:185–189, 1965.
35. Jensen, J.S.: Middle third femoral fractures treated with medullary nailing or AO compression plating. Injury *8*:174–181, 1977.
36. Kamdar, B.A., Arden, G.P.: Küntscher nail for fractured femoral shaft. J. Bone Joint Surg. *55B*:882, 1973.
37. Kovacs, A., Richard, L.B., Miller, J.: Infection complicating intramedullary nailing of the fractured femur. J. Bone Joint Surg. *55A*:1306, 1973.
38. Nichols, P.J.R.: Rehabilitation after fractures of the shaft of the femur. J. Bone Joint Surg. *45B*:96–102, 1963.
39. Patterson, A.H., Scott, W.N.: Ten years' experience with femoral shaft fractures. J. Trauma *15*:348–355, 1975.
40. Peace, P.K.: Five year review of Küntscher nailing for femoral shaft fractures with emphasis on complications. Acta Orthop. Belg. *41*:346–354, 1975.
41. Rokkanen, P., Slätis, P., Vankka, E.: Closed and open intramedullary nailing of femoral fractures. A comparison with conservatively treated cases. J. Bone Joint Surg. *51B*:313–323, 1979.
42. Sage, F.P.: The second decade of experience with the Küntscher medullary nail in the femur. Clin. Orthop. *60*:77–85, 1968.
43. Schneider, H.W.: Use of the four-flanged self-cutting intramedullary nail for fixation of femoral fractures. Clin. Orthop. *60*:29–39, 1968.

44. Warmbrod, J.G., Helton, C.L., Weiss, A.B.: Intramedullary nailing of femoral shaft fractures. Clin. Orthop. *114*:282–286, 1976.
45. Wickstrom, J., Corban, M.S., Vise, G.T., Jr.: Complications following intramedullary fixation of 324 fractured femurs. Clin. Orthop. *60*:103–113, 1968.
46. Küntscher, G.: Practice of Intramedullary Nailing. Springfield, IL, Charles C. Thomas, 1967.
47. Aginsky, J., Reis, N.D.: The present state of medullary nailing of the femur: Biomechanical limitations and problems of blood supply to the fractures due to reaming. Injury *11*:109–197, 1980.
48. Charnley, J., Guindy, A.: Delayed operation in the open reduction of fractures of the long bones. J. Bone Joint Surg. *43B*:664–671, 1971.
49. Rand, J.A., An, K.N., Chao, E.Y., Kelly, P.J.: A comparison of the effect of open intramedullary nailing and compression-plate fixation on fracture-site blood flow and fracture union. J. Bone Joint Surg. *63A*: 427–442, 1981.
50. Rhinelander, F.W.: Effects of medullary nailing on the normal blood supply of diaphyseal cortex, AAOS. Instructional Course Lectures. St. Louis, C.V. Mosby Co., 1973.
51. Rush, L.V.: Atlas of Rush Pin Technics. Meridian, Berivon Co., 1976.
52. Street, D.M.: One hundred fractures of the femur treated by means of the diamond-shaped medullary nail. J. Bone Joint Surg. *33A*:659–669, 1951.
53. Grontvedt, R., Wilhelmsen, T.: One hundred ASIF-plated fractures of the femoral shaft. Acta Orthop. Scand. *48*:344, 1977.
54. Müller, M.E., Allgöwer, M., Schneider, R., Willenegger, H.: Manual of Internal Fixation. New York, Springer-Verlag, 1979.
55. Rüedi, T.P., Luscher, J.N.: Results after internal fixation of comminuted fractures of the femoral shaft with DC plates. Clin. Orthop. *138*:74–76, 1979.
56. d'Aubigne, R.M., Maurer, P., Zucman, J., et al.: Blind intramedullary nailing for tibial fractures. Clin. Orthop. *105*:267, 1974.
57. Bayne, L.G., Morris, H., Wickstrom, J.: Evaluation of intramedullary fixation of the tibia with the Lottes nail. South. Med. J. *53*:1429, 1960.
58. Lottes, J.O.: Medullary nailing of the tibia with the Triflange Nail. Clin. Orthop. *105*:253, 1974.
59. Sedlin, E.D., Zitner, D.T.: The Lottes nail in the closed treatment of tibia fractures. Clin. Orthop. *192*:185, 1985.
60. Solheim, K., Bo, O.: Intramedullary nailing of tibial shaft fractures. Acta Orthop. Scand. *44*:323, 1973.
61. Velazco, A., Whitesides, T.E., Fleming, L.L.: Open fractures of the tibia treated with Lottes nail. J. Bone Joint Surg. *65A*:879, 1983.
62. Court-Brown, C.M., McQueen, M.M., Quaba, A.A., Christie, J.: Locked intramedullary nailing of open tibial fractures. J. Bone Joint Surg. *73B*:959–964, 1991.
63. Melcher, G.A., Ryf, C., Leutenegger, A., Ruedi, T.: Tibial fractures treated with the AO unreamed tibial nail. Injury, *24*:407–410, 1993.
64. Piccioni, L., Guanche, C.A.: Clinical experience with unreamed locked nails for open tibial fractures. Orthop. Rev. *21*:1213–1219, 1992.
65. Whittle, A.P., Russell, T.A., Taylor, J.C., Lavelle, D.G.: Treatment of open fractures of the tibial shaft with the use of interlocking nailing without reaming. J. Bone Joint Surg. *74A*:1162–1171, 1992.
66. Kerr, P.S., Jackson, M., Atkins, R.M.: Cardiac arrest during intramedullary nailing for femoral metastases. J. Bone Joint Surg. *75B*:972–973, 1993. (UI: 94064745)
67. Pell, A.C., Christie, J., Keating, J.F.: Sutherland GR. The detection of fat embolism by transoesophageal echocardiography during reamed intramedullary nailing. A study of 24 patients with femoral and tibial fractures. J. Bone Joint Surg. *75B*:921–925, 1993.
68. Blitzer, C.M.: Hamilton L. Oxygen saturation during reaming and intramedullary nailing of the femur. Orthopedics *15*:1403–1405, 1992. Abstract available. (UI: 93096717)
69. Pape, H.C., Auf'm'Kolk, M., Paffrath, T., Regel, G., Sturm, J.A., Tscherne H.: Primary intramedullary femur fixation in multiple trauma patients with associated lung contusion—a cause of posttraumatic ARDS? J. Trauma *34*:540–547; discussion 547–548, 1993.
70. Pape, H.C., Dwenger, A., Regel, G., et al.: Pulmonary damage after intramedullary femoral nailing in traumatized sheep—is there an effect from different nailing methods? J. Trauma *33*:574–581, 1992.
71. Pape, H.C., Regel, G., Dwenger, A., et al.: Influences of different methods of intramedullary femoral nailing on lung function in patients with multiple trauma. J. Trauma *35*:709–716, 1993.
72. Bucholz, R.W., Ross, S.E., Lawrence, K.L.: Fatigue fracture of the interlocking nail in the treatment of fractions of the distal part of the femoral shaft. J. Bone Joint Surg. *69A*:1391–1399, 1987.
73. Adair, I.V.: The use of plaster casts in the treatment of fractures of the femoral shaft. Injury *7*:194–201, 1976.
74. Andersen, R.L.: Conservative treatment of fractures of the femur. J. Bone Joint Surg. *49A*:1371–1375, 1967.
75. Carr, C.R., Wingo, C.H.: Fractures of the femoral diaphysis. A retrospective study of the results and costs of treatment of intramedullary nailing and by traction and a Spica cast. J. Bone Joint Surg. *55A*:690–700, 1973.
76. Colley, J.D.: Experience in the treatment of femoral shaft fractures using a vitrathene cast-brace. Prosthet. Orthot. Int. *2*:76–78, 1928.
77. Connolly, J.F., Dehne, E., Lafollette, B.: Closed reduction and early cast-brace ambulation in the treatment of femoral fractures. J. Bone Joint Surg. *55A*: 1581–1599, 1973.
78. Crotwell, W.A.: The thigh lacer: Ambulatory nonoperative treatment of femoral shaft fractures. J. Bone Joint Surg. *60A*:112–117, 1978.
79. Gillquist, J., Liljedahl, S.O., Rieger, A.: Fracture of the femur diaphysis. Traction or nailing? Acta Chir. Scand. *137*:515–520, 1971.
80. Griffith, T.G., Albertson, C.E., Lafollette, D.F.: Hinged cylinder cast management of femoral shaft fractures. Presentation at Western Orthopaedic Association. October 1975.
81. Hardy, A.E., Nicholson, O.R.: Cast brace application and early ambulation as a treatment for femoral shaft fractures. N. Z. Med. J. *83*:111–114, 1976.
82. Hardy, A.E., White, P., Williams, J.R.: The treatment of femoral fractures by cast-brace and early walking. J. Bone Joint Surg. *61B*:151–154, 1979.
83. Heater, R.D., Christensen, J.L., Riggins, R.S.: Review of management of fractures of the femur. J. Bone Joint Surg. *57A*:135, 1975.
84. Lafollette, B.F., Cantu-Lara, R.: The nonoperative early ambulatory management of adult femoral shaft fractures. J. Bone Joint Surg. *56A*:1309, 1974.
85. Alawneh, I.: Immediate management of femoral shaft fracture in multiply injured children. Med. Welt *27*: 1895–1899, 1976.
86. Beam, H.P., Jr., Seligson, D.: Nine cases of bilateral femoral shaft fractures: A composite view. J. Trauma *20*:399–402, 1980.
87. Bone, L., Johnson, J., Weigelt, J., et al.: Early versus delayed femoral fracture stabilization: A prospective randomized study. J. Bone Joint Surg. *71A*:336, 1989.

88. Border, J.R., Hassett, J., LaDuca, J., et al.: The gut origin septic states in blunt multiple trauma (ISS-40) in the ICU Ann. Surg. *206*:427, 1987.
89. Johnson, K.D., Cadambi, A., Seibert, G.B.: Incidence of adult respiratory distress syndrome in patients with multiple musculoskeletal injuries: Effect of early operative stabilization of fractures. J. Trauma *25*:375, 1985.
90. Seibel, R., LaDuca, J., Hassett, J.M., et al.: Blunt multiple trauma (ISS 36), femur traction, and the pulmonary failure-septic state. Ann. Surg. *202*:283, 1985.
91. Liebergall, M., Lowe, J., Whitelaw, G.P., Wetzler, M.J., Segal D.: The floating hip. Ipsilateral pelvic and femoral fractures. J. Bone Joint Surg. *74B*:93–100, 1992.
92. Pintore, E., Maffulli, N., Petricciuolo, F.: Interlocking nailing for fractures of the femur and tibia. Injury *23*: 381–386, 1992.
93. Anastopoulos, G., Assimakopoulos, A., Exarchou, E., Pantazopoulos, T.: Ipsilateral fractures of the femur and tibia. Injury *23*:439–441, 1992.
94. Langer, R.H., Foster, R.J.: Skeletal management of humeral shaft fractures associated with forearm fractures. Clin. Orthop. *195*:173, 1985.
95. Bergman, M., Tornetta, P., Kerina, M., et al.: Femur fractures caused by gunshots: Treatment by immediate reamed intramedullary nailing. J. Trauma *34*: 783–785, 1993.
96. Brumback, R.L., Ellison, P.S., Jr., Poka, A., Lakatos, R., Bathon, G.H., Burgess, A.R.: Intramedullary nailing of open fractures of the femoral shaft. J. Bone Joint Surg. *71A*:1324, 1989.
97. Grosse, A., Christie, J., Taglang, G., Court-Brown, C., McQueen, M.: Open adult femoral shaft fracture treated by early intramedullary nailing. J. Bone Joint Surg. *75B*:562–565, 1993.
98. Lhowe, D., Hansen, S.T., Jr.: Immediate nailing of open fractures of the femoral shaft. J. Bone Joint Surg. *70A*:812, 1988.
99. Wright, D.G., Levin, J.S., Esterhai, J.L., Heppenstall, R.B.: Immediate internal fixation of low-velocity gunshot-related femoral fractures. J. Trauma *35*:678–681; discussion 681–682, 1993.
100. Tornetta, P. III, Bergman, M., Watnik, N., Berkowitz, G., Steuer, J.: Treatment of grade-IIIb open tibial fractures. A prospective randomized comparison of external fixation and non-reamed locked nailing. J. Bone Joint Surg. *76B*:13–19, 1994.
101. Court-Brown, C.M., Christie, J., McQueen, M.M.: Closed intramedullary tibial nailing: Its use in closed and type I open fractures. J. Bone Joint Surg. *72B*:605, 1990.
102. Johnson, E.E., Simpson, L.A., Helfet, D.L.: Delayed intramedullary nailing after failed external fixation of the tibia. Clin. Orthop. *253*:251, 1990.
103. Siebenrock, K.A., Schillig, B., Jakob, R.P.: Treatment of complex tibial shaft fractures. Arguments for early secondary intramedullary nailing. Clin. Orthop. *290*: 269–274, 1993.
104. Wu, C.C., Shih, C.H.: Complicated open fractures of the distal tibia treated by secondary interlocking nailing. J. Trauma *34*:792–796, 1993.
105. Mauter D.J., Morkow, R.L., Gustilo, R.B.: Infection after intramedullary nailing of severe open tibial fractures initially treated with external fixation. J. Bone Joint Surg. *71A*:835, 1989.
106. Riemer, B.L., Butterfield, S.L.: Comparison of reamed and nonreamed solid core nailing of the tibial diaphysis after external fixation: A preliminary report. J. Orthop. Trauma *7*:279–285, 1993.
107. Wheelwright, E.F., Court-Brown, C.M.: Primary external fixation and secondary intramedullary nailing in the treatment of tibial fractures. Injury *23*:373–376, 1992.
108. Miller, C.W., Anderson, L., Grossman, J.: Comparison of three treatments for fractures of the diaphysis of the femur. Surg. Gynecol. Obstet. *146*:572–576, 1978.
109. Lesin, B.E., Mooney, V., Ashby, M.E.: Cast bracing for fractures of the femur. J. Bone Joint Surg. *59A*: 917–923, 1977.
110. Mital, M.A., Bonadio, O.: Fractures of the shaft of the femur: Progress in treatment (1961–1971) experience with conservative traction with ambulatory cast-brace treatment in seventy-five patients. Am. J. Surg. *127*: 434–441, 1974.
111. Moll, J.: The cast-brace walking treatment for open and closed femoral fractures. South Med. J. *66*:345, 1973.
112. Mooney, V.: Cast bracing. Clin. Orthop. *102*:159–166, 1974.
113. Mooney, V., et al.: Cast-brace treatment for fractures of the distal part of the femur. J. Bone Joint Surg. *52A*: 1563–1578, 1970.
114. Ramey, E.E., Jr.: Femoral shaft fractures. A study of closed reduction and open treatment. California Med. *92*:150–154, 1960.
115. Sarmiento, A., Latta, L.L.: Closed Functional Treatment of Fractures. New York, Springer-Verlag, 1981.
116. Scully, T.J.: Ambulant, nonoperative management of femoral shaft fractures. Part II. Clin. Orthop. *100*: 204–210, 1974.
117. Schweigel, J.F., Gropper, P.T.: A comparison of ambulatory versus nonambulatory care of femoral shaft fractures. J. Trauma *14*:474–481, 1974.
118. Seligson, D., Harman, K.: Negative experiences with pins-in-plaster for femoral fractures. Clin. Orthop. *138*:243–245, 1979.
119. Wardlaw, D.: The cast-brace treatment of femoral shaft fractures. J. Bone Joint Surg. *59B*:411–416, 1977
120. Weiss, A.B.: Cast bracing for femoral shaft fractures. South Med. J. *69*:326–330, 1976.
121. Cameron, C.D., Meek, R.N., Blachut, P.A., O'Brien, P.J., Pate, G.C.: Intramedullary nailing of the femoral shaft: A prospective, randomized study. J. Orthop. Trauma, *6*:448–451, 1992.
122. Lhowe, D.W., Hansen, S.T.: Immediately nailing of open fractures of the femoral shaft. J. Bone Joint Surg. *70A*:812, 1988.
123. Browner, B.: Pitfalls, errors, and complications in the use of locking Küntscher nails. Clin. Orthop. *212*:192, 1986.
124. Brumback, R.J., Reilly, J.P., Poka, A., Lakatos, R.P., Bathon, G.H., Burgess, A.R.: Intramedullary nailing of femoral shaft fractures. Part I. Decision making errors with interlocking fixation. J. Bone Joint Surg. *70A*: 1441, 1988.
125. Brumback, R.J., Uwagie-Ero, S., Lakatos, R.P., Poka, A., Bathon, G.H., Burgess, A.R.: Intramedullary nailing of femoral shaft fractures. Part II. Fracture-healing with static interlocking fixation. J. Bone Joint Surg. *70A*:1453, 1988.
126. Winquist, R., Clawson, D.K., Hansen, S.T.: Closed intramedullary nailing of femoral fractures. J. Bone Joint Surg. *66A*:529, 1984.
127. Kempf, I., Grosse, A., Beck, G.: Closed locked intramedullary nailing. J. Bone Joint Surg. *67A*:709, 1985.
128. Klemm, K., Schellmann, W.D.: Dynamische und Statische Verriegelung des Marknagels. Monatsschr. Unfallheilk. *75*:568, 1972.
129. Bennett, F.S., Zinar, D.M., Kilgus, D.J.: Ipsilateral hip and femoral shaft fractures. Clin. Orthop. *296*: 168–177, 1993.

130. Leung, K.S., So, W.S., Lam, T.P., Leung, P.C.: Treatment of ipsilateral femoral shaft fractures and hip fractures. Injury *24*:41–45, 1993.
131. Wiss, D.A., Brien, W.W.: Subtrochanteric fractures of the femur. Results of treatment by interlocking nailing. Clin. Orthop. *283*:231–236, 1992.
132. Lucas, S.E., Seligson, D., Henry, S.L.: Intramedullary supracondylar nailing of femoral fractures. A preliminary report of the GSH supracondylar nail. Clin. Orthop. *296*:200–206, 1993.
133. Sanders, R., Koval, K.J., DiPasquale, T., Helfet, D.L., Frankle, M.: Retrograde reamed femoral nailing. J. Orthop. Trauma *7*:293–302, 1993.
134. Schewitsch, E.H., Kowalski, W.J., Swiontkowski, M.F., Hamington, R.M., Senft, D.: Effects of reamed versus unreamed locked nailing on collus blood flow and early strength of union in a fractured sheep tibia model. J. Bone Joint Surg. *18*:145, 1994.
135. Reis, N.D., Aginsky, J.: A double-compression medullary nail: Preliminary report of an early clinical trial. Injury *11*:197–202, 1980.
136. Mast, J.W., et al.: Fractures of the humeral shaft. Clin. Orthop. *112*:254, 1975.
137. Weseley, M.S., Barenfeld, P.A., Eisenstein, A.L.: Rush pin intramedullary fixation for fractures of the proximal humerus. J. Trauma *17*:29, 1977.
138. Christensen, N.O.: Küntscher intramedullary reaming and nail fixation for nonunion of the humerus. Clin. Orthop. *116*:222, 1976.
139. Barnes, C.E., Shuler, T.E.: Complications associated with the Seidel nail. Orthop. Rev. *22*:699–706, 1993.
140. Crolla, R.M., de Vries, L.S., Clevers, G.J.: Locked intramedullary nailing of humeral fractures. Injury *24*: 403–406, 1993.
141. Dalton, J.E., Salkeld, S.L., Satterwhite, Y.E., Cook, S.D.: A biomechanical comparison of intramedullary nailing systems for the humerus. J. Orthop. Trauma *7*: 367–374, 1993.
142. Ingman, A.M., Waters, D.A.: Locked intramedullary nailing of humeral shaft fractures. Implant design, surgical technique, and clinical results. J. Bone Joint Surg. *76B*:23–29, 1994.
143. Watanabe, R.S.: Intramedullary fixation of complicated fractures of the humeral shaft. Clin. Orthop. *292*: 255–263, 1993.
144. Mazul, R.: Intramedullary fixation in the arm and the forearm. Clin. Orthop. *2*:75, 1958.
145. Rush, L.V., Rush, H.L.: A technique for longitudinal pin fixation of certain fractures of the ulna and of the femur. J. Bone Joint Surg. *21*:619, 1939.
146. Sage, F.P.: Medullary fixation of fractures of the forearm: A study of the medullary canal of the radius and a report of 50 fractures of the radius treated with a prebent triangular nail. J. Bone Joint Surg. *41A*:1489, 1959.
147. Sage, F.P.: Fractures of the Shaft of the Radius and Ulna in the Adult. *In* Current Practice in Orthopaedic Surgery. 1st Ed. Edited by J.P. Adams. St. Louis, C.V. Mosby Co., 1963.
148. Smith, H., Sage, F.F.: Medullary fixation of forearm fractures. J. Bone Joint Surg. *39A*:91, 1957.
149. Chapman, M.W., Gordon, J.E., Zissiumos, A.G.: Compression plate fixation of acute fractures of the diaphysis of the radius and ulna. J. Bone Joint Surg. *71A*: 139, 1989.
150. Maruenda-Paulino, J.I., Sanchis-Alfonso, V., Gomar-Sancho, F., Darder-Prats, A., Gasco-Gomez de Membrillera, J.: Küntscher nailing of femoral shaft fractures in children and adolescents. Int. Orthop. *17*: 158–161, 1993.
151. Timmerman, L.A., Rab, G.T.: Intramedullary nailing of femoral shaft fractures in adolescents. J. Orthop. Trauma *7*:331–337, 1993.
152. Heinrich, S.D., Drvafic, D., Darr, K., MacEwen, G.D.: Stabilization of pediatric diaphyseal femur fractures with flexible intramedullary nails (a technique paper). J. Orthop. Trauma *6*:452–459, 1992.

3

The Vascular Response of Bone to Internal Fixation

J. Dean Cole

Healing of long-bone fractures is a dynamic process that is influenced by numerous, often interrelated variables. Among these variables, stabilization of the fracture and maintenance or restoration of an adequate blood supply are the two most important aspects of fracture repair.[1] The attainment of osseous union is, therefore, ultimately dependent on the biologic milieu and mechanical environment of the fracture site.

Clinicians have the ability to control many of the conditions that affect the biology and mechanics of bone healing through their choice of operative or nonoperative interventions. Treatment decisions regarding the type and timing of intervention, soft-tissue management, surgical approach, and the method of fixation affect both the mechanical environment of the fracture site and bone vascularity. Ultimately, these treatment decisions affect the patient's outcome, fracture healing, or the development of complications.

Therefore, a thorough understanding of bone blood flow and the mechanics of fracture stabilization is necessary and should serve as a cornerstone of knowledge to guide orthopedists in their selection of treatment options for long-bone fractures. The effect of any intervention on bone blood flow must be considered when determining the optimal treatment plan. Educated decisions should be based on an understanding of the basic scientific studies relating to bone vascularity, as opposed to reliance on creative thinking, results of uncontrolled case series and nonexperimental study designs, "expert" opinion, or the surgical experience of our mentors and ourselves.[2,3] With these points in mind, this chapter has been designed to serve as a reference guide to basic bone vascularity research that is applicable from a clinician's viewpoint.

NORMAL BONE BLOOD SUPPLY

An understanding of the normal blood supply of long bones forms the foundation for comprehension of the vascular response to fracture. Bone blood supply may be classified according to the physiology of flow or in terms of the anatomic vasculature of the long bone. Both a number of similarities and differences exist in the anatomic vasculature of the human long bones. Yet, this disparity does not preclude generalization of a discussion on long-bone blood supply and the vascular response of long bones to fracture and intramedullary nailing. In general, all long bones have separate, yet anastomotic metaphyseal and diaphyseal blood supplies; the diaphysis is supplied primarily by one or more nutrient arteries; and an extraosseus soft-tissue sleeve provides an abundant source of periosteal vessels that are concentrated around fascial attachments. However, in the tibia, a single, principle nutrient artery supplies approximately 70% of the arterial blood to the diaphysis.[4] Numerous nutrient vessels supply arterial blood to the femur and humerus. The femur and humerus also have an abundant, circumferential extraosseous soft-tissue sleeve. The anterior tibia, on the other hand, lacks this additional vascular source. (This is of particular importance in open fractures.)

Rhinelander advocated classification (of normal bone blood supply) in terms of physiologic blood flow. Foremost, he recognized the direction of normal bone blood flow through the diaphyseal cortex of a long bone as centrifugal, flowing from medulla to periosteum. He described three functional components of bone blood supply: (1) the afferent vascular system carries nutrients and oxygen to all parts of bone, (2) the efferent vascular system carries waste products away from bone, and (3) the intermediate vascular system, which functions as a connecting link between the afferent and efferent systems within cortical bone. The function of the intermediate vascular system is similar to the capillary network of soft tissue or cancellous bone.

"The afferent vascular system has three components: the nutrient artery system, metaphyseal arterioles and periosteal vessels."[1] The principal nutrient artery supplies approximately 70% of the blood supply to the tibial diaphysis. The principal nutrient artery, or nutrient arteries, traverse the cortex of the long bone, enter the medullary cavity, and divide into ascending and descending branches. The ascending and descending branches give rise to radially arranged lateral conduits, which may enter the endosteal surface of the diaphyseal cortex or branch off into short segments of ascending or descending paraendosteal vessels that parallel the longitudinal axis of the long bone.[5] The lateral conduit arteries and arterioles penetrate the endosteal surface of the cortex to varying degrees and give rise to ascending and descending furcations that enter the surrounding osteons (osteal circulation of the entire cortex.) In humans, these furcated segments tend to be only a few millimeters in length. This is in contrast to similar vessels in hoofed animals in which the arterioles entering the cortex branch into long segments of ascending and descending vessels within the osteal circulation.

In the tibia, periosteal arterioles enter the cortex at firm fascial attachments along the longitudinal axis of the long bone. These vessels penetrate the cortex at variable depths, supplying arterial blood to the outer one-third of the cortex (Fig. 3–1). Although diaphyseal periosteal circulation is largely independent of

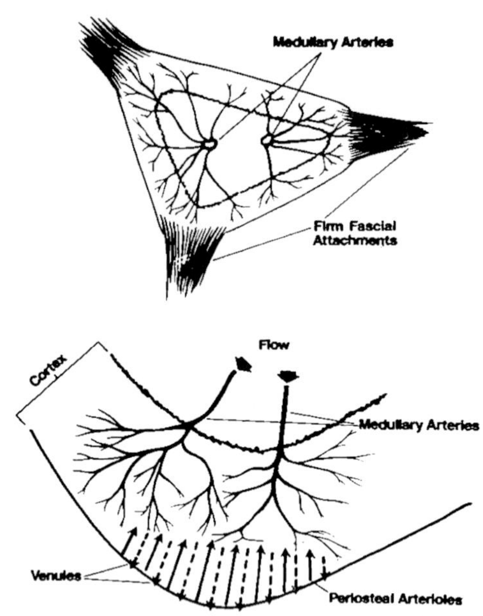

Fig. 3–1. Cross-section drawings of an idealized mature long bone. Observe that branches of the medullary arteries supply the full thickness of the cortex everywhere except at firm fascial attachments, which are typically at the corners. The enlargement demonstrates that periosteal arterioles (solid arrows) supply approximately the outer third of the cortex at these fascial attachments. All venous drainage (broken arrows) is to the periosteal surface. (From Rhinelander, F.W., Wilson, J.W.: Blood supply to developing, mature and healing bone. *In* Bone in Clinical Orthopaedics. Edited by G. Sumner-Smity. Philadelphia, W.B. Saunders, 1982.)

endosteal circulation, these two systems are able to supplement each other if one of the routes is compromised. However, it is important to understand that this process does not occur immediately. Nor does the process involve a reversal of periosteal flow through anastomoses between the two systems. Rather, there is a delay in time during which neovascularization and ingrowth of periosteal vessels towards the endosteum, or endosteal vessels towards the periosteum, must occur (Fig. 3–2).[6]

Metaphyseal circulation is quite different from diaphyseal blood flow. A concentrical arrangement of metaphyseal arterioles enter the metaphysis at firm fascial attachments in the proximal and distal ends of the long bone. Other arteries around the joint may directly penetrate the metaphysis. The vessels that enter this cancellous bone form an arcade pattern, completely supplying the metaphysis. This epi-

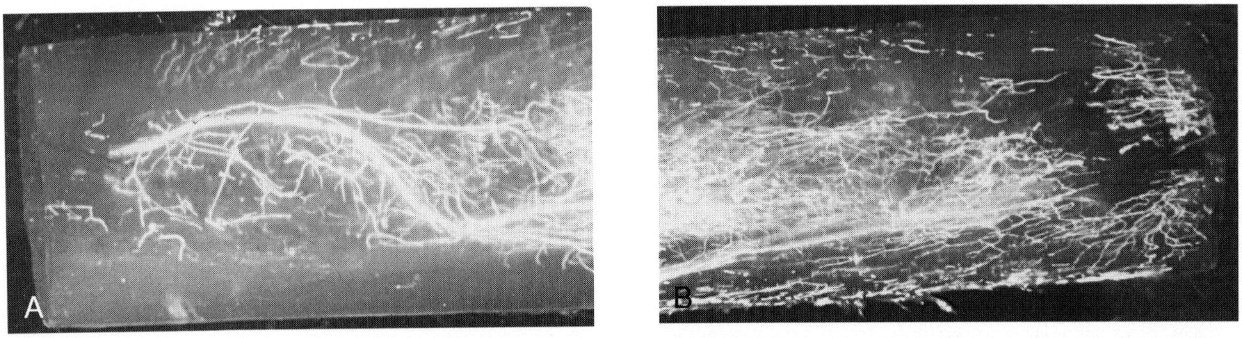

Fig. 3–2. *A,* Distal segment of a 14-day canine tibial osteotomy performed with minimal stripping and a cooled saw. Three descending branches of intact intramedullary vessels are visible. There is filling of the vessels, as well as filling of periosteal vessels. There is some avascular bone adjacent to the fracture area. *B,* Proximal segment of a 3-day canine tibial osteotomy. The nutrient system and intramedullary system are intact with increased filling. Increased filling of the periosteal vasculature is also noted.

physeal-metaphyseal system anastomoses with the nutrient artery system of the diaphysis, supplying a source of additional arterial blood to the cortical circulation. Thus, a reversal of flow or centripetal circulation (from periosteum to medulla) is seen in the metaphyseal regions of long bones.

The intermediate vascular system is the connecting link between the afferent and efferent systems. The intermediate or intracortical vascular system is composed of thin-walled vessels of capillary size which arise from segmental branches of the lateral conduit and periosteal arterioles. In cortical bone, these capillary-like vessels occupy both the Haversian and Volkmann canals. Surrounding each haversian canal are concentric layers of osteocytes. Each osteocyte occupies a space called a lacuna. Radiating from each lacuna are numerous minute canals called canaliculi, which traverse the dense matrix of the bone tissue and connect adjacent lacunae (Fig. 3–3).

The capillaries within the haversian and Volkmann canals of the cortical bone function in a manner similar to capillaries within other body tissues in regard to movement of ions and molecules. Narrow intercellular channels allow the passage of water-soluble ions and molecules between the capillary blood and the extracellular fluid within the osteon. Intracellular transport via pinocytotic vesicles may be used to transport larger ions, while lipid-soluble substances diffuse across the endothelial cells and into the interstitial fluid of the haversian canal.[7] Nutrients and fluid are then transported to the osteocyte via the canaliculi. The mechanism for afflux of ions and molecules from the extravascular space of bone back to the general circulation through the bone capillaries may be controlled by a concentration-dependent binding mechanism. Excess interstitial fluid may be absorbed by capillaries further along the osteon, but it is returned to the gen-

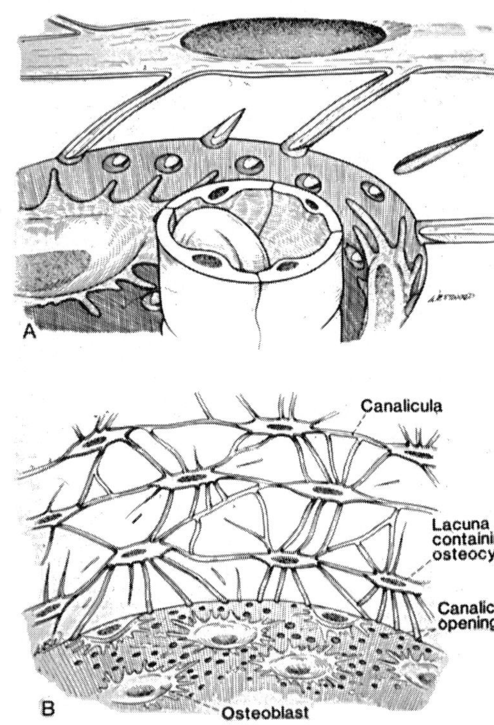

Fig. 3–3. *A,* The relationship of capillary to canaliculi. Fluid leaves the capillary via slits between the endothelial cells of the wall to reach the extracellular fluid space. *B,* Diagram of osteocytes and osteoblasts. (From Kelly, P.J.: Pathways of transport in bone. *In*: Handbook of Physiology. Edited by Shephard and Abboud. Baltimore, Williams & Wilkins, 1983.)

eral circulation primarily through lymphatic vessels within the Volkmann canals.[8]

The efferent vascular system drains blood from the long bone via metaphyseal and diaphyseal pathways. In the metaphysis, multiple veins that accompany the metaphyseal arteries freely drain blood from the ends of the long bone. Cortical diaphyseal bone is drained almost entirely by efferent venules that connect with periosteal veins.[4,7] Abundant periosteal veins also drain interstitial fluid and "waste" products from perivascular prelymphatic vessels.[8] However, the mechanism of diaphyseal marrow drainage is not fully understood. Some investigators believe that sinusoids within the medullary cavity empty into a large, central medullary sinus.[4,7,9] Oni et al. suggested that the marrow is an open circulatory system with ill-defined boundaries.[8] From the central sinus or marrow cavity, medullary wastes are believed to be drained centrifugally by large, transcortical emissary veins that connect directly to the periosteal venous system at either end of the long bone or by nutrient veins.[4,7–9] Thus, a direct link may exist between the intramedullary canal and the venous system.

EXPERIMENTAL METHODS

Raskob et al. have warned against premature, enthusiastic introduction of new therapies into clinical practice. Often, they suggest, these therapies are later shown to be only partially effective, ineffective, or even harmful.[2] Two major reasons for the premature acceptance of a surgical therapy into clinical practice have been outlined. First, a new therapy may be assumed to be of clinical benefit based on pathophysiological knowledge, which is uncritically accepted as hard evidence of clinical efficacy. A second reason may be a lack of awareness among clinical investigators of the essential study design features that are required to adequately evaluate the effectiveness of a procedure.

Numerous experimental and clinical studies have documented that fracture site vascularity is a key component of fracture healing, and that the success of any therapeutic regimen may depend on its effect on fracture site vascularity. A wealth of information is available on the subject of bone blood supply and the vascular response of bone to fracture. These experimental studies form the foundation for evaluation of therapeutic regimens on fracture site vascularity. However, the applicability of these basic scientific studies to clinical practice must be evaluated closely prior to their widespread acceptance (and clinical use). An understanding of the advantages and limitations of experimental methods for assessing bone blood supply in a fracture model assists the clinician in evaluating various clinical studies in the pursuit of the best treatment method for any given long-bone fracture.

In order to apply the results of basic scientific research to a clinical situation, it is important that the investigator is aware of essential study design variables that may impede extrapolation or generalization of results. Study features which must be considered in bone blood flow studies include the animal model, fracture model, and the experimental method that is used.

Animal Model

The animal model that is chosen for study may greatly affect the applicability of results to a human clinical situation. The most commonly used animal models for bone vascularity studies are rats, rabbits, sheep, and dogs. In bone blood flow studies, the type of bone and anatomic vasculature of the animal should resemble, as closely as possible, these same features in humans.

Cortical bone may differ greatly from one species to another. In small animals, the conical bone consists of layers of lamellar bone called compact bone. In this compact bone, there is no special arrangement of the vascular network.[5] In hoofed animals, the cortical bone is termed plexiform bone. Plexiform bone consists of layers of lamellar and woven bone with an abundance of vascular channels located mainly in the woven bone.[5] Rapid bone growth, with the accumulation of large amounts of bone over a short period of time, may be inherent to the arrangement of plexiform bone. An elaborate intracortical vascular plexus is also seen in the models of larger, hoofed animals.[5] Canine cortical bone consists of a complex arrangement of lamellar bone circumferentially surrounding a neurovascular or haversian canal. This type of cortical bone is similar to the cortical bone in humans, and is much more complex than that of hoofed animals, rats, or rabbits. The differences in cortical bone structure and vascularity between various animal species and humans may limit the applicability to humans of studies involving these animals. The canine is thus an excellent model for experimental bone vascularity procedures. The canine tibia is similar to the human tibia in medullary and cortical vasculature and the differentiation of haversian bone. Canal shape, presence of a fibula, and degree of remodeling are also comparable.

The patterns of bone healing and remodeling in the animal model must also be considered. Fracture healing in any mammal model occurs both periosteally and endosteally.[7,10] Remodeling in the human may occur on the endosteal or periosteal surfaces of the bone or interstitially.[7] This in contrast to bone remodeling in rats and rabbits. In these species, no significant interstitial (haversian) remodeling occurs. Rodents models may thus be inappropriate for bone blood flow studies that are intended to apply directly to humans. The dog, on the other hand, is a good model for such studies, as bone healing and remodeling are quite similar to that of humans.[7,11]

Fracture Model

Results of experimental research studies should guide clinicians in managing fractures which they encounter in the patient population. The fracture model used in animal experiments must therefore be appreciated when determining the applicability of these studies to human clinical situations. Among the fracture site variables that the clinician must consider are the energy of the injury, mechanism of the fracture or osteotomy, and the condition of the soft-tissue sleeve, including periosteum, muscle, fascia, subcutaneous tissues, and skin.

In general, production of experimental fractures may be considered low energy. In rats or rabbits, the fracture site is often created by driving an awl percutaneously through the bone, followed by manual breakage of the weakened bone.[12] Most studies of bone blood flow in a large animal fracture model monitor healing of a transverse osteotomy in the diaphysis of a long bone.[13,14] Study bias is minimized by using these types of reproducible fracture models; however, the applicability of results of these studies to problematic fractures that may be encountered in a clinical situation, is limited. Although low-energy, transverse diaphyseal fractures do occur in the human population, management of these injuries is usually routine.

On the other hand, management of problematic high-energy, open or closed injuries with comminuted fracture patterns remains controversial. Experimental exclusion studies are extremely helpful for studying and understanding healing, blood flow, and the effects of various fixation methods in these types of injuries. Exclusion studies employ surgical trauma that mimics the potential damage to tissue that may occur in clinical injuries at the time of fracture or fixation.[15] One or more circulatory pathways (periosteal, extraosseous, endosteal, or metaphyseal) are blocked, and the compensatory vascular mechanisms of the intact pathways are evaluated. Both qualitative and quantitative bone blood flow studies have been conducted in this manner.

Qualitative Methods

A historical review of long-bone fracture vascularity research reveals a progression in methodology from qualitative histologic and microangiographic analysis to the use of sophisticated quantitative techniques. Microangiography, as pioneered by Trueta and his associates, has been used extensively over the past 30 years to investigate the revascularization of bone in different stages of fracture repair and the use of implants of various types.[16] Preparation of tissues for microangiography involves intravascular injection of micropaque (finely divided barium sulfate) into the limb under study. The host animal is then sacrificed and the limb harvested. One millimeter slices of decalcified specimens of the fracture site are used for microangiography.[17] Histologic evaluation of the cellular and matrical response to fracture and various fixation types is often performed concurrently to correlate with the microangiographic investigation of the specimens.

Although microangiography and histology have been used extensively in fracture site vascularity studies, there are numerous limitations to these techniques. Studies using these techniques are generally designed to analyze specimens over a continuum of time, for example, at 1 day, 7 days, 14 days, and 21 days postoperatively. Preparation of specimens at each given point, in time requires sacrifice of the host animal. Qualitative differences in blood flow at various time intervals can only be inferred from the amount of vessel branching or differences in vessel size from specimen to specimen. Host differences, including animal age and heterogeneity of blood flow, may bias results. Another limitation of the technique is that direction of flow can only be determined by examining patterns of vessel branching. Thin section analysis required for microangiography limits visualization of the three-dimensional anastomotic patterns responsible for bone blood flow in the fracture model. Vessels frequently branch perpendicular to the plane of the microscopic section and therefore are not appreciable using these two-dimensional techniques.

Stereoscopic dissection using Microfil (FlowTek; Boulder, CO) injecting and casting techniques may offer some advantages over two-dimensional microangiography for defining neovascular fracture site architecture and circulatory flow patterns. The procedure involves injection of Microfil into the animal under study. Specimens are then harvested, decalcified, and dehydrated for analysis. Stereoscopic dissection of the specimen allows adequate recognition of the three-dimensional network of the osteotomy site and surrounding callus. Yet, despite this advantage over two-dimensional techniques, Microfil studies, like microangiographic and histologic studies, are qualitative and may be biased by host differences such as heterogeneity of blood flow or animal age.

Intravital staining has also been used to indirectly evaluate the effects of various fixation methods on cortical circulation. The technique involves intravenous infusion or oral administration of chemical stains that have an affinity for bone in a healing state. Staining may be performed once or sequentially over a period of several days using two or more different dyes. Following staining, the limb is harvested, and bone specimens are sectioned into 0.1-mm increments for evaluation under a fluorescence microscope. Fluorescence photomicrographs are taken for digital contrast enhancement of the stained specimens. Ideally, researchers using vital staining attempt to quantitatively identify differences in the amount of (cortical destruction or) callus formation at the fracture site over a period of time.

However, this type of quantitative analysis has several limitations. In addition to the unavoidable host differences, bone uptake of the stain may be variable. Although most of the injected stain will be absorbed by new bone, it is difficult to estimate the uptake of stain by old bone. This is of particular importance in studies of multiple dye injections. Fracture site mass may change significantly over the course of several days. Although the majority of this change may be secondary to osteoblastic activity, osteoclastic activity may also occur, rendering it impossible to evaluate the amount of remodeled bone at the fracture site.[7] Although qualitative changes in fracture mass may be analyzed with this technique, attempts to quantitate results of intravital staining studies may be unreasonable.

Quantitative Methods

Although microangiographic, histologic, and vital staining studies are useful for identifying fracture site vessels, they are of little value for determining blood flow differences in various fracture models. Sophisticated radiolabled microsphere techniques and laser doppler flowmetry may be more appropriate for quantitative analysis of fracture site blood flow.

Radiolabeled Microspheres

Since the late 1940s, microspheres of various composition have been used to study circulatory patterns.[18] The first radioactive microspheres were produced by neutron bombardment of glass microspheres which transformed the glass sodium into radioactive sodium-24.[19] The introduction of radiolabeled ceramic microspheres soon followed in the study of circulatory patterns.[20] These heavy microspheres tended to settle rapidly as their specific gravities were much higher than that of red blood cells.[21,22] This limitation was overcome by the development of plastic microspheres in which a specific radionuclide label (such as ^{46}Sc, ^{85}Sr, ^{141}Ce, ^{95}Nb, ^{113}Sn, and ^{125}I) was incorporated into the inert plastic.[21,23]

The technique for measuring bone blood flow using radiolabeled microspheres has been described in detail.[21,24] In brief, the technique first involves placement of three long-term catheters. One intracardiac catheter, placed into the left ventricle via the right carotid artery, serves as the microsphere injection site. Another catheter is positioned in the descending aorta, and a third is placed into the jugular system for venous access. Microspheres 15 μm in diameter are injected into the left ventricle of the experimental animal. Ideally, the microspheres should be evenly mixed with blood in the left ventricle, and, following dispersion, the microspheres are completely trapped within the microcirculation of all tissues. Immediately prior to injection, and at subsequent intervals continuing until a few minutes after microsphere injection, samples of arterial blood are withdrawn from the descending aorta. (Cardiac output is measured using the first reference sample.) The reference samples are placed in counting vials for radionuclide assay. At the end of the experiment, the host animal is sacrificed and the limb under study is harvested. Samples are cleaned and placed in counting vials. Additional tissue samples (including liver, kidney, lung, bowel, muscle, etc.) are obtained for comparison of the vascular response in other organs. A gamma spectrometer is used to assay the specimens. Blood flow to the bone and tissue samples is then quantitated. The distribution of microspheres in the bone and tissues reflects the distribution of the cardiac output and allow measurement of blood flow throughout the bone or reference organ under study.

Over the past few years, methodological improvements in microsphere techniques have led to the widespread use of the method for quantitatively evaluating bone blood flow. Yet, it is not without its limitations. Methodologic principles *must* be followed to minimize variation between blood flow measurements: (1) the microspheres must be of an appropriate size to prevent shunting through arteriovenous anastomoses in bone;[25–28] (2) the spheres must be uniform in size and in radioactivity per sphere;[21,24] (3) the spheres must be adequately mixed with arterial blood;[22,25,29,30] and (4) the sphere dosage should not obstruct the normal microvascular circulation of the bone to the extent that artifactual distortion of the blood flow occurs.[29]

Microsphere injection and counting methods are thus undoubtedly demanding and not without technical error. McGrory and his associates evaluated the reproducibility of serial microsphere injections in an anesthetized canine model and reported the overall error (i.e., random error plus error caused by counting, mixing, and sampling) using their most reliable samples as 10%.[24] This concurs with error calculations reported by other investigators.[30–32] Expense in another factor which must be considered if microspheres are used to quantitatively evaluate bone blood flow. Not only are the microspheres expensive, but elaborate laboratory setups with sophisticated computer software programs and nuclear scanning equipment are necessary to decrease technical error.

The inherent heterogeneity among different experimental animals must also be controlled. Numerous factors affect the animal's vascular response to an investigational stimulus, and many of these factors are specific for the animal studied. These include age, general health and nutritional status, the animal's sympathetic response to anesthesia and the environment, and emotional responses. In a canine model, bone formation and resorption varies greatly depending on the age of the dog.[7,33] For these reasons, age must be standardized in order to accurately measure fracture healing, bone remodeling, and bone blood flow in a canine model. Variability resulting from multiple animals may be minimized if paired comparisons (using the contralateral limb) of a single experimental animal are used to obtain flow calculations throughout the study.

One of the major advantages of the microsphere technique is that it allows, if desired, multiple blood flow determinations over a specified time period in a single experimental animal. As many as six separate measurements of blood flow in one animal are possible.[24,29] If serial measurements are desired, microspheres with varying radioisotope labels are used, and the gamma-emitting isotopes are separated by differential spectroscopy. This significantly decreases the inherent bias of intergroup comparisons. One must still consider the systemic effect that occurs following fracture and the potential increase in normal blood flow to the contralateral limb in studies that use paired comparisons. In studies that use serial injections of microspheres, the physical and psychological effects of treatment on the experimental animal may be significant; yet, the method requires that the condition of the animal remains stable during the experiment.[34]

Although blood flow measurements can be obtained in conscious animals, the results may vary significantly. True basal levels may be difficult to obtain in conscious animals. Nervousness, excitement or animal discomfort may introduce hemodynamic variations.[27] Jones et al. hypothesized that physiologic variables that affect bone blood flow may be controlled by anesthetizing the animal.[27] However, although anesthesia may yield the most reproducible and reliable data, the effect of anesthesia must be considered. Jones et al. reported bone blood flow measurements that were slightly lower in anesthetized dogs than in conscious dogs.[27] McGrory et al. also found a significant decrease in bone blood flow over time in an anesthetized canine model.[24] They suggested that serial estimates of bone blood flow can only be interpreted if the results are normalized to the contralateral limb or a control group of bones. They further suggested that a control group of animals should be included in microsphere experiments of bone blood flow. Bone blood flow measurements may also vary depending on the animal's state of consciousness.

Laser Doppler Flowmetry

Laser doppler flowmetry (LDF) is another quantitative tool for measuring bone blood flow in vivo. LDF is based on the conversion of the Doppler shift of a monochromatic beam of light that is reflected from moving blood cells into an electric signal.[35] Most bone probes consist of three optical fibers; one efferent fiber is for the laser source and two afferent fibers lead the reflected light to photodetectors that convert it into electrical signals.[36] A flushing channel prevents thrombus formation at the viewing chamber.

LDF has been used for measuring cancellous bone blood flow in a number of experimental studies using porcine, ovine, and canine models.[36–39] Lausten and his colleagues found a high correlation between LDF and the microsphere method for measuring cancellous blood flow in a porcine model. LDF has also been used as a clinical tool for assessing regional bone blood flow in humans. Since Swiontkowski and his colleagues first studied femoral head osteonecrosis in humans in 1985, LDF has been used to intraoperatively evaluate anterior cruciate ligament blood flow, nonunion vascularity, and bone perfusion during debridement in patients with osteomyelitis.[40–42]

The usefulness of LDF for measuring cortical bone blood flow, however, may be limited by the depth at which the laser Doppler probe can evaluate flow. Nötzli et al. reported the maximum depth at which the laser Doppler probe can evaluate flow in cortical bone to be 2.9 ± 0.2 mm.[36] Furthermore, the procedure requires repeated exposure of bone to obtain measurements. This may adversely affect the new callus that has formed. Therefore, although LDF provides a simple technique for estimation of changes in the microvascular perfusion of bone, additional studies or modifications in the design of the Doppler probes may be necessary prior to widespread acceptance of this method as an experimental tool for evaluating cortical bone blood flow.

BONE BLOOD SUPPLY IN A FRACTURE MODEL

Because there is an intimate and dynamic relationship between bone and its blood flow, with interruption of the bone (fracture), the bone blood supply is also affected. In general, the vascular response of bone to fracture occurs in five phases: (1) blood flow is interrupted secondary to tearing or crush of the vessels following fracture; (2) vasoconstriction occurs in response to the injury; (3) heightened blood flow secondary to recruitment and/or vessel hypertrophy are noted; (4) the bone is revascularized; and (5) remodeling occurs.

Immediately following an injury and interruption of the bone vasculature, blood flow to the fracture site is significantly reduced. This is demonstrated in a number of studies. Grundnes and Reikerås studied blood flow in rat femurs using radiolabeled microspheres.[12,43] Following transverse mid-diaphyseal osteotomy, they found a reduction in total bone blood flow by 50%, and a reduction in cortical flow by 40%. They attributed this reduction to a physiological vasoconstriction of the periosteal and endosteal vessels in response to the trauma. Smith et al. also reported a 50% reduction in bone blood flow 10 minutes after osteotomy in a dog, and a 29% reduction after four hours.[44] Gross et al. demonstrated similar vasomotor responsiveness in a canine model responding to hemorrhage.[26] Although the duration of this initial decrease in flow may vary depending on the nature of the injury and preexisting host variables, in general, it is short-lived.

One of the most noted sequela of injury is the increase in blood supply observed at the fracture site, which peaks 5 to 14 days after the fracture.[45] Initially, within the first 1 to 3 days after injury, the increase in bone blood flow results from recruitment (perfusion of resting capillaries) and dilatation of existing components of the normal vasculature. This has been demonstrated in a number of in vivo experiments. Hughes et al. used indicator dilution studies in canine tibiae to demonstrate that the pattern of blood flow in bone is nonuniform, and after fracture increased flow to bone is achieved by recruitment.[46] In a large series of canine experiments, Kelly and Bronk studied the relationship of increased venous pressure to formation of periosteal new bone.[47] Common to all of their studies was dilatation of capillaries and sinusoids in the bone in response to increased venous pressure. Rhinelander's microangiographic studies on displaced canine radius fractures studies allow qualitative assessment of vessel dilatation in response to fracture (Fig. 3–4).

Microcirculatory neovascularization also contributes to the increase in bone blood flow following fracture. Traditionally, our understanding of neoangiogenesis is descriptive in nature. That is to say, we are able to identify neoangiogenesis as it occurs following fracture. However, the triggering mechanism responsible for neoangiogenesis is not well understood. Although a well-regulated sequence of vascular responses have been documented, the mediators responsible for eliciting revascularization have not yet been defined. Local biochemical factors are thought to be responsible for augmentation of cortical bone revascularization following fracture.[13,48–50] Endothelial cell stimulating factor (ESAF) is one example of a tissue growth factor which appears to be specific for promoting capillary angiogenesis in vivo. Wallace, et al. found increased levels of ESAF in a small group of patients with tibial fractures who were compared to a cohort of healthy volunteers.[49] Prostaglandins E1 and E2 (PGE1 and PGE2) have the capacity to induce capillary sprouting from veins and may contribute to angiogenesis.[51] Basic fibroblast growth factor (βbFGF), transforming growth factor beta-(TGFβb) angiogenin, and SIKAV have also been found to induce formation of new blood vessels.[52–56] However, to my knowledge, the role of these biochemical factors in cortical revascularization has not been previously investigated.

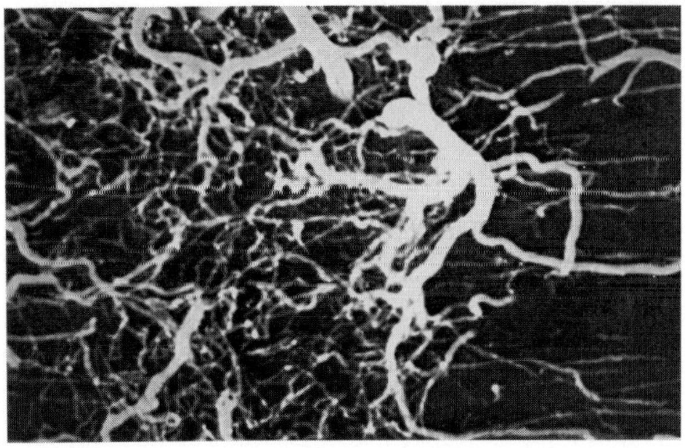

Fig. 3–4. Mature canine radius 2 weeks after undisplaced closed diaphyseal fracture. Enlarged microangiogram showing the great vascular response in the narrow fracture gap (×35). (From Rhinelander, F.W., Baragry, R.A.: Microangiography in bone healing. I. Undisplaced closed fractures. J. Bone Joint Surg, 44A:1273, 1962.)

In addition to biochemical stimuli, the response of bone vasculature to physiologic, neurologic, and humeral stimuli, and venous stasis have been studied.[26,47] Venous stasis, resulting in increased venous pressure has been associated with an increase in periosteal new bone formation in a fracture model. A direct link has not been found, however, between venous stasis, increased venous pressure, PO2, PCO2, or pH, and fracture site revascularization.[47] Clearly, more extensive investigations are required to determine the precise mediators that may stimulate neoangiogenesis and increased fracture site blood flow.

Fracture Site Revascularization

Fracture site revascularization is possible by a number of modes; periosteal, endosteal, or intracortical revascularization may occur. In addition, a new and transitory extraosseous blood supply may be derived from the soft tissues surrounding the fracture. The extraosseous blood supply is entirely distinct from the normal periosteal blood supply, and it serves to nourish the periosteal callus and detached fracture fragments.[1] The response of these individual vascular pathways to fracture may be studied using experimental exclusion techniques. Exclusion studies employ surgical trauma that inhibits periosteal, extraosseous, or endosteal circulation, in order to evaluate the compensatory vascular mechanisms of the intact pathways.[15] From the results of such studies, a number of investigators have hypothesized that the increased blood supply to a healing diaphyseal fracture is derived principally from the periosteum and extraosseous tissues during the period of early fracture repair.[15,17,57,58] Qualitative studies conducted at my institution support the early contribution of the periosteal circulation to the

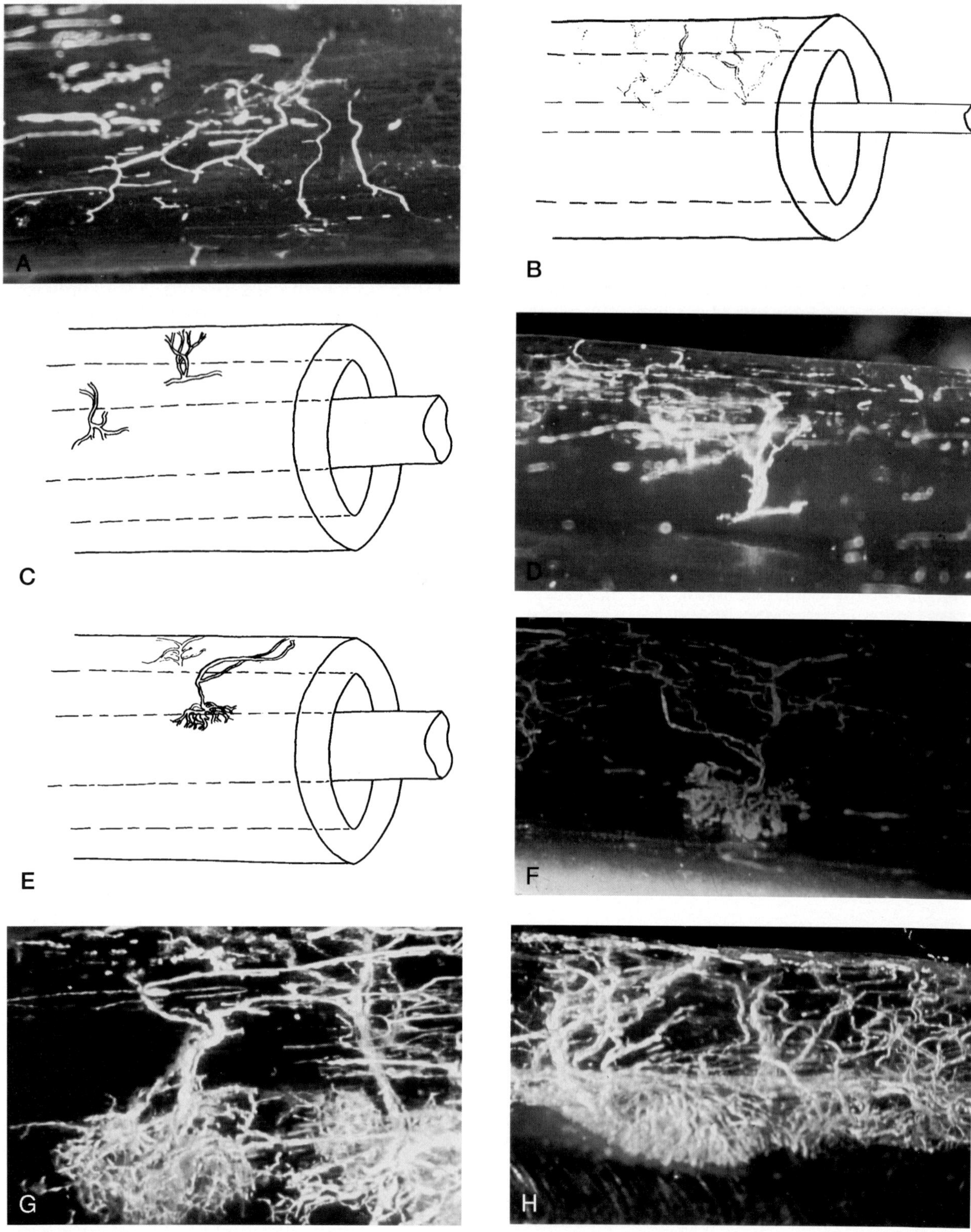

Fig. 3–5. Stages of revascularization following reamed nailing. *A,B,* Stage I: Three days post-osteotomy, increased filling of the periosteal vessels, and penetration of the periosteal vessels into the cortex are observed. Blood flow in a centripetal direction is initiated. *C,D,* Stage II: Six days post-osteotomy, early branching of periosteal vessels is observed. Multiple small branches of the periosteal vessels begin to carry blood centripetally towards the intramedullary canal where new endosteal callus is being produced. *E,F,* Stage III: Six to 9 days post-osteotomy, vascular island formations are noted where the centripetally directed periosteal branches enter the intramedullary canal. *G,* Stage IV: Twelve days postoperatively, interconnections are formed between vascular islands. *H,* Stage V: Reestablishment of larger-diameter intramedullary vessels occurs.

revascularization process. Microfil injection studies allow qualitative assessment of the revascularization process as early as the third day after fracture. Under normal conditions, the periosteal vessels supply blood centripetally to the outer one-third of the cortex. Following fracture, there exists a lag time during which the periosteal vessels undergo neoangiogenesis and ingrowth into the endosteal surface of the cortex. The microvascular situation at 14 days in the cortex of a canine osteotomy treated with casting is shown in Figure 3–2A. These injected vessels represent pre-existing periosteal, or new extraosseous vessels that have grown to traverse the tibial cortex and supply the endosteal surface of the fractured bone. In addition to the periosteal neovascularization demonstrated here, endosteal neovascularization may also occur, as illustrated in Figure 3–2B. New endosteal vessels traverse the cortex to supply the periosteal surface. Thus, the periosteal and endosteal systems supplement each other, not by immediately reversing the direction of their flow, but through revascularization across the cortex of the long bone. This provides evidence against the theory that the periosteal and endosteal systems are anastomotic and immediately supplement each other through a reversal in flow when one of the routes is compromised.[59]

The metaphyseal and endosteal diaphyseal vascular systems, although largely independent, are anastomotic and can also supplement each other when one of the routes is compromised.[1,6]

Qualitative Studies

The effects of reamed and unreamed nailing on fracture site revascularization were studied in a series of experiments on canine tibiae. Microfil injection studies were used to identify the anastomotic patterns responsible for maintenance and/or restoration of endosteal vascularity following intramedullary nailing. The three-dimensional Microfil vessel casts provided an illustrative model of fracture site vascularity. In this series of canine experiments, bilateral tibial osteotomies were performed. One tibia was treated with a reamed 6.4-mm slotted intramedullary nail, and the contralateral tibia was treated with an unreamed 4-mm solid nail. The nails were interlocked using proximal and distal locking screws. Microfil injections were performed 1, 3, 6, 9, and 12 days post-osteotomy. Additional flow studies were conducted on one dog at 18 and 23 days post-osteotomy. Vascular casts of the canine tibial fractures revealed that unreamed nailing spared the paraendosteal vessels, assuring continuous cortical diaphyseal blood flow.[6]

Although the medullary vessels were completely destroyed in the reamed diaphyseal fractures, revascularization of the endosteum occurred rapidly. Figure 3–5A is the stereoscopic photograph and Figure 3–5B is the corresponding line diagram of a reamed osteotomy site 3 days after surgery. Although the endosteal vasculature has been eliminated, a number of periosteal vessels partially penetrate the periosteal cortex. By 6 days post-osteotomy, the periosteal vessels continue to penetrate across the cortex, but still have not reached the endosteal surface. However, by 9 days post-osteotomy, neovascularization occurred completely across the tibial cortex. Periosteal vessels penetrate the endosteal cortex; their terminating branches are newly formed vascular buds. Figure 3–5G shows the microvascular situation 12 days post-osteotomy and reamed nailing. An abundance of periosteal vessels have penetrated completely through the cortex

Table 3–1. Inner cortex blood flow following intramedullary fixation

Dog #	Fixation Method	Blood Flow in mL/min/100 gm								
		Baseline	*Day 1*	*Day 3*	*Day 6*	*Day 9*	*Day 12*	*Day 15*	*Day 18*	*Day 23*
2617	Reamed	4.34	0.40	1.05		53.81			57.64	45.49
	Unreamed	4.18	0.96	3.62		118.04			50.51	20.42
2743	Reamed	1.19	0.24	0.81	23.58	2.68	1.50	1.49		
	Unreamed	1.23	0.69	3.95	86.88	10.50	6.14	6.49		
2805	Reamed	5.04	1.07	1.46	3.09	3.20	14.22			
	Unreamed	5.74	2.03	5.10	8.91	7.19	14.95			

Table 3–2. Outer cortex blood flow following intramedullary fixation

Dog #	Fixation Method	Blood Flow in mL/min/100 gm								
		Baseline	*Day 1*	*Day 3*	*Day 6*	*Day 9*	*Day 12*	*Day 15*	*Day 18*	*Day 23*
2617	Reamed	4.02	0.89	4.31		305.25			141.40	64.27
	Unreamed	4.15	0.97	5.33		191.31			77.02	41.96
2743	Reamed	1.95	1.01	6.89	208.87	27.69	13.88	10.15		
	Unreamed	2.15	1.29	5.97	232.67	20.72	12.55	13.56		
2805	Reamed	5.36	1.48	2.75	6.60	5.02	16.49			
	Unreamed	5.21	1.61	1.62	3.63	3.41	12.54			

to the endosteal surface. The terminating branches of these vessels demonstrate a plethora of new vascular buds. Early reestablishment of a longitudinal flow is observed between the new vascular branches in the endosteal cortex. Figure 3–5H shows another 12-day fracture. Observe the large longitudinal vessels that have been established in the canal. Numerous microvascular buds are also apparent at the nail-bone interface.

Two significant conclusions were drawn from these experiments. First, it was apparent that blood flow through the cortex of fractures treated with reamed nailing did not involve an immediate reversal from a centrifugal to a centripetal direction through anastomoses between periosteal and endosteal vascular pathways. Significant vascular anastomoses between the two systems were not observed, even in the 1-day postosteotomy specimens. Instead, the reversal of normal bone blood flow involves neovascularization or the formation of new periosteal vessels that penetrated through the cortex and gave rise to formation of a new medullary circulation.

Furthermore, although the medullary vessels were completely destroyed by the reaming process, revascularization of the medullary canal was well underway as early as 12 days post-osteotomy. In this series of experiments, rapid revascularization was facilitated by the creation of a low-energy fracture with an intact soft-tissue sleeve. Thus, in fractures with an abundant soft-tissue supply, as is found clinically in the femur or humerus, reluctance to ream may be unjustified. Reamed nailing of tibial fractures, particularly in the face of open injuries, may be associated with high rates of infection and subsequent nonunion. Because of the lack of soft tissues covering the anterior tibia, the periosteal and extraosseous vascular responses may be inhibited. Thus, the fixation method should spare the endosteal vasculature. For these reasons, unreamed nailing may be advantageous in diaphyseal tibial fractures.

Quantitative Studies

Quantitative studies of fracture site blood flow following reamed and unreamed nailing in a canine model were conducted using the radiolabeled microsphere method. Bilateral tibial

Table 3–3. Whole cortex blood flow following intramedullary fixation

Dog #	Fixation Method	Blood Flow in mL/min/100 gm								
		Baseline	*Day 1*	*Day 3*	*Day 6*	*Day 9*	*Day 12*	*Day 15*	*Day 18*	*Day 23*
2617	Reamed	4.11	0.75	3.37		223.36			117.12	58.83
	Unreamed	4.16	0.97	4.78		69.79			68.51	35.04
2743	Reamed	1.70	0.76	4.89	147.88	9.80	9.80	7.30		
	Unreamed	1.78	1.05	5.16	174.41	9.99	9.99	7.40		
2805	Reamed	5.22	1.30	1.93	5.06	15.50	15.50			
	Unreamed	5.44	1.79	3.05	5.85	13.57	13.57			

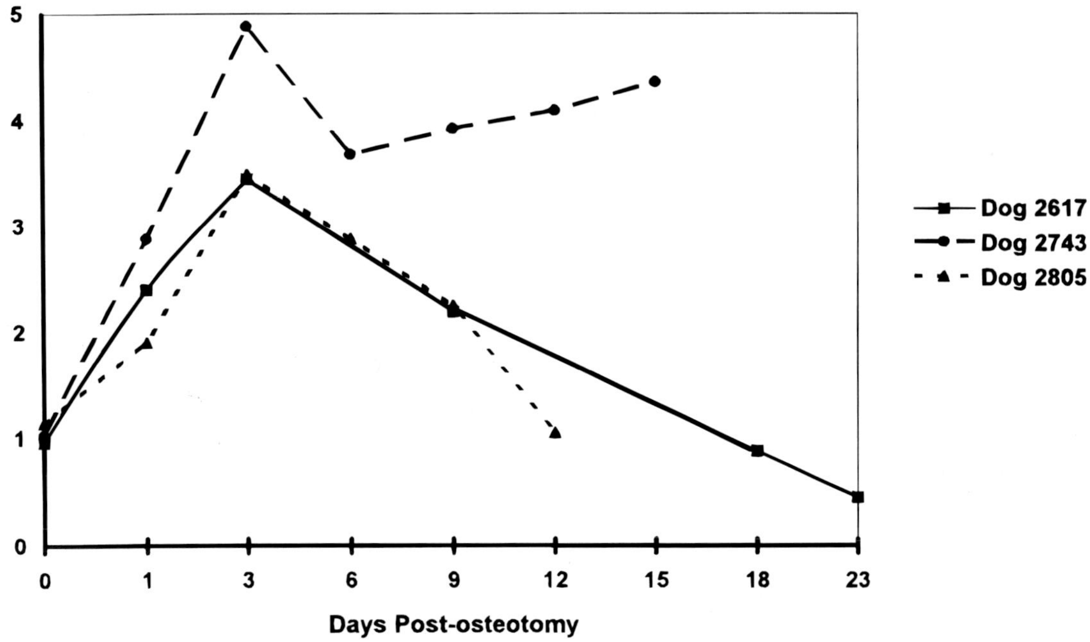

Fig. 3–6. Inner cortex blood flow following intramedullary fixation (unreamed/reamed).

osteotomies were performed on five mature mongrel dogs. Again, one tibia was treated with a reamed 6.4-mm slotted intramedullary nail, and the other was treated with an unreamed 4-mm solid nail. Proximal and distal locking screws were employed. Serial microsphere injections were performed with the animal under intravenous sedation at baseline, immediately after the osteotomy procedure, at 24 hours, and at 3, 6, 9, and 12 days postoperatively. Results of these blood flow studies are shown in Tables 3–1 through 3–3. Blood flow to the endosteal cortex was similar at baseline in three of the dogs. Immediately following nailing, bone blood flow decreased in both models, with flow in the reamed tibia equal to approximately one

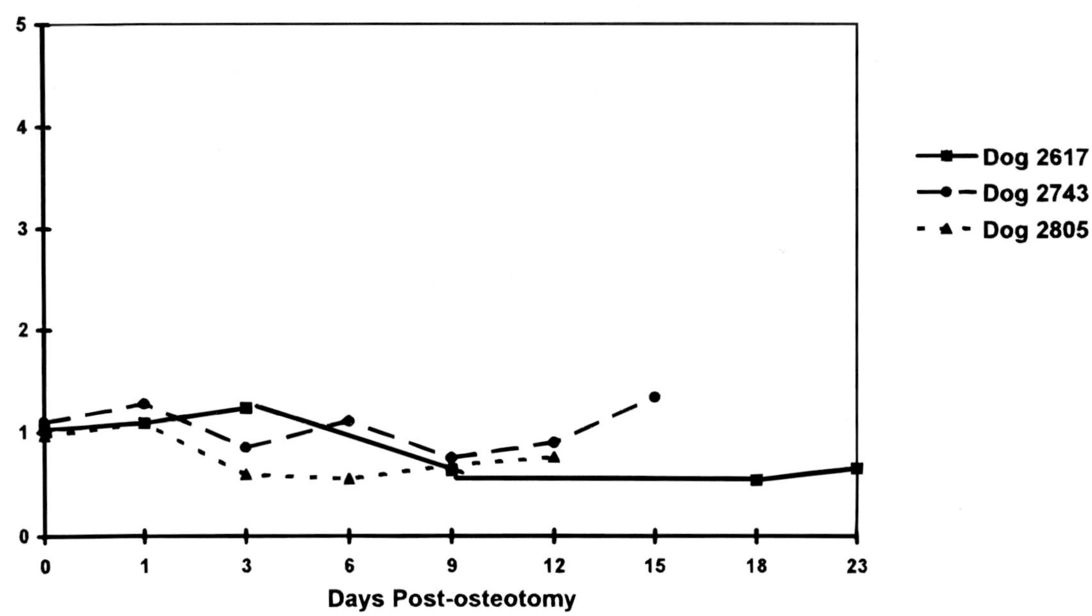

Fig. 3–7. Outer cortex blood flow following intramedullary fixation (unreamed/reamed).

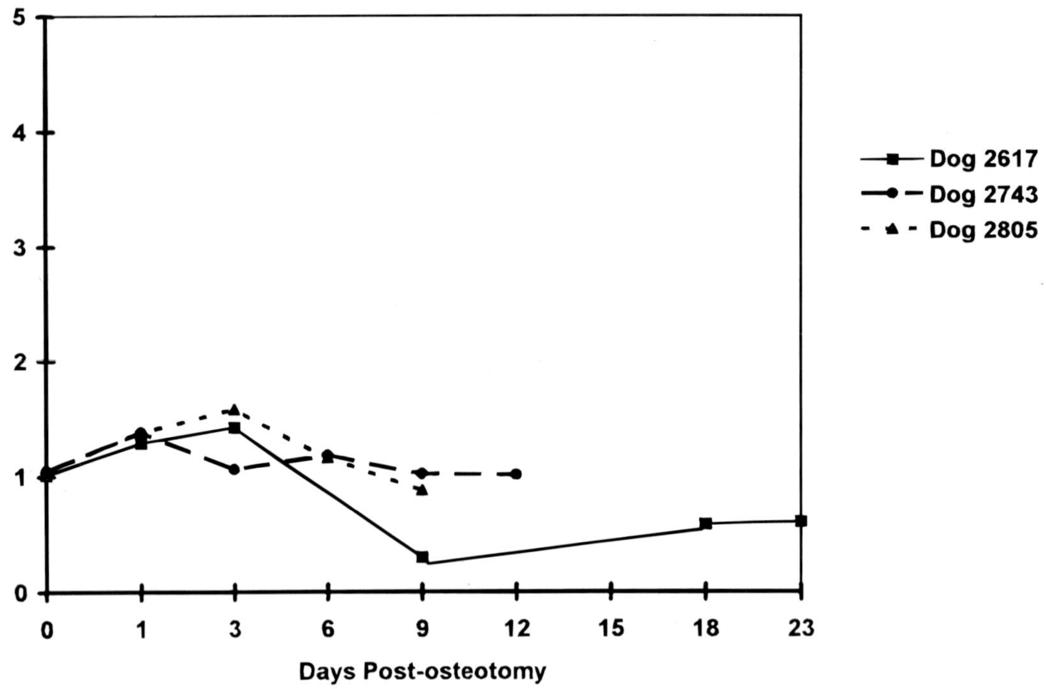

Fig. 3–8. Whole cortex blood flow following intramedullary fixation (unreamed/reamed).

half of that to the unreamed bone. Early in the experiments, blood flow to the inner cortex was significantly lower in the fractures treated with reamed nailing. After 2 weeks, endosteal flow was essentially equal between the two groups.

Blood flow to the outer cortex also decreased immediately following reamed and unreamed nailing. However, by the sixth postoperative day, periosteal cortical blood flow was greater in the reamed fractures as compared to the unreamed bones. In effect, a greater periosteal reaction was elicited in response to the increased medullary destruction caused by reaming. In all models, by the sixth postoperative day, whole bone blood flow was greater than or equal to baseline values. Furthermore, the differences in bone blood flow between the reamed and unreamed fractures were not long-lasting in the canine tibial osteotomy models that were studied.

The ratios of unreamed to reamed bone blood flow were also compared (Figs. 3–6 through 3–8). Comparing the ratios of unreamed to reamed bone blood flow in the inner cortex, a significant difference was noted initially (early), with flow two to four times greater in the unreamed nails. In the outer cortex, bone blood flow was clearly dominated by the periosteal reaction in response to reamed nailing. Looking at the ratio of bone blood flow in unreamed versus reamed fractures (examining the whole bone) little difference was noted.

FACTORS AFFECTING FRACTURE SITE BLOOD FLOW

Attainment of osseous union following fracture is ultimately dependent on stabilization, and maintenance or restoration of an adequate blood supply to the fracture site. Because revascularization is an important aspect of fracture healing, an understanding of factors that affect fracture site blood flow should guide clinicians in their selection of treatment regiments for long-bone fractures. A number of interrelated variables affect the revascularization process. These include injury-related variables, host factors, local biologic factors implicit to neoangiogenesis and the healing process, and treatment variables.[59]

The biomechanical environment of any fracture site and, ultimately, healing of the fracture are affected by the clinician's treatment decisions regarding the method of fixation, soft-tissue management, surgical approach, and timing of intervention. Although clinicians presently possess the ability to control only the treatment-related variables, the effect of local and host factors on fracture site vascularity must be considered when determining a treatment plan for any long-bone fracture.

Host-Related Variables

Preexisting or concurrent host conditions may negatively or positively affect bone blood supply and fracture healing. Hormones, including estrogens, corticosteroids, thyroid hormone, and calcitonin may have an inhibitory effect on fracture healing. The presence of a pathologic condition such as diabetes, vascular insufficiency, or a metabolic disorder may elicit a systemic decrease in the patient's "normal" bone blood flow and may inhibit heightened blood flow. The existence of a catabolic state secondary to trauma may result in decreased blood flow, while in severe head injured patients, increased revascularization and bone formation has been documented (Fig. 3–9).[60]

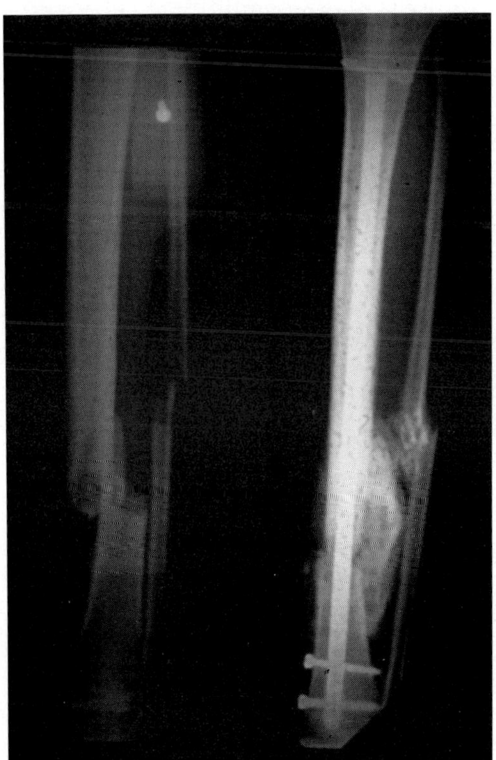

Fig. 3–9. Abundant callus formation 8 weeks postoperatively in a patient with a diaphyseal tibial fracture and closed head injury.

Injury-Related Variables

The mechanism and energy of the injury, fracture location, degree of comminution, and the condition of the surrounding soft-tissue sleeve affect fracture site blood flow. In open injuries, stripping of the periosteum and soft tissues not only interrupts the periosteal blood supply to the cortex but may also affect revascularization of the fracture site. Periosteal tissues play a primary role in the revascularization process and disruption of the periosteal circulation or extensive excision of the periosteum impairs formation of periosteal callus.[15,59,61,62] Whiteside and Lesker studied the effects of muscle transection and extraperiosteal or subperiosteal dissection on the healing of tibial osteotomies in rabbits and found that damage to extraosseous tissues, such as muscle, may also retard fracture healing.[59]

Open fractures are generally more susceptible to infection than closed injuries. Trauma alters the arterial, venous, and lymphatic circulations of the bone and surrounding soft tissues.[63] Capillary leakage causes edema, which in turn decreases vascular resistance. Venous blood flow is diminished and the immune response is delayed, resulting in rapid colonization of unattended open wounds.

Current Controversies: Reamed versus Unreamed Nailing

A great deal of controversy centers around the topic of reamed versus unreamed nailing of long-bone fractures. I believe that a consensus on the appropriate use of a particular nailing technique has not been reached, in part, because of difficulties encountered in studying the effects of reamed versus unreamed nailing in a clinical setting. Although vascular damage occurs any time a nail is driven down the medullary cavity of a long bone, the extent and significance of the vascular varies depending on a number of variables. It is difficult to determine the effect of individual variables on changes in fracture site blood flow, fracture healing, and the development of complications. Blood flow, time to healing and the development of complications thus may be influenced by factors not related to the nailing technique. Second, the parameters available for measuring blood flow and healing times in a clinical setting require qualitative interpretation by the investigator. For these reasons, it is particularly difficult to study the effects of reamed versus unreamed nailing in a clinical situation.

Furthermore, because the disputed advantages of one technique over another are quite different depending on the particular long bone which is being studied, it is beneficial to discuss the advantages and disadvantages of each technique in terms of the bone under study. Most current controversies recognize the effects of reamed versus unreamed nailing techniques for the tibia or femur.

Since the advent of small-diameter, unreamed interlocking nails, surgeons have been embroiled in arguments over the optimal surgical technique for assuring superior healing of tibial fractures. In deliberations over tibial fracture management, the most important factors for the surgeon to consider are the "local" effects of the reamed or unreamed surgical technique on (1) skeletal vascularity, (2) healing, and (3) the susceptibility to (development of postoperative) infection. The surgeon must also be cognizant of the fact that the effects of reamed and unreamed nailing vary depending on the location of the fracture in the tibial diaphysis or metaphysis.

In the femur, current controversy centers on "extraskeletal" factors such as the systemic effects of reaming on pulmonary function, and the potentially less deleterious effects of unreamed nailing. However, the local effects of reaming must also be considered.

Reaming Advantages: Tibial Fractures

As with any surgical procedure, the potential risks and benefits of reamed versus unreamed nailing must be weighed prior to their widespread acceptance or rejection. Reaming may offer a number of mechanical, anatomical, biological, and technical advantages over use of unreamed nails. One of the primary advantages of reaming is that it allows insertion of a larger-sized implant. In treating any long-bone fracture, the diameter of the nail should be large enough to allow weight bearing and joint function during the healing process. This is of particular importance in metaphyseal fractures of the tibia. The majority of hardware failures in patients treated with tibial nails occur in patients with metaphyseal fractures that are treated with smaller-diameter nails. Nine millimeters should be considered the minimal acceptable nail diameter for treating metaphyseal fractures. If possible, 10-mm nails should be used. This is necessary to decrease the possibility of hardware failure and to increase function during healing. With insertion of a larger nail, implant failure, except at screw holes, is uncommon. Screws may also be less prone to failure because the ratio of screw hole size to nail is increased, allowing the use of larger screws. Insertion of a larger implant often has a positive effect on patients' abilities to work and perform activities of daily living during healing, by decreasing the possibility of implant failure. A good reduction fixed with a strong, locked implant may improve patient function and satisfaction during early healing.

Reaming of long-bone fractures also improves nail-bone cortical contact across the working length of the implant, and directs fracture fragments into a more anatomic position. This anatomical advantage is of particular importance in infraisthmal fractures where reaming may be necessary to achieve the best bone to implant contact.

From a biologic standpoint, reaming is advantageous in that systemic factors which promote mitosis of osteogenic stem cells, and stimulate osteogenesis are released in the reaming debris. Finally, canal reaming offers a technical advantage over unreamed techniques by decreasing the risk of iatrogenic fracture, or fracture extension which may result from driving too large an implant down the patient's medullary canal, or from inserting the nail without the direction of a guide wire.

Reaming Disadvantages: Tibial Fractures

While there are no mechanical or technical disadvantages to using an unreamed intramedullary nail, there are anatomic and biologic factors that may favor the use of unreamed nailing in tibial fractures. If a tibial fracture is not properly reduced during reaming, eccentric reaming may cause malreduction of the fracture (Fig. 3–10). Reaming also destroys all medullary blood vessels, resulting in an initial decrease in endosteal blood flow. This initial decrease in blood flow will result in a decreased immune response, and may delay early healing of the involved cortices.

Reaming may also be disadvantageous in the face of certain open injuries. Because direct interruption of the blood supply occurs with ev-

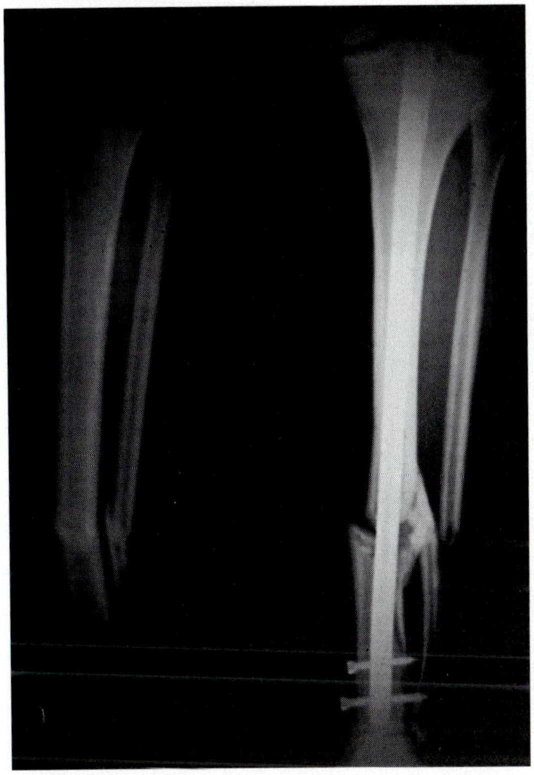

Fig. 3–10. Thirty-year-old man sustained a closed tibial diaphyseal fracture in a motorcycle accident. Eccentric reaming during canal preparation resuled in malreduction of his fracture.

ery long-bone fracture, to some extent, avascular or nonviable (dead) bone is present at every fracture site (Fig. 3–11). The amount of nonviable bone depends upon the degree of vascular interruption at the fracture site. Unreamed nails have been advocated as a relatively safer method of fixation (as compared to reamed nailing) for the management of open fractures. Although reaming is a standard treatment for femur and closed tibial fractures, when the indications for reamed nailing are extended to all open fractures, high complication rates have been documented. These complications most likely result from the increase in nonviable bone that is unable to resist infection. Figures 3–11B and 3–11C are an example of a high-energy injury associated with extensive soft-tissue stripping. In the face of such a large quantity of nonviable bone, the tibia is particularly susceptible to infection. By performing an adequate debridement and covering the fracture acutely, the possibility of infection is significantly decreased. By using an unreamed nail, the endosteal circulation remains viable in the face of compromised periosteal circulation. This, along with opposition of the fracture fragments increases the possibility of rapid revascularization and primary healing of the fracture.

However, it is not safe to assume that because unreamed nails spare the endosteal vasculature to a greater degree than reamed nails, that fewer complications will result. In a study at my institution, cortical bone biopsies were performed on 10 patients who sustained grade IIIB tibial fractures. All patients were treated with acute soft-tissue coverage and acute unreamed intramedullary nailing. Specimens used for study were taken from the mid-diaphysis 7 to 10 days postoperatively. Standard histologic analysis of the specimens was performed. Although all fractures had been treated with unreamed nailing, three of the patients had avascular bone along the entire length of their biopsy specimens (from the periosteal to endosteal cortices).

When reaming disrupts the intramedullary circulation, nonviable bone will be present at the fracture site. Conversely, unreamed nailing with insertion of a loose-fitting implant may spare the cortical blood supply and decrease the amount of nonviable bone at the fracture site. This intuitively implies that unreamed nailing may be appropriate for management of open fractures in which contamination is likely, and that reamed nailing, which is associated with extensive nonviable cortex, may be inappropriate for managing open tibial fractures. However, one must exercise judgement and caution when applying unreamed nailing in high-energy open fractures.

As demonstrated by the empty lacunae in Figure 3–11A, regardless of whether or not an unreamed nail and excellent surgical technique is used, in the face of an open fracture, the surgeon must deal with a dead bone that may likely serve as a nidus for infection. It has been hypothesized that implant infections occur because of contamination of the prosthesis with very small numbers of bacteria.[64,65] These bacteria may be protected in the interstices of the intramedullary nail by a glycocalyx biofilm where they are unlikely to be exposed to parenteral antibiotics or affected by debridement.[64,65] Therefore, when an injury results in massive amounts of dead bone, it is far better to acutely cover the wound to reduce the risk of further nosocomial contamination, and aid the

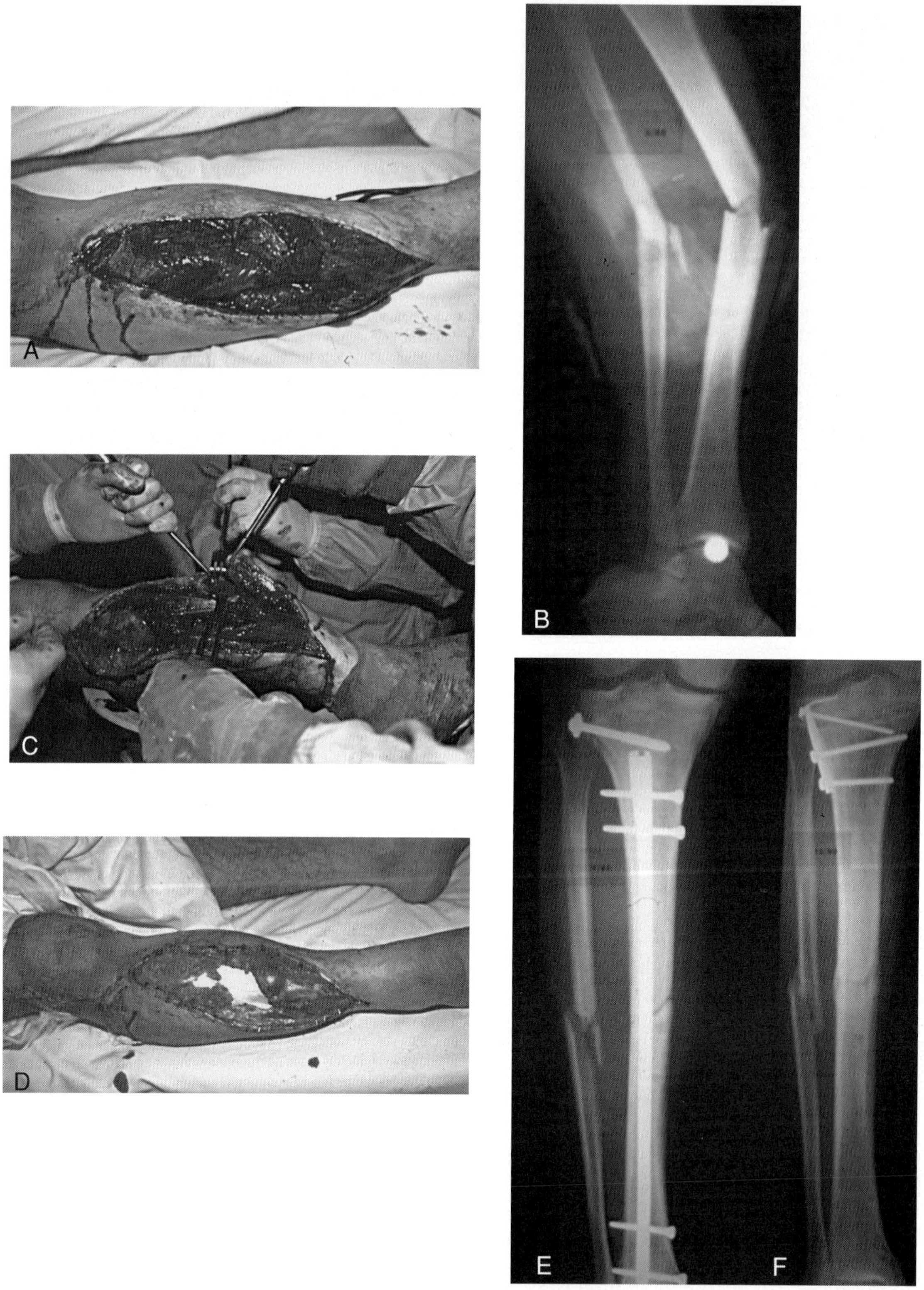

Fig. 3–11. *A,* Tibial specimen harvested 7 days after fracture and nailing shows cortical bone with empty lacunae. A marked amount of nonviable bone is present, despite acute coverage and use of a small-diameter nail inserted using an unreamed technique. *B,* Acute preoperative radiograph shows noncomminuted diaphyseal fracture pattern associated with severe soft-tissue injury. *D,* Acute wound coverage was obtained using medial gastrocnemius and medial hemisoleus flaps. *E,F,* Postoperative AP radiograph demonstrating intramedullary nail fixation; 16-month postoperative radiograph shows fracture with minimal callus formation. *(Figure continues)*

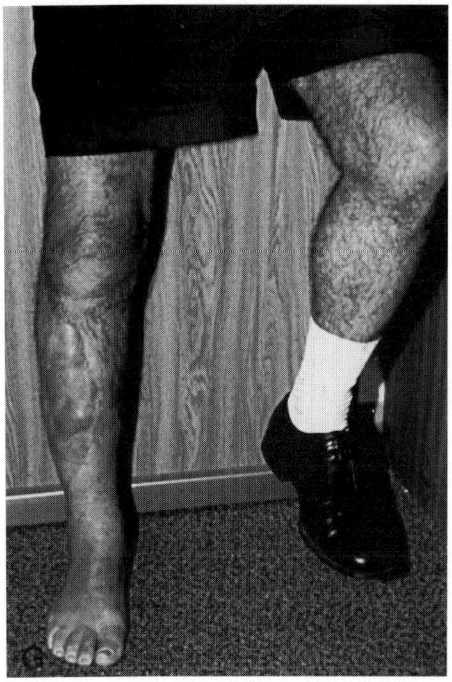

Fig. 3–11. *(continued) G,* Patient had a good functional outcome 8 months after injury.

immune response by allowing for healing of the soft-tissue sleeve prior to fixation of the fracture.

Reamed versus Unreamed Tibial Nailing: Metaphyseal Versus Diaphyseal Circulations

The vascular effects of reaming a metaphyseal fracture are quite different from those encountered after reaming a diaphyseal fracture. To demonstrate the differences between metaphyseal and diaphyseal circulations and the vascular response of each to nailing, the tibia of two mature canines were completely divided in the distal metaphysis by osteotomy with a Stryker saw. Figure 3–12 presents the vascular findings 3 days post-osteotomy and nailing. Figure 3–12A presents a metaphyseal osteotomy treated with unreamed intramedullary nailing. The stereoscopic microvascular anatomy is similar to that of the metaphyseal osteotomy treated with reamed nailing. The flow of blood through the metaphysis was not severely compromised by nailing or canal reaming.

Metaphyseal cortical blood flow differs greatly from diaphyseal cortical flow. This is of particular significance to the clinician managing metaphyseal tibial fractures. The diameter of the tibial nail should be large enough to allow weight bearing and decrease the possibility of implant failure. Use of larger intramedullary nails often necessitates reaming of the intramedullary canal. However, this should not be considered unfavorable. The effects of reaming a metaphyseal fracture are considerably different from those observed with reaming of a diaphyseal fracture. Because metaphyseal fractures are located largely in cancellous bone, they are less likely to suffer circulatory deficiency or necrosis from overheating following reaming.[66] Furthermore, whereas diaphyseal blood flow is centrifugal, metaphyseal arteries supply blood centripetally to the entire metaphysis. Metaphyseal arteries also play a major role in cortical revascularization by maintaining perfusion of the intramedullary canal following reaming and subsequent disruption of the nutrient artery.[67] For these reasons, reluc-

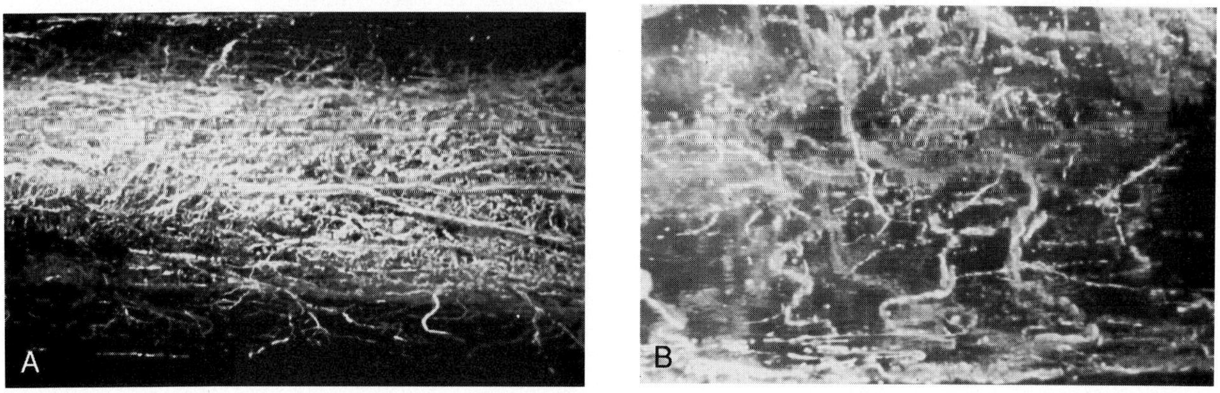

Fig. 3–12. *A,* Mature canine tibial metaphysis 3 days post-osteotomy and unreamed intramedullary nailing. Metaphyseal blood flow is intact. *B,* Mature canine tibial metaphysis 3 days post-osteotomy and reamed intramedullary nailing (enlarged view). Metaphyseal blood flow is not severely compromised by reaming and nail insertion.

tance to ream proximal or distal metaphyseal fractures is not justified.

Femoral Fracture Reaming: Advantages and Disadvantages

The mechanical, anatomic, biologic, and technical advantages of intramedullary reaming that were outlined for tibial fractures, are equally as applicable to reaming of femur fractures. Yet, despite the advantages of reamed nailing, unreamed femoral nailing has gained popularity, becoming a vogue procedure in the 1990s. Reaming obliterates the endosteal vasculature and has been associated with significant rises in intramedullary pressure and cortical thermal necrosis. Reaming has also been cited as the cause of systemic complications, most notably fat embolism syndrome and ARDS.

Pape and his colleagues investigated the effects of primary intramedullary femoral nailing with and without reaming on lung function and pulmonary hemodynamics in 31 multiple-trauma patients.[68] Patients included in the study did not have significant thoracic trauma and underwent surgical fracture stabilization within 24 hours. The investigators found that lung function deteriorated intraoperatively during reaming, and oxygenation ratios improved only after 48 hours. Pulmonary artery pressures (PAP) also increased in the reamed femoral nail patients but returned to normal after 1 hour. No changes in PAP or oxygenation ratios were seen in patients submitted to unreamed nailing. In light of these results, the investigators suggested that unreamed intramedullary stabilization of femur fractures has less deleterious effects on the lung. In the presence of concurrent pulmonary contusion, unreamed nailing might reduce the incidence of postoperative ARDS. However, in multiple-trauma patients subjected to surgical intervention, one must judge carefully the pathogenic significance of reaming. Although reaming may have a negative effect on oxygenation ratios and PAP, biochemical and immunologic factors may also contribute to development of ARDS in multiple trauma patients.

Pell et al. intraoperatively monitored the effects of fracture fixation using reamed intramedullary nailing in a human clinical study of 17 tibial and 7 femoral fractures.[72] Using transesophageal echocardiography, they reported three different groups of patients: (1) those with little or no evidence of embolic phenomena, (2) those with intermittent showers of echogenic material 1 to 10 mm in diameter, and (3) those in whom there was sonographic evidence of emboli 1 to 8 cm in diameter. At first glance, these figures painted a grim picture of diaphyseal fracture reaming. However, closer examination of the results revealed that in Group II emboli usually appeared in the right atrium within 10 seconds of starting closed reduction of the fracture. Successive emboli showers were also associated with canal entry, reaming, and nail insertion. This lends support to the hypothesis that, in patients who have not suffered concurrent pulmonary injuries, the development of fat embolism syndrome may be attributed to the fracture or fracture reduction, rather than reaming.[70] Certainly, additional studies are necessary to determine the individual contributions of fracture, reduction, and reamed or unreamed nail insertion on the development of fat embolism syndrome or ARDS.

As with any surgical procedure, the potential risks and benefits of reamed versus unreamed nailing must be weighed prior to their widespread acceptance or rejection. Recognition of the potentially harmful effects of reamed nailing does not justify the conclusion that unreamed nailing is a preferential form of treatment for all long-bone fractures. Rather, the decision to ream or not to ream any given fracture must be based on a number of considerations, including the infection risk, functional demands of the patient, revascularization potential, bone quality, and fracture pattern. Use of good reaming techniques may also decrease the incidence of complications associated with femoral fracture reaming.

REAMING TECHNIQUE

Passage of a reamer down a tight medullary canal must be thought of as a piston in a cylinder. Heat and hydraulic pressure are produced as the reamer advances into the medullary cavity, destroying the endosteal surface and depressing marrow contents. Reaming may also damage cortical bone, with the amount of destruction being largely dependent on the surgeon's reaming technique. The amount of pressure that develops during reaming depends on the flow rate of medullary contents out of the medullary cavity. Good reaming techniques facilitate passage of medullary contents out of the canal, prevent cortical temperature increases, and avoid significant increases in intramedullary pressure.

In femur fractures, insertion of a larger, reamed nail achieves greater fracture site contact and decreases the risk of cortical penetration of fracture resulting from insertion of a solid, unreamed nail (Fig. 3–13). However, care must be taken to avoid overreaming, as this may deform the fracture site. Reaming should be continued not only for passage of the guide wire, but also during each reamer passage. This is necessary to avoid eccentric reaming and nonanatomic alignment. Figure 3–14 presents radiographs of a 21-year-old man who sustained a diaphyseal fracture that was treated with reamed intramedullary nailing. Rapid reaming using blunt reamers resulted in a significant periosteal reaction away from the fracture site, but limited periosteal reaction at the fracture. A lack of reactive osteopenia is also noted. Over time, the presence of resorptive changes on radiographs signified that a vascular supply was being reestablished. However, it was occuring in a nonuniform fashion. The fracture went on to nonunion and healed after treatment with autogenous bone grafting.

Theoretically, a number of interventions may lower the pressure and temperature increases associated with reaming:

1. Sharp cutting heads should be used, as blunt reamers increase both the intramedullary pressure and cortical temperature and produce a higher tangential strain on the diaphysis.[71–72]
2. Reamer heads should be designed to propagate, limit the amount of debris that remains trapped in the cutting flutes, and disperse a large amount of medullary fluid. Long, deep flutes facilitate passage of a larger volume of marrow contents past the cutting head (reamer), as compared to reamers with shorter flutes.[71] Flow rate is directly proportional, while the increase in intramedullary pressure is inversely proportional to the diameter of the reamer and the diameter of the drive shaft. Thus, as the difference in diameters decreases, the flow rate decreases, resulting in increased intramedullary pressure (while intramedullary pressure increases).[71–73]
3. Axial advancement of the reamer should proceed slowly with the reamer rotating at full speed. This may prevent cortical necrosis and crack propagation. If a great deal of resistance is encountered, reaming should be stopped and the reamer backed out slightly. Gentle reaming proceeds with a repeated back and forth movement based on the amount of friction that is encountered. As the reamer approaches the fracture site, the speed of rotation and ad-

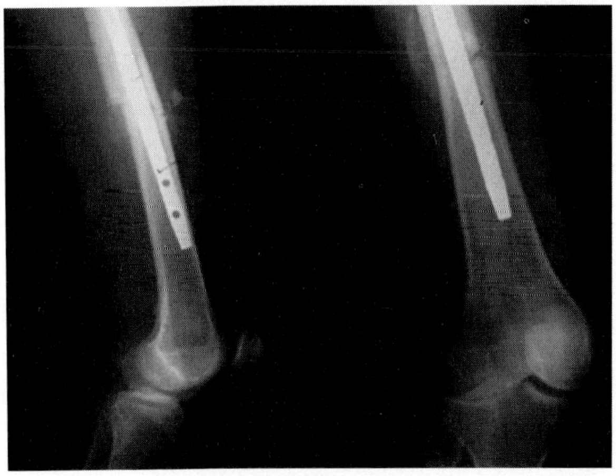

Fig. 3–13. The unreamed femoral nail penetrated the anterior cortex and initiated an intercondylar fracture. Canal reaming is necessary to adequately prepare the femur for nailing.

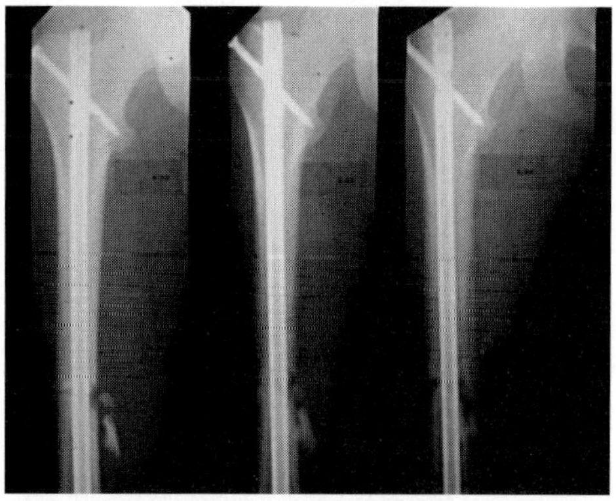

Fig. 3–14. Comminuted femoral diaphysis fracture in a 21-year-old man was treated with a reamed nail with impaction at the fracture site. Subsequent radiographs show obvious nonviable femoral cortex with increased density and periosteal cortical resorption. Overreaming killed cortical bone and resulted in a nonunion.

vancement are slowed to ensure that the fracture fragments are anatomically aligned to prevent eccentric reaming.

4. The fracture site itself offers an effective vent for release of medullary contents. Use of a distal vent hole may also contribute to pressure reduction. However, the viscosity of medullary contents determines their ability to pass through the vent hole. The vent must be monitored continuously to prevent clogging of the reaming debris.
5. Finally, vascular tourniquets should remain down (deflated) during reaming to allow circulating blood to cool the medullary canal. Inflated tourniquets impede this vital blood flow.

Current Controversies: Bone Blood Flow in Nonunions

Adequate vascularity has been deemed one of the most important aspects of fracture repair.[1] Consequently, fractures with an inadequate blood supply may not heal or may result in delayed union. However, what is an inadequate blood supply? Or for that matter, what is adequate vascularity? Does the presence of an adequate blood supply assure healing? Do fractures with decreased bone blood flow always result in delayed healing or nonunion? At what point is decreased bone blood flow significant enough to delay healing? Clearly, a number of important questions remain unanswered.

Although few reviews or research studies are available on the vascular supply of long-bone nonunions, I have found that the presence of an adequate blood supply to the fracture site does not always assure healing (Fig. 3–15). Accessory factors are obviously involved in the healing process. Intuitively, these factors are released at the time of fracture and circulate systemically for an indefinite period of time before they are metabolized. If a fracture has progressed to nonunion, more than likely, the systemic factors which stimulate fracture healing have dissipated. Reaming of fracture nonunions is advantageous in that it may once again release the factors necessary for union to occur.

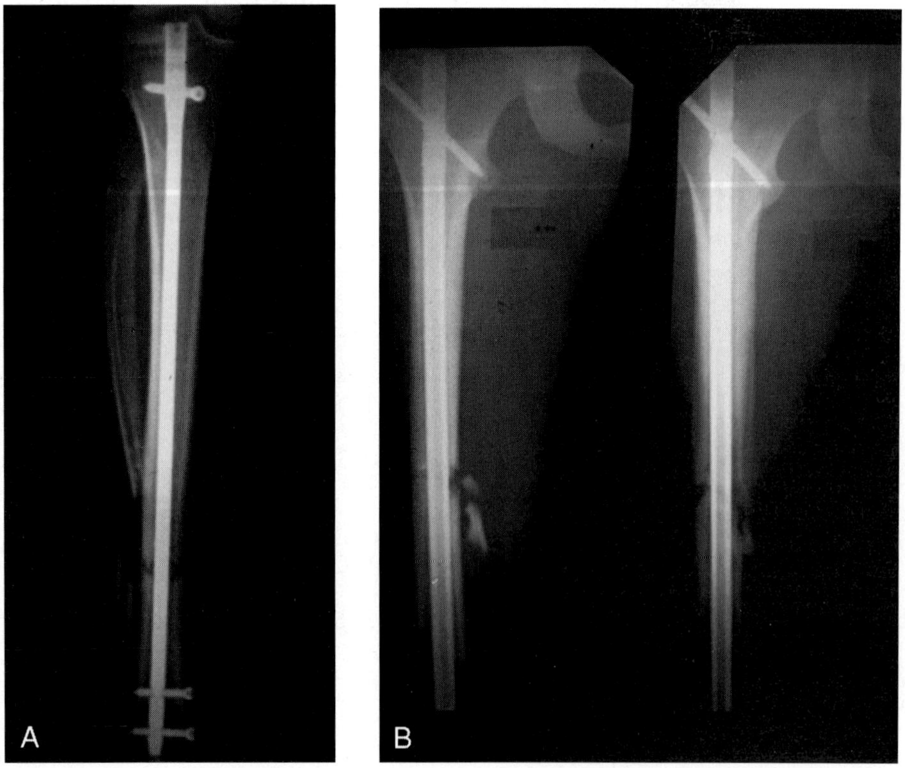

Fig. 3–15. *A*, Postoperative radiograph of high-energy open tibial fracture which resulted in a nonunion. *B*, Abundant cortical blood flow was noted at the fracture site. Presence of adequate vascularity did not assure healing of the fracture.

The effects of reaming a nonunion, particularly a diaphyseal nonunion, are much different than reaming a fresh fracture. The cortical bone surrounding the nonunion site may not be as susceptible to reaming. This may be caused by the altered vascular situation at the nonunion site. The cortical bone of nonunions is not necessarily avascular. In fact, the cortex of nonunions may be more vascular than that of uninjured bones as a result of ingrowth of periosteal vessels across the cortex or the presence of an intracortical network of vascular channels. A centripetal blood flow pattern, similar to the metaphyseal circulation pattern, may exist in long-bone nonunions. Reaming of a diaphyseal nonunion may therefore be associated with decreased blood flow compromise because of the centripetal flow of blood from the periosteal to endosteal cortices.

Current Controversies: Acute versus Delayed Nailing—Acute Fractures

The timing of reaming may affect fracture site vascularity, healing, and the development of systemic complications. For a simple fracture, fixation should be performed acutely. With a problematic fracture (i.e., an open fracture, with excessive periosteal stripping or contamination, or a closed fracture with severely crushed soft tissues), internal fixation should be delayed. As the periosteal and extraosseous circulations are vital for cortical revascularization, definitive fixation should be delayed in these types of injuries until coverage of the fracture site with a viable soft-tissue sleeve has been accomplished, thus optimizing the biologic milieu at the fracture site.

If reaming is indicated, it may be advantageous to ream at a time when neo-angiogenesis of periosteal vessels growing toward the endosteum has taken place. Reaming releases factors that stimulate neo-osteogenesis and fracture healing. Intuitively, if reaming is delayed for 9 or 10 days, an increased number of soft-tissue and cortical vessels will be available to transport the biochemical mediators that may be released during reaming. Furthermore, because revascularization of the fracture is readily apparent as early as the third day after injury, a delay in reaming may decrease the load of nonviable bone at the fracture site. Decreasing the amount of nonviable bone is particularly important in the face of contamination.

The vascular advantages of delayed reamed nailing must be weighed against the potential complications associated with the procedure. The timing of reaming or fixation is of particular importance in patients with long-bone fractures (particularly those of the femur) and associated pulmonary injuries. Pell et al. used transesophageal echocardiography to intraoperatively monitor embolic phenomena during fracture reduction and intramedullary nailing with reaming.[69] Large quantities of echogenic material and the most severe clinical symptoms were seen in 2 patients who had nailing delayed more than 48 hours (3 and 10 days). In a prospective, randomized study comparing the results of early versus delayed stabilization of acute femur fractures, Bone et al. documented a higher incidence of ARDS and fat embolism syndrome, longer hospital stays, an increased number of intensive-care days and increased hospital costs when stabilization of the femur fracture was delayed more than 48 hours after injury.[74] In retrospective studies, a number of other investigators, including Riska and Myllynen, Border, Goris et al., Jonson et al., LeDuca, and Seibel also documented a relationship between a delay in fracture stabilization and an increased incidence of respiratory complications.[73–79] These factors must be considered when determining the optimum treatment plan for any given long-bone fracture.

Current Controversies: Open versus Closed Procedure

The surgical technique that is used during intramedullary nailing may also have an effect on the bone's vascularity. Use of an open technique allows direct manipulation and reduction of fracture fragments. However, open reduction and fixation requires increased dissection and stripping of bone fragments. The impact on bone blood flow and healing using an open versus closed procedure was studied in rats by Grundnes and Reikerås.[12] They found that femoral fractures treated by closed nailing healed better in the first 12 weeks, compared with those that were openly nailed. Interestingly, bone blood flow to the callus was increased at 4 and 8 weeks in bones treated with an open procedure.

Current Controversies: Soft-Tissue Management

The effects of periosteal devascularization have been studied using techniques of tissue exclusion. Wallace et al. quantitatively examined the effect of periosteal devascularization on the healing of osteotomized sheep tibia held in an instrumented external fixation system.[13,58] They found significantly lower cortical flow at the osteotomy sites in the devascularized group as compared to the standard group. Postmortem mechanical testing found that the well-vascularized osteotomies exhibited increased torsional strength, suggesting that devascularization may delay early healing. Oni et al. studied the contributions of the periosteum and bone marrow as sources of fracture callus in rabbits.[61] They observed a progressive reduction in medullary vascularization after the periosteum was elevated and a Silastic sheath wrapped around the tibial shaft. At the end of 4 weeks, no osteotomy had united. In contrast, intense periosteal proliferative activity resulting in union occurred as early as 2 weeks in rabbits treated with preservation of the periosteum and initial exclusion of the endosteal circulation by reaming and nailing. The work of Triffitt et al. further supports the significance of the periosteum and extraosseous tissues during the early period of diaphyseal fracture healing.[15]

Nowhere is an adequate knowledge of the effects of soft-tissue damage on fracture site vascularity more important than in the management of fractures of the tibia. The anterior tibia, in particular, lacks abundant musculocutaneous (extraosseous) coverage. As the periosteal vessels and extraosseous soft tissues play a vital role in reestablishment of cortical circulation, fracture site vascularity and union may be affected by extensive periosteal stripping as seen in open fractures. Richards and Schemitsch suggested that early muscle flap coverage may effect the bone blood flow of devascularized tibial fractures.[80] In contrast, Paeimont et al. demonstrated that early free flap coverage does not substantially increase periosteal blood flow. In open tibia fractures, perhaps, even more important than early reestablishment of periosteal blood flow and fracture fixation is the prevention of infection. Adequate debridement and acute wound coverage using interventions that do not further sacrifice periosteal or extraosseous blood flow may be more useful in preventing nosocomial contamination or colonization of tissues contaminated by injury.

Current Controversies: Effects of Weight Bearing and Surgical Technique on Fracture Site Blood Flow

The vascular response of bone to fracture and internal fixation has been described in a number of clinical and experimental research studies. However, despite this wealth of information, a number of important questions remain unanswered. Foremost, the exact mechanisms that stimulate the revascularization process remain obscure and somewhat controversial

Several investigators have suggested that blood flow to the fracture site is an indicator of the metabolic rate of the tissue.[14,82] In other words, bone blood flow is determined by the patient's metabolic needs, with the amount of blood flow being proportionate to the amount of anabolic activity at the fracture site. The anabolic activity at the fracture site depends on a number of factors, most notably, the degree of stability afforded by the fixation method during weight bearing. In studies conducted at the Mayo clinic, investigators found blood flow to canine fractures fixed with intramedullary rods greater than blood flow to plate-fixed fractures.[81] They noted that a strong, external bridging callus formed in response to the decreased stability afforded by the rods as compared to those treated with plates. Initially, the investigators suggested that this increase represented a compensatory mechanism to increase blood flow to the bone because the medullary circulation was blocked by an intramedullary rod.

In a later report, the increased blood flow to the rod-fixed fractures was attributed to the higher metabolic demands of nourishing the callus.[81,82] Interestingly, despite the increase in blood flow observed in fractures treated with rods, a corresponding delay in biomechanical maturation was documented. Similar results were reported by Wallace et al. after studying the effects of axial micromovement in sheep treated with osteotomies and external fixators of varying axial stiffness.[13] At 14 days, they documented increased periosteal callus size and a fourfold increase in fracture site blood flow in the semirigid group, when compared to the rigid fixation group. The early vascular response is thus very sensitive to the initial mechanical environment of the fracture site.[13]

In separate studies conducted at the Mayo Clinic, O'Sullivan, et al. compared the effects of decreased, increased and baseline mechanical loading on early fracture healing in an adult canine tibia model.[14] Both periosteal bone formation and blood flow were increased in the increased-loading fracture site compared with the decreased-loading and baseline-loading fracture sites. These experiments did not elicit the exact biophysical or biochemical mechanisms that stimulate and regulate the vascular response to changes in metabolism, micromovement, or other stimuli at the fracture site. Clearly, additional studies in this area are necessary. However, results of the Mayo studies further support the view that increased blood flow may be secondary to increased metabolic demands at the fracture site. Such findings are particularly relevant to clinical practice as they point to the importance of weight bearing in promoting an increased vascular response to fracture and, quite possibly, healing. In summary, the researchers demonstrated that the mechanical environment of the fracture site affects bone blood flow and that mechanical loading of fractures increases anabolic activity at the fracture site. In the presence of an adequate, viable extraosseous sleeve, fixation methods that maintain cortical contact but allow limited motion in response to mechanical stress (such as weight bearing) optimize callus formation and fracture healing. Thus, the surgical treatment of any long-bone fracture should allow for weight bearing and promotion of fracture healing.

Through their choice of fixation method, the surgeon affects the mechanical environment at the fracture site and, ultimately, the patient's outcome. In light of this, surgeons should strive to attain and maintain fracture reduction and choose an implant that allows early weight bearing in a wide variety of long-bone fractures. With the use of interlocking intramedullary nails for long-bone fracture fixation, it is possible to obtain adequate fixation for promotion of weight bearing and to maintain cortical contact while allowing limited fracture site motion.

ACKNOWLEDGEMENT

The author gratefully acknowledges Samuel Weirich, MD for his invaluable contribution to the animal studies that were performed at the University of Texas, Houston and Lori J. Ansel, RN for her assistance with preparation of this chapter. This research was funded in part by educational grants from Smith and Nephew Richards and Howmedica, Inc.

REFERENCES

1. Rhinelander, F.W.: Vascular response of bone to internal fixation. *In* The Science & Practice of Intramedullary Nailing. 1st Ed. Edited by B.D. Browner and C.C. Edwards. Philadelphia, Lea & Febiger, 1987.
2. Cowell, H.R., Curtiss, P.H.: Editorial. The randomized clinical trial. J. Bone Joint Surg. *67A*:1151–1152, 1985.
3. Rudicel, S., Esdaile, J.: The randomized clinical trial in orthopaedics: Obligation or Option? J. Bone Joint Surg. *67A*:1284–1293, 1985.
4. Wilson, J.W.: Vascular supply to normal bone and healing fractures. Semin. Vet. Med. Surg. (Small Anim) *6*: 26–30, 1991.
5. Kaplan, F.S., Hayes, W.C., Keaveny, T.M., Boskey, A., Einhorn, T.A., Iannotti, J.P.: Form and function of bone. In Orthopaedic Basic Science. Edited by S. R. Simon. American Academy of Orthopaedic Surgeons, 1994.
6. Cole, J.D.: The effects of reamed and unreamed intramedullary nailing on fracture site vascularity. Proceedings of the Japanese Orthopaedic Association. Kobe, Japan. April, 1994.
7. Kelly, P.J., Montgomery, R.J., Bronk, J.T.: Reaction of the circulatory system to injury and regeneration. Clin Orthop. *254*:275, 1990.
8. Oni, O.O., Stafford, H., Gregg, P.J.: An investigation of the routes of venous escape from the diaphyseal marrow of the canine and rabbit long bones. Int. J. Microcirc. Clin. Exp. *7*:31–41, 1988.
9. Brookes, M.: The blood supply of bone. An approach to bone biology. London, Butterworths, 1971.
10. McLean, F.C., Urist, M.R.: Fracture healing. *In* An Introduction to the Physiology of Skeletal Tissue. 2nd Ed. Edited by P.P.H. DeBruyn. Chicago, University of Chicago Press, 1961.
11. Morris, M.A., Kelly, P.J.: Use of tracer microspheres to measure bone blood flow in conscious dogs. Calcif. Tissue Int. *32*:69–76, 1980.
12. Grundnes, O., Reikerås, O.: Closed versus open medullary nailing of femoral fractures. Blood flow and healing studied in rats. Acta Orthop. Scand. *63*: 492–496, 1992.
13. Wallace, A.L., Draper, E.R.C., Strachan, R.K., McCarthy, I.D., Hughes, S.P.F.: The vascular response to fracture micromovement. Clin. Orthop. *301*:281–290, 1994.
14. O'Sullivan, M.E., Bronk, J.T., Chao, E.Y.S., Kelly, P.J.: Experimental study of the effect of weight bearing on fracture healing in the canine tibia. Clin. Orthop. *302*: 273–283, 1994.
15. Triffitt, P.D., Cieslak, C.A., Gregg, P.J.: A quantitative study of the routes of blood flow to the tibial diaphysis after an osteotomy. J. Orthop. Res. *11*:49–57, 1993
16. Trueta, J.: Blood supply and the rate of healing of tibial fractures. Clin. Orthop. *105*:11–26, 1974.
17. Rhinelander, F.W.: Microangiography in bone healing. I. Undisplaced closed fractures. J. Bone Joint Surg. *44A*: 1273–1298, 1962.
18. Prinzmetal, M., Simkin, B., Bergman, H.C., Kruger, H.E.: Studies on the coronary circulation. The collat-

eral circulation of the normal human heart by coronary perfusion with radioactive erythrocytes and glass spheres. Am. Heart J. 33:420–442, 1947.
19. Grim, E., Lindseth, E.O.: Distribution of blood flow to the tissues of the small intestines of the dog. Univ. Minn. Med. Bull. *30*:138–145, 1958.
20. Hamlin, R.L., Marsland, W.P., Smith, C.K., et al: Fractional distribution of right ventricular output in the lungs of dogs. Circ. Res. *10*:763–766, 1962.
21. Heymann, M.A., Payne, B.D., Hoffman, J.I.E., Rudolph, A.M.: Blood flow measurements with radionuclide-labeled particles. Prog. Cardiovasc. Dis. *20*:55–79, 1977.
22. Hoffbrand, B.I., Forsyth, R.P.: Validity studies of the radioactive microsphere method for the study of the distribution of cardiac output, organ blood flow, and resistance in the conscious rhesus monkey. Cardiovasc. Res. *3*:426–432, 1969.
23. Rudolph, A.M., Heymann, M.A.: The circulation of the fetus in utero. Circ. Res. *21*:163–184, 1967.
24. McGrory, B.J., Moran, C.G., Bronk, J., Weaver, A.L., Wood, M.B.: Canine bone blood flow measurements using serial microsphere injections. Clin. Orthop. *303*: 264–279, 1994.
25. Buckberg, G.D., Luck, J.C., Payne, D.B., Hoffman, J.I.E., Archie, J.P., Fixler, D.E.: Some sources of error in measuring regional blood flow with radioactive microspheres. J. Appl. Physiol. *31*:598–608, 1971.
26. Gross, P.M., Heistad, D.D., Marcus, M.L.: Neurohumoral regulation of blood flow to bones and marrow. Am. J. Physiol. *237*:H440–H448, 1979.
27. Jones, L.C., Niv, A.I., Davis, R.F., Hungerford, D.S.: Bone blood flow in the femora of anesthetized and conscious dogs in a chronic preparation, using the radioactive tracer microsphere method. Clin. Orthop. *170*:286–295, 1982.
28. Tothill, P., Hooper, G., McCarthy, I.D., Hughes, S.P.F.: The pattern of distribution of blood flow in dog limb bones measured using microspheres. Clin. Phys. Physiol. Meas. *8*:239–247, 1987.
29. Gross, P.M., Marcus, M.L., Heistad, D.D.: Measurement of blood flow to bone and marrow in experimental animals by means of the microsphere technique. J. Bone Joint Surg. *63A*:1028–1031, 1981.
30. Kaihara, S., Van Heerden, P.D., Migita, T., Wagner, H.N.: Measurement of distribution of cardiac output. J. Appl. Phys. *25*:696–700, 1968.
31. Li, G., Bronk, J.T., Kelly, P.J.: Canine bone blood flow estimated with microspheres. J. Orthop. Res. *7*:61–76, 1989.
32. Neutze, J.M., Wyler, F., Rudolph, A.M.: Use of radioactive microspheres to assess distribution of cardiac output in rabbits. Am. J. Physiol. *215*:486–495, 1968.
33. Pinto, M.R., Gorski, J.P., Penniston, J.T., Kelly, P.J.: Age-related changes in composition and Ca^{2+}- binding capacity of canine cortical bone extracts. Am. J. Physiol. *255*:H101–H110, 1988.
34. Davis, T.R.C., Holloway, I., Pooley, J.: The effect of anaesthesia on the bone blood flow of the rabbit. J. Orthop. Res. *8*:479–484, 1990.
35. Lausten, G.S., Kiaer, T., Dahl, B.: Laser Doppler flowmetry for estimation of bone blood flow: Studies of reproducibility and correlation with microsphere technique. J. Orthop. Res. *11*:573–580, 1993.
36. Nötzli, H.P., Swiontkowski, M.F., Thaxter, S.T., Carpenter, G.K., Wyatt, R.: Laser doppler flowmetry for bone blood flow measurements: Helium-neon laser light attenuation and depth of perfusion assessment. J. Orthop. Res. *7*:413–424, 1989.
37. Hellem, S., Jacobsson, L.S. Nilsson, G.E., Lewis, D.H.: Measurement of microvascular blood flow in cancellous bone using laser Doppler flowmetry and ^{133}Xe-clearance. Int. J. Oral Surg. *12*:165–177, 1983.
38. Schemitsch, E.H., Kowalski, M., Swiontkowski, M.F., Senft, D.: Effects of reamed versus unreamed locked intramedullary nailing on bone blood flow in a fractured sheep tibia model. Orthop. Trans. *17*:1042, 1993–1994.
39. Schuurman, A.H., Bos, K.E.: Laser Doppler bone probe: An experimental study in dogs. Microsurgery *12*: 246–251, 1991.
40. Sanders, R.W., Swiontkowski, M.F., Schlehr, F.: The evaluation of non-union using LDF. Orthop. Trans. *11*: 464–465, 1987.
41. Schlehr, F., Limbird, T., Swiontkowski, M.F., Keller, T.: The use of laser Doppler flowmetry in evaluating anterior cruciate blood flow. J. Orthop. Res. 5:150–153, 1987.
42. Swiontkowski, M.F., Tepic, S., Ganz, R., Perren, S.M.: Laser Doppler flowmetry for measurement of femoral heal blood flow: Experimental investigation and clinical application. Helv. Chir. Acta. *53*:55–59, 1986.
43. Grundnes, O., Reikerås, O.: Blood flow and mechanical properties of healing bone. Femoral osteotomies studied in rats. Acta Orthop. Scand. *63*:487–491, 1992.
44. Smith, S.R., Bronk, J.T., Kelly, P.J.: Effect of fracture fixation on cortical bone blood flow. J. Orthop. Res. *8*: 471–478, 1991.
45. Paradis, G.R., Kelly, P.J.: Blood flow and mineral deposition in canine tibial fractures. J. Bone Joint Surg. *57A*: 220–226, 1975.
46. Hughes, S., Khan, R., Davies, R., Lavender, P.: The uptake by the canine tibia of the bone-scanning agent ^{99}mTc-MDP before and after an osteotomy. J. Bone Joint Surg. *60B*:579–582, 1978.
47. Kelly, P.J., An, K., Chao, E.Y.S., Rand, J.A.: Fracture healing: Biomechanical, fluid dynamic and electrical considerations. *In* Bone and Mineral Research. 3rd Ed. Edited by W. A. Peck. New York, Elsevier, 1985.
48. Hughes, S., Davies, R., Khan, R., Kelly, P.J.: Fluid space in bone. Clin Orthop. *134*:332–341, 1978.
49. Wallace, A.L., McLaughlin, B., Weiss, J.B., Hughes, S.P.F.: Increased endothelial cell stimulating angiogenesis factor in patients with tibial fractures. Injury. *22*: 375–376, 1991.
50. Zetter, B.R.: Angiogenesis. State of the art. Chest. *93*: 1595-1665, 1988.
51. Diaz-Flores, L., Gutierrez, R., Valladares, F., Varela, H., Perez, M.: Intense vascular sprouting from rat femoral vein induced by prostaglandins E1 and E2. Anatomic Record *238*:68–76, 1994.
52. Eppley, B.L., Doucet, M., Connolly, D.T., Feder, J.: Enhancement of angiogenesis by bFGF in mandibular bone graft healing in the rabbit. J. Oral Maxillofac. Surg. *46*:391–398, 1988.
53. Fett, J.W., Olson, K.A., Rybak, S.M.: A monoclonal antibody to human angiogenin. Inhibition of ribonucleolytic and angiogenic activities and localization of the antigenic epitope. Biochemistry *33*:5421–5427, 1994.
54. Gajdusek, C.M., Luo, Z., Mayberg, M.R.: Basic fibroblast growth factor and transforming growth factor beta-1 synergistic mediators of angiogenesis in vitro. J. Cell. Physiol. *157*:133–144, 1993.
55. Kibbey, M.C., Corcoran, M.L., Wahl, L.M., Kleinman, H.K.: Laminin SIKVAV peptide-reduced angiogenesis in vivo is potentiated by neutrophils. J. Cell. Physiol. *160*:185–193, 1994.
56. Phillips, G.D., Whitehead, R.A., Knighton, D.R.: Inhibition by methylprednisolone acetate suggests an indirect mechanism for TGF-B induced angiogenesis. Growth Factors *6*:77–84, 1992.
57. Strachan, R.K., McCarthy, I., Fleming, R., Hughes, S.P.F.: The role of the tibial nutrient artery. Microsphere estimation of blood flow in the osteotomised canine tibia. J. Bone Joint Surg. *72B*:391–394, 1990.
58. Wallace, A.L., Draper, E.R.C., Strachan, R.K., Mc-

Carthy, I.D., Hughes, S.P.F.: The effect of devascularization upon early bone healing in dynamic external fixation. J. Bone Joint Surg. *73B*:819–825, 1991.
59. Whiteside, L.A., Lesker, P.A.: The effects of extraperiosteal and subperiosteal dissection on fracture healing. J. Bone Joint Surg. *60A*:26–30, 1978.
60. Goitz, R.J., Goitz, H.T., Armstrong, L.J., Tisdale, N.A., Wang, G.J., Jane, J.A.: Severe head injury and fracture healing—a quantitative assessment. Orthop. Trans. *15*: 639,1991.
61. Oni, O.O.A., Stafford, H., Gregg, P.J.: A study of diaphyseal fracture repair using tissue isolation techniques. Injury. *23*:467–470, 1992.
62. Rhinelander, F.W.: Tibial blood supply in relation to fracture healing. Clin. Orthop. *105*:34–81, 1974.
63. Oestern, H.J., Tscherne, H.: Pathophysiology and classification of soft tissue injuries associated with fractures. *In* Fractures with Soft Tissue Injuries. Edited by H. Tscherne and L. Gotzen. New York, Springer, 1984, 10-32.
64. Gristina, A.G., Costerton, J.W.: Bacterial adherence to biomaterials and tissue: The significance of its role in clinical sepsis. J. Bone Joint Surg. *67A*:264–273, 1985.
65. Gristina, A.G., Naylor, P.T., Myrvik, Q.N.: Musculoskeletal infection, microbial adhesion, and antibiotic resistance. Infect Dis. Clin. North. Am. *4*:391–408, 1990.
66. Cole, J.D., Latta, L.L.: Fatigue failure of interlocking tibial nail implants. Orthop. Trans. *16*:663, 1992.
67. Court-Brown, C.M., Keating, J.F., McQueen, M.M.: Infection after intramedullary nailing of the tibia. Incidence and protocol for management. J. Bone Joint Surg. *74B*:770–774, 1992.
68. Pape, H., Regel, G., Dwenger, A., Krumm, K., Schweitzer, G., Krettek, C., Sturn, J.A., Tscherne, H.: Influences of different methods of intramedullary femoral nailing on lung function in patients with multiple trauma. J. Trauma *35*:709–716, 1993.
69. Pell, A.C.H., Christie, J., Keating, J.F., Sutherland, G.R.: The detection of fat embolism by transoesophageal echocardiography during reamed intramedullary nailing. A study of 24 patients with femoral and tibial fractures. J. Bone Joint Surg. *75B*:921–925, 1993.
70. Rokkanen, P., Slätis, P., Vankka, E.: Closed or open intramedullary nailing of femoral shaft fractures: A comparison with conservatively treated cases. J. Bone Joint Surg. *51B*:313, 1969.
71. Müller, C., Rahn, B.A., Pfister, U., Weller, S.: Extent of bluntness and damage to reamers from hospitals. Injury *24*:S31–S35, 1994.
72. Müller, C., McIff, T., Rahn, B.A., Pfister, U., Weller, S.: Intramedullary pressure, strain on the diaphysis and increase in cortical temperature when reaming the femoral medullary cavity-a comparison of blunt and sharp reamers. Injury *24*:S22–S30, 1994.
73. Peter, R.E, Selz, T., Koestli, A.: Influence of the reamer shape on intraosseus pressure during closed intramedullary nailing of the unbroken femur: A preliminary report. Injury *24*:S48–S55, 1994.
74. Bone, L.B., Johnson, K.D., Weigelt, J., Scheinberg, R.: Early versus delayed stabilization of femoral fractures. A prospective randomized study. J. Bone Joint Surg. *71A*:336–340, 1989.
75. Border, J., LaDuca, J., Seibel, R.: Priorities in the management of the patient with polytrauma. Prog. Surg. *14*: 84–120, 1975.
76. Goris, R., Gimbrere, J., Van Neikerk, J., et al.: Early osteosynthesis and prophylactic mechanical ventilation in the multitrauma patient. J. Trauma *22*:895–903, 1982.
77. Johnson, K.D., Cadambi, A., Seibert, G.B.: Incidence of adult respiratory distress syndrome in patients with multiple musculoskeletal injuries: Effect of early operative stabilization of fractures. J. Trauma *25*:375–385, 1985.
78. LaDuca, J., Bone, L., Seibel, R., et al.: Primary open reduction and internal fixation of open fractures. J. Trauma *20*:580–586, 1980.
79. Riska, E.B., von Bonsdorff, H., Hakkinen, S., Jaroma, H., Kiviluoto, O., Paavilainen, T.: Prevention of fat embolism by early internal fixation of fractures in patients with multiple injuries. Injury. *8*:110–116, 1976.
80. Richards, R.R., Schemitsch, E.H.: Effect of muscle flap coverage on bone blood flow following devascularization of a segment of tibia. An experimental investigation in the dog. J. Orthop. Res. *7*:550–557, 1989.
81. Rand, J.A., An, K.N., Chao, E.Y.S., Kelly, P.J.: A comparison of the effect of open intramedullary nailing and compression-plate fixation on fracture-site blood flow and fracture union. J. Bone Joint Surg. *63A*:427–442, 1981.
82. Smith, S.R., Bronk, J.T., Kelly, P.J.: Effect of fracture fixation on cortical bone blood flow. J. Orthop. Res. *4*: 471–478, 1990

4

The Effects of Intramedullary Reaming

Sven Olerud

Intramedullary reaming naturally causes total destruction of the contents of the marrow cavity. Empirically, this medullary trauma does not seem to have any major adverse effects. However, if we look at the process more closely, several pathophysiologic aspects of interest emerge. Such close observation might produce a better and safer way of performing nailing procedures. Because medullary trauma, for obvious reasons, must be extensive in total joint replacement, it must have implications in both hip and knee procedures as long as the medullary cavity is involved.

The medullary cavity contains blood vessels and marrow. The function of this tissue will cease after total medullary destruction. Concerning its role as a blood-generating organ, marrow reserves in other bones are so great that the damage to one medullary cavity has no significant overall impact on the human body.

Direct injury to the medullary canal will affect the circulation of the cortical bone in the immediate vicinity and will cause more or less complete avascularity of the inner layer of this cortical bone. This side effect, which was extensively discussed by Rhinelander in 1982,[1] will not be dealt with here.

Reaming also disrupts all vascular connections where vessels penetrate cortical bone. After disruption, there must be wide openings into the vascular bed. Closure of these open vessels only occurs when the blood has coagulated in the canals of the cortical bone. Before this happens, it is quite possible that there will be free communication and interchange between the medullary cavity, on the one hand, and the vascular bed and the general circulation, on the other.

During a reaming procedure, there are several factors that have to be considered. The two main factors are the pressure within the medullary cavity (and its variation) and the damaged medullary tissue, consisting of blood components, crushed cells, and free fat.

Consideration of these two factors combined gives reason to ask the question: Will these debris products enter the general circulation during phases of elevated intramedullary pressure? Such an event seems highly possible. Two more questions may then be asked:

1. If such intravasation does occur, to what extent does it take place and what significance does it have?
2. Will it only have a local effect on the cortical bone, or will it have a distant, more general effect on the body, or both?

INTRAMEDULLARY PRESSURE

The medullary cavity has stiff inflexible walls, and when a reamer is pushed down into it, it will function like a piston. If the reaming is not performed gently, pressure will increase and will continue to do so as the reamer speed is increased. This pressure has been calculated during reaming in rabbit experiments,[2] and pressure figures as high as 300 mm Hg have been recorded. The intramedullary pressure has also been estimated in human beings during the process of inserting the femoral component during total hip replacement.[3] Pressure increases of more than 1000 mm Hg easily occur in such cases. The use of a vent, in the form of a distal hole leading into the medullary cavity, has been found to reduce this pressure in both animals and in humans.

MEDULLARY CONTENT

The increased pressure and the mechanical abrasion of the reamers will destroy the medullary contents, reducing them to liquefied cellular debris, proteins, and enzymes. After the first reaming, air will also be present in the cavity.

The ease and readiness with which these marrow elements are able to enter and to pass through the cortical bone can be proved experimentally in two ways:

1. By observing a rabbit's tibia with intact periosteum during reaming. As soon as some pressure is generated within the medullary cavity, the periosteum will become separated from the bone by a subperiosteal hematoma.[4]
2. By watching the blood drain from the leg in rabbits during reaming. This has been done by visually examining the bloodstream passing through a transparent plastic catheter placed in the femoral vein. Just after reaming, conglomerates of medullary components and air passed through.[4]

These experiments have demonstrated that there can be two important adverse effects of reaming the medullary cavity, namely, a local effect on the cortical bone, where some medullary contents will be trapped, and a generalized effect, with entry of medullary contents into the general circulation. Once in the general circulation, marrow elements may become trapped in the filter-like vascular bed of the lung.

EFFECTS ON CORTICAL BONE AFTER REAMING

Following reaming of the medullary cavity in rabbits and dogs without reduction of the intramedullary pressure with a distal vent, Danckwardt-Lilliestrom (1969) searched the cortex for fat. In many areas, he found all cortical canals filled with fat droplets. A considerable amount of fat had also accumulated subperiosteally (Fig. 4–1). To test the hypothesis that fat will be resorbed much more slowly than thrombi, the revascularization time of the cortical bone was calculated in the rabbit tibia. Rabbits in which reaming had been performed with a distal vent (i.e., those in which there was probably no entrapment of medullary material in the cortical bone) were compared with rabbits that had undergone reaming without any precautions (Fig. 4–2).[5] It was found that the cortical circulation was restored about 4 weeks earlier in the vented tibiae than in the nonvented tibiae (Fig. 4–3). In two such groups of rabbits, the healing was smooth and uneventful, in contrast to the nonvented group, where pseudarthrosis was common (Fig. 4–4). In the latter group, sequestra were frequently formed from the inner side of the cortex (Fig. 4–5). This was never seen in the vented group.

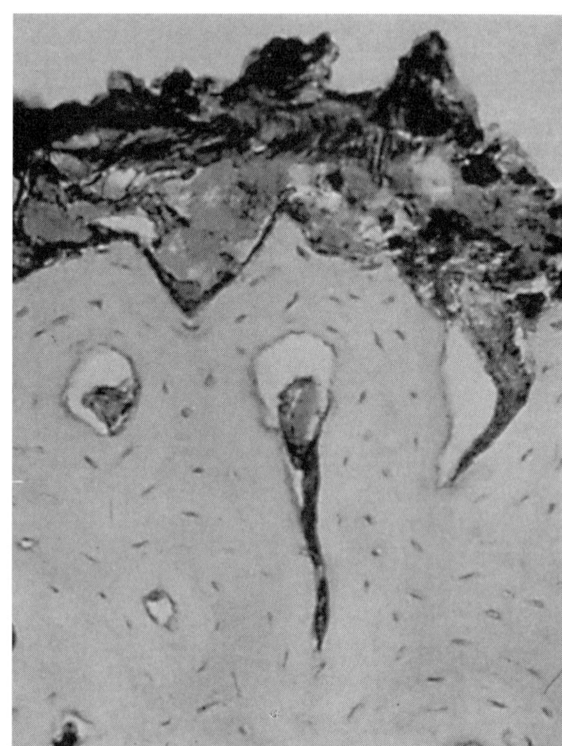

Fig. 4–1. Transverse section of cortical bone including the corresponding periosteum. Fat material is seen both in the haversian vascular systems and subperiosteally.

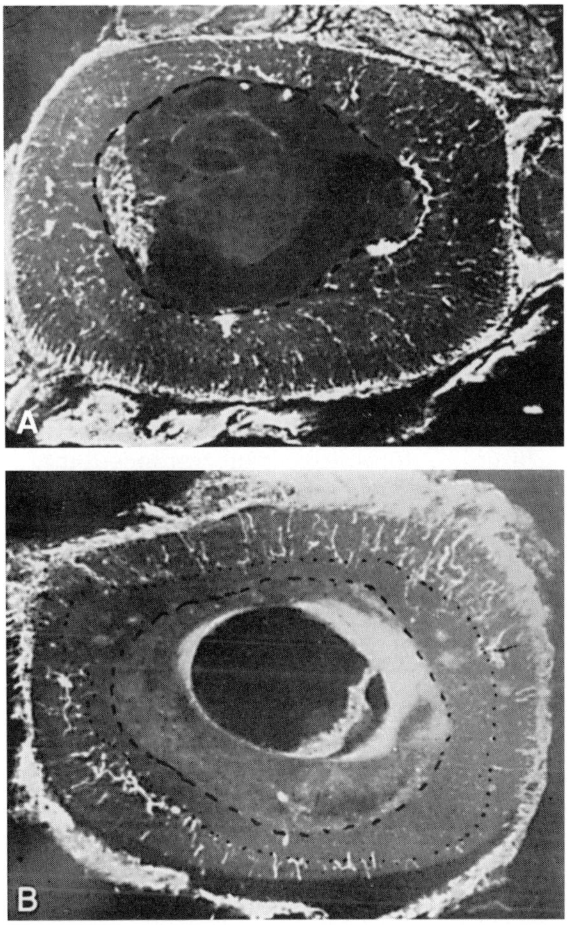

Fig. 4–2. Microangiography of 100-μm-thick preparations of a transverse section of the distal third of a rabbit tibia that had undergone intramedullary reaming 2 weeks before sacrifice. *A,* After reaming of the cavity with use of a pressure-releasing distal vent, there is only a small avascular area. *B,* Here no venting procedure was used and there is a large area of avascularity located between the dotted lines.

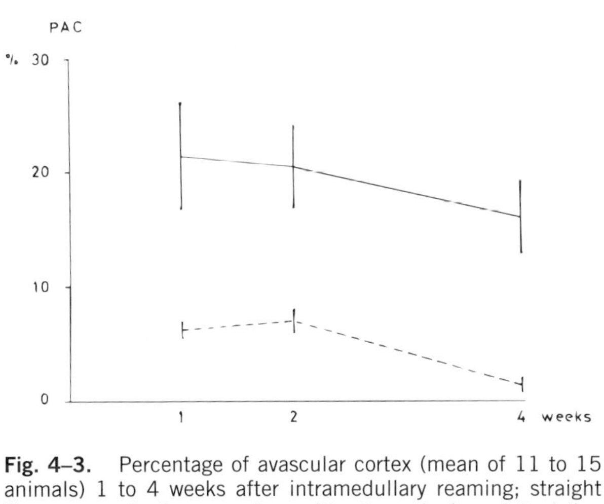

Fig. 4–3. Percentage of avascular cortex (mean of 11 to 15 animals) 1 to 4 weeks after intramedullary reaming; straight line represents the procedure without suctioning; dotted line represents simultaneous suction of the medullary cavity. The bars indicate standard errors of the mean.

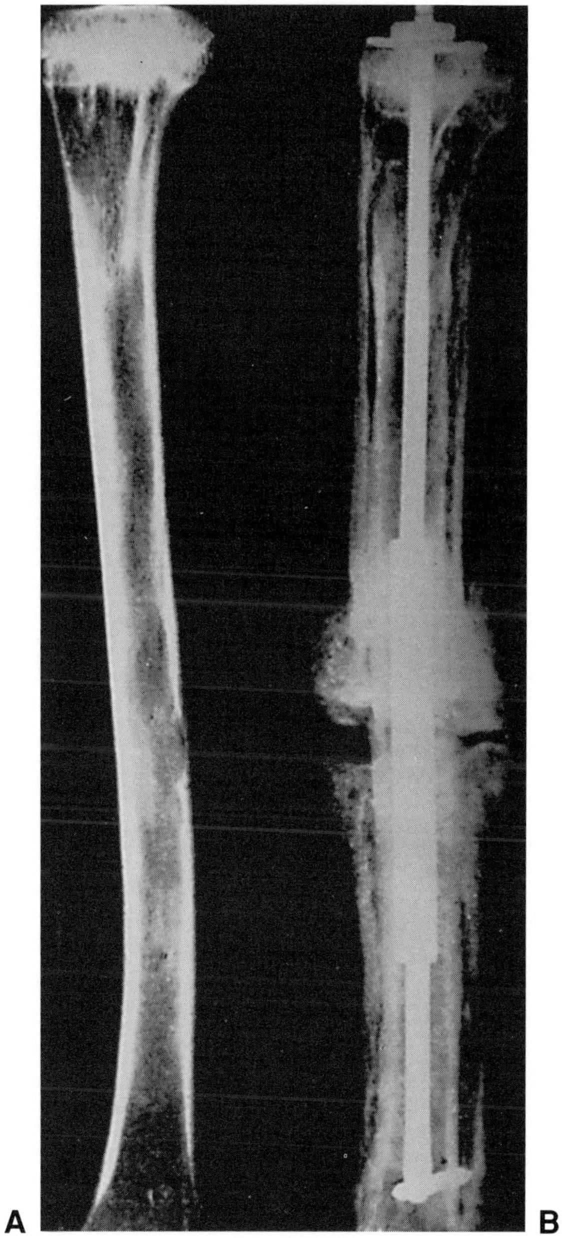

Fig. 4–4. Healing of osteotomies of rabbit tibiae. *A,* Eight weeks after surgery (the compression nail extracted) in a rabbit in which suction was performed during the reaming procedure. *B,* The same experiment as shown in "A." The compression nail fixing the osteotomy is still in place. Rich periosteal callus formation has developed, but there is no union of the cortical bone because of avascularity after reaming.

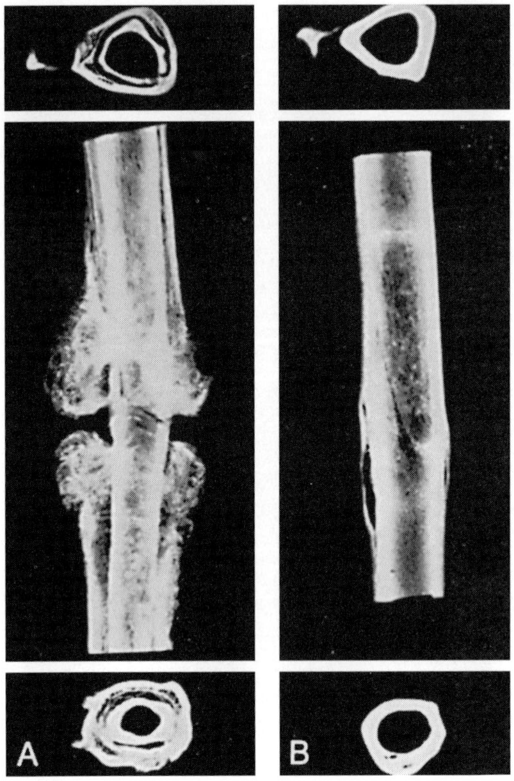

Fig. 4–5. *A,* A rabbit tibia 12 weeks after reaming of the medullary cavity without a distal venting hole. The osteotomy was fixed by a compression nail as in Figure 4–4. There was no cortical bone healing. A pseudoarthrosis (elephant foot) developed. The inner cortical layer, which probably became avascular during the reaming, is found as sequestra throughout the entire medullary cavity. *B,* Corresponding rabbit tibia after reaming with simultaneous suction. The same nailing fixing device was used as in Figure 4–4B. Good, almost invisible healing of the osteotomy is seen. No sequestra have formed inside the cavity.

INDIRECT EFFECTS OF REAMING

As already mentioned, medullary debris is easily forced into the general circulation. In the first part of a series of experiments on rabbits with tibial nailing after intramedullary reaming, in which the reaming was not performed with a distal vent hole,[4] the mortality rate was 25%. However, in the second part of the series, such a vent hole was used, there was no mortality at all. The deaths might have been caused either by the emboli when these were trapped in the lungs or by a reaction from enzymes. Suspicion of the latter possibility was aroused when we were studying the amount of fat that could be collected from the blood during reaming of a femoral fracture in humans. The femoral vein was cannulated in a patient and blood samples were taken prior to and during the last moments of every reaming procedure. After 5 reamings, we had 10 test tubes filled with 20 mL of blood. We then noted that the blood in every second test tube was coagulated (i.e., in those samples that were taken just after reaming). It was concluded that the medullary debris must be rich in thromboplastin products.[6] This might have explained the high mortality rate in the rabbit series of experiments with reaming without a distal vent hole.

Based on the hypothesis that medullary debris might cause such a high thromboplastin effect, an investigation was started in patients undergoing total hip joint replacement. In many respects, the medullary trauma was similar to the reaming procedures in the femoral fractures. In these cases, high intramedullary pressures were generated.[3]

In this experimental series, the pulmonary artery was catheterized in order to obtain prepulmonary blood samples. The thromboplastin level was evaluated as the recalcification time of the blood. The amount of fat globules in the blood was also assessed, along with various marrow cell types on blood smear glasses. The samples were collected during five different steps of the hip operation[6] in 13 patients (see Table 4–1). During the cementing of the femoral component without a venting catheter (Charnley's original procedure), which was period four of the procedure (i.e., the occasion when the intramedullary pressure was at its maximum), the recalcification time of the blood was very fast. The reason for this was that a large amount of thromboplastin-active enzymes had entered the bloodstream, which would also cause hypercoagulability. The arterial oxygen tension in the blood, which was monitored throughout the operation, was also very low during period four, the phase cementing the femur (Fig. 4–6). When a vent was used during this femoral cementing phase, with a pressure-releasing catheter placed at the bottom of the intended bed for the femoral component, there was a statistically significant better oxygen uptake by the blood. This finding proved that with the use of a vent to prevent high intramedullary pressure less medullary debris was pressed out, and consequently, a smaller amount of thromboplastin enzymes.

From smears of blood from the pulmonary artery, even medullary cells, including mitotic cells, were found. This was considered to be

Table 4–1. Measurement of coagulability (recalcification time) during various phases of total hip replacement

Number of Patients *13*	*Reaming the Acetabulum* *I*	*Cementing the Acetabulum* *II*	*Reaming the Femur* *III*	*Cementing the Femur* *IV*	*Following Reduction and Test of Hip Motion* *V*
Mean	147	135	138	123.3	139.8
Standard Deviation	13.9	21.1	19.3	23.6	23.1
Difference in Mean to that of Period I		−12.0	−9.5	−23.3	−7
Difference in Mean to that of Previous Period		12.6	2.5	15.7	16.5

definite proof that medullary contents had been forced out of the medullary cavity into the general circulation during reaming. However, there was no correlation between the amount of fat found in pulmonary arterial blood and the thromboplastin effect.[7] This investigation also demonstrated a close relationship between the hypercoagulability (i.e., the decreased recalcification time of the blood) and a fall in blood pressure during the phase of cementing of the femur. Sudden deaths described after cementing of the femoral component in total hip replacements may be explained better by the rapid effect of thromboplastin products, generating the pulmonary microembolism syndrome with ensuing pulmonary and circulatory dysfunction.[8] A pulmonary microembolism syndrome has been shown to occur in connection with impaction of the femoral prosthesis.[6] Both clinical[7] and experimental studies[9] provide firm evidence against methylmethacrylate monomer as the cause of these reactions.

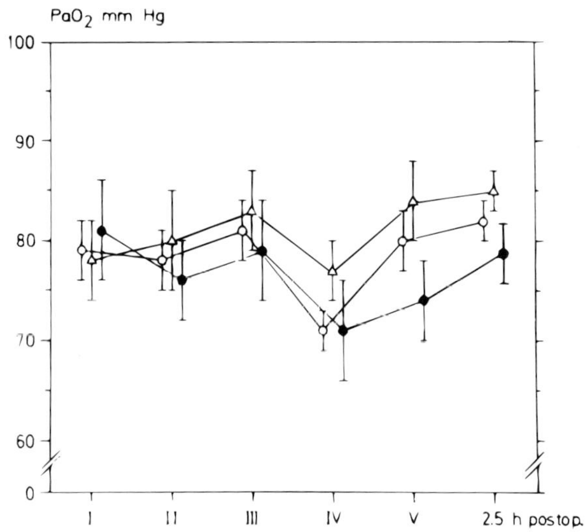

Fig. 4–6. Serial arterial oxygen tension (PaO_2) measurements made during total hip replacement show a statistically significant decrease in PaO_2 during femoral component cementing (IV) in two cases (● and ○) without venting as compared to the third case (△) with venting.

The high mortality rate in the earlier described series where the rabbit tibiae were reamed without a venting hole may also be explained by this sequence of events. The physiologic explanation for cause of death seems to be caused by an increased pulmonary vascular resistance leading to a decreased left ventricular output simultaneously with a systemic vasodilation, both giving rise to a profound decrease in coronary blood flow. To this should be added the increased pulmonary venous admixture (i.e., increased intrapulmonary shunting of blood) leading to a decrease in arterial oxygenation. All these events taken together give rise to a severe myocardial ischemia and cardiac failure.[10]

In most fracture cases where the femur is reamed, the described events may occur, although probably only with minor and not especially obvious effects. On the other hand, in fresh multitrauma cases in which shock and hypercoagulability may be present, intramedullary reaming may be dangerous if the surgeon is not fully aware of the possible adverse effects of medullary trauma. Before such reaming is undertaken, the patient must be in good hemodynamic balance, as otherwise the negative effects of the reaming procedure will add to the already poor microcirculation and jeopardize the outcome.

CONCLUSIONS

1. Medullary trauma on reaming of the marrow cavity may generate high intramedullary pressure. A distal venting hole diminishes this occurrence.
2. High intramedullary pressure causes medullary components to be forced into the cortical bone and to enter the general circulation.
3. Medullary components, including fat, will be entrapped in the cortical wall. There is experimental evidence that revascularization of the cortical bone under such circumstances is slow and also that normal bone healing is disturbed.
4. With a high intramedullary pressure, medullary components will enter the bloodstream, causing the pulmonary microembolism syndrome with ensuing low arterial oxygenation and circulatory dysfunction. It may therefore be advisable to vent the medullary space in the distal fragment during reaming unless a cannulated reaming system is employed that provides adequate decompression of the intramedullary canal.

REFERENCES

1. Rhinelander, F.W., Wilson, J.W.: Blood supply to developing, mature, and healing bone. *In* Bone in Clinical Orthopaedics. A Study in Comparative Osteology. Edited by G. Sumner-Smith. Philadelphia, W.B. Saunders Co., 1982.
2. Danckwardt-Lilliestrom, G.: Reaming of the medullary cavity and its effect on diaphyseal bone. A fluorochromic, microangiographic and histologic study on the rabbit tibia and dog femur. Acta Orthop. Scand. Suppl. *128,* 1969.
3. Hallin, G., Modig, J., Nordgren, L., Olerud, S.: The intramedullary pressure during the bone marrow trauma of total hip replacement surgery. Ups. J. Med. Sci. *79*: 51–54, 1974.
4. Danckwardt-Lilliestrom, G., Lorenzi, G.L., Olerud, S.: Intramedullary nailing after reaming. An investigation on the healing process in osteotomized rabbit tibias. Acta Orthop. Scand. Suppl. *134,* 1970a.
5. Danckwardt-Lilliestrom, G., Lorenzi, G.L., Olerud, S.: Intracortical circulation after intramedullary reaming with reduction of pressure in the medullary cavity. A microangiographic study on the rabbit tibia. J. Bone Joint Surg. *52A*:1390–1394, 1970b.
6. Modig, J., Busch, C., Olerud, S., Saldeen, T.: Pulmonary microembolism during intramedullary orthopaedic trauma. Acta Anesthesiol. Scand. *18*:133–143, 1974.
7. Modig, J., Busch, C., Olerud, S., Saldeen, T., Waernbaum, G.: Arterial hypotension and hypoxemia during total hip replacement: The importance of thromboplastic products, fat embolism and acrylic monomers. Acta Anaesthesiol. Scand. *19*:28–43, 1975a.
8. Modig, J., Olerud, S., Maimberg, P.: Sudden pulmonary dysfunction in prosthetic hip replacement surgery. A case report. Acta Anaesthesiol. Scand. *17*:276–282, 1973.
9. Modig, J., Busch, C., Waernbaum, G.: Effects of graded infusions of monomethylmethacrylate on coagulation, blood lipids, respiration, and circulation. Clin. Orthop. *113*:187–197, 1975b.
10. Modig, J., Malmberg, P.: Pulmonary and circulatory reactions during total hip replacement. Acta Anaesthesiol. Scand. *19*:219–237, 1975.

5

Pulmonary Complications After Intramedullary Stabilization of the Femur

Hans Christophe Pape, Gerd Regel, and Harald Tscherne

Intraoperative side effects in patients with femur fractures treated by intramedullary reaming and nailing were described in detail by Küntscher. He assumed, that intraoperative cardiovascular complications could be attributed to liberation of bone marrow contents and therefore advised to stop the reaming procedure if arrhythmias appeared on the electrocardiogram tracing or if hypotension occurred.[1] In the following years, flexible drills were developed. Along with further technical improvements of drills and reaming systems and along with improved intraoperative management of ventilation by anesthesiologists, bone marrow embolism was no longer considered a risk for the patient, if suffering an isolated injury.

Within the last decade, reports of intraoperative cardiovascular complications attributed to embolization of bone marrow contents and/or bone cement, were made in patients undergoing total hip replacement. Intraoperative sudden hypotension, cardiac arrhythmias, signs of pulmonary embolism, and subsequent right heart failure were reported, sometimes representing a fatal complication.[2–5] Three main factors were thought to be responsible for these intraoperative events:

1. Monomer products of bone cement (methylmethacrylate) are likely to cause vasodilatation in the systemic circulation ([6]I).
2. A direct toxic effect of methylmethacrylate is said to occur and be responsible for cardiopulmonary disturbances.[2,7]
3. Mechanical occlusion of the pulmonary arterial system has also been discussed in association with deteriorations of lung function.[7]
4. In addition, it was shown that obviously reflectory changes within the pulmonary circulation play a role in acute intraoperative complications.[8]

It must be stressed that in the case of femoral fractures, complications from reaming of the medullary canal do represent an exception. In our department, within the last decade we have had one case of acute lethal complication in a young and otherwise healthy patient. Reaming of the medullary canal for improvement of vascularization in posttraumatic pseudarthrosis of the femur intraoperatively caused the clinical syndrome of pulmonary arterial obstruction, impaired oxygenation, and cardiac failure refractory to vigorous resuscitation. Postmortem histologic examination revealed extensive embolization of bone marrow fat as well as osseous material obstructing even large size vessels (Fig. 5–1). In this specific case, a combination of an unusually narrow medullary canal and medullary contents prone to loosening (spongious bone) must be assumed. Similar reports from other centers do exist.[7,9]

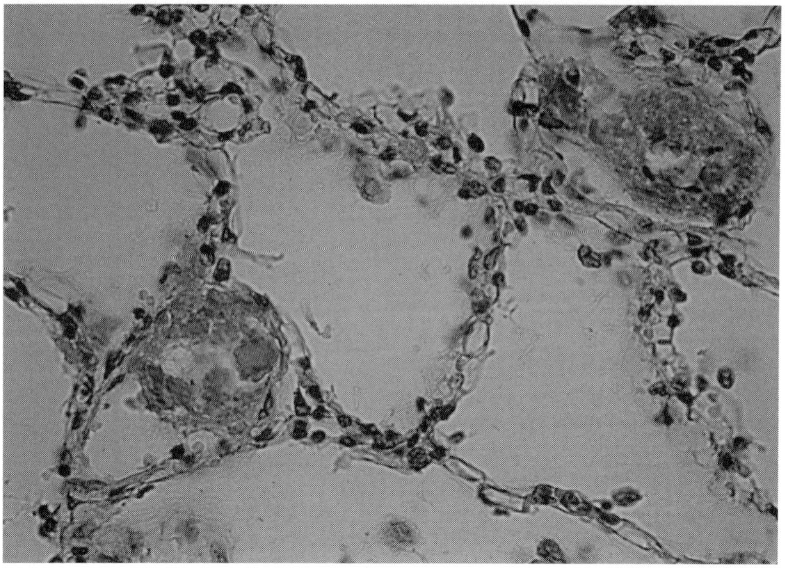

Fig. 5–1. Staining of a lung section in a patient who died of intraoperative cardiovascular failure after reaming of the closed medullary canal. Extensive embolization is present with blocking of a majority of pulmonary vessels. Findings found throughout several lung sections explain the development of right heart failure despite the absence of previous cardiopulmonary disease.

These reports clarify that a potential risk appears to be present in surgical methods involving opening of the medullary canal. However, in the case of isolated femoral fractures the lung usually appears to be able to cope with the potentially damaging effect.

INTRAOPERATIVE VERSUS POSTOPERATIVE COMPLICATIONS: DIFFERENCES IN PATHOGENESIS?

The sequelae of acute intraoperative changes, as described in patients undergoing alloarthoplasty, has to be attributed to cardiac failure rather than pulmonary failure (arrhythmia being a sign of right ventricular overload). Hip surgery patients represent a specially sensitive group because they are of old age and thus are prone to develop cardiovascular failure. Likewise, the introduction of sealing maneuvers of the medullary canal has almost abolished the risk of intraoperative cardiovascular failure in these patients.

In patients with multiple trauma, the acute intraoperative changes as described above have also been found.[10] However, no comparable sequelae have been described in the literature. Instead, an unusually high number of patients developed pulmonary deterioration and progressive ARDS. The relationship between ARDS development and stabilization of the femur was not readily found. Only in single reports a possible relationship between intramedullary nailing and the development of pulmonary failure days after surgery was described. Recently, in a retrospective analysis of a large group of multiple-trauma patients the conditions of pulmonary failure were investigated. Two factors were found to be responsible for the increased risk of ARDS: (1) the timing of intramedullary stabilization and (2) the presence of additional lung contusion.

Patients with thoracic trauma, if submitted to intramedullary nailing within 24 hrs posttrauma, developed ARDS more frequently than those operated secondarily.[11] There was no further cause of ARDS in these patients and the degree of pulmonary injury (lung contusion) present at the time of surgery was comparable in both patient groups. In contrast, those patients without thoracic trauma had a low incidence of ARDS regardless of the time of surgery (Fig. 5–2).

If no lung injury was present, intramedullary nailing was associated with shorter ventilation time and a lower risk of infectious complications (Fig. 5–3). This finding corresponds to the current principles of fracture stabilization in multiple trauma. Early stabilization is regarded

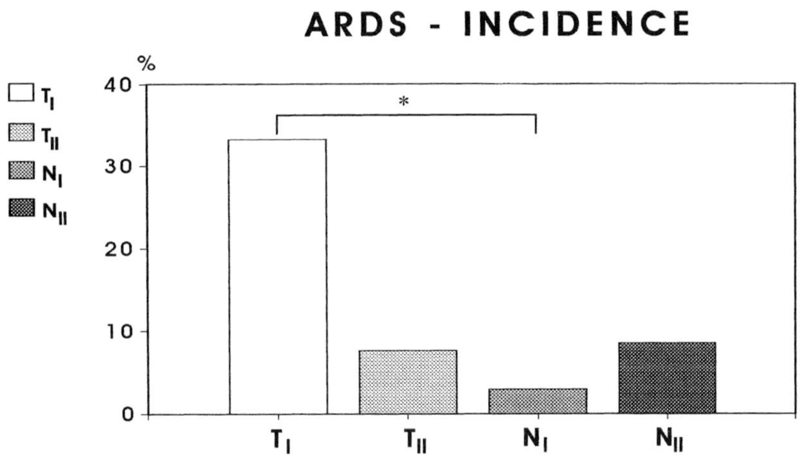

Fig. 5–2. ARDS incidence in severely traumatized patients undergoing intramedullary nailing. T represents the groups with thoracic trauma; N represents the group without thoracic trauma and I = primary (<24 hrs) and II = secondary (>24hrs) stabilization. Primary intramedullary nailing in the presence of lung contusion is associated with increased incidence of ARDS.

as an important principle.[12–15] A disadvantage of primary intramedullary nailing of the femur therefore is an unexpected phenomenon implying the necessity of further investigation.

Prior to discussing the pathogenetic factors leading to ARDS in polytrauma associated with intramedullary nailing, it appears important to differentiate definitions of *intraoperative* versus *postoperative* complications. These differences are summarized in Table 5–1.

The pathogenesis of acute intraoperative complications in alloarthroplasty patients is made obvious by mechanisms discussed previously and by the specific vulnerability of this group of patients. However, the relationship between ARDS and intramedullary nailing cannot be readily explained by the same mechanisms. Generally, the development of complications apparently requires the presence of additional susceptibility. In patients with a single type in-

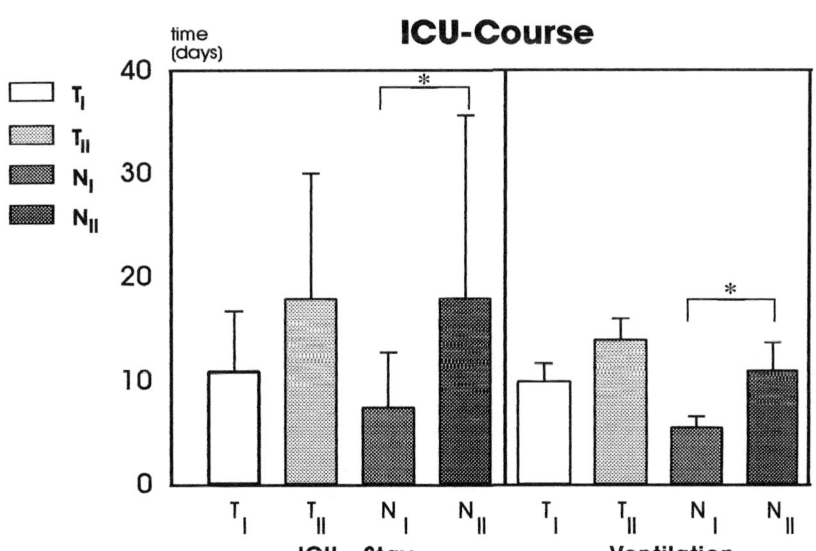

Fig. 5–3. Duration of intensive care therapy in severely traumatized patients undergoing intramedullary nailing. T represents the groups with thoracic trauma; N represents the group without thoracic trauma and I = primary (<24 hrs) and II = secondary (>24hrs) stabilization. In patients without thoracic trauma secondary stabilization is associated with increased ICU stay and should be avoided.

Table 5–1. Intraoperative vs. postoperative complications

	Acute Changes	*Subacute Changes*
Time pattern	Intraoperative, (minutes)	Postoperative, (days)
Pathophysiology	Right heart failure	Lung failure (ARDS)
Population	Prone to cardiac complications (hip alloarthroplasty, old age)	Lung contusion (young, no disease)
Sequelae	If treatable, no sequelae	Long-term ICU-stay
	Low mortality	High mortality
Cause	Acute fat embolization	Fat embolization and further mechanisms

jury such as an isolated femoral fracture or undergoing hip surgery, the lung usually should be able to cope with a moderate degree of additional damage.

It therefore appears necessary to consider all mechanisms occuring during intramedullary nailing sequentially and to correlate these with the posttraumatic course. The following questions are of specific importance:

1. What kind of local changes occur during reaming and nailing of the femur with respect to fat embolization into the lung?
2. Is pulmonary dysfunction a result of pure mechanical occlusion of pulmonary vessels and microvessels, or are other factors involved?
3. What effect does additional lung contusion in the presence of multiple trauma have on the susceptibility of developing ARDS after intramedullary nailing?
4. Can timing of surgery influence the clinical course and is it able to play a role as a "priming factor" of pulmonary complications?

PATHOGENESIS OF ARDS AFTER INTRAMEDULLARY NAILING IN MULTIPLE-TRAUMA PATIENTS

Influence of Intramedullary Femoral Nailing

Intramedullary Pressure

An intramedullary pressure increase upon reaming of the medullary canal has been demonstrated both in experimental and clinical studies. Experimentally, pressure increases up to 300 mm Hg were seen.[16] In a sheep model using the tibia, Stürmer found pressure increases of up to 1000 mm Hg.[17] In patients with femur fractures, elevations of intramedullary pressure between 140 and 830 mm Hg were found.[18] Wehner described pressures of about 120 mm Hg in the medullary canal, rising from 30 to 40 mm Hg baseline values.[19]

The mechanisms occurring during reaming were discussed by Küntscher as "compression of bone marrow by the reamer in a piston like fashion."[1] Questions therefore arise concerning the fate of the intramedullary contents. It appears obvious that some kind of compression takes place. In a sheep model, a constant pressure of 300 mm Hg was applied to mimic this situation. Embolization of bone marrow contents into the pulmonary circulation was demonstrated. In the presence of an intact intramedullary canal, fat and bone marrow thus can be exprimed by increased intramedullary pressure.[20]

It might be assumed that the reaming procedure, as it destroys the subcortical bone, also destroys venous outflow. In several animal studies, a blockage of intracortical canal systems has been described with fat and osseous material.[16] A further possible site for medullary content to escape would be the area of the fracture, thus mingling with the fracture hematoma and already exuded fat, as has been shown by Harms et al.[21] If a complete blockage was the case, no more fat should enter the general circulation as soon as the bone distal of the fracture site is reamed.

However, in clinical investigations evidence of bone marrow embolism, as determined by pulmonary artery pressure increases, was present especially when reaming of the distal fragment was performed. During this time, elevations of pressure in the medullary canal were most pronounced. Similar pressure dynamics were described in experimental investigations. Stürmer found the highest pressure increases upon opening of the medullary canal as well as during reaming of the distal fragment. The insertion of the nail did not cause a further pressure increase.[16] In patients undergoing reamed intramedullary nailing, transesophageal echocardiography was applied intraoperatively. The investigators describe several bursts of material floating through the right atrium into the lung. Embolization occurred during the entire reaming procedure. Also, when higher diameter reamers were applied, there was still evidence of floating material.[19] It therefore appears proven that despite severe destruction of the medullary canal by the reaming procedure, still a significant outflow from the femoral canal occurs. The significance of the local specifics of venous blood flow thus appear to play an important role.

Femoral Venous Blood Drainage

Two main vascular systems are responsible for drainage of the femoral bone. One consists of periosteal capillaries and veins that drain into the surrounding soft tissues and further into large extremity veins (the centrifugal system). The other system, the centripetal system, is represented by sinusoids confluing into a large intramedullary sinus. This confluates into large emissary veins located diaphyseally, as well as proximally and distally. It is important to consider that under normal circumstances (i.e., no fracture) the centrifugal venous system is responsible for the majority of venous outflow from the femur.[22]

Experimental investigations in dog tibiae revealed complete destruction of the medullary venous system by reaming of the medullary canal. In contrast to what might be expected, the centrifugal direction of venous outflow remained intact. Microangiography 4 weeks following experimental intramedullary nailing showed numerous subperiosteal vessels draining into widely filled periosteal vessels; the centrifugal system thus appears to be able to cover all necessary drainage.[20]

In summary, the outflow of marrow material can conceivably derive from three different sites: (1) the fracture, (2) the remnants of emissary veins, and (3) the centrifugal venous system. It appears likely that upon reaming again the majority of material might be transported by the centrifugal system, as seen under normal circumstances.

Influence of Host Response to Intramedullary Nailing

Multiple Trauma—Predisposing for Pulmonary Failure (ARDS)

> Recent emphasis on the pulmonary complications of *nonthoracic trauma* has increased usage of the term "shock lung" and given the implication that the lung is a target organ in instances of shock.[23]

In recent years, extensive investigations have been undertaken to evaluate pathogenetic factors triggered by multiple trauma. Hypovolemic shock and associated hypoxemia causes extensive microvascular damage. In animal studies, an increase of pulmonary capillary permeability, which represents the hallmark of ARDS,[24] has been measured during hemorrhagic shock.[25] Clinically, patients with severe trauma who later developed ARDS were found to have increased microvascular permeability regardless of the distribution of injury. Microvascular damage has been said to be responsible for later development of ARDS and multiple organ failure. These late complications, ARDS and multiple organ failure, presently represent the main problems limiting survival in the severely traumatized.[26]

The microvascular endothelial damage triggers circulating neutrophils to regard autologous endothelial cells as antigens, leading to activation of the immune system. The neutrophil therefore becomes activated, adheres to the endothelium, and will initiate phagocytosis. Because this cannot be achieved, so-called "frustrane phagocytosis" occurs, in which proteolytic enzymes and oxygen radicals are liberated into the bloodstream and aggravate the degree of endothelial damage. Thus a vicious cycle begins, with the neutrophil playing a pivotal role in this setting. Increased amounts of proteases from neutrophils (e.g., Elastase), have been demonstrated in several clinical studies. Neutrophils isolated from multiple-trauma patients have been shown to be highly activated.[27] These mechanisms prime for a variety of further cascade mechanisms, such as activation of the complement system, the prostaglandin system, the specific immune system, and others.[28]

Activation of these cascade systems leads to a generalized inflammatory reaction, adding to the increased endothelial and vascular permeability caused by initial hemorrhagic shock. Because the lung contains by far the highest amount of vessels in the body, ARDS might as well be regarded as a quantitative problem caused by specific anatomic features. The major problem in the development of ARDS is, however, the self-maintaining nature of the cascade systems which have been activated initially. This also renders difficult the efficacy of several currently discussed therapeutic strategies. Instead, any procedure or therapeutic intervention has to be strictly avoided that might add to further activation of these cascade systems. In summary, severe multiple trauma and associated shock, regardless the distribution of injury, is known to be a risk factor for ARDS and outcome.

Lung Contusion Predisposing for Pulmonary Failure (ARDS)

> The *progressive nature* of pulmonary contusion ...[29]

It appears obvious at first glance that direct or indirect injury to the lung will have negative effects on pulmonary function. In a series of 203 patients with pulmonary contusion, out of which 60% required mechanical ventilation, an overall mortality rate of 20% was found. The presence of shock, additional injury and old age substantially increased mortality.[30] Johnson et al. found comparable results, in addition the number of blood units exceeding three was found be of predictive importance.[31]

The importance of the degree of impact velocity in determining the character and the severity of nonpenetrating thoracic injury have been stressed.[32] In a rabbit model, Lau et al. were able to demonstrate that a low impact velocity mainly causes bronchial injury, while high energy impact leads to alveolar injury.[33] In further experimental studies Fulton reports that despite severe pulmonary injury dysfunction is not fully detectable early after trauma. He found only a moderate decrease of pulmonary blood flow and an increase of pulmonary vascular resistance and pulmonary edema. However, all of these changes continue to deteriorate as time proceeds.[28] Oppenheimer investigated the effects of a right lower lobe contusion in a dog model. According to his results, hypoxemia also increases with time, which was explained by intrabronchial bleeding and flooding of air spaces with blood and plasma.[34] All of these studies coincide concerning the fact that there is "a progressive nature of pulmonary contusion."[29]

The problem in the daily care of the multiple-trauma patient is mainly to recognize the severity of pulmonary damage. Soon after trauma, the overall degree of pulmonary injury is difficult to assess, because blood gas parameters are still within normal limits and the chest radiograph also will be falsely negative in most cases. To date, only computed tomography has been discussed to adequately reveal the overall degree of destruction.[35] For practical and economical reasons, a routine chest CT scan on admission of a multiple-trauma patient does not appear justified.

In this context, it is important to mention that the mechanisms initiated by pulmonary contusion are comparable as seen after severe injury; in patients with pulmonary contusion an unusually high incidence of interstitial edema has been found. Mechanisms as known to be present in patients with severe injury are present, leading to activation of the immune response systems.[36,37] Thus, even though triggered differently, the host response to pulmonary contusion is similar as to nonpulmonary injury, resulting in an increased risk of ARDS.

Pathogenesis of ARDS after Intramedullary Nailing: A Combination of Mechanic vs Systemic Effects

The main clinical features of ARDS are (1) a low pressure permeability edema and (2) an increased pulmonary artery pressure.

These features also occurred upon intramedullary reaming and nailing.

The pulmonary artery pressure rise is among the acute, intraoperative dysfunctions experimentally, as well as clinically.[7,18,20,21,38] This increase hints at blockage effect of fat. It might, however, be argued whether the fat content of a single femur might be able to produce an increase of this degree. Compared to the capillary system of the general circulation, pulmonary capillaries are much shorter (about 3 mm) and the pressure gradient between arterioles and capillaries in the lung is only 5 mm Hg. Because of this fact and because of the extreme size of the pulmonary capillary bed, the pulmonary resistance is small compared to other systems in the body (11 Pa $\times$ ml^{-1} $\times$ sec. for the lung; 740 Pa $\times$ ml^{-1} $\times$ sec. for the kidney).[39,40] In theory, a huge amount of material therefore is necessary to create measurable differences of pulmonary artery pressure. In addition, it is known that part of the material mobilized out of the bone marrow cavity remains in the area of the fracture.[41] For these reasons, mechanical occlusion alone does not explain the rise of pulmonary artery pressure. In contrast, reflectory changes occuring after pulmonary embolization have been described. Invasion of an embolus into a lung with preserved nervous supply caused an acute rise of pulmonary artery pressure in the contralateral lung.[8]

Also, mediators appear to play a role. The pulmonary perfusion is in part regulated by the antagonists Prostacyclin (vasodilatation) and Thromboxan (vasoconstriction). In patients undergoing intramedullary nailing, increased levels of thromboxane have been measured in blood withdrawn from the femoral vein.[42] Thus, in addition to the mechanic and reflectory mechanisms described above, the release of humoral mediators obviously plays a role.

The same applies to the mechanisms causing increased pulmonary permeability. As discussed previously, the development of ARDS after severe trauma is largely triggered by inflammatory mediators liberated by neutrophils. Several cascade mechanisms seem to play a role. Jakobovitz-Derks et al., in a thorough investigation performed in dogs, looked at the time pattern of pulmonary morphology after experimental fat infusion. They found increasing evidence of invasion of inflammatory cells and signs of increased pulmonary permeability until 3 days after the infusion. During the same period signs of capillary congestion and neutral fat embolism diminished, thus pointing out a clearing mechanism within the lung. The study therefore gives a further clue that fat infusion may well be a primary trigger mechanism, however, during the further time course, on-going pulmonary injury is mediated by activation of inflammatory cells.[43]

Doerschuk also found clear-cut evidence for a definite influence of neutrophils. The pulmonary damage induced by fat infusion was preventable by induction of neutropenia.[40] Investigators further researched the role of fat embolization in animal experiments. In order to investigate whether neutral fat was able to provoke ongoing pulmonary damage, one group receiving an infusion of neutral fat was compared to a group with multiple fractures. Pulmonary dysfunction was more sustained in the multiple fracture group.[44] All of these studies show that pulmonary vascular occlusion, even though it might occur after intramedullary nailing, is not the only mechanism causing pulmonary damage. Instead, a variety of systemic effects are activated, representing an additional potential to induce pulmonary damage.

COMBINED EFFECTS—ADDITIVE PULMONARY DAMAGE?

Because the incidence of ARDS occurs especially in those patients suffering from combined multiple trauma and pulmonary injury (lung contusion), it appears likely that both factors, which independently carry a risk of ARDS, might have additive effects.

Several animal investigations have focused on additive effects of several damaging stimuli. Nuytinck applied the combination of zymosan activated plasma and a period of systemic hypoxia in rabbits. The pulmonary changes such as interstitial edema and the systemic inflammatory changes were much more severe if both stimuli were applied.[45] Nerlich tried to mimic the embolization of bone marrow fat by a continuous intravenous infusion. If fat infusion was performed following an I.V. bolus of endotoxin, an accepted model of acute lung injury, the combination caused not only additive lung injury, but a potentiation of damage.[46,47]

In a further investigation using the Staub sheep model, effects of intramedullary reaming and nailing on pulmonary injury were investigated. Nailing was done in a group of sheep undergoing previous hemorrhagic shock (2 hrs, 50 mm Hg) and lung contusion in the right-middle and lower lobe (in control animals no shock and lung contusion was present. Intramedullary nailing caused acute intraoperative disturbances in both groups. An acute rise of pulmonary artery pressure was associated with an increase of central venous triglyceride levels (Figs. 5–4 and 5–5). However, the effects of the subacute postoperative complications were different between groups. Intramedullary nailing only caused pulmonary damage in those animals previously submitted to additional injury (i.e., shock and lung contusion)(Fig. 5–8). Obviously, in accordance to clinical observations, a lung without previous damage was able to withstand the effects of the trigger factors caused by intramedullary nailing.

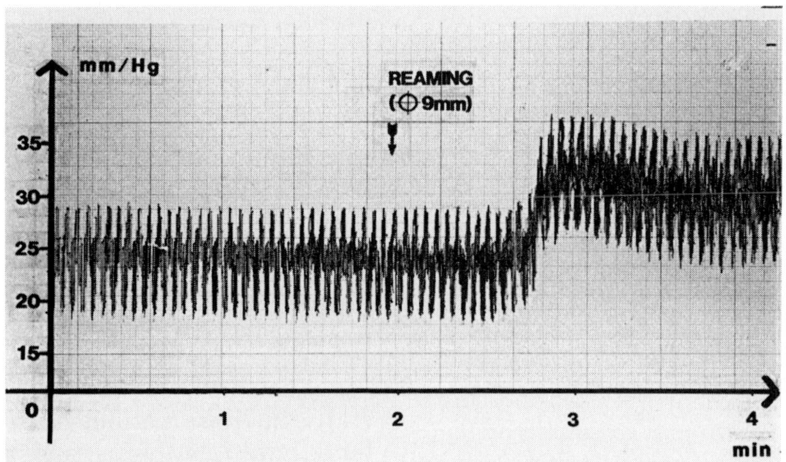

Fig. 5–4. Rise of pulmonary artery pressure in a sheep model after reaming of the medullary canal. This rise did not occur after unreamed femoral nailing.

THERAPEUTIC ASPECTS

Experimental Investigations

In experimental investigations using the model of lung contusion, hemorrhagic shock and a nailing procedure after reaming it was then evaluated to determine whether the use of a procedure without prior reaming of the intramedullary canal using a small-diameter nail might prevent pulmonary damage (Fig. 5–6). In fact, in the animals receiving nonreamed intramedullary nailing, no increase of pulmonary artery pressure occurred and the degree of microvascular pulmonary damage was significantly less. Obviously, the lung of these animals, despite previous systemic (hemorrhage) and pulmonary (lung contusion) damage, was able to withstand the operative procedure. The amount of fat liberation obviously seems to play an important role. This might be caused

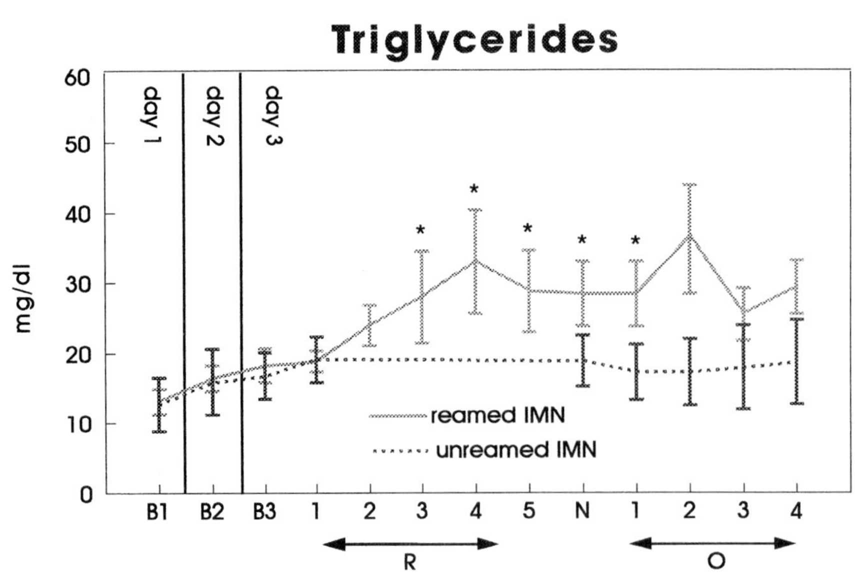

Fig. 5–5. Rise of central venous triglyceride levels in a sheep model after reaming of the medullary canal. This occurred regardless of the presence or absence of previous shock and lung contusion.

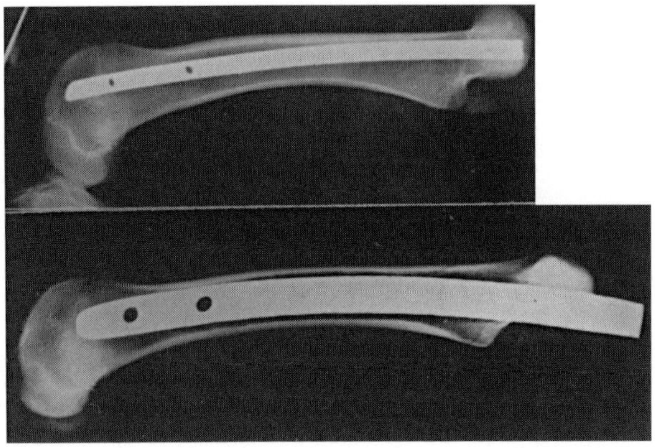

Fig. 5–6. Comparison of a reamed and unreamed nail in a sheep femur.

less by compression than by reduced reamer diameter or by less outflow out of intact intramedullary vasculature.[37] Again, cellular activation of neutrophils plays an important role. In animals submitted to nonreamed nailing less activation of neutrophils was present after intramedullary nailing.[38]

Clinical Studies

An unreamed femoral nail also is available for clinical use (Fig. 5–7). Studies in multiple-trauma patients revealed that no pulmonary artery pressure increase (intraoperative effect) occurs, and recuperation from disturbed oxygenation (postoperative effect) occurs more rapidly if unreamed femoral nailing is performed (Fig. 5–9). Experimentally, using an external fixateur also did not cause pulmonary damage despite shock and lung contusion.

In addition to the effects caused by reaming itself, the degree of pulmonary damage from intramedullary nailing is also dependent on the timing of surgery. As could be shown retrospectively, multiple-trauma patients suffering lung contusion do not develop ARDS if femoral reaming and nailing is performed later than 24 hours after injury. Because the surgical method is the same and intraoperative changes are comparable, differences of the host response must be responsible. The activation of neutrophils is most severe during the first days after injury. The threshold for influencing the clinical condition of the patient's lung function is most sensitive during this period of time. Care must be taken in order not to provoke further damage (i.e., inadequate activation of the body's defense systems which then will act in an autoaggressive manner). Reaming of the medullary canal represents an important factor with respect to activation capacity.

Instead, if the acute postinjury period has passed in the presence of adequate oxygenation and tissue perfusion, the subacute period after injury does no more represent a high risk.

The present status of knowledge of pulmonary impairment in multiple trauma patients submitted to reamed intramedullary nailing can be summarized as follows:

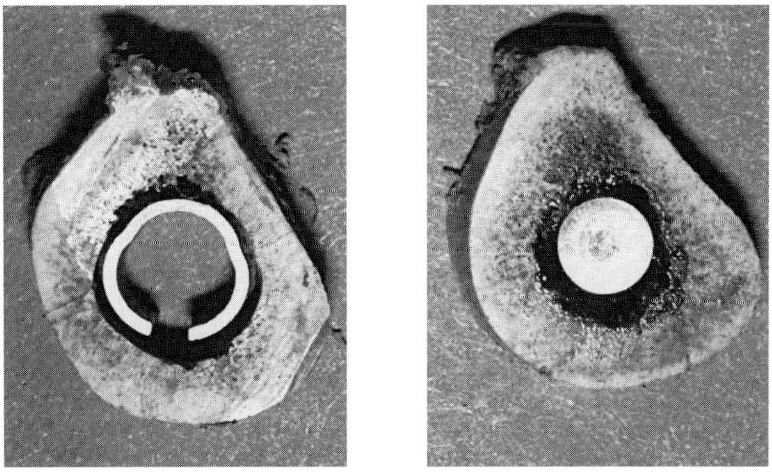

Fig. 5–7. Femur specimen in midshaft area following reaming and nailing; (left: 14 mm o) unreamed nailing and solid nail (right, 9 mm o).

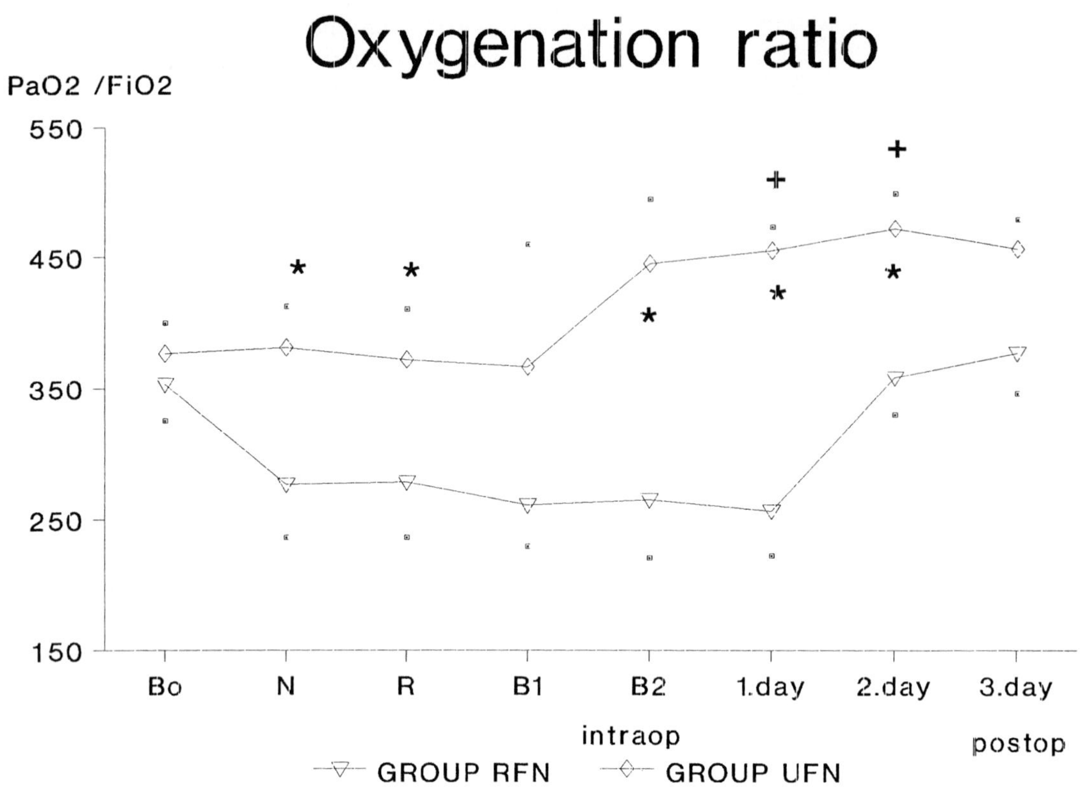

Fig. 5–8. Deterioration of pulmonary function (PaO_2/FiO_2) during reamed and unreamed intramedullary femoral nailing in multiple-trauma patients. Patients submitted to unreamed nailing recuperated more rapidly.

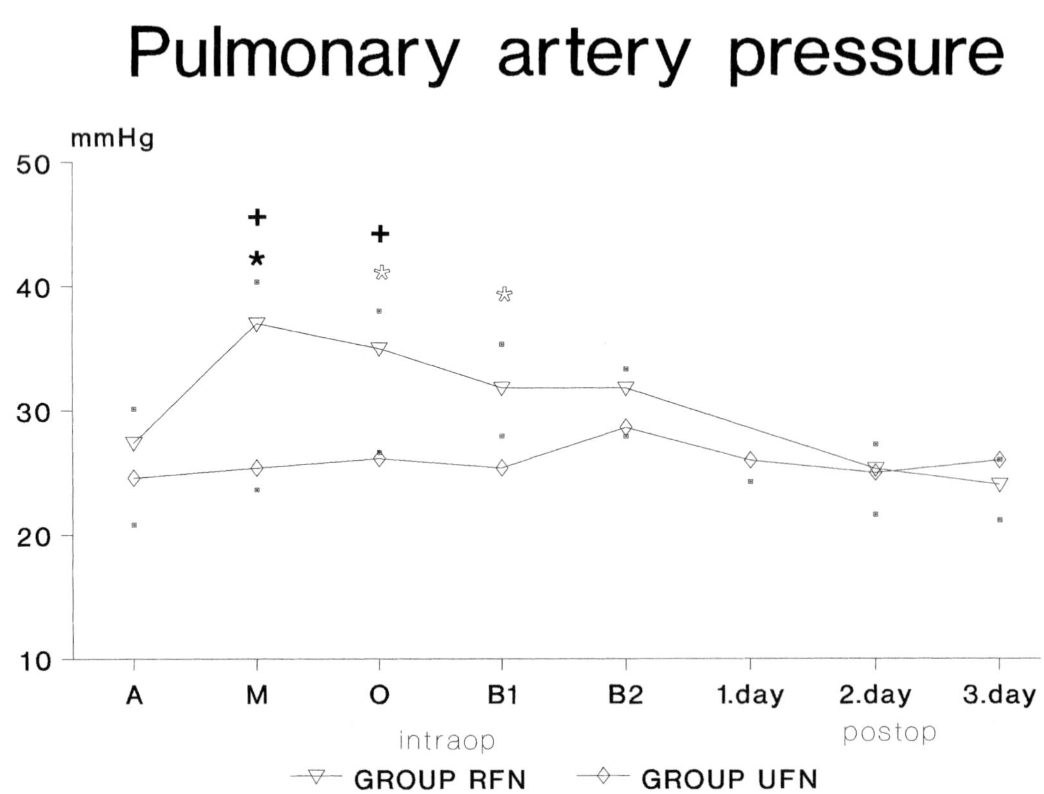

Fig. 5–9. Pulmonary artery pressure only rises in patients submitted to reamed femoral nailing (group RFN). Patients undergoing unreamed femoral nailing (group UFN) did not show a comparable rise during surgery.

1. The local changes inside the medullary canal caused by reaming are a pressure increase, destruction of vascular supply, and subsequent facilitation of bone marrow outflow into the systemic circulation.
2. Subsequent embolization of fat into the lung, which represents a filter organ, causes an acute increase of pulmonary artery pressure and a transient impairment of oxygenation. Because of anatomical and physiological rules, a pure blockage effect is not able to cause pulmonary damage alone. Instead, fat embolization is able to trigger the release of further mediators by activating the release of vasoactive transmitters (TXB_2) and neutrophils. The activated neutrophils trigger self-maintaining cascade mechanisms that can damage pulmonary vascular endothelium.
3. In the case of multiple trauma and lung contusion, a combination of disturbed oxygenation capacity and of increased immune response mechanisms is present. Because the degree of pulmonary injury cannot be judged adequately early after injury, the caution necessary with respect to the therapeutic measurements the lung can withstand might be easily misjudged. Thus, a potentially damaging surgical procedure such as reamed intramedullary nailing can represent the factor leading the crossing of the "threshold of pulmonary capacity."[48]
4. In view of the pathogenetic principles discussed above, the following therapeutic strategies might appear adequate to prevent pulmonary failure after intramedullary nailing. If severe trauma with additional pulmonary damage is present, reaming of the medullary canal should be avoided. For temporary stabilization in the presence of a critical patient condition, the use of an external fixateur could be of value. However, delaying surgery will cause further problems such as an increased risk of infection and prolonged intensive care stay. Primary stabilization of fractures continues to a major goal in the care of the multiple-trauma patient. Unreamed procedures might be a future alternative in the special situation of additional lung injury. Further clinical studies remain to be undertaken in order to evaluate more specifically the indication for its use.

REFERENCES

1. Küntscher, G.: Praxis der Marknagelung. Hrsg. Klaus Klemm, Frankfurt, Main, 1972.
2. Brittain, G.J.C., Ryan, D.J.: Hypotension and Methylmethacrylate Cement. Br. Med. J.*3*:667, 1972.
3. Modig, J., Busch, G., Olerud, S., Saldeen, T., Waernbaum, G.: Arterial hypotension and hypoxemia during total hip replacement: The importance of thromboplastic products, fat embolism and acrylic monomers. Acta Anaesthesiol. Scand. *19*:28, 1975.
4. Orsini: Cardiopulmonary function and pulmonary microemboli during arthroplasty using cemented or noncemented components. J. Bone Joint Surg. *69*:822, 1987.
5. Burgess, D.M.: Cardiac arrest and bone cement. Br. Med. J. *3*:588, 1970.
6. Schlag, G., Schliep, H.J., Dingeldein, E., et al.: Sind intraoperative Kreislaufkomplikationen bei Alloarthroplastiken durch Methylmethacrylat bedingt? Anaesthesist *25*:60, 1976.
7. Frost, P.M.: Systemic effects of acrylic cement. *In* Arthroplasty of the hip. Edited by G. Chapchal. Stuttgart, Thieme, 1973.
8. Weidner, M.G., Light, R.A.: Role of the autonomic nervous system in the control of the pulmonary vascular bed III. Further studies in experimental pulmonary embolism. Ann. Surg. *147*:895, 1958.
9. Peltier, L.: Fat embolism following intramedullary nailing. Surgery *32*:719–722, 1952.
10. Pape, H.-C.: Chronisthe therapie retrabtäre osteomyelitis langer Röhren Guoden-Möglichkeiten und Risiden der Markrammbohrung, Unfallchirurg, in press.
11. Pape, H.-C., Paffrath, T., Regel, G., Sturm, J.A., Tscherne, H.: Primary intramedullary fixation in polytrauma patients with associated lung contusion—a cause of posttraumatic ARDS? J. Trauma *34*,540–548, 1993.
12. Johnson, K.D., Cadambi, A., Seibert, B.: Incidence of adult respiratory distress syndrome in patients with multiple musculoskeletal injuries: Effect of early operative stabilization of fractures. J. Trauma *25*:375, 1985.
13. Lhowe, D.W., Hansen, S.T.: Immediate nailing of fractures of the femoral shaft. J. Bone Joint Surg. *70*: 812–816, 1988.
14. Behrman, S.W., Fabian, T.C., Kudsk, K.A., et al.: Improved outcome with femur fractures: Early vs delayed fixation. J. Trauma *30*:792 1990.
15. Bone, L.B., Johnson, K.D., Weigelt, J., et al.: Early versus delayed stabilization of fractures. J. Bone Joint Surg. *71*:336–339, 1989.
16. Danckwardt-Liljestrom, G.: Reaming of the medullary canal and its effects on diaphyseal bone. Acta Orthop. Scand. 1969.
17. Stürmer, K.M., Schuchardt, W.: Neue Aspekte der gedeckten Marknagelung und des Aufbohrens im Tierexperiment—Der intramedulläre Druck beim Aufbohren der Markhöhle. Unfallheilkunde *83*:346–352, 1980.
18. Wenda, K.: Habilitationsschrift, Unfallchirurgische Klinik, Johannes Gutenberg Unviversitaet Mainz, 1988.
19. Wehner, W., Morgenstern, C., Zeumer, G.: Das Verhalten des intramedullären Drucks bei der Markbohrung und-nagelung. Zentralbl Chir. *91*:209, 1966.
20. Wenda, K., Ritter, G., Ahlers J., et al.: Nachweis und Effekte von Knochenmarkemschwemmungen bei Operationen im Bereich der Femurmarkhöhle. Unfallchirurg *93*:56–61, 1990.
21. Harms, J., Berg, van den, P.A.: Die venöse Drainage des langen Röhrenknochens nach Aufbohrung und Marknagelung. Eine experimentelle Untersuchung an der Hundetibia. Arch. Orthop. Unfallchir. *82*:93, 1975.

22. Brooks, M.: The blood supply of bone. 1971.
23. Horovitz, J.H., Carrico, C.H., Shires, T.: Pulmonary response to major injury. Arch. Surg. *108*:349, 1974.
24. Staub, N.C.: Pulmonary edema. Physiol. Rev. *543*: 679–811, 1974.
25. Todd, T.T.J., Baile, E., Hogg, J.C.: Pulmonary capillary permeability during hemorrhagic shock. J. Appl. Physiol. *45*:298, 1978.
26. Weiland, J.E., Davis, B., et al.: Lung neutrophils in the adult respiratory distress syndrome. Am. Rev. Respir. Dis. *133*:218, 1986.
27. Dwenger, A., Regel, G., Schweitzer, G.: Pathomechanisms of the adult respiratory distress syndrome (ARDS)—Chemiluminescence analysis of polymorphonuclear leukocytes. Fresenius Z. Anal. Chem. *324*: 360–365, 1986.
28. Dwenger, A., Regel, G., Ellendorf, B., Sturm, J.A., Tscherne, H.: Alvelor cell pattern and chemiluminescence response of blood neutrophils and alveolar macrophages. J. Clin. Chem. Clin. Biochem. *28*: 163–168, 1990.
29. Fulton, R.L., Peter, E.T.: The progressive nature of pulmonary contusion. Surgery *67*:499, 1970.
30. Stellin, G.: Survival in trauma victims with pulmonary contusion. Am. Surg. *57*:780, 1991.
31. Johnson, J.A., Cogbill, T.H., Winga, E.R.: Determinants of outcome after pulmonary contusion. J. Trauma *26*: 695, 1986.
32. Viano, D.C.: Evaluation of biomechanical response and potential injury from thoracic impact. Aviat. Space. Environ. Med. *49*:125, 1978.
33. Lau, V.K., Viano, D.C.: Influence of impact velocity and chest compression on experimental pulmonary injury severity in rabbits. J. Trauma *21*:1022, 1981.
34. Oppenheimer, L., Craven, K.D., Forkert, L., et al.: Pathophysiology of pulmonary contusion in dogs. J. Appl. Physiol. *47*:718, 1979.
35. Schild, H.H., Strunk, H., Weber, W., et al.: Pulmonary contusion: CT vs plain radiograms. J. Comput. Assist. Tomogr. *13*:417, 1989.
36. Tate, R.M., Repine, J.E.: Neutrophils and the adult respiratory distress syndrome. Am. Rev. Respir. Dis. *128*: 552, 1983.
37. Pape, H.-C., Dwenger, A., Grotz, M., et al.: Does the reamer type influence the degree of lung dysfunction after femoral nailing following severe trauma? J. Orthop. Trauma *8*:300-309, 1994.
38. Pape, H.-C., Dwenger, A., Regel, G., et al.: Pulmonary damage due to intramedullary femoral nailing in severe trauma in sheep—is there an effect from different nailing methods? J. Trauma *33*:574 1992.
39. Schmidt, R.F., Thews, G.: Physiologie des Menschen. 20. Aufl., Springer-Verlag Berlin, Heidelberg, New York, 1980.
40. Doerschuk C.M., Allard, M.F., Hogg J.: Neutrophil kinetics in rabbits during infusion of zymosan-activated plasma. Am. Physiol. Soc. *7*:88–95, 1989.
41. Manning, J.B., Bach, A.B., Herman, C.M., et al.: Fat release after femur nailing in the dog. J. Trauma *23*:322, 1983.
42. Oettinger, W., Bach, A.: Thromboxanfreisetzung während intramedullärer Nagelung von Femurschaftfrakturen bei Patienten. Chir. Forum *233*, 1984.
43. Jacobovitz-Derks, D.O., Derks, C.: Pulmonary neutral fat embolism in dogs. Am. J. Pathol. *95*:29, 1979.
44. Jacobs, R.R., Wheeler, E.J., Jelenko, C., McDonald, T.F., Bliven, F.E.: Fat embolism: A microscopic and ultrastructure evaluation of two animal models. J. Trauma *13*:980-993, 1973.
45. Nuytinck, J., Goris R., Weerts, J., Schillings, P., Schuurmans, S.J.H.: Acute generalized microvascular injury by activated complement and hypoxia: The basis of the adult respiratory distress syndrome and multiple organ failure? Br. J. Exp. Pathol. *67*:537–548, 1986.
46. Nerlich, M.L., Albes, J.M., Wisner, et al.: Combined effects of fat embolism and endotoxemia in sheep. Circ. Shock *16*:47–48, 1985.
47. Regel, G., Nerlich, M.L., Dwenger, A., et al.: Induction of pulmonary injury by polymorphonuclear leucocytes after bone marrow injection and endotoxemia: A sheep model. Theor. Surg. *101*:1–9, 1989.
48. Pape, H.-C., Regel, G., Dwenger, A., et al.: Influences of intramedullary femoral nailing on lung function in patients with multiple trauma. J. Trauma *35*:709–715, 1993.

6

Biomechanics of Intramedullary Nailing

Joan E. Bechtold, Richard F. Kyle, and Stephan M. Perren

Intramedullary nails first came into usage during World War II. Dr. Gerhard Küntscher inserted these devices into soldiers with femur fractures. These soldiers were able to return to the field, and after the war some of them returned to the United States, through whom their local surgeons learned of the new technique.

Intramedullary nails basically act as an internal splint for a fractured bone. The nails are best at controlling bending loads, and they do not provide substantial resistance to axial shortening or rotation unless there is auxiliary fixation such as interlocking screws or fins. The following discusses biomechanical factors critical to the successful application of intramedullary nails, beginning with a review of terminology.

REVIEW OF TERMINOLOGY

Stress

Stress is defined as a load divided by the area over which it acts (Fig. 6–1). If a load acts over a small area, the stress is higher than if the same load acts over a larger area. The units of stress are load/area; N/m^2 = Pascal (Pa) or lb/in^2 = psi. 1.0 pound = 4.45 Newtons, and 1.0 psi = 6.90 kPa.

Strain

Strain is defined as the change in deformation divided by the original deformation. In the case of a bone, the strain in the fracture gap is defined as the gap width divided by the motion of the bone ends in that gap. Thus, a motion of 1 mm in a 2-mm gap results in 50% strain, whereas the same motion of 1 mm in a larger 4-mm gap results in 25% strain. Similarly, a motion of 0.5 mm in a 2-mm gap results in 25% strain. Because a smaller gap results in a larger strain, there is a trade-off between (a) reducing the fracture as well as possible and (b) creating too large a strain in the fracture gap for the cells to mature without exceeding their fracture strain. Plating a fracture under compression results in zero strain, because there is no fracture gap or relative displacement.

Strain in a bone is similarly defined as the localized deformation of the bone divided by its original length (locally). The units of strain are mm/mm or in/in; hence it is unitless. Strain is often referred to in terms of percentage.

Modulus of Elasticity

The modulus of elasticity (E), also known as Young's modulus, is the slope of the linear portion of the stress-strain curve. It represents the stiffness of a material. It is a property of a material that denotes how brittle (high modulus) or ductile (low modulus) the material is. The units of the modulus of elasticity are the same as stress, because strain has no units. Thus, the units of (E) are Pa or psi.

Force

Force is a load (Fig. 6–2). A force vs. deformation diagram is the result of mechanical test-

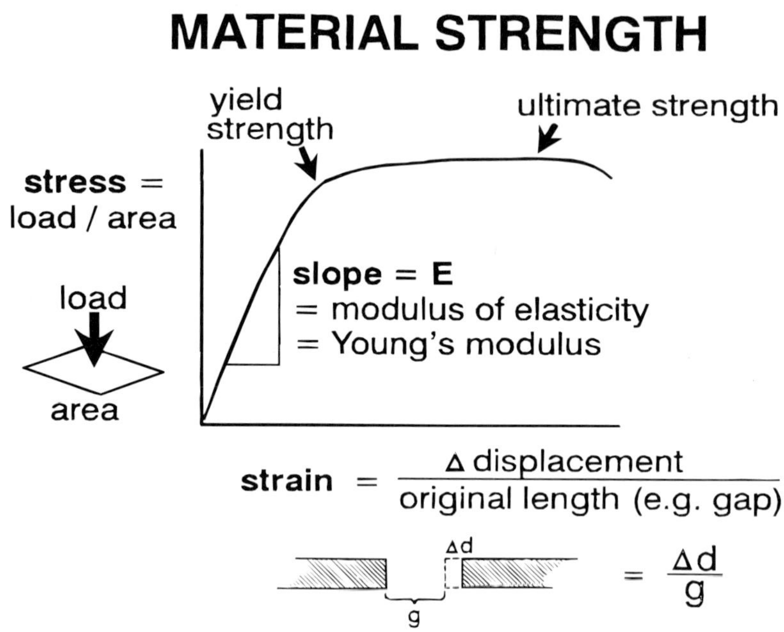

Fig. 6–1. Mechanical properties of materials. Stress is defined as load divided by the area over which it acts. Strain is defined as a change in deformation over an original length (i.e., strain in the fracture gap is the gap width divided by the amount of motion between bone ends). The modulus of elasticity (E) is defined as the slope of the stress-strain curve. Yield strength is the strength at which the stress-strain curve deviates from the linear (i.e., the deformation is no longer elastic, or recoverable). The ultimate strength is the highest stress sustained prior to fracture.

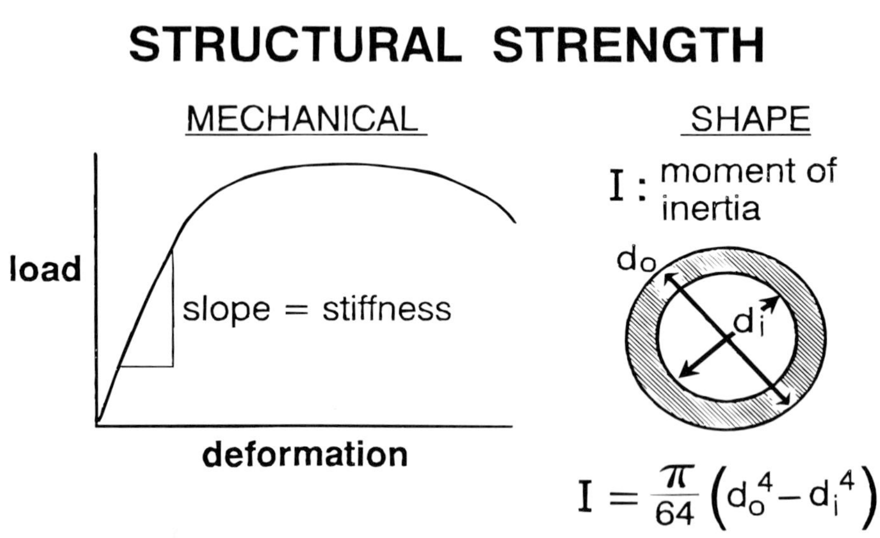

Fig. 6–2. Structural properties of materials. Load is the force applied to an object, and deformation is the amount of displacement under that load. Stiffness is the slope of the load/deformation diagram. Shape is represented by the moment of inertia, (I). (I) describes the distribution of material in an object, and the material furthest from the center does the most to increase (I).

ing of a structure such as an intramedullary nail. The units of force (load) are Newtons or pounds; 1.0 lb = 4.45 N. In an intramedullary nail, the material properties represent the material out of which the nail is made (e.g., titanium or stainless steel). The structural properties are influenced by the shape of the nail (in cross section) as well as the material out of which it is fabricated.

Displacement

Displacement is the deformation of a structure under mechanical testing or physiologic loading. The units of displacement are mm or inches (1.0 in = 25.4 mm).

Torque

Torque is a force acting at a distance from the center of rotation (i.e., moment) and is defined as the force multiplied by its distance from the center of rotation. The units of torque are N-m or in-lb (1.0 in-lb = 0.113 N-m).

Rotation is displacement about a central point. The units of rotation are degrees.

Stiffness

The *stiffness* of a structure is the slope of the load/deformation or torque/rotation diagram from mechanical testing. Rigidity is a termed used analogously to stiffness. The units of axial stiffness are N/mm, lb/in, and the units of torsional stiffness are N-m/mm or in-lb/in.

Moment of Inertia

The moment of inertia is a mathematical representation of the distribution of material in an object. A high moment of inertia contributes to the structural strength of an object. For a circular tube (e.g., long bone or intramedullary nail), the moment of inertia (I) equals $\pi/64\ (d_o^4 - d_i^4)$. For circular objects, because the diameter is raised to the fourth power, it is apparent that the outer material contributes most to the moment of inertia. Thus, reaming a bone spares the material that is most responsible for the bone's strength (this is discussed in more detail in a later section of this chapter). Similarly, a hollow intramedullary nail does not have a substantially smaller moment of inertia than a solid nail, because the material which is removed contributes the least to (I). The units of moment of inertia are mm^4 or in^4.

Flexural Rigidity

The flexural rigidity of a structure is the moment of inertia multiplied by the modulus of elasticity of the material out of which the structure is made (EI). The flexural rigidity of the femur at midshaft is its moment of inertia (I) multiplied by (E) of cortical bone. The flexural rigidity of an intramedullary nail is its moment of inertia multiplied by E of stainless steel or titanium. The units of flexural rigidity are N-mm or in-lb.

Stability

The stability of a fractured bone refers to the amount of relative motion between the bone fragments. A lack of relative motion is termed a stable configuration; the presence of relative motion is termed an unstable configuration.

INTRINSIC MECHANICAL FEATURES OF AN INTRAMEDULLARY NAIL

Internal Splint

An intramedullary nail functions as an internal splint. It is termed a flexible gliding implant.[1] This is in contrast to compression plates that achieve completely rigid fixation across a fracture site. As a gliding implant, the unaugmented intramedullary nail is not able to control shortening, axial loading or rotation. However, it is good at controlling bending loads.

Geometry

The geometry of an intramedullary nail is responsible for its strength, rigidity, and fixation with the bone. The major geometric features of an intramedullary nail are its longitudinal (anterior) bow, the cross-sectional shape, transverse diameter, slot characteristics, material properties, and structural stiffness (Fig. 6–3). Each of these are discussed in detail below.

Longitudinal (Anterior) Bow

The longitudinal curvature of the intramedullary nail governs how easily it can be inserted, as well as the bone/nail mismatch. The

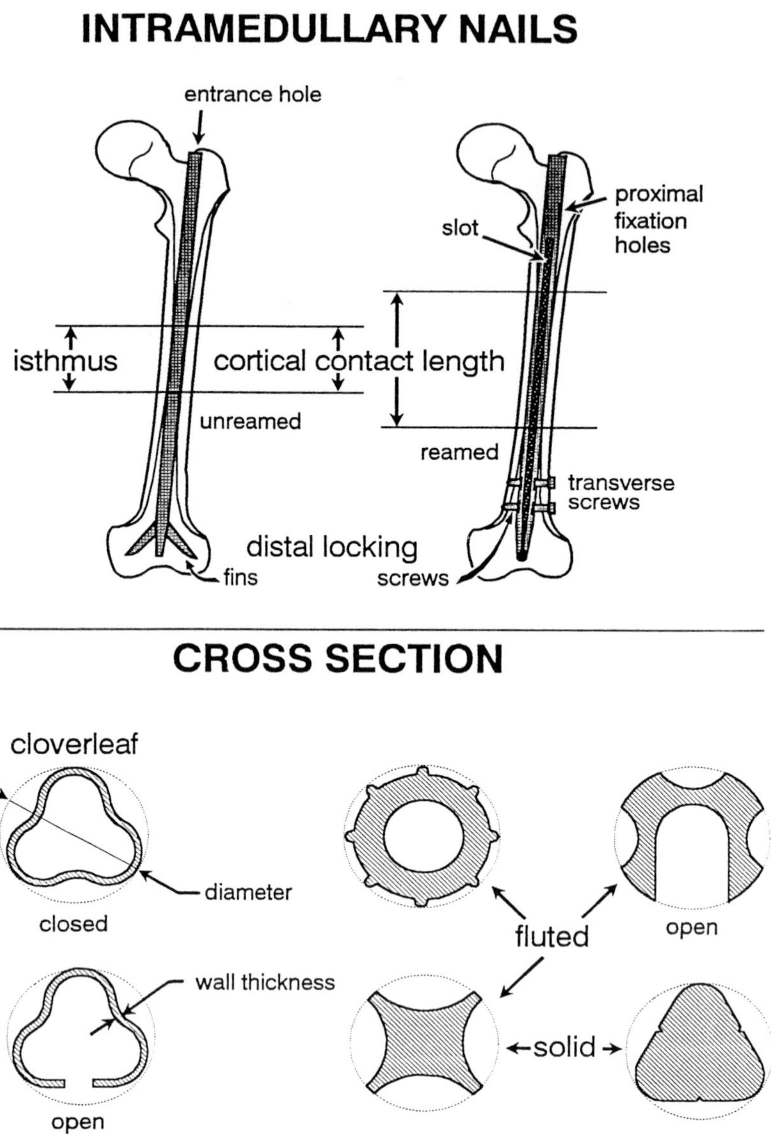

Fig. 6–3. Geometric features of an intramedullary nail which influence its performance.

mismatch in shape between the intramedullary nail and the intramedullary canal influences the stability of the fixation of the intramedullary nail in the bone. Complete congruency between the intramedullary nail and bone minimizes normal forces between the nail and bone, and hence offers little frictional component to the nail's fixation. Conversely, gross mismatch between the intramedullary nail and bone (such as a straight nail in the curved femur) will increase the frictional component of fixation but may inadequately reduce the fracture.

Most femoral intramedullary nails are designed with a curvature that is less than the curvature of an average femur. This eases insertion and results in some bone/nail mismatch to improve frictional fixation. The curvature of an intramedullary nail of 109 cm^2 accommodates the normal curvature of a femoral intramedullary canal. The bone/nail mismatch is also a function of the starting hole, which will be discussed in a later section.

Tibial nails are designed with a proximal bend, to ease insertion into the straight tibial canal. The location of the bend influences the mismatch between the bone and nail, and is particularly critical for proximal tibial fractures. If the fracture is proximal to the bend, the nail can wedge into the distal fragment upon insertion, and drive the distal fragment further distally.[3] It is not recommended to use a tibial nail for fractures proximal to the bend.

Cross-Sectional Shape

The cross-sectional shape of a particular size of intramedullary nail determines its moment of inertia, (I). There are several cross-sectional shapes of commercially available intramedullary nails. The most common is a variant of the basic cloverleaf of the original Küntscher nail. The purpose behind a cloverleaf shape is to avoid totally occluding the intramedullary canal and to provide channels for revascularization. Different cloverleaf designs have deeper channels (e.g., Grosse-Kempf nail) or shallower channels (AO/ASIF Universal nail and Russell-Taylor nail), and different wall thicknesses. The moment of inertia of each of these nails are within 15% of each other for medial-lateral and anterior-posterior directions.[4] Combining (I) with the modulus of elasticity of the nail (E), determines its stiffness or flexural rigidity (EI).

Other shapes which have been used clinically are a diamond cross section, and fluted cross sections (Schneider, Sampson). Cross sections with sharp flutes have the advantage of providing superior torsional stability. However, designs with flutes or flanges have been found difficult to extract clinically, because the bone grows around the protrusions and anchors the nail.

Size—Diameter

The size or diameter of a particular cross-sectional shape of the intramedullary nail also contributes to its moment of inertia, I. A smaller intramedullary nail has a smaller (I). Because of the dependence of (I) on the fourth power of the diameter, (I) increases rapidly for each millimeter increase in diameter (Table 6–1).[5] Consequently, larger-diameter intramedullary nails with the same cross-sectional shape are both stiffer and stronger than smaller-diameter intramedullary nails.

Some intramedullary nails are designed so that the stiffness does not substantially vary with diameter, or so that all size nails are approximately the same stiffness.[4] As an example, the wall thickness for the Russell-Taylor nail is increased to 1.2 mm for the smaller 12-mm intramedullary nail and kept at 1 mm for the 13- to 16-mm intramedullary nails.[4]

Table 6–1. Flexural rigidity (EI) of slotted cloverleaf intramedullary nails (1.0 mm wall thickness) (Nmm^2)

Nail Diameter (mm)	*Stainless Steel (× 10^6)*	*Titanium (× 10^6)*
10	40.0	20.0
11	52.0	26.0
12	69.0	34.5
13	88.8	44.4
14	112.1	56.4
15	139.1	69.6
16	170.1	75.1
17	241.4	120.7

It should be noted that intramedullary nails of the same diameter from different manufacturers have shown a twofold difference in flexural rigidity and a threefold difference in torsional modulus.[6] In addition, nails of the same nominal diameter may not result in the same clearance for a given amount of reaming; that is, the nominal diameter is not always the circumscribed diameter. It may be worthwhile to physically determine the circumscribed diameter of a nail and compare it to the circumscribed diameter of the reamer heads prior to reaming. (Reamer heads can change diameter as they become duller.)

Slot

Most intramedullary nails are hollow except for smaller unreamed nails (e.g., Lottes nail). Hollow intramedullary nails are designed either with open cross sections (i.e., slotted) or with closed sections (i.e., nonslotted). The purpose of a slot in an intramedullary nail is to allow radial compression upon nail insertion, thereby accommodating minor bone/nail geometric mismatch. An increased frictional component of fixation is also gained through radial compression of the nail and a corresponding increase in hoop stresses in the bone.

It has been observed that an intramedullary nail undergoes substantial twisting as it is inserted into the bone,[7] as evidenced by the displacement of distal locking holes. A slot markedly reduces the torsional rigidity from 1/30[4] to 1/50[8] the rigidity of a closed section nail.

It is unknown whether the torsional rigidity of a closed section nail is of clinical advantage, because both open and closed section nails yield excellent clinical results.[4]

The tip of the slot is known to be a site of stress concentration as evidenced by the preponderance of partial and complete cracks emanating from the tip. In a study to determine if an optimum slot-tip geometry exists, it was possible to reduce maximum stress in a theoretical model by 40% by simply widening the slot tip.[9] However, this reduction in stress did not occur for all loading modes. Until in vivo loading modes of the intramedullary nail at the slot tip have not been adequately characterized, an improved slot tip cannot be recommended. The AO/ASIF universal nail with its proximal keyhole slot extension addresses the concentration at the slot tip by eliminating the slot tip altogether and making a fully slotted nail. The proximal keyhole is important to maintain the thread alignment of the proximal extraction hole.

Material Properties

The material properties of an intramedullary nail influence its stiffness and strength. Most intramedullary nails are fabricated from stainless steel, with a smaller number of titanium nails. Titanium's modulus of elasticity (E_{Ti} = 110 GPa) is approximately half that of 316L stainless steel (E_{ss} = 200 GPa). The ultimate strength of titanium (U_{Ti} = 800 MPa) is approximately 1.6 times that of stainless steel (U_{ss} = 500 MPa).

Structural Stiffness: Flexural Rigidity

As discussed previously, both the shape of the intramedullary nail and its material influence how stiff and strong it is. Table 6–1 details the change in flexural rigidity for slotted cloverleaf intramedullary nails of diameter from 10 to 17 mm, with 1-mm wall thickness (ASTM F339-71) and fabricated from stainless steel and titanium. For each nail diameter, the flexural rigidity of the titanium nail is half the flexural rigidity of the stainless steel nail (since E_{Ti} is half of E_{ss}).

For each millimeter increment in nail diameter, there is an exponential increase in the flexural rigidity (because of the dependence of the moment of inertia on the fourth power of the diameter). For example, increasing by an increment of 1 mm from 10 mm to 11 mm in diameter increases the flexural rigidity of a stainless steel nail from 40 Nmm^2 to only 52 Nmm^2. However, increasing 1 mm from 16 mm to 17 mm increases the flexural rigidity of a stainless steel nail from 170.1 Nmm^2 to 241.4 Nmm^2.

Intramedullary Nail Fatigue Strength

Fortunately, intramedullary nails rarely break in service. If they do break, it rarely compromises the success of the fracture healing. If the nail is noninterlocking, failure is usually confined to the slot-tip. If the nail is interlocking, it usually fails through one of the interlocking holes. The more proximal of the two distal screw holes is the most common site.[10] The previous section on intramedullary nail slots and the following section on screws details problems associated with nail or screw fracture.

Occasionally nail breakage occurs after the fracture has healed. In this case, either the fatigue loading during the process of fracture healing continues to a lesser extent after the fracture has healed, or a defect or pre-existing microcrack is the site for the eventual crack elongation and fracture.[11]

PATIENT-RELATED AND SURGEON-RELATED FEATURES OF INTRAMEDULLARY NAILING

Reaming

Reaming a bone serves several purposes. It creates a larger contact area between the nail and the bone, thereby improving fracture site stability by increasing the frictional component of fixation. Reaming also allows insertion of a larger-diameter, stronger intramedullary nail, and reaming can stimulate fracture healing by providing a source of autologous bone graft at the fracture site.

Disadvantages of reaming include the risk of fat embolism and that it temporarily disrupts the endosteal blood supply. However, the periosteal blood supply has been found to adequately compensate until the endosteal blood supply reconstitutes itself. Another disadvantage is that reaming can weaken the bone by thinning the cortex.

Increase in Contact Area

Reaming increases contact area because it enlarges the isthmus, the midshaft region of the bone with constant diameter. Table 6–2 presents the increase in contact area with sequential reaming of an average femur.[12] The second column shows the percentage of the bone with constant diameter, for each millimeter incrementally reamed. The third column shows the incremental increase in percentage of contact area, for each additional millimeter reamed. It is apparent that the incremental benefit of increased contact area is small if a bone is reamed more than 2 mm. Another feature noted was that the contact increases disproportionately more distally than proximally, because the taper of the isthmus is more gradual distally.

The contact area of an intramedullary nail with the bone depends on the original size of the bone and on how much was reamed, as is illustrated in Figure 6–4.[5] A mathematical description of an average femur with two different original medullary canal diameters, both implanted with an identical 13-mm intramedullary nail (ASTM F339-71), is depicted in this figure. Six midshaft sections, separated by 1 cm are shown. The top femur has a medullary canal diameter of 12 mm and is reamed to 14 mm. The bottom femur has a medullary canal diameter of 14 mm and is unreamed. Although the same 13-mm diameter nail is implanted in both femurs, there is greater contact area for the femur that has been reamed by 2 mm from 12 mm to 14 mm. Thus, the nail/bone contact area for a given diameter of intramedullary nail depends on both the original diameter of the canal and how much it has been reamed.

Nail Diameter

Reaming allows insertion of a larger diameter, stronger intramedullary nail. Table 6–1 lists the increase in flexural rigidity for an increase in nail diameter. Flexural rigidity is related to the structural strength of the intramedullary nail, hence a larger flexural rigidity reflects a stronger construct. As was discussed previously, because flexural rigidity depends on the moment of inertia, which is proportional to the nail diameter to the fourth power, small increases in nail diameter can lead to dramatic increases in flexural rigidity. Reaming 2 mm to insert a larger intramedullary nail will substantially increase its strength and reduce its chance of breakage.

Table 6–2. Increase in nail/femur contact with reaming

mm Reamed	*% of Bone With Constant Diameter*	*% Increase in Contact Area (For Each Additional mm)*
0	26	—
1.0	36	38
2.0	46	26
3.0	51	11
4.0	56	7

(Adapted from Hoeltzel, D.A.: The contribution of an implanted intramedullary nail to the load carrying capacity of a fractured femur. Ph.D. Thesis, University of Minnesota, 1984.)

It is generally recommended that the bone be reamed 1 mm larger than the diameter of the nail to be inserted. Because the fixation of the nail with the bone is achieved in the isthmus through mismatch between the nail and the bone, the relative difference in nail diameter and reamed diameter dictates the degree of frictional fixation. An increase in the reamed diameter of 1 mm larger than the intramedullary nail diameter decreased the pushout force in cadaver femora eightfold.[6]

Effect of Reaming on Bone Strength

The positive benefits of reaming as outlined above bring with them a disadvantage. For every millimeter the bone is enlarged to allow insertion of a larger stronger intramedullary nail with a longer contact area and more secure fixation, there is a concomitant decrease in bone strength. Fortunately, reaming removes the bone which contributes least to its strength. That is, the endosteal bone contributes least to the bone's moment of inertia and hence its flexural rigidity and strength.

A finite element structural model of a sequentially reamed femur was created to examine the decrease in bone strength with reaming.[13] The outer cortex of a cadaver femur which had been instrumented with strain gauges was used as a basis for a finite element mesh. The model's canal was enlarged to represent sequential reaming, and the strains generated under torsional load were calculated. In

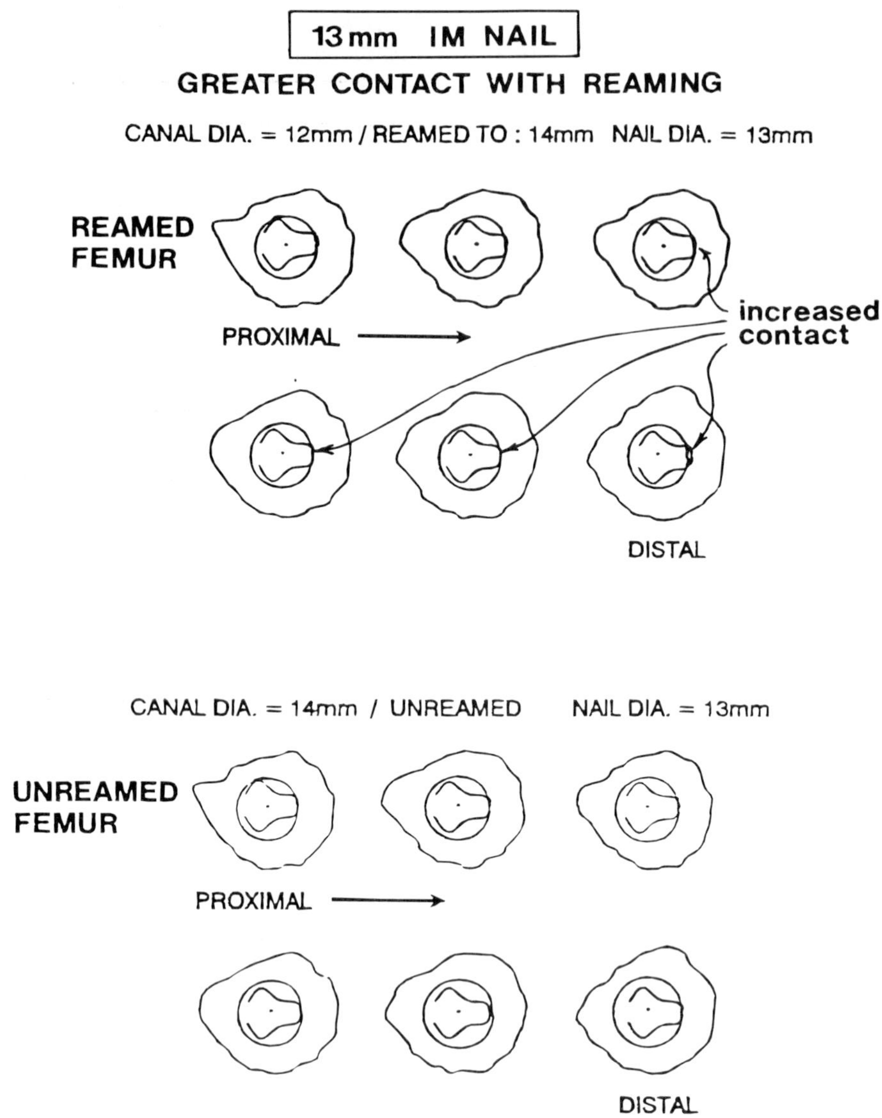

Fig. 6–4. The effect of reaming to increase contact area between nail and femur. Six midshaft sections separated by 1 cm are shown for (top) femur with original medullary diameter of 12 mm, reamed to 14 mm, and (bottom) femur with medullary diameter of 14 mm, unreamed. Although both reamed and unreamed bones are implanted with a 13-mm intramedullary nail, the reamed bone has greater contact with the intramedullary nail.

this particular bone, reaming from 10 to 12 mm increased the maximum bone strain 13%, reaming to 14 mm increased the bone strain 25.5% (compared to 12 mm), and reaming to 16 mm increased the bone strain 70% (compared to 14 mm). An increase in strain for a given applied torque is indicative of a decrease in strength.

Because the moment of inertia depends on both the endosteal and periosteal diameters, the overall size of the bone is important not just the amount reamed. For a constant endosteal diameter of 12 mm, a femur with a 22-mm medial-lateral periosteal diameter showed 66% more strain than a bigger femur with a 26-mm medial-lateral diameter, and a femur with only a 19-mm medial-lateral periosteal diameter showed 93% more strain than the femur with a 22-mm medial-lateral diameter.

It is important to note, however, that in the experimental portion of this study, it was not possible to ream the bones to large enough inner diameter to achieve a marked decrease in their strength. Theoretical models show that strain is related to moment of inertia in an exponential manner, but the clinically relevant portion of the curve is flat. That is, concern of weakening a bone by reaming should be secondary to other factors.

Starting Hole

The starting hole for inserting a femoral nail should be in the anterior portion of the piriformis process, just medial to the greater trochanter.[2,14] If the hole is placed too anteriorly, it will cause splitting of the anterior femoral cortex.[6] Placement of the starting hole 6 mm anteriorly from the neutral axis of the medullary canal causes high-hoop stresses at the fracture site and eventual bursting of the anterior cortex.[15] In this study, the hoop stresses were less sensitive to medial or lateral deviation from the ideal starting hole. Stiffness and load to failure of cadaver femora with different sizes of starting holes, and starting hole locations showed that the location of the starting hole was more important in maintaining the strength of the bone. Large but correctly placed holes caused less strength reduction than correctly sized but inappropriately placed holes.[14]

The location of the starting hole dictates the amount and location of mismatch between the intramedullary nail's curvature and the curvature of the femur. Correct placement of the starting hole allows the implanted nail's curvature to match the bone's anterior curvature. Improper placement (particularly in the anterior-posterior plane) can result in severe nail distortion and/or malposition of the fragments and possible comminution upon insertion.

Loading

An intramedullary nail is subjected to a combination of loads during activities of daily living (Fig. 6–5). The major loading mode is bending; however, compressive loading occurs throughout the gait cycle, and torsional loading occurs when arising from a chair and when climbing stairs.

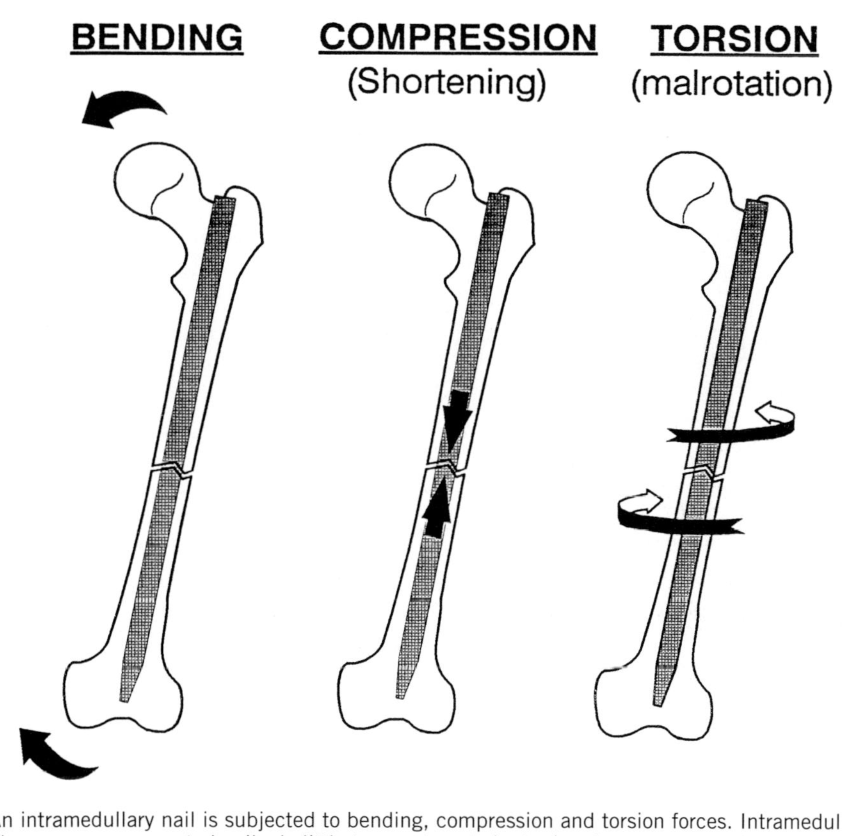

Fig. 6–5. An intramedullary nail is subjected to bending, compression and torsion forces. Intramedullary nails are good at resisting bending, however, unaugmented nails do little to counteract shortening due to compression and malrotation due to torsion.

Bending

Bending is the major loading mode which an intramedullary nail is expected to resist. It turns out that intramedullary nails are good at counteracting bending forces. There is little difference in the bending strength between different types of cloverleaf intramedullary nails,[4,16] because their basic cross sections are similar. In bending, the lateral femoral cortex is subjected to tension and the medial cortex is subjected to compression. Similarly, the lateral wall of the nail is subjected to tension and the medial wall to compression.

Compression

Compression forces are generated across a fracture site because of the action of muscles and the superimposed body weight. Because intramedullary nails are gliding implants, they do not resist axial compression. Interlocked nails are an exception and are discussed in a later section. If a nail is not interlocked, the fracture should be relatively transverse and noncomminuted, so it has intrinsic stability against axial shortening.

Torsion

Torsional forces are generated across a fracture site during specific activities such as arising from a chair and climbing stairs. Again, because intramedullary nails are gliding implants, they have little resistance against torsional forces and can result in malrotation of the bone. Interlocking the nail provides for torsional stability, as does casting (particularly tibial fractures). A fracture with interlocking fragments will offer some intrinsic stability against malrotation.

Fracture Configuration and Location

The configuration and location of the fracture influences the function of the intramedullary nail (Fig. 6–6). The configuration of the fracture determines the intrinsic stability at the fracture site, and the location of the fracture determines how much isthmus contact the bone has with the intramedullary nail on either side of the fracture.

Fracture Configuration

Transverse midshaft fractures provide the ideal indication for a routine intramedullary nailing. With reaming, there is adequate bone/nail contact proximal and distal to the fracture site, allowing the intramedullary nail to sufficiently stabilize the fracture (against all loading modes) for healing to occur.

Oblique and comminuted fractures do not provide the intrinsic fracture site stability needed to control shortening against axial loads or torsional loads. Some type of auxiliary fixation, such as interlocking or a brace or cast, is needed to provide adequate stabilization for healing to occur.

Fracture Location

Midshaft fractures are the optimal location for routine intramedullary nailing, because there is bone contact with the nail above and below the fracture site. This contact provides the frictional component of fixation stability, which allows the fracture to heal.

Fractures which are proximal or distal to the isthmus are more difficult to treat with intramedullary nails, because they only have cortical contact with the nail on one side of the fracture site. Proximal and distal fractures benefit from interlocking, which serves to immobilize each of the fragments against shortening and rotation. Interlocking is discussed in the following section.

Interlocking Intramedullary Nails

The introduction of interlocking intramedullary nails in the early 1980s greatly expanded the indications for intramedullary nailing. Interlocking intramedullary nails have a means for achieving positive fixation with the proximal and distal fragments and allow fixation of comminuted, proximal, and distal fractures. The most common means for interlocking are with screws that pass through one cortex, through a hole in the nail, and thread into the far cortex. Other means for interlocking include fins.

Static nailing refers to intramedullary nails which have both proximal and distal interlocks with the bone. Statically locked intramedullary nails do not allow gliding of the nail within the bone and control both axial shortening and malrotation. Because of the loads being placed on the interlocking screws as they control shortening and rotation, there have been relatively common reports of screw breakage. For

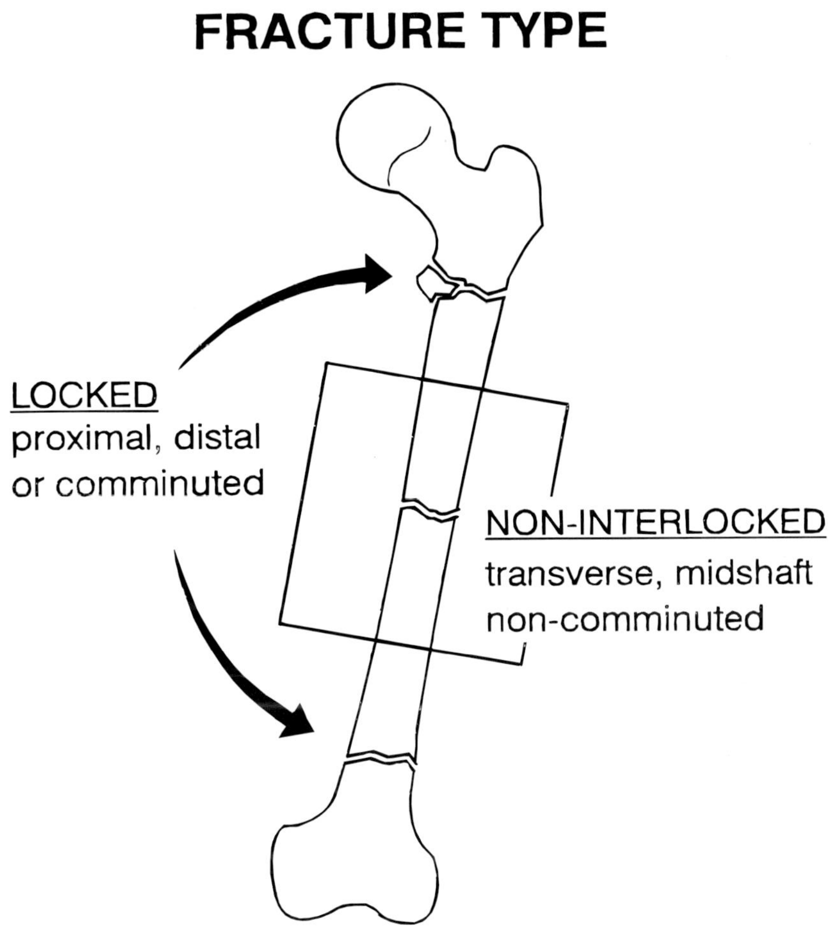

Fig. 6–6. Fracture configuration and location influence the success of the intramedullary nailing. Transverse, midshaft fractures are ideal for routine intramedullary nailing. Comminuted or oblique fractures, or those proximal or distal to the isthmus require some type of auxiliary fixation such as interlocking.

this reason, weight bearing with statically locked intramedullary nails is not recommended until fracture consolidation has begun to occur, allowing load to be carried across the fracture site.

Dynamic nailing refers to intramedullary nails which have either a proximal or a distal interlock. Dynamically locked intramedullary nails do allow gliding of the nail within the bone. Dynamic locking is usually reserved for cases where one of the fracture fragments is felt to achieve adequate fixation with the isthmus. Dynamically locked nails have the advantage of allowing early weight bearing, because there is not a concern over screw breakage. Dynamically locked nails with proximal interlock are easier to insert surgically and require less operative time, because the distal interlocking holes do not have to be radiographically determined.

When interlocking nails were first in clinical use, there was concern that static locking would be a "nonunion machine." It was felt that static locking may function to keep fracture fragments apart, and would impede the healing while controlling shortening and rotation. To avoid potential nonunions, nail dynamization was often performed, where either the proximal or distal screws were removed. Removal of screws would theoretically allow the nail to glide and provide coaptation force. The fears of nonunions have turned out to be unfounded, and routine dynamization is no longer common.

Type of Interlock—Effect on Fixation Strength

Bending. The biomechanical performance of most currently available interlocking nails with

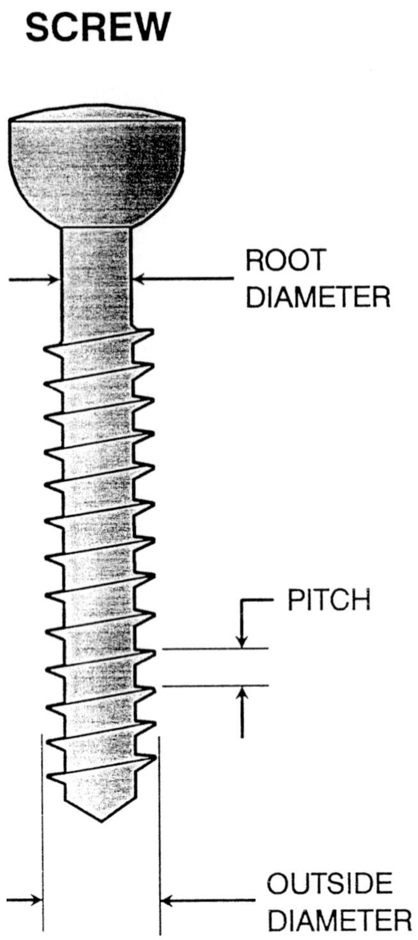

Fig. 6–7. Screw strength is exponentially dependent upon its root diameter. Holding power is dependent on outer diameter. Pitch also influences holding power.

hollow cross section are similar, particularly in bending.[16,17] Femoral shaft fractures interlocked with screws have approximately 75% the bending rigidity of an intact femur.[2] Distal fourth fractured tibiae with slotted cloverleaf intramedullary nails without interlocking were approximately twice as stiff in bending as tibiae fixed with Lottes nails in bending, and they were over seven times stiffer than tibiae fixed with multiple Ender nails.[18]

Torsion and Axial Compression. In torsion and axial compression, the differences among nail designs are more apparent. The type of fixation which most reliably stabilizes a fractured femur against compression and torsion is proximal and distal interlocking screws.[16,19] Such nails can axially support up to 400% of normal body weight.[2] Intermediate in torsional fixation is an interlocking with fins, such as with the Brooker-Wills nail. [16,17] However, distal fins do not provide predictably stable fixation against compression.[19] Multiple Ender rods or noninterlocked Küntscher-type rods provide only minimal protection against shortening or rotation.[17] In distal fourth fractured tibiae, multiple Ender's nails were almost twice as stiff in rotation as slotted cloverleaf intramedullary nails without interlocking, which were twice as stiff as tibiae fixed with Lottes nails.[18]

Screw Strength

A screw is characterized by an outer diameter (the circumscribed diameter of the threads), a root diameter (the diameter at the base of the threads), and the pitch (distance between threads) (Fig. 6–7). The shape of the threads at their base determines their stress concentrating factor, with a sharp base being more likely to lead to screw breakage than a rounded base.

The strength of the screw is dependent upon the root diameter. Similar to the other tubular structures discussed here (i.e., bone and intramedullary nails) the strength is a function of the moment of inertia. Because the moment of inertia is proportional to the fourth power of the diameter, a small increase in diameter results in a large increase in strength.

The pullout strength of a screw is dependent upon its outer diameter. A larger outer diameter can engage more bone, and effect a stronger fixation. Similarly, the more threads which can engage in the bone, the more secure the fixation. Interlocking screws are limited to the cortical thickness as the amount of bone which can be engaged; however, as mentioned previously, bicortical threads will be more secure than unicortical.

It is a design goal to improve the strength of the locking screws, because they are the most common site of nail failure. The largest diameter of screw which can be used in an interlocking nail is limited by the diameter of the nail. Increasing the diameter of the screws reduces the cross section of the intramedullary nail at its screw hole, which can predispose it to failure. Also, an attempt to improve bone purchase and hence screw fixation by fully threading the screw for bicortical fixation reduces the screw strength as compared with a partially threaded screw allowing only unicortical fixation.[4]

REFERENCES

1. Cornell, C.N., Lane, J.M.,: Newest factors in fracture Healing. Clin. Orthop. *277*:297–311, 1992.
2. Johnson, K.D., Tencer, A.: Mechanics of intramedullary nails for femoral fractures. Unfallchirurg *93*:506–511, 1990.
3. Henley, M.B., Meier, M., Tencer, A.F.: Influences of some design parameters on the biomechanics of the unreamed tibial intramedullary nail. J. Orthop. Trauma *7*: 311–319, 1993.
4. Russell, T.A., Taylor, J.C., LaVelle, D.G., Beals, N.B., Brumfield, D.L., Durham, A.G.: Mechanical characterization of femoral interlocking intramedullary nailing systems. J. Orthop. Trauma *5*:332–340, 1991.
5. Bechtold, J.E.: Anatomic Design of Orthopaedic Implants: Parametric design analysis of an intramedullary nail using techniques of computer aided geometric design and analytic beam theory, Ph.D. Thesis, University of Minnesota, 1987.
6. Tencer, A.F., Sherman, M.C., Johnson, K.D.: Biomechanical factors affecting fracture stability and femoral bursting in closed intramedullary rod fixation of femur fractures. J. Biomech. Eng. *107*:104–111, 1985.
7. Hunter, S.G.: Deformation of femoral intramedullary nails. Clin. Orthop. *171*:83–86, 1982.
8. Allen, W.C., Piotrowski, G., Burstein, A.H., Frankel, V.H.: Biomechanical principles of intramedullary fixation. Clin. Orthop. *60*:13, 1968.
9. Beaupré, G.S., Schneider, E., Perren, S.M.: Stress analysis of a partially slotted intramedullary nail. J. Orthop. Res. *2*:369–376, 1984.
10. Bucholz, R.W., Ross, S.E., Lawrence, K.L.: Fatigue fracture of the interlocking nail in the treatment of fractures of the distal part of the femoral shaft. J. Bone Joint Surg. *69A*:1391–1399, 1987.
11. Surdo, V., Dalla, P.P.: Breakage of the Küntscher nail in fractures of the femur after healing has occurred. Ital. J. Orthop. Traumatol. *17*:125–130, 1991.
12. Hoeltzel, D.A.: The contribution of an implanted intramedullary nail to the load carrying capacity of a fractured femur. Ph.D. Thesis, University of Minnesota, 1984.
13. Sandvig, S.: Effect of reaming on the torsional strength of femora. Master's Thesis, University of Minnesota, 1995.
14. Miller, S.D., Burkart, B., Damson, E., Shrive, N., Bray, R.C.: The effect of the entry hole for an intramedullary nail on the strength of the proximal femur. J. Bone Joint Surg. *75B*:202–206, 1993.
15. Johnson, K.D., Tencer, A.F., Sherman, M.C.: Biomechanical factors affecting fracture stability and femoral bursting in closed intramedullary nailing of femoral shaft fractures, with illustrative case presentations. J. Orthop. Trauma *1*:1–11, 1987.
16. Kyle, R.F., Schaffhausen, J.M., Bechtold, J.E.: Biomechanical characteristics of interlocking femoral nails in the treatment of complex femoral fractures. Clin. Orthop. *267*:169–173, 1991.
17. Johnson, K.D., Tencer, A.F., Blumenthal, S., August, A., Johnston, D.W.: Biomechanical performance of locked intramedullary nail systems in comminuted femoral shaft fractures. Clin. Orthop. *206*:151–161, 1986.
18. Nagano, J., Hoeltzel, D.A., Simon, F.D., Gustilo, R.B.: The rotational and bending stability of intramedullary nailing in distal fourth tibia fractures. Transactions, Orthop. Res. Soc. *8*:305, 1983.
19. Bankston, A.B., Keating, E.M., Saha, S.: The biomechanical evaluation of intramedullary nails in distal femoral shaft fractures. Clin. Orthop. *276*:277–282, 1992.

7

Proximal Femoral Locking Nails: The Intramedullary Hip Screw Concept

James F. Kellam

The operative treatment for subtrochanteric and/or intertrochanteric fractures has commonly required either a sliding compression hip screw or a 95° angled plate.[1,2] Depending on the fracture pattern and the technique of fixation, variable union rates have been achieved.[3–7] With a better understanding of the impact of the soft tissue on fracture healing and the theoretical improvement in biomechanics of intramedullary fixation, an attempt to use intramedullary fixation to treat these fractures has occurred. The first attempt was by Küntscher with his trochanteric nail or Y nail. Küntscher's goal was to stabilize the trochanteric area with a flanged nail inserted into the femoral head and neck. Then a thin intramedullary nail was introduced through the flanged nail and into the femur. Recent use of the Y nail by Seligson has shown that up to 80% of patients can enjoy good to excellent results with this device. The investigators had a 9% major complication rate that effected clinical results and a 15% minor complication rate.[8] It was determined that this device was suitable for unstable intertrochanteric fractures, as there was not a truly effective treatment for this fracture pattern.

Hans Ender popularized the use of thin flexible intramedullary nails inserted in a retrograde fashion for stabilization of intertrochanteric and subtrochanteric fractures.[9] This technique of flexible retrograde nailing, although theoretically good, did not produce a consistent acceptable result in clinical review. In a review by Jeffries of 225 hips, 84% had good to excellent results and 98% of patients returned to preinjury ambulation status. They had one nonunion in this series and a 3% malunion rate. An overall reoperation rate of 7% was present.[10] However, these results could not be reproduced by North American surgeons and because of unacceptable external rotation deformities and considerable knee pain at the insertion site, the concept of retrograde flexible nailing lost popularity.

During the mid-1960s, Zickel developed a subtrochanteric nail to provide intramedullary fixation for subtrochanteric fractures. This was a long nail that locked into the femoral head and neck. This nail required an open procedure and usually adjunctive methods of fixation to maintain the reduction. Still, 97% union rates were obtained by Zickel.[11] These good results have been reproduced by surgeons skilled in intramedullary nailing. However, the inability to lock distally eliminates unstable fracture patterns. Because of the double curve in the nail, significant fracture problems occurred at the time of nail removal.

To maximize the benefits of the theoretical biomechanical advantages of intramedullary nailing in the proximal femur and to take advantage of closed techniques, Halder in Halifax, England and Grosse in Strasbourg, France independently developed a short intramedullary nail with a sliding compression hip screw. This was based upon the Küntscher Y nail, and their experience with Ender's intramedullary fixation.[12–14] The mechanical construction of the nail was reversed so that a lag screw could be placed through a short intramedullary nail which was designed to match the proximal femoral anatomy and thus avoid the double bend of the Zickel nail. Two distal holes provided for static locking. After initial successful results at the Center for Traumatology and Orthopedics in Strasbourg, France and Halifax, England, this device has become an alternative for the treatment of intertrochanteric/subtrochanteric and high-subtrochanteric fractures of the hip. Further modifications of this nail, in order to change its proximal configuration, have occurred through the work of Asian orthopaedic surgeons in attempt to make this nail fit the Asian population.

DESIGN

The design of the intramedullary nail is based upon the anatomical structure of the

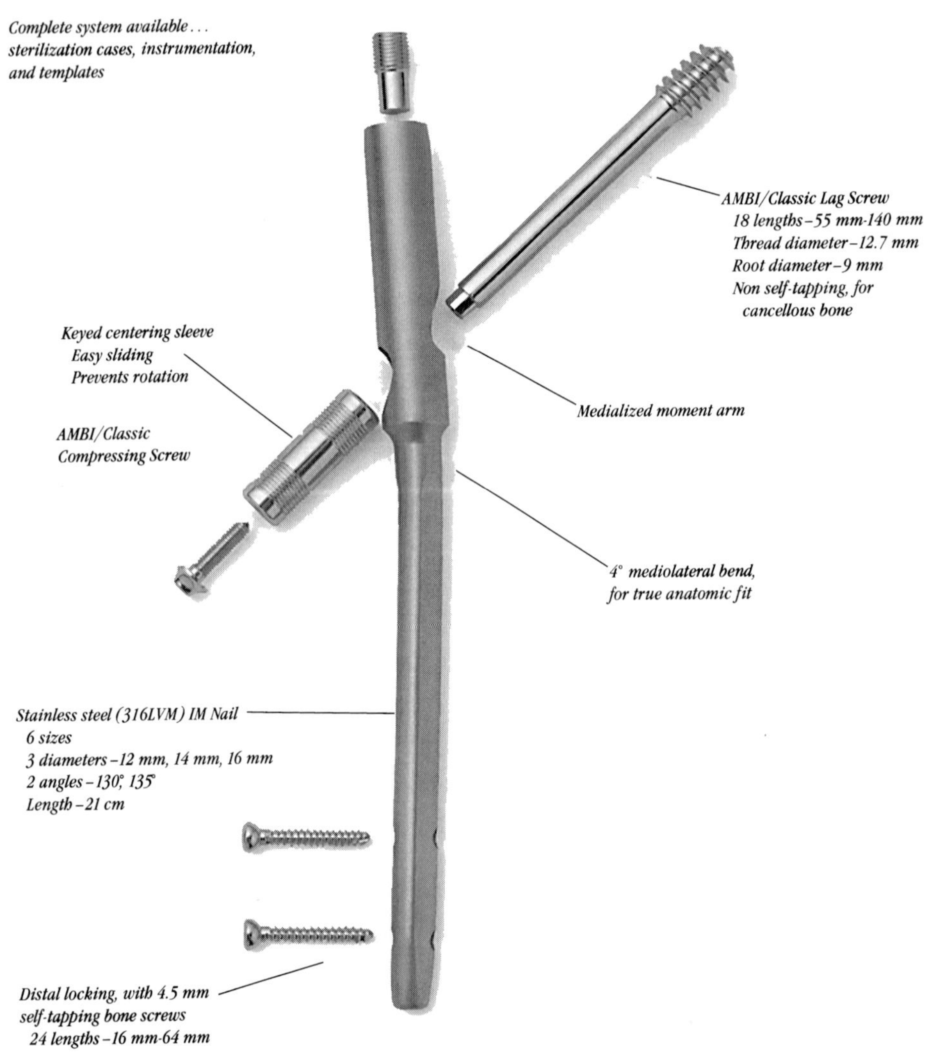

A

Fig. 7–1. Two intramedullary hip screws are available. *A*, The Richards Intramedullary Hip Screw This represents a cannulated 20-cm intramedullary device with a 4° medial to lateral bend in the AP projection in the proximal one-third of the nail. It uses 4.5-cm self-tapping screws for locking, as well a keyed centering sleeve to allow the use of the compression hip screw. (*Figure continues*)

proximal femur. The nail in its anterior posterior view has a medial lateral bow of 4 to 10° in its proximal portion to allow it to be inserted through the greater trochanteric region (Fig. 7–1). The nail is a closed cylinder. It is 20 cm in length with 3 diameters of 12, 14, and 16 mm, although a smaller 11-mm nail is under clinical evaluation for the Asiatic population. The nail's proximal hole has the angles of 125°, 130°, 135°, and 140° for centering the sliding compression hip screw into the femoral head. Commonly 125° to 130° will reproduce the CCD angle at the head and neck region. Various mechanisms of keying the nail to the lag screw to prevent rotation are available. These will not abolish sliding.

In order to understand the biomechanics of intramedullary hip screws, a study was undertaken by Mahomed at the Biomechanical Laboratory at Sunnybrook Medical Centre.[15] Using 10 pairs of fresh frozen adult cadaveric proximal femurs, testing of intertrochanteric and subtrochanteric fractures in stable and unstable configurations was undertaken. The intramedullary hip screw system was compared to a standard 4-hole or 8-hole compression hip screw plate system. There appeared to be no significant difference in axial stiffness between the compression hip screw system and the intramedullary hip screw system, when tested in the intact femur, two-part and four-part intertrochanteric fracture patterns. At failure, however, the intramedullary hip screw nail-bone composite was 30% stiffer but failed at a similar value (4 to 5 times body weight). Strain gauge data showed that both devices reduced the strain pattern on the medial femoral cortex, but there were significantly greater lateral ten-

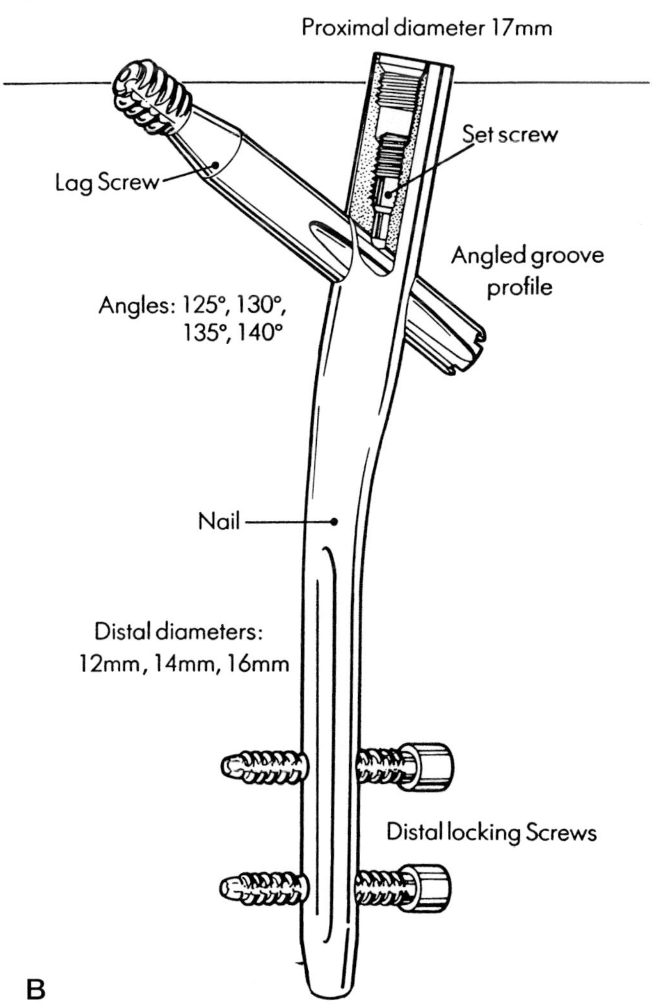

Fig. 7–1. (*continued*) *B*, The Gamma nail is a 20-cm cannulated nail, which has a 10° medial-lateral bend in the anterior posterior plane in the proximal one-third of the nail. It has a sliding screw which fits through the proximal nail, and is locked or keyed by a set screw. It uses 6.5-cm fully threaded distally locking screws. (Courtesy of Howmedica; Rutherford, NJ.)

sile strains from the plate system than the nail system. In the subtrochanteric model, axial stiffness was comparable for stable fracture patterns. However, the intramedullary hip screw had statistically significant greater axial stiffness than the compression hip screw in the unstable situation. In the stable subtrochanteric mode, both compression and tensile strains were noted in the medial and lateral femoral cortex of the implant bone composite. However, in the unstable situation no significant compressive strains could be seen on the medial femoral cortex with the plate device; compressive strains were seen with the intramedullary hip-screw device. Maximum load to failure of both devices occurred at about the same level with no statistically significant difference. The compression hip screw failed by pull-out of the screws or by fracturing of the femur distal to the side plate, while the intramedullary hip screw failed each time by fracturing of the femur through the distal locking screw holes. In conclusion, the study showed that both implants were able to withstand loads greater than three times body weight, and that both implants seemed mechanically able to stabilize both intertrochanteric and subtrochanteric fractures. It appeared that the intramedullary hip screw was stiffer then the compression hip screw and was therefore better able to stabilize the fracture site in the unstable situation.

In a biomechanical study, Rosenblum confirmed the decreased medial strained patterns using a intramedullary hip screw and concluded that this may be disadvantageous to bone healing.[16]

Repeating his classic experiments on sliding of the screw in the barrel of a compression hip screw, Kyle showed that with the intramedullary hip screw it did not slide nearly as well. This is related to the smaller area of contact between the nail and the screw.[17] However, this is not a physiological test situation, and in the clinical situation, it appears that sliding occurs. In the bone model testing, Shaw has shown again that there may not be as much sliding, and that there may be a jamming of the compression screw in the nail creating a rocking mechanism between the proximal fracture fragment and the shaft. This may lead to failure, particularly with cut out, as the screw will not slide and will be acting as a fixed angled device.[18]

It appears from the biomechanical studies that the so-called theoretical rationale for improved biomechanics by placing the nail in the intramedullary canal may not hold true. Certainly it appears that there may be increased axial stiffness with the nail in the unstable situation so that the intramedullary device may have some potential advantages.

INDICATIONS

The proximal femoral intramedullary devices are proposed to treat intertrochanteric fractures, high subtrochanteric fractures, and combination of these fractures.

Stable intertrochanteric fractures can be adequately treated with this device. It is probably most advantageous in treating unstable intertrochanteric fractures, in which the posterior medial comminution is greater then 50% leading to minimal contact between the proximal fracture fragment and the shaft. This device may act as a calcar replacement or posterior fracture fragment reduction supplement. Because of the nail's intramedullary placement, the proximal fragment will abut against the nail as it collapses and thus give it stability (Fig. 7–2).

Subtrochanteric fractures located in and about the region of the lesser trochanter are suitable for the treatment with this device. If there is greater than 5 cm of extension below the level of the lesser trochanter, this device should probably not be used. It is very difficult to determine subtle cracks that may extend down to the tip of the nail. Consequently, in a subtrochanteric region only those fractures that occur within 5 cm of the lesser trochanter should be treated. This obviously will eliminate any shaft extension of subtrochanteric fracture that may occur in a high-energy injury in a young individual (Fig. 7–3).

This device is very useful for the treatment of isolated pathological lesions in the intertrochanteric/subtrochanteric region that are confined to this region and not below the lesser trochanter. Certainly metastatic deposits within the trochanteric area can be adequately handled by this device, as long as the surgeon has ruled out other metastatic deposits that are occurring in the remainder of the distal femoral shaft, supracondylar region, and femoral head (Fig. 7–4).

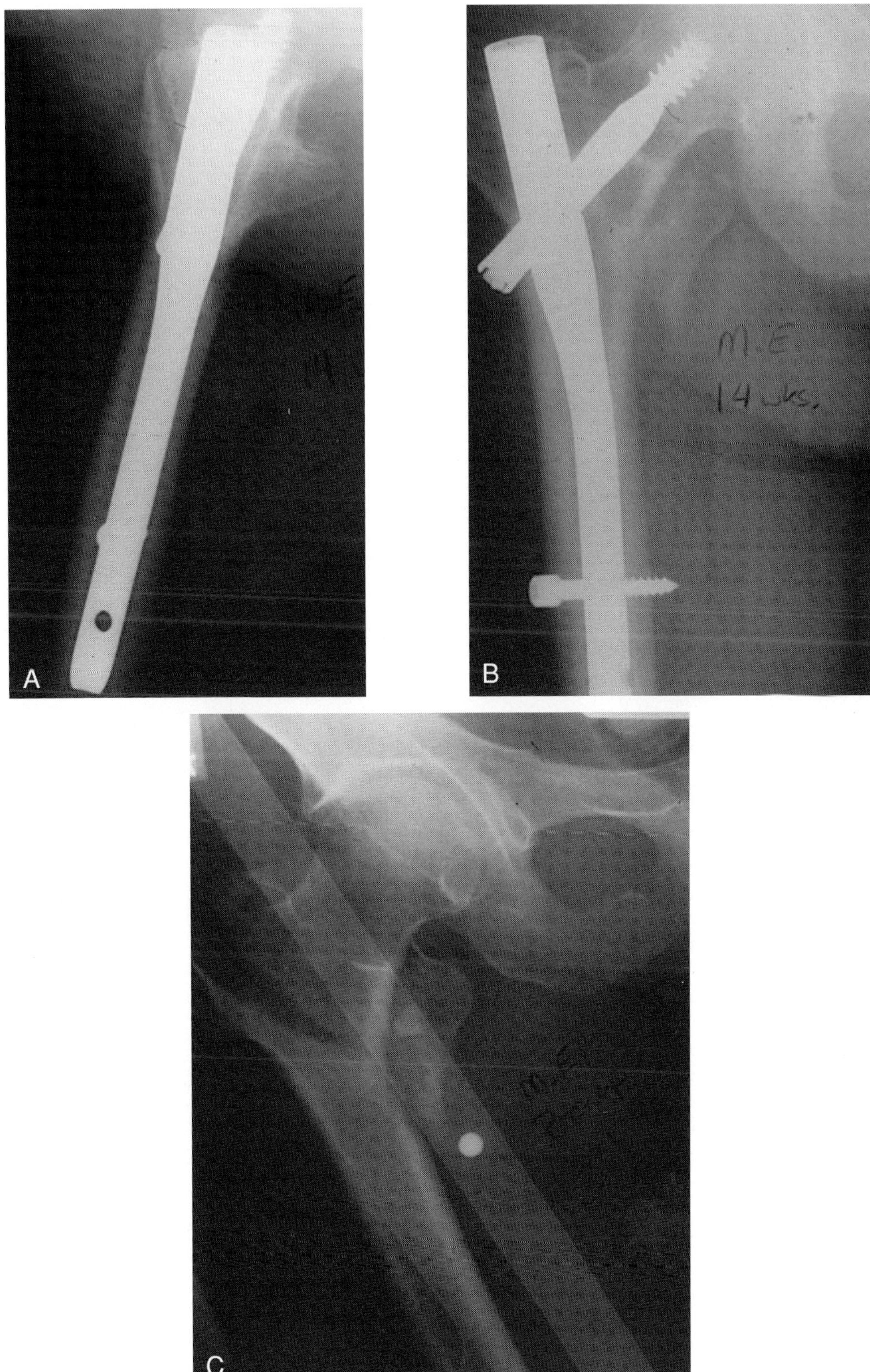

Fig. 7–2. *A,* This represents an unstable intertrochanteric fracture with a large posterior medial wedge (lesser trochanteric displaced) and the hip in varus. *B,* This has been treated with an intramedullary hip screw with a reasonable reduction. *C,* The patient went on to an uneventful recovery and was able to fully bear weight postoperatively.

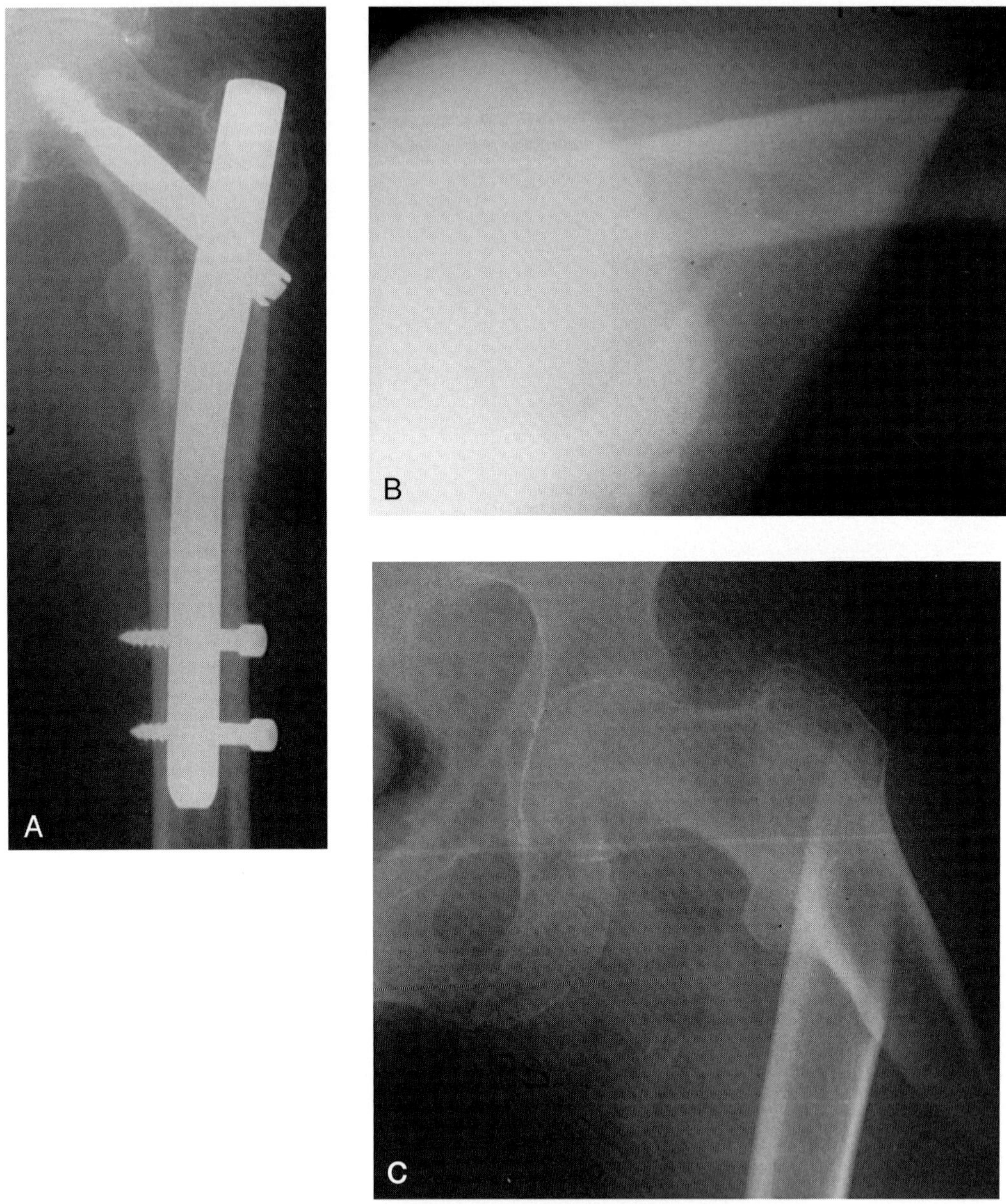

Fig. 7–3. *A,* This is a long spiral subtrochanteric fracture in the region of the lesser trochanter. This fracture may extend the indications of the use of the intramedullary hip screw as it does to extend further than 5 cm below the lesser trochanter; however, it was adequately immobilized with intramedullary hip screw. *B,C,* The fracture united.

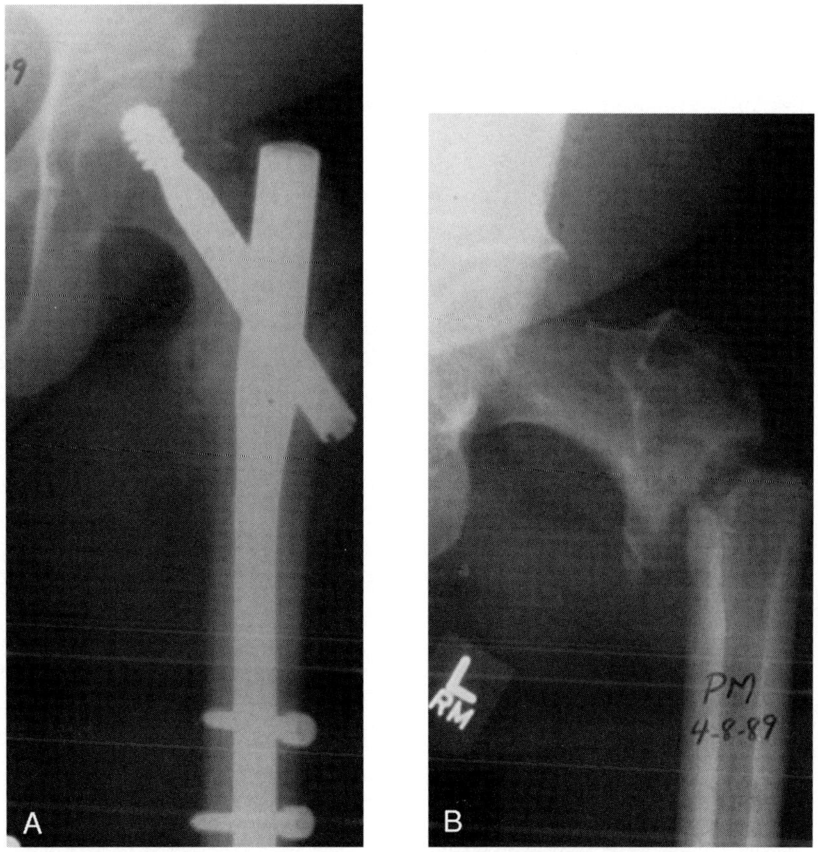

Fig. 7–4. *A,* This represents a pathological subtrochanteric fracture in a 35-year-old woman with breast cancer. The fracture was reduced and stabilized with an intramedullary hip screw. *B,* Radiation subsequently followed this, and the patient went on to uneventful union. *C,* The postoperative radiograph is after 3 months and union can be seen.

This device has no role to play in the treatment of ipsilateral femoral neck and shaft fractures or in the treatment of isolated femoral neck injuries fractures. In fact, it may be very important to evaluate a comminuted fracture in the intertrochanteric-subtrochanteric region to make sure that one is not dealing with a low femoral neck fracture. If this is the case, this device may not be the ideal device to treat this type of fracture pattern.

TECHNIQUE

Preoperative Planning

If an intramedullary hip screw device is selected, then it is important to understand that there are certain imperative preoperative planning technique steps that must be undertaken. First, adequate AP and lateral radiographs of the uninjured hip must be obtained. Using the appropriate intramedullary hip screw templates, the ideal implant angle to reconstitute the normal hip CCD angle can be determined (Fig. 7–5). As well, the medullary canal of the proximal 20 cm must be evaluated for its size to determine the need for reaming. Any deformity of the proximal femur can be assessed. The common implant is a 130° angle using a 12-mm diameter nail. However, certain individuals may have a varus or valgus hip and it is important to note this so that a slightly lower or higher angled nail will be chosen. The nail must never be hammered in, consequently the diameter of the medullary canal must be evaluated in the proximal 20 cm. The canal diameter must be 2 cm greater than nail size planned. This will determine how much reaming will be necessary.

However, most important is the determination of any proximal femoral deformity. As the device cannot be contoured and is being in-

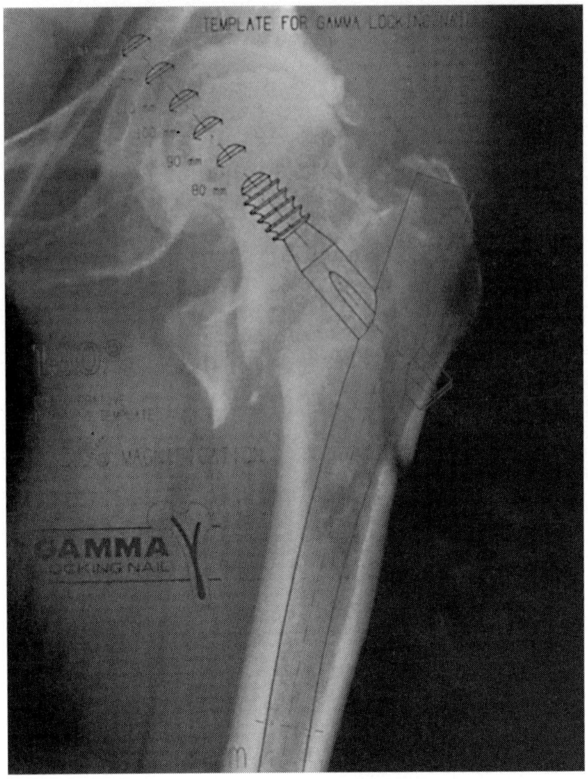

Fig. 7–5. Preoperative planning is essential. There are templates that will provide the operating surgeon with the appropriate guide to size of nail, medullary canal, and appropriate angle of fixation. These are imperative to be used in order to confirm the availability of implant material. They can either be done on a normal hip radiograph from the opposite side or on a reduction film taken from the C-arm during the reduction. This picture shows a C-arm reduction picture used for templating. (Courtesy of Howmedica; Rutherford, NJ.)

serted down the intramedullary canal, the canal must be able to accept this device. If there is any deformity secondary to metabolic bone disease or old injury, then this device may not be appropriate for the treatment of this fracture. Obviously, old fractures that have healed in this region that do not have a medullary canal may make this implant insertion extremely difficult.

The other step of preoperative planning is to assure that the appropriate instrumentation and implants are available for use. It is wise to check this prior to entering into the procedure and to make sure that one has reviewed the technique.

OPERATIVE PROCEDURE

The supine position on a fracture table is preferred for this operation. The patient's injured hip is placed in extension with traction through the foot. The opposite uninjured leg can be placed either in 90° hip and knee flexion in a well-leg holder or may be placed in extension and abduction with slight traction. With extension and abduction and slight traction, the pelvis will be stabilized making a reduction more easily accomplished. However, it does make it difficult if one needs to freehand distal screw fixation. Only with a difficult reduction is the use of this position recommended (Fig. 7–6). The trunk should be pushed away from the injured side to allow easy access to the trochanteric region (Fig. 7–7). The image intensifier or C-arm must be positioned to give a true AP view as well as a true lateral view of the hip. On the lateral view, it is important to understand the amount of anteversion that is present. If one can internally rotate the hip during the reduction so that the neck is parallel with the floor, there will then be no anteversion (15 to 20° of internal rotation). However, if this cannot be obtained, then one must look at the amount of rotation of the C-arm that will give the true lateral of the hip. This is when the femoral neck is lined up along the shaft and there is no angulation between the junction of the neck and the shaft. This will determine the amount of anteversion required when the nail is inserted (Fig. 7–8).

REDUCTION

Reduction is extremely important. The first step of reduction is in the anterior posterior plane and is accomplished through traction. Once it appears that the appropriate CCD angle has been obtained and that the tip of the trochanter is at the center of the femoral head, then a lateral view is obtained. At this point, rotation is then carried out in an attempt to reduce the fracture on the lateral. If the fracture is not reducible in the lateral view without disturbing the AP view, then the leg should be placed in the normal anatomical position of approximately 15° external rotation and the position in the lateral be accepted and reduced manually at the time of insertion of the guide wire. The most important reduction maneuver in this situation is the maintenance of length and obtaining the right CCD angle of the hip on the anteroposterior view.

Subtrochanteric fractures can be particularly difficult to reduce because of the muscle forces

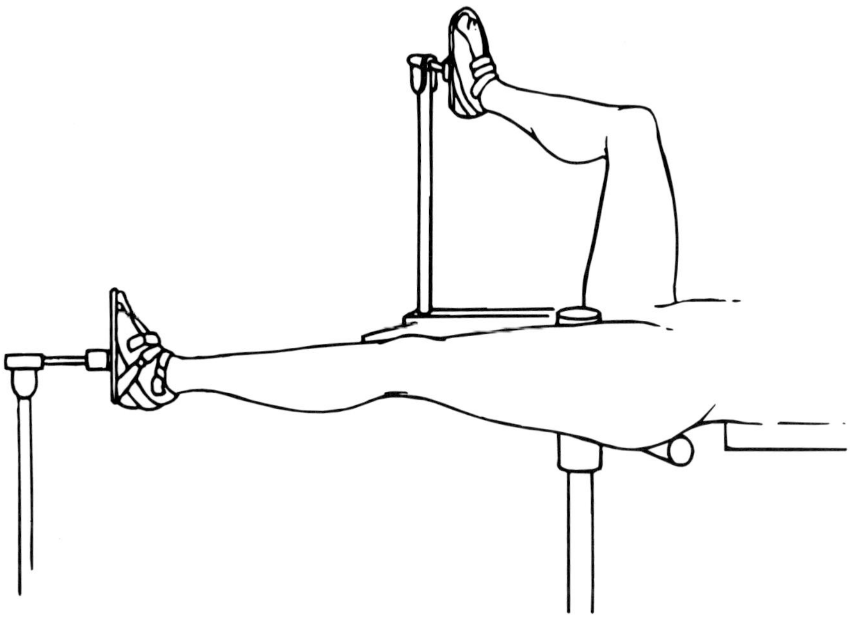

Fig. 7–6. Positioning of the patient is very important. This figure demonstrates the use of a well-leg holder to flex and abduct the hip. This technique is particularly useful in order to get a true lateral of the hip and to get a right angle view of the femur for distal locking in a freehand manner. (Courtesy of Smith & Nephew Richards; Memphis, TN.)

causing abduction, external rotation, and flexion of the proximal fracture fragment. This must be considered at the time of reduction, making it impossible to reduce the proximal fracture fragment to the distal. The most important aspect is the maintenance of length, so that at the time of surgical intervention the lateral view may be reduced manually through a small nail or a clamp upon the greater trochanter fracture fragment. Reduction must be confirmed with the C-arm. Otherwise, the surgeon must be confident that he or she will be able to achieve any further reductive manipulations during the operation.

ENTRY HOLE

With the fracture appropriately reduced, an incision of about 8 cm is made starting at the tip of the trochanter and extending proximally (Fig. 7–9). It is important to realize that the nail will not be inserted in the piriformis fossa as a standard intramedullary nail is but will be inserted into the center of the greater trochanteric area. The tip of the trochanter is exposed. Taking a curved awl and placing it upon the tip of the trochanter, an AP view on the C-arm is taken. The position of the awl should reproduce what the implant should look like as it enters into the greater trochanteric region. One should not worry about the comminution in this region, as with reduction ligamentotaxis will pull the fragments back together and lock them in position. Broaching a hole through the comminution is important so that the nail and reamers will not disrupt the reduction. With the appropriate position on the AP at the tip of trochanter and not sliding to the medial side or off the lateral aspect, a lateral view is then obtained. This should be a true lateral view remembering the amount of rotation to get this from the original preoperative reduction. At this time the awl should be noted to be bisecting the femoral neck. This means that the nail is inserted into the anterior half of the greater trochanteric region. The normal anatomy of the proximal femur has the neck originating from the anterior half of the greater trochanter and there is usually a large posterior overhang covering the piriformis fossa. On insertion, the awl will line up in the center of the femoral neck on the lateral view and will appear on the AP view to be reproducing the gentle 10° valgus curve that is present in the nail. Once the awl has been placed in the greater trochanter, it can be removed and the beaded guide wire is inserted (Fig. 7–10).

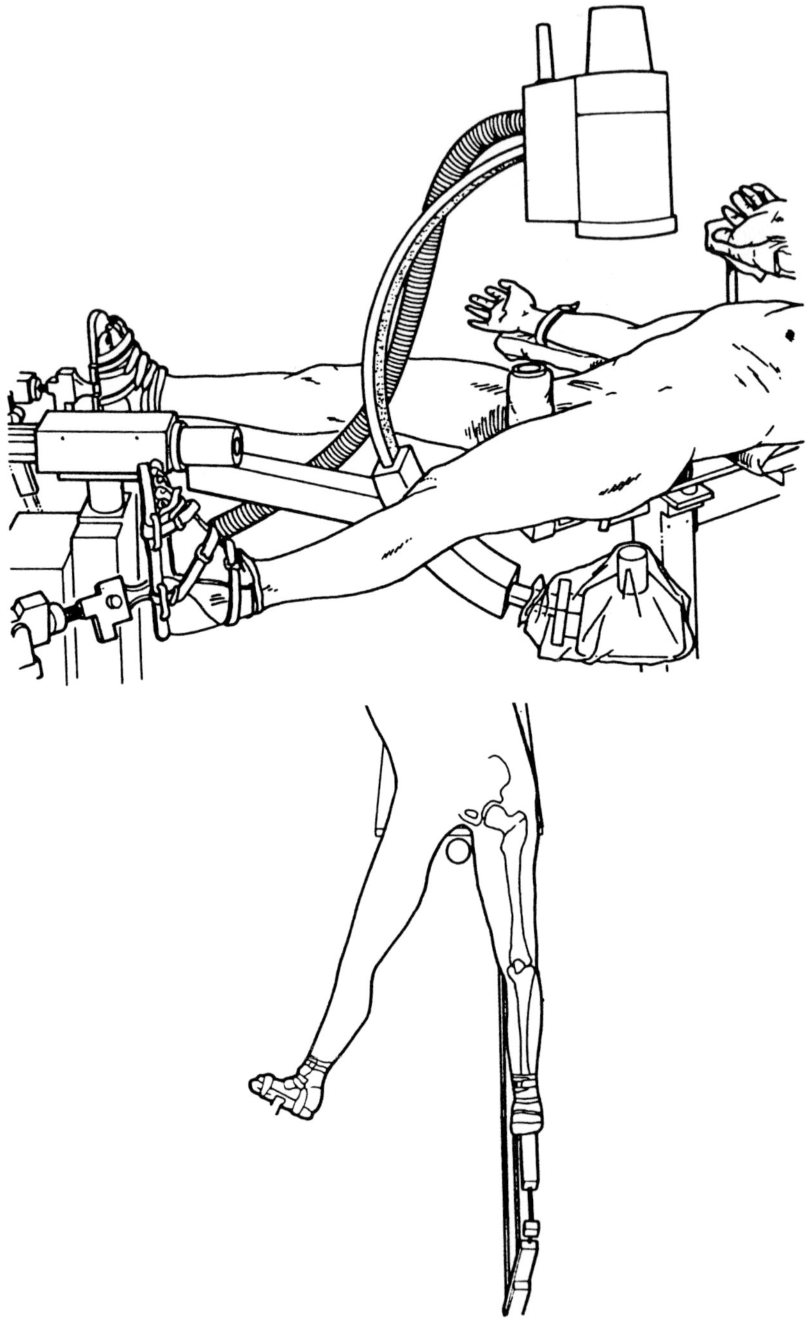

Fig. 7–7. This figure shows a supine position for nailing with the leg in a extended and abducted position. This is also a very helpful position, particularly in the traumatic situation where the other leg may be injured. The disadvantage of this positioning is that it does not allow a true lateral of the shaft, therefore freehand locking is difficult. (Courtesy of Howmedica; Rutherford, NJ.)

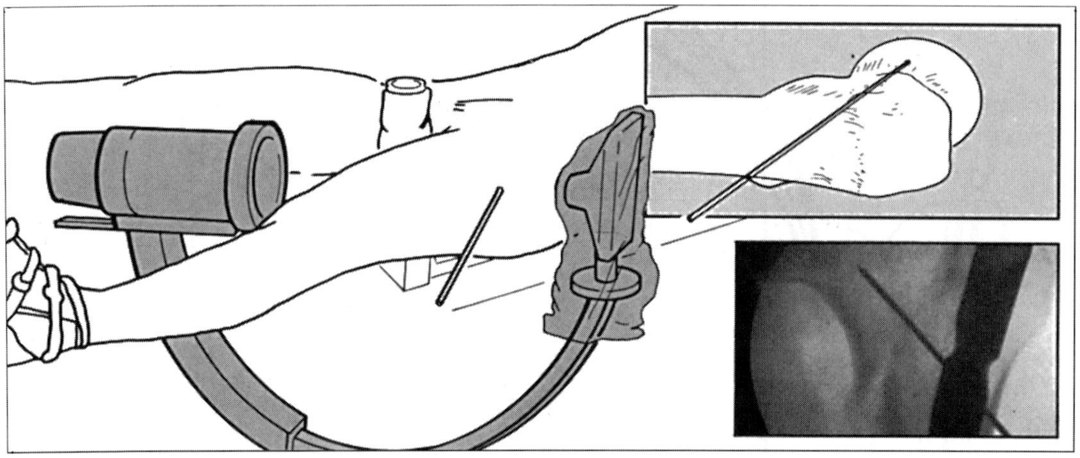

Fig. 7–8. This figure shows the use of the C-arm in the lateral position to determine anteversion. Either the use of a guide wire up the anterior aspect of the neck and impaled into the head neck junction or the tilting of the C-arm to get a true lateral can be useful. This will provide a view which shows the femoral head and the neck and shaft all in one line or collinear. The degree of rotation of the C-arm will determine the amount of anteversion the nail must be placed in. (Courtesy of Howmedica; Rutherford, NJ.)

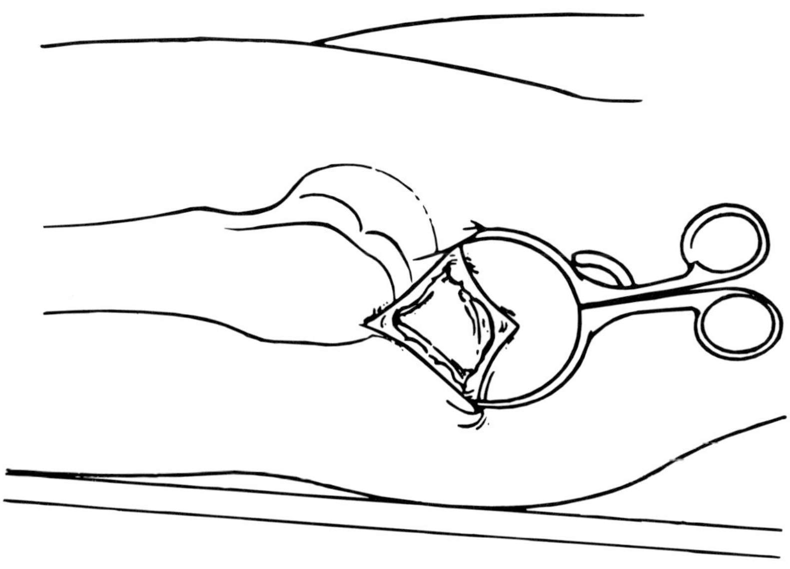

Fig. 7–9. An 8-cm incision is made starting at the tip of trochanter and directed in a linear fashion above the trochanteric region. (Courtesy of Howmedica; Rutherford, NJ.)

that the threaded portion be placed right into the subchondral bone, so it does not migrate when using the lag screw reamer. Usually an awl is necessary to broach the outer cortex, so that the guide wire can pass in easily. Care should be taken as this is done not to push the nail back out or to push the cannula up into a more proximal position.

Once the guide wire position is confirmed on the C-arm in both AP and lateral views, then the reamer is used. The reamer should first be started by hand. The reamer is available in two sizes of increasing diameter. If there has been any proximal shifting of the cannulas, the reamer will bind between the guide wire and the nail, consequently making passage difficult. If power is being used, there is potential to destroy the nail, the reamers, or both and to amputate the guide wire. Consequently, insertion should be carried out by hand until all stages of the reamer have passed through the hole in the nail, and then power may be added to advance the reamer. This maybe necessary in young individuals who have very dense bone in the femoral head. Adequate reaming is confirmed by the pre-set stop on the shaft of the reamer or when the tip of the reamer just reaches the threads of the guide wire. Once the double channel has been reamed, the compression lag screw is inserted into the proximal femoral head. Position is confirmed by C-arm (Fig. 7–12).

The set screw is then inserted. In unstable fracture patterns, the insertion of the distal screws should be carried out. The guides are very accurate if used appropriately. With the awl inserted through the appropriate cannula, the lateral femoral cortex is manually broached. At no time is a hammer used to tap the awl into the cortex. This may cause microfractures and jeopardize fixation. At this point the drill is then placed through the cannula, and advanced under C-arm visualization through the profile of the hole in nail. It is important to watch this to make sure that one does not deflect posteriorly or anteriorly and create extra holes that will cause stress risers. Following drilling through both cortices, screw length is measured and a fully threaded screw is inserted through the hole. It is probably unnecessary to use more then one screw distally, unless the nail has been used to treat very distal subtrochanteric fractures (Fig. 7–13).

IMPACTION

These devices allow mechanical compression following screw insertion. However, with poor bone quality there is the potential for this to tear the thread out of the head or, more importantly, the impaction device tends to go through the lateral lag screw hole and migrate into the bone. Consequently, manual impaction by releasing the traction and pushing on the greater trochanteric region is a good alternative method of achieving impaction of the fracture.

CLOSURE

The instruments are removed and the wounds are closed. At this time review of the position of the screw should be undertaken to make sure that there is no interarticular penetration.

POSTOPERATIVE COURSE

Biomechanically, the nail can withstand between 3 to 5 times body weight; the only limiting factor for weight bearing postoperatively is the weakness of the bone. As most bone will be able to withstand this weight bearing, one is able to allow the patient to be weight bearing as tolerated on the first postoperative day. One contraindication to this is where a distal screw hole has been missed. A small fall or twist of the leg may lead to a femoral shaft fracture at the tip of the nail. Also, full weight bearing or weight bearing as tolerated is limited in those fractures which are in the subtrochanteric region and extend downward to within 4 to 5 cm of the proximal distal locking screw. In this situation it maybe more advisable to prescribe toe touch with crutches. In standard fracture patterns in the intertrochanteric subtrochanteric region of all patients, other than the above, weight bearing as tolerated is allowed.

Follow-up of radiographs between 7 to 10 days are imperative to make sure that the implant is in a good position, there is no evidence of loosening or cut out, and impaction is occurring. Follow-up at 6 weeks is carried out with radiograph control to again confirm position of the implant and appropriate healing. By 3 months, follow-up radiograph control should show consolidation. If at this time there is some question about delayed union in the intertrochanteric-subtrochanteric region, then se-

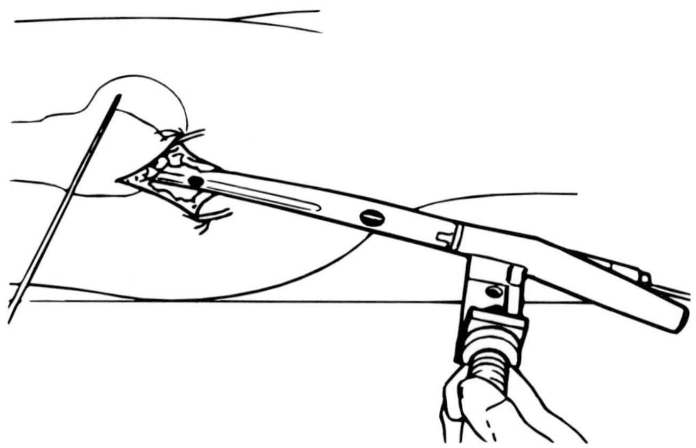

A

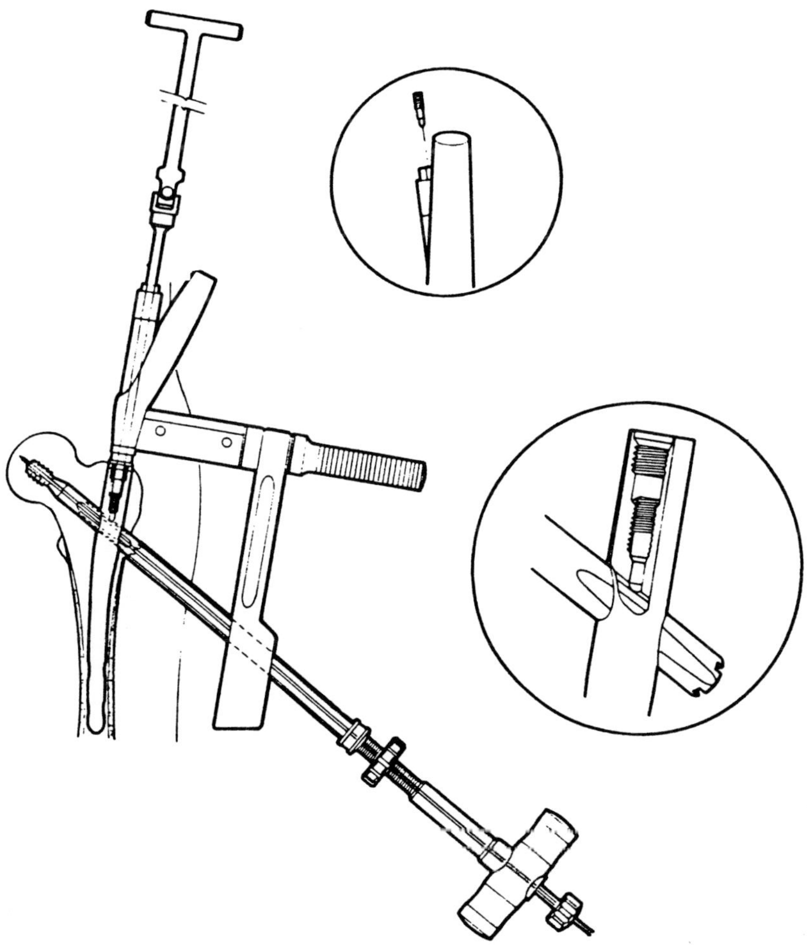

B

Fig. 7–12. *A,* The nail is then inserted by hand. If there is any resistance to nail insertion then further reaming of the canal or correction of the deformity or position of the nail in the anterior posterior or lateral view should be carried. *B,* As the nail is seated, the top of the nail sits on the trochanter and the anterior posterior view of the outline of the proximal locking screw hole sits just below the inferior aspect of the neck. In the lateral view, the nail should bisect the femoral head. Following this view, using the appropriate device the screw is then inserted up into the head. (Courtesy of Howmedica; Rutherford, NJ.)

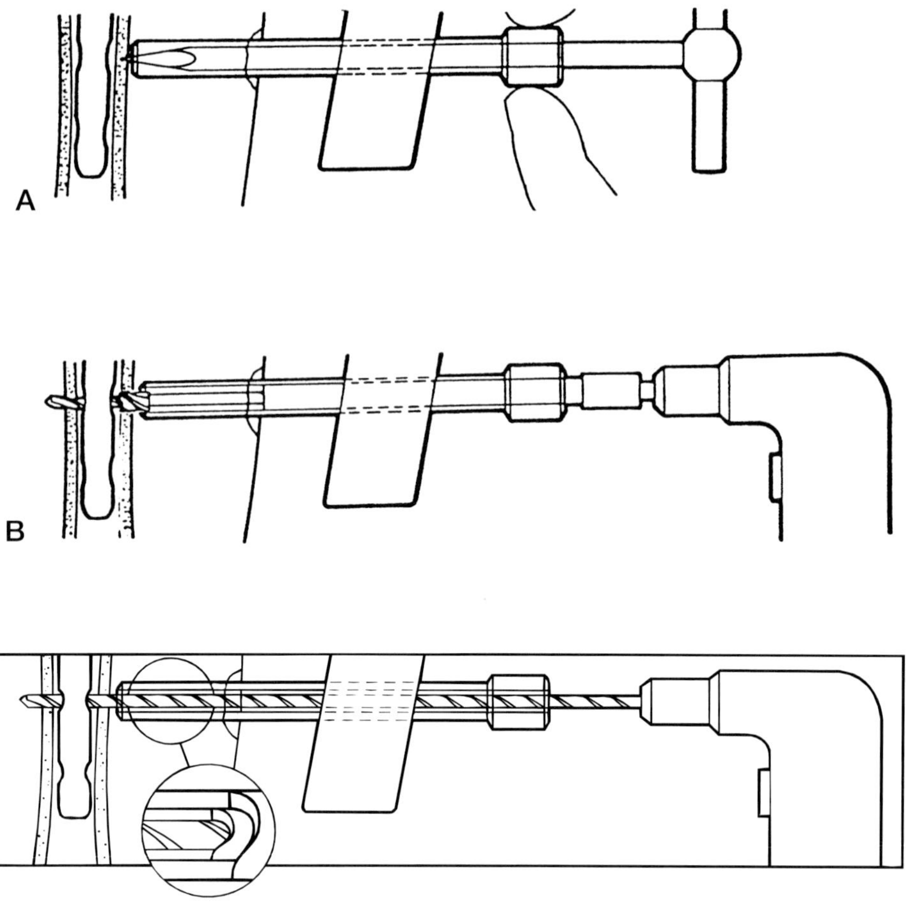

Fig. 7–13. Distal locking is then performed after the proximal screw has been inserted. Take care not to use an awl and hammer through the cortex for the fear of fracturing. Care should be taken as the drill is placed through to make sure it goes through the appropriate cannulas and the hole in the nail. (Courtesy of Howmedica; Rutherford, NJ.)

rious consideration should be given to dynamization of a statically locked nail. In the vast majority of situations, these fractures will be healed or on their way to healing and this is not necessary. Further follow-up at 6 months and 1 year is done with radiograph control to ascertain union. It is important that at 6 months and 1 year that appropriate functional evaluation of the patient be obtained. This includes subjective satisfaction, the ability to handle activities of daily living, the impact of the fracture upon their activities through work, sports, and recreation, and range of motion, shortening, and strength of the extremity.

PITFALLS AND POSTOPERATIVE COMPLICATIONS

As with any device, there are significant pitfalls and problems that are inherent in their use. It is imperative that the surgeon be aware of these prior to undertaking the implantation of this device. First and foremost, this is a closed intramedullary technique. Consequently, all the rules and guidelines of closed intramedullary nailing of the femur apply: (1) the patient must be positioned correctly on the table, (2) a closed reduction must be obtainable or obtained, and (3) the appropriate equipment and radiograph control are present in a good working order. The major aim in this procedure is bringing the neck and head into correct relationship with the femoral shaft, in essence, to restore length the correct CCD angle and avoid rotational deformity. As mentioned before, one must obtain an anatomical reduction of the CCD angle and length and rotation in the AP plane. Any final control for reduction in the lateral plane can be done intraoperatively, either by a closed technique or with the introduction of appropriate instruments to help reduce and control its position.

Intraoperative pitfalls are only those that occur if the technique is not followed exactly. This is a very unforgiving technical operation. It is not like a sliding compression hip screw in which there can be some room for error in the implant and lag screw positioning. With this device, this is not allowed. Consequently, three key points should be observed: (1) the insertion of this device requires no hammering, (2) insertion of the lag screw must be done manually, and (3) there should be no attempt to achieve a tight canal fit with the nail. The canal must be reamed 2 to 2.5 mm greater than the nail diameter chosen for insertion.

The major postoperative complication of this device has been the occurrence of femoral shaft fractures at the tip of the nail. The cause of this has been unclear. However, it appears to be related to several technical problems. The first is the use of the awl to broach the lateral cortex when putting in the distal locking screws. If the awl is hammered, this will tend to create microfractures in the bone, which will proliferate with a small twist within the first several weeks and lead to a spiral fracture around the tip of the nail. It can be theorized that the greater the canal fill of the distal portion of the nail, the greater the stress riser at the end of the nail; this will increase the risk of femoral shaft fracture as well. In order to avoid this, one should not hammer the awl and one should use the smallest nail possible for the diameter of the femur that is present. Distal screw fixation may also be omitted, but when this is done one must realize that there is no rotational control on the nail; therefore, in the postoperative course there may be increasing pain and discomfort, as well as inability to control the rotational position of the leg, thus leading to external rotation deformity. It probably is adequate enough to use only one distal screw in the proximal hole. Another cause is proximal femoral deformity that will make it difficult to insert the nail.

Superior cut out of the lag screw has been reported. This is a technical error on behalf of the operating surgeon. The screw must be placed in the center portion of the femoral head on both the AP and lateral within 5 to 10 mm of the subchondral plate. If this is done the chance of screw cut out is minimized. This is the same as with a compression hip screw. The device itself is not more prone to this. Careful attention when placing the screw into the head through the nail must be observed. If the rotation of the nail is wrong, the nail must be extracted and then rerotated and reinserted. The reason for this is that once the medial lateral bow of the nail has been fully implanted, rotation is limited by the proximal angle of the device. Attempts to rotate the nail may crack or lever off the greater trochanter. Consequently, one has to back the nail out until the bend is out of the femur and then reinsert in a different position to correct the rotational abnormality.

Another concern is the length of the lag screw. The length of this screw must extend from 5 to 10 mm of the subchondral boney surface to the outer aspect of the lateral femoral cortex. If for some reason the screw falls inside the lateral cortex, there is the potential that it will not slide as it will be caught on the cortex. Care must be taken to choose the right length of screw, so that the inferior distal end is left outside the lateral cortex. This may lead to discomfort in thin patients over the prominence of the screw at times, but this has not been a major concern.

CLINICAL EXPERIENCE

The original clinical experience of the nail has been reported by Kempf.[19] He reported on 120 patients, 90% of which had acute fractures with an average operating time of 38 minutes. All fractures consolidated and in 84.5% the results were good or very good. Complications included 3 cut outs of the lag screw from the femoral head, 2 fractures of the superior part of the femoral diaphysis caused by excessive force during nail introduction, 2 cases of varus greater than 10°, 1 case late consolidation, and 1 case of infection. The investigators felt the use of this nail was better than the use of Ender's nails for the treatment of intertrochanteric and high subtrochanteric fractures and allowed earlier weight bearing and better rehabilitation. In a large series of 648 cases from a multicenter Italian study reported by Boriani, the investigators found that 70% of the patients were able to bear weight in the first postoperative week, and 78% of the patients had returned to their preinjury walking ability.

Complications included shaft fractures in 3% of the cases, lag screw cut out in 3% of the cases, and a 0.5% nail failure. These shaft fractures all occurred when excessive force was used to insert the nail. No fracture occurred with 2 mm of over reaming and introduction by hand. Postoperative shaft fracturing occurred in 5 of 419 cases; all were caused by significant trauma.

Another large multicenter trial reported by Chen has shown that in 331 cases this has been a reliable technique.[20] Their average operating time was 58 minutes with a 10.8% intraoperative complication rate involving 7 cases of fracture in the lateral cortex, 3 jamming of the nail, and 5 failures to lock the distal screws. Three cases of distal diaphyseal fracturing did occur. In 15.2% general postoperative complications were noted with a common complication being chest infections. In this series there was a 7.5% complication in the postoperative phase. This series had 5 cases of shaft fracture and 5 cases of compression lag screw failure for a rate of less then 1.8% for either of these complications. By 6 months all fractures were healed, and sliding of the screw was 5.96 mm on average. At 6 months, follow-up was good with regards to pain, function, and motion. They concluded that this device is an effective implant for the Asian Pacific patient with peritrochanteric fractures when the appropriate surgical techniques were followed.

Two randomized prospective trials have been published with regards to the comparison of the intramedullary hip screw concept with compression sliding screw nails. Bridle reviewed 100 patients in a prospective fashion randomizing them to an intramedullary hip screw group and a compression hip screw group.[21] Fifty cases were in each group. They showed there was no significant difference in their groups between age, sex, mental testing, and anesthesia severity and fracture pattern. In the results there was no significant difference with regard to set up time, anesthesia complications, blood loss, postoperative hemoglobin, transfusion requirements, and hospital stay. As well, there was no significant difference with regard to mortality, complications, and morbidity. The only significant difference between the two systems was the position of the lag screw with the compression hip screw being worse, but there still was an equal cut out rate between the two techniques. The major problem was femoral shaft fractures in the postoperative phase. One of these was iatrogenic and three were secondary to trauma. The conclusion from this study was that there was no difference between the intramedullary hip screw nail and the compression hip screw in a randomized prospective trial. However, the study did emphasize the concern of the femoral shaft fracture complication and suggested redesign of the implant.

Leung presented a randomized prospective trial of 225 fractures of which 186 were followed for 7 months.[22] These were randomized into 93 compression hip screws and 93 intramedullary hip screws. In this study the only significant differences between the 2 systems showed that the intramedullary hip screws had significantly decreased C-arm time, blood loss, and time to full weight bearing, but they experienced an increased intraoperative complication rate. However, these complications were not significant in the long term. They felt that the nail itself did not really show any major difference over the use of the compression hip screw, but there appeared to be a tendency for this nail to work better in the more unstable intertrochanteric-subtrochanteric fractures. Further cohort or randomized prospective studies have shown that there is very little difference in operative technique, blood loss, and outcome. The major concern in all studies has been the incidence of femoral shaft fracture. This does require a significant operation to correct this complication. Consequently, this device has not gained full popularity. However, it should be pointed out that in all studies the cause of this in the intraoperative phase or early postoperative phase can probably be directly related to inappropriate technical use. Long-term femoral shaft fractures appear to be unrelated to the nail and are probably no greater than those that occur associated with stress rising effect of a plate on the lateral cortex of the femur.

OVERVIEW

As can be seen by the randomized prospective trials done to date, there is no significant difference between the intramedullary hip screw concept and the sliding compression screw. Although it may be stronger biomechanically and provides some increased axial stiffness in the more unstable situation, the intramedullary hip screw concept is equal to the sliding compression hip screw.

So, where is the role of this concept in the present treatment of proximal femoral fractures? It appears from clinical experience and the articles written that more unstable fractures have a tendency to do better with the intramedullary hip screw concept. A randomized prospective trial will be necessary to prove this. However, in those fractures in which reduction is difficult and where there is significant instability, this intramedullary hip screw technique offers a consistent technical procedure with minimal blood loss which will give a reasonable anatomical alignment and consistent healing. This is probably not so of the compression hip screw at this time. Presently, based on clinical experience the best indication for this device is in the unstable intertrochanteric fracture with significant posterior medially comminution and in the intertrochanteric-subtrochanteric fracture that does not extend more than 5 cm below the subtrochanteric region. Although it is no better than a sliding compression hip screw, this does not prevent the surgeon from using this for all intertrochanteric fractures if he is well skilled in the use of intramedullary devices in a closed fashion, and follows the technical aspects of this device properly. There is no doubt that this a less forgiving implant than the sliding compression hip screw and therefore must be treated with much more respect and care when implanted.

REFERENCES

1. Levy, R.N.: Intertrochanteric hip fractures. In Skeletal Trauma. Edited by Browner, B., Jupiter, J., Levine, A., & Trafton, P., Philadelphia, W.B. Saunders Co., 1992.
2. Russell, A., Taylor, C.: Subtrochanteric fractures of the femur. *In* Skeletal Trauma. Edited by B. Browner, J. Jupiter, A. Levin, & P. Trafton. Philadelphia, W. B. Saunders Co., 1992.
3. Larsson, S. Frieberg, S., Hensson, L.: Trochanteric fractures influence of reduction implant position on impaction and complications. Clin. Orthop. *259*:130, 1990.
4. Parker, M.J., Myles, J.W., Anand, J.K., Drewet, R.: Cost benefit analysis of hip fracture treatment. J. Bone Joint Surg. *74B*:261, 1992.
5. Senter, B., Kendig, R., Savoie, F.H.: Operative stabilization of subtrochanteric fractures of the femur. J. Orthop. Trauma *4*:399, 1990.
6. Waddell, J.T.: Subtrochanteric fractures of the femur: A review of 130 patients. J. Trauma *29*:582, 1979.
7. Wu, C., Sheih, C., Lee, Z.: Subtrochanteric fractures treated with interlocking nailing. J. Trauma. *31*:326, 1991.
8. Seligson, D., Henry, S., Hemple, D.: Küntscher Y-nailing. In the Science and Practice of Intramedullary Nailing, Ed. Browner, B. and Edwards, C.: Philadelphia, PA, Lea & Febiger, 1986.
9. Ender, H.: The treatment of pertrochanteric and subtrochanteric fixation with Ender nails. In the Science and Practice of Intramedullary Fixation. Ed. Browner: B. and Edwards, C., Lea & Febiger, Philadelphia, 1987.
10. Jeffries, J.E., Schaumburg, P.W., Weissfeld, S.C.: Clinical experience with Ender nailing of proximal femur. In the Science and Practice of Intramedullary Fixation, Ed. Browner, B. and Edwards, C.: Page 115. Lea & Febiger: 1987 Philadelphia.
11. Zickel, R.E.: An intramedullary fixation device for proximal part of the femur: 9 years' experience J.Bone Joint Surg. *58A*:866, 1976.
12. Grosse, E.A., Taglang, G.: Gamma Locking Nail: Surgical technique. London: Howmedica. 1990.
13. Halder, S.C.: The gamma nail for peritrochanteric fractures. J. Bone Joint Surg. *74B*:340, 1992.
14. Küntscher, G.: The Practice of Intramedullary Nailing. Springfield, Illinois short form. Charles C. Thomas, 1967.
15. Mahomed, N., Hearn, T., Kellam, J.: Biomechanical Analysis of the Gamma Nail and Sliding Hip Screw. Presented at Annual Orthopaedic Trauma Association Meeting 1990, Toronto Ontario Canada.
16. Rosenblum, S.F., Zukerman, J.D., Kummer, F.J., Tamb, S.: A biomechanical evaluation of the gamma nail. J. Bone Joint Surg. *74B*:352, 1992.
17. Kyle, R.: Biomechanical Analysis of the Sliding Characteristics of the Gamma Nail. Presented at Orthopaedic Trauma Association Annual Meeting, Minneapolis, MN 1992.
18. Shaw, J.: Treating Stable and Unstable Intertrochanteric Fractures and Subtrochanteric Fractures with Compression Hip Screw and Gamma Nail. Presented at Orthopaedic Trauma Association, Minneapolis, MN 1992.
19. Kempf, I. Grosse, A., Taglang, G.: The Gamma Nail. In Proximal Femoral Fractures.: Ed. Marti, R.K. and Dunki-Jacobs, P.B. Page 439 Medical Press Limited, London, 1993.
20. Chen, C.M., Leung, K.S.: Multicentric trial with the AP gamma nail in east Asia. Presented at Strausburg Annual Trauma Course, March 31 through April 2, 1993. Strausburg, France.
21. Bridle, S.H., Patel, A.D, Bircher, M., Calvert, P.T.: Fixation of intertrochanteric fractures of the femur: A randomized prospective comparison of the gamma nail and the dynamic hip screw. J. Bone Joint Surg. *73B*: 330, 1991.
22. Leung, K.S., So, W.S, Shen, W. Y., Hui, P.W.: Gamma nail and dynamic hips screws for pertrochanteric fractures. J. Bone Joint Surg. *74B*:345, 1992.
23. Boriani, S.: Results of the multicentric Italian experience on the gamma nail: A report of 640 cases. Orthopedics. 1307, 1991.

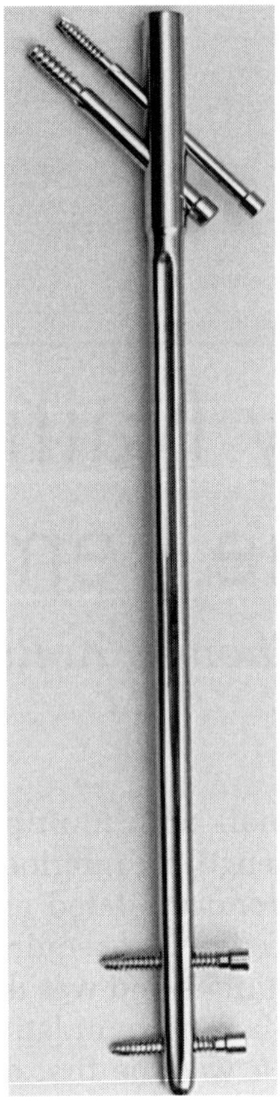

Fig. 8–1. Russell-Taylor Reconstruction nail courtesy of Smith & Nephew Richards, Memphis, Tennessee.

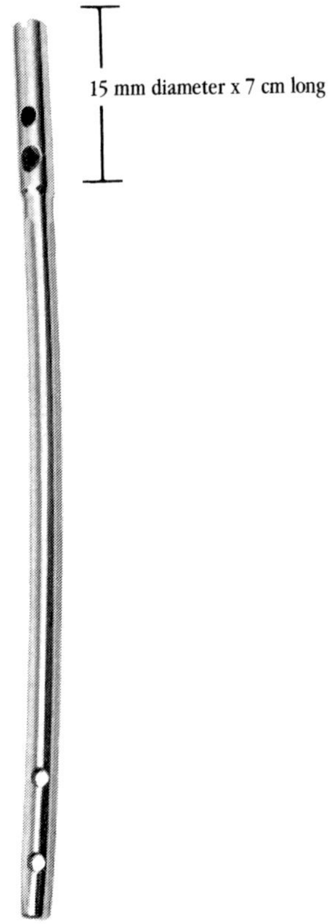

Fig. 8–2. Russell-Taylor Reconstruction nail proximal expansion to 15 mm over 7 cm segment to maximize fatigue strength in subtrochanteric area.

study confirmed that nail stiffness is proportional to the fourth power of the outer diameter of the nail **minus** the inner diameter of the nail to the fourth power. Similarly, strength relates to the third power of the outer diameter **minus** the third power of the inner diameter. This proportionality allowed modification of each Reconstruction nail to a specified stiffness by varying the wall thickness.

Strength and stiffness characteristics are also related to nail curvature and cross section (slotted or nonslotted). By increasing the proximal diameter of the first 7 cm of the Reconstruction nail to 15 mm and using a closed section design throughout the nail, the highly stressed proximal region is maximally reinforced (Fig. 8–2). This did not increase the effective nail stiffness, because this proximal section is not in an area requiring nail elastic deformation during insertion.

The next area of biomechanical concern involved the perforations within the nail proximally and distally. Interlocking intramedullary nails have been shown by Bucholz et al. to be subject to fatigue failure, preferentially through the locking holes in the nail.[2] Methods to minimize this stress concentration about the perforations yielded two modifications. First in the proximal hole region, the nail is reinforced to 15 mm in diameter as stated and the neck shaft angle for the holes was selected at 135°, which allows the best sliding characteristics for the proximal screw fixation. A new technique of cold-working the distal holes, borrowed from the aerospace industry, involves cold-working the distal locking holes to leave residual compressive stresses at the distal perforations, greatly increasing the fatigue life of the implant.[3] This combination of varying wall thickness, cross section modification, and perforation reinforcement maximizes the strength and fatigue characteristics of the nail while maintaining ample flexibility for ease of nail insertion.

The interlocking screws are of three different types. Proximally, an 8-mm sliding lag screw and/or a 6.4-mm sliding lag screw are used. Similar to a 135° hip compression screw, proximal fixation uses a sliding lag screw that allows compression across the fracture in femoral neck

So, where is the role of this concept in the present treatment of proximal femoral fractures? It appears from clinical experience and the articles written that more unstable fractures have a tendency to do better with the intramedullary hip screw concept. A randomized prospective trial will be necessary to prove this. However, in those fractures in which reduction is difficult and where there is significant instability, this intramedullary hip screw technique offers a consistent technical procedure with minimal blood loss which will give a reasonable anatomical alignment and consistent healing. This is probably not so of the compression hip screw at this time. Presently, based on clinical experience the best indication for this device is in the unstable intertrochanteric fracture with significant posterior medially comminution and in the intertrochanteric-subtrochanteric fracture that does not extend more than 5 cm below the subtrochanteric region. Although it is no better than a sliding compression hip screw, this does not prevent the surgeon from using this for all intertrochanteric fractures if he is well skilled in the use of intramedullary devices in a closed fashion, and follows the technical aspects of this device properly. There is no doubt that this a less forgiving implant than the sliding compression hip screw and therefore must be treated with much more respect and care when implanted.

REFERENCES

1. Levy, R.N.: Intertrochanteric hip fractures. In Skeletal Trauma. Edited by Browner, B., Jupiter, J., Levine, A., & Trafton, P., Philadelphia, W.B. Saunders Co., 1992.
2. Russell, A., Taylor, C.: Subtrochanteric fractures of the femur. *In* Skeletal Trauma. Edited by B. Browner, J. Jupiter, A. Levin, & P. Trafton. Philadelphia, W. B. Saunders Co., 1992.
3. Larsson, S. Frieberg, S., Hensson, L.: Trochanteric fractures influence of reduction implant position on impaction and complications. Clin. Orthop. *259*:130, 1990.
4. Parker, M.J., Myles, J.W., Anand, J.K., Drewet, R.: Cost benefit analysis of hip fracture treatment. J. Bone Joint Surg. *74B*:261, 1992.
5. Senter, B., Kendig, R., Savoie, F.H.: Operative stabilization of subtrochanteric fractures of the femur. J. Orthop. Trauma *4*:399, 1990.
6. Waddell, J.T.: Subtrochanteric fractures of the femur: A review of 130 patients. J. Trauma *29*:582, 1979.
7. Wu, C., Sheih, C., Lee, Z.: Subtrochanteric fractures treated with interlocking nailing. J. Trauma. *31*:326, 1991.
8. Seligson, D., Henry, S., Hemple, D.: Küntscher Y-nailing. In the Science and Practice of Intramedullary Nailing, Ed. Browner, B. and Edwards, C.: Philadelphia, PA, Lea & Febiger, 1986.
9. Ender, H.: The treatment of pertrochanteric and subtrochanteric fixation with Ender nails. In the Science and Practice of Intramedullary Fixation. Ed. Browner: B. and Edwards, C., Lea & Febiger, Philadelphia, 1987.
10. Jeffries, J.E., Schaumburg, P.W., Weissfeld, S.C.: Clinical experience with Ender nailing of proximal femur. In the Science and Practice of Intramedullary Fixation, Ed. Browner, B. and Edwards, C.: Page 115. Lea & Febiger: 1987 Philadelphia.
11. Zickel, R.E.: An intramedullary fixation device for proximal part of the femur: 9 years' experience J.Bone Joint Surg. *58A*:866, 1976.
12. Grosse, E.A., Taglang, G.: Gamma Locking Nail: Surgical technique. London: Howmedica. 1990.
13. Halder, S.C.: The gamma nail for peritrochanteric fractures. J. Bone Joint Surg. *74B*:340, 1992.
14. Küntscher, G.: The Practice of Intramedullary Nailing. Springfield, Illinois short form. Charles C. Thomas, 1967.
15. Mahomed, N., Hearn, T., Kellam, J.: Biomechanical Analysis of the Gamma Nail and Sliding Hip Screw. Presented at Annual Orthopaedic Trauma Association Meeting 1990, Toronto Ontario Canada.
16. Rosenblum, S.F., Zukerman, J.D., Kummer, F.J., Tamb, S.: A biomechanical evaluation of the gamma nail. J. Bone Joint Surg. *74B*:352, 1992.
17. Kyle, R.: Biomechanical Analysis of the Sliding Characteristics of the Gamma Nail. Presented at Orthopaedic Trauma Association Annual Meeting, Minneapolis, MN 1992.
18. Shaw, J.: Treating Stable and Unstable Intertrochanteric Fractures and Subtrochanteric Fractures with Compression Hip Screw and Gamma Nail. Presented at Orthopaedic Trauma Association, Minneapolis, MN 1992.
19. Kempf, I. Grosse, A., Taglang, G.: The Gamma Nail. In Proximal Femoral Fractures.: Ed. Marti, R.K. and Dunki-Jacobs, P.B. Page 439 Medical Press Limited, London, 1993.
20. Chen, C.M., Leung, K.S.: Multicentric trial with the AP gamma nail in east Asia. Presented at Strausburg Annual Trauma Course, March 31 through April 2, 1993. Strausburg, France.
21. Bridle, S.H., Patel, A.D, Bircher, M., Calvert, P.T.: Fixation of intertrochanteric fractures of the femur: A randomized prospective comparison of the gamma nail and the dynamic hip screw. J. Bone Joint Surg. *73B*: 330, 1991.
22. Leung, K.S., So, W.S, Shen, W. Y., Hui, P.W.: Gamma nail and dynamic hips screws for pertrochanteric fractures. J. Bone Joint Surg. *74B*:345, 1992.
23. Boriani, S.: Results of the multicentric Italian experience on the gamma nail: A report of 640 cases. Orthopedics. 1307, 1991.

8

Cephalomedullary Nailing of the Femur

Thomas A. Russell

Cephalomedullary nails or "second generation" interlocking intramedullary nails were introduced in 1986 in North America. The prototype for this class of intramedullary nail system is the Russell-Taylor Reconstruction nail (Smith & Nephew Richards, Memphis, Tennessee)(Fig. 8–1). It was designed in 1985 to expand the benefits of closed interlocking intramedullary nailing into the more proximal femoral region. Subsequently, the Delta Reconstruction nail and Delta II Reconstruction nails were designed for use in smaller femoral anatomy situations.

The Reconstruction nail combines a closed antegrade intramedullary nail technique with interlocking screws that permit fixation into the femoral head. Interlocking screws distally in the epiphyseal area provide rotational and axial stability of the femoral shaft. The nail is curved slightly less than the average curvature of the femoral shaft. The nail design is altered throughout its length with variations in cross section to maximize its strength and to minimize its stiffness.

Historically, the Küntscher Y nail, the Huckstep nail, and the Zickel nail are the predecessors of the Russell-Taylor Reconstruction nail. The stainless steel Küntscher Y nail employed a U-shaped blade inserted into the femoral head and neck that wedged into the intramedullary nail through a proximal perforation. The Küntscher Y nail did not control length and rotation very well and was prone to implant fatigue failure. The Huckstep nail consisted of a solid titanium nail with multiple perforations throughout its length for interlocking screws. The nail was noncannulated and straight in design. The Huckstep nail required insertion using an open technique and was difficult to insert because of its lack of cannulation and physiologic curvature. It was the first design with lag screws that could be inserted through the nail into the femoral head for sliding compression fixation of femoral neck fractures; however, there are no published reports of its use for this indication.

BIOMECHANICAL DESIGN RATIONALE

The Reconstruction nail was the first computer-assisted designed intramedullary nail. The specific design goals altered the nail geometry in order to achieve two goals. First, fatigue performance was maximized because of the high demands and stresses placed on this implant in the area of the proximal femur. Secondly, the proportional bending stiffness of the implant was disassociated from the external diameter to minimize stiffness for ease of nail insertion. In the case of the Reconstruction nail, this modification yielded a stiffness comparable to most 14-mm diameter interlocking femoral nails.

Biomechanical studies by Russell et al. confirmed the ability of the implant manufacturers to affect the stiffness and strength characteristics of commercially available nails by section modulus and wall thickness variations.[1] This

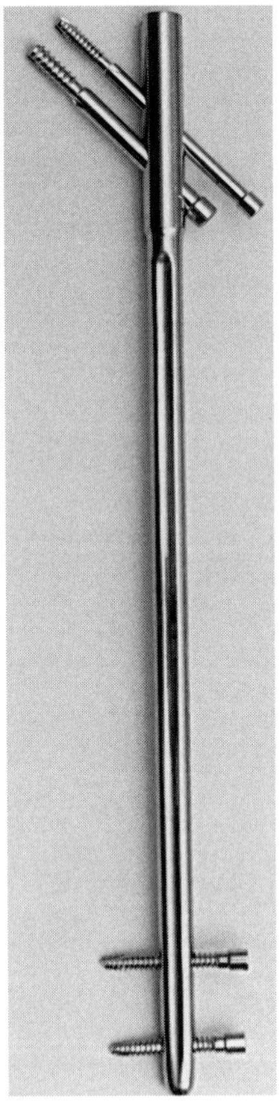

Fig. 8–1. Russell-Taylor Reconstruction nail courtesy of Smith & Nephew Richards, Memphis, Tennessee.

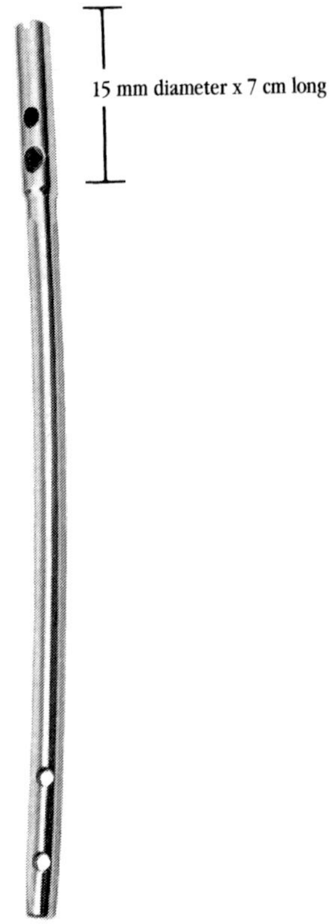

Fig. 8–2. Russell-Taylor Reconstruction nail proximal expansion to 15 mm over 7 cm segment to maximize fatigue strength in subtrochanteric area.

study confirmed that nail stiffness is proportional to the fourth power of the outer diameter of the nail **minus** the inner diameter of the nail to the fourth power. Similarly, strength relates to the third power of the outer diameter **minus** the third power of the inner diameter. This proportionality allowed modification of each Reconstruction nail to a specified stiffness by varying the wall thickness.

Strength and stiffness characteristics are also related to nail curvature and cross section (slotted or nonslotted). By increasing the proximal diameter of the first 7 cm of the Reconstruction nail to 15 mm and using a closed section design throughout the nail, the highly stressed proximal region is maximally reinforced (Fig. 8–2). This did not increase the effective nail stiffness, because this proximal section is not in an area requiring nail elastic deformation during insertion.

The next area of biomechanical concern involved the perforations within the nail proximally and distally. Interlocking intramedullary nails have been shown by Bucholz et al. to be subject to fatigue failure, preferentially through the locking holes in the nail.[2] Methods to minimize this stress concentration about the perforations yielded two modifications. First in the proximal hole region, the nail is reinforced to 15 mm in diameter as stated and the neck shaft angle for the holes was selected at 135°, which allows the best sliding characteristics for the proximal screw fixation. A new technique of cold-working the distal holes, borrowed from the aerospace industry, involves cold-working the distal locking holes to leave residual compressive stresses at the distal perforations, greatly increasing the fatigue life of the implant.[3] This combination of varying wall thickness, cross section modification, and perforation reinforcement maximizes the strength and fatigue characteristics of the nail while maintaining ample flexibility for ease of nail insertion.

The interlocking screws are of three different types. Proximally, an 8-mm sliding lag screw and/or a 6.4-mm sliding lag screw are used. Similar to a 135° hip compression screw, proximal fixation uses a sliding lag screw that allows compression across the fracture in femoral neck

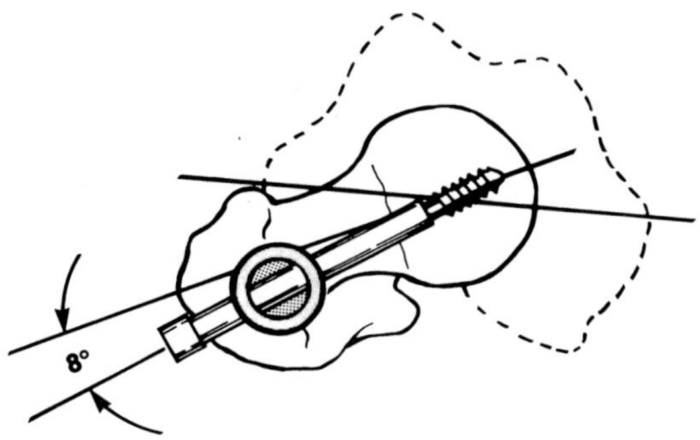

Fig. 8–3. Rotational anteversion of proximal screws are 8° reference to the distal locking screw alignment to facilitate proximal and distal locking.

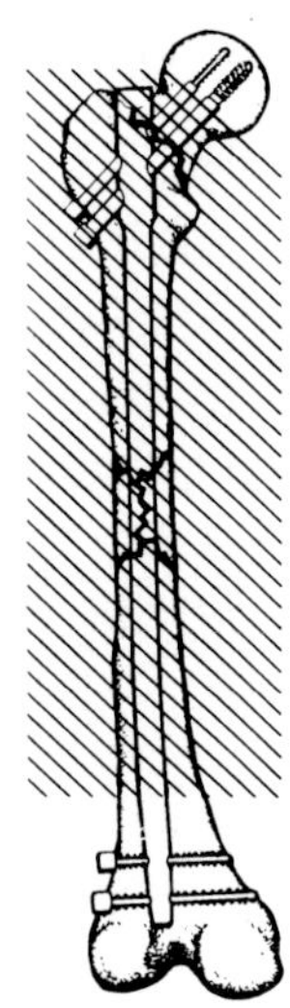

Fig. 8–4. Zone of application of Reconstruction nail to mid femoral neck to within approximately 6 cm of intercondylar notch of the distal femur.

and the basicervical fractures of the hip. Conceptually, two-screw fixation proximally minimizes rotational shear in the pertrochanteric area and in the femoral neck. Distally, 6.4-mm fully threaded cortical-type screws are used for interlocking in the standard Reconstruction nail.

Currently, standard Reconstruction nail sizes range from 12 to 14 mm in shaft diameter with a length of 36 cm to 48 cm. The nails are right and left sided. This was necessitated because of the anteversion of the femoral neck shaft axis. The proximal locking screw holes are oriented 8° anteriorly in relation to the distal screw holes to facilitate screw entry into the femoral head (Fig. 8–3). The Delta Reconstruction nail has a shaft diameter of 10 or 11 mm, lengths of 32 cm to 48 cm, and uses two 6.4-mm sliding lag screws proximally and 5-mm cortical screws distally; its proximal expansion is downsized to 13 mm. The Delta II Reconstruction nail has 8- or 9-mm shaft diameters with lengths of 24 to 38 cm and a 13-mm proximal expansion with 6.4-mm proximal sliding lag screws and 4.5-mm cortical screws distally.

INDICATIONS FOR RECONSTRUCTION NAILS

The Reconstruction interlocking nail was originally designed for the treatment of complex subtrochanteric femoral fractures and ipsilateral hip and shaft fractures. Mechanically, the Reconstruction nail in a static lock mode can be used to stabilize injuries and deformities from the midfemoral neck to approximately 4 cm above the knee (Fig. 8–4). This is occasionally quite useful for the treatment of pathologic fractures in the subtrochanteric area, because of possible later extension of the disease into the distal femur. We have also used the Reconstruction nail for the treatment of malunions and nonunions of the femur in which a long fatigue life will be required. The Reconstruction nail should not be considered as a nail of first choice for conventional diaphyseal fractures of the femur, as it introduces the further complexity of targeting and femoral head fixation with proximal sliding screws. Multiple studies have confirmed satisfactory results using conventional interlocking nails with diagonal interlocking screws, and we would prefer a conventional interlocking nail for true diaphyseal shaft fractures over the Reconstruction nail.

PREOPERATIVE PLANNING[4]

Preoperative radiographs should visualize the entire femur including the femoral head, neck, and knee on AP and lateral views. Inspect the radiographs carefully to detect intrarticular propagation of fractures or disease. Preoperative radiographs of the uninjured femur may be used to estimate proper nail diameter, expected amount of reaming, and final nail length for severely comminuted fractures. Radiograph templates for preoperative planning for the Reconstruction nail are available (Smith & Nephew Richards, Memphis, Tennessee). Distraction of the diaphyseal fracture must be obtained with traction before initiating closed antegrade intramedullary nailing (except in acute cases). Excessive intraoperative traction can lead to pudendal and sciatic nerve injuries.

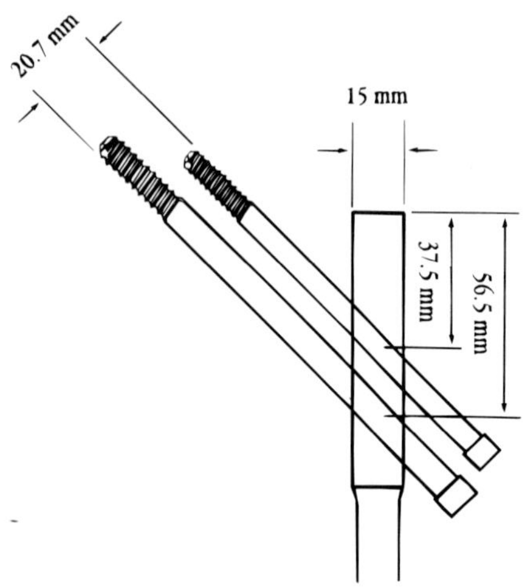

Fig. 8–5. Spacing of proximal fixation in 12, 13, 14 mm shaft diameters in the Russell-Taylor Reconstruction nail.

Proximally, measure the femoral neck width to determine the maximum spacing of the interlocking screws. The 12-, 13-, and 14-mm diameter Reconstruction nails have a 20.7-mm effective outer diameter (Fig. 8–5). The Delta and Delta II Reconstruction nails have a 17.4-mm effective outer diameter of the proximal locking screws (Fig. 8–6).

The nail size used depends on the size of the patient and the extent of femoral comminution. However, it should be noted that a small but consistent percentage of complications caused by nail fatigue failure remains. Therefore, it is always recommended that the largest implant suitable for the patient be used. The nail should fill the medullary canal at the isthmus to minimize translational deformation even when interlocking is employed. Further impaction is occasionally seen if severely comminuted fractures are later dynamized. This risk should be considered during selection of nail length to prevent later nail migration into the knee or nail protrusion out of the proximal femur.

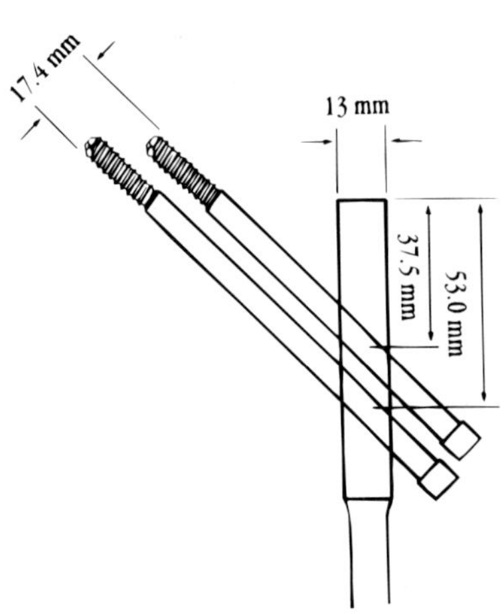

Fig. 8–6. Spacing of proximal fixation in 10 and 11 mm shaft diameters in the Russell-Taylor Delta reconstruction nail.

Surgical Technique

Patient Positioning

With the patient in the supine position, abduct the unaffected limb while adducting the trunk and affected extremity. Flex the affected hip 15°. Maintain the "heel-to-toe" relationship (Fig. 8–7). Apply traction through a skeletal pin or special foot holder through the fracture table. Determine rotational alignment of the proximal fragment with the image intensifier. Rotate the distal fragment to match the proximal fragment. Remember that the femoral neck anteversion in adults averages 15° in most North Americans but may be up to 30° in Oriental populations. In the supine position, correct rotation of the leg will usually place the foot in 0 to 15° of external rotation. Always check the uninvolved hip for rotational range of motion. The more restricted hip motion is preoperatively, the more critical

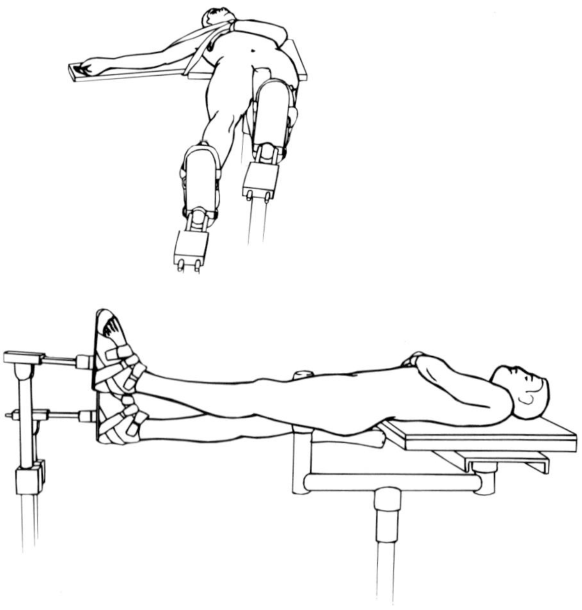

Fig. 8–7. Supine position recommended for Reconstruction nailing.

correct rotational alignment will be in the postoperative rehabilitation phase.

The lateral decubitus position is not recommended for the Reconstruction nail because of the necessity to view the femoral head and neck on AP and lateral radiographic projections. Some newer fracture tables may permit radiographic visualization in the lateral decubitus position, but open reduction of the femoral neck region, if required, would be difficult in the lateral position.

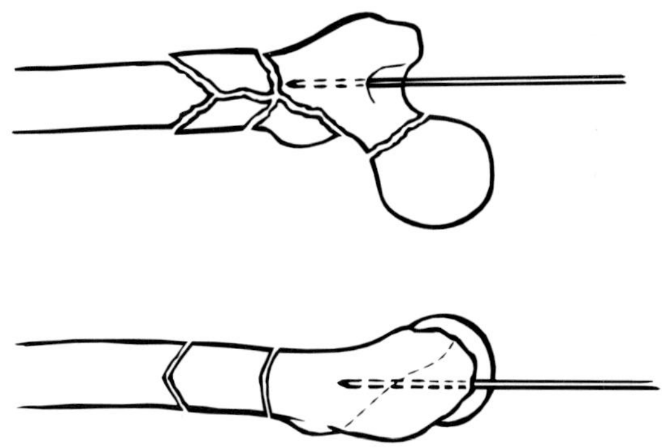

Fig. 8–9. Entry portal in line with medullary canal on AP and lateral radiographic views.

Patient Preparation

Scrub and prepare the patient in the standard manner. Drape the buttocks and lateral thigh to the popliteal crease. Cover the image intensifier arm with a sterile isolation drape.

Surgical Approach

Make an oblique skin incision just proximal to the greater trochanter and continue the incision proximally and medially for 9 to 10 cm (Fig. 8–8). Incise the fascia of the gluteus maximus in line with its fibers. Identify the subfascial plane of the gluteus maximus and palpate the trochanteric fossa.

Femoral Preparation

In all intramedullary nailing, determining the proper entry portal is crucial. This is especially important in extremely high subtrochanteric and femoral neck fractures, as an opening too laterally may create a varus reduction.

In the supine position, determine the entry site by using a 3.2-mm-tip threaded guide pin inserted at the trochanteric fossa, which will place the pin in the midplane of the femur in both AP and lateral views (Fig. 8–9). Enlarge the entry portal with the cannulated reamer. An alternative technique is to introduce the curved awl at the trochanteric fossa, though this technique is more suited for the lateral decubitus positioning. Make the opening directly in the midplane of the femur, verified on the AP and lateral views. Ream the proximal 8 cm of the femur to 15 mm in diameter. (Use the skin protector when reaming.)

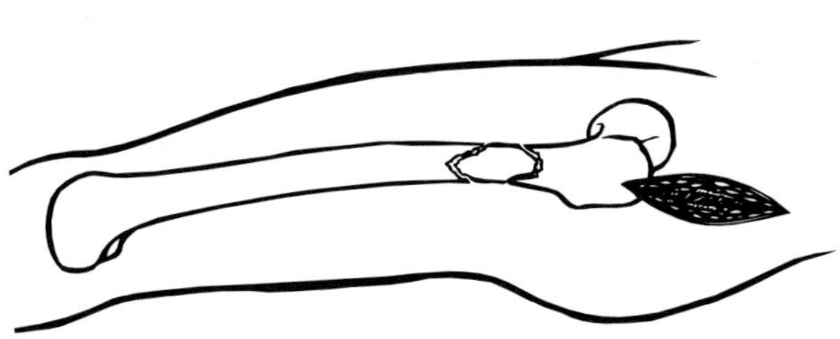

Fig. 8–8. Proximal incision. Avoid exposure of the piriformis fossa directly.

In the treatment of femoral neck fractures, obtaining and maintaining reduction of the femoral head and neck is primary and critical. The femoral neck fracture takes first priority and anatomic reduction is required, through open reduction and provisional fixation if necessary. Use the tapered straight medullary reamer as a "nail blank" in the metaphyseal canal, and insert Kirschner wires and/or cannulated screws anteriorly to posteriorly into the femoral head to stabilize the femoral neck fracture during reaming and nail insertion.

In some subtrochanteric fractures, the proximal femoral fragment is flexed, externally rotated, and adducted to such a degree that the entry portal cannot be visualized. Some fracture tables will allow a counter pad to elevate the affected hip, which will help position the hip into a more accessible position (Fig. 8–10).

Guide Rod Insertion

To assist in reduction of shaft fractures, three different 3.2-mm guide rods are available. Standard fractures will require a straight guide rod, although more severely displaced fractures may require the use of a curved-tip guide rod. For obstructed intramedullary canals, the cutting edge of a spade-tip guide rod may be helpful.

Introduce the selected guide rod by means of a T-handle chuck to the level of the fracture

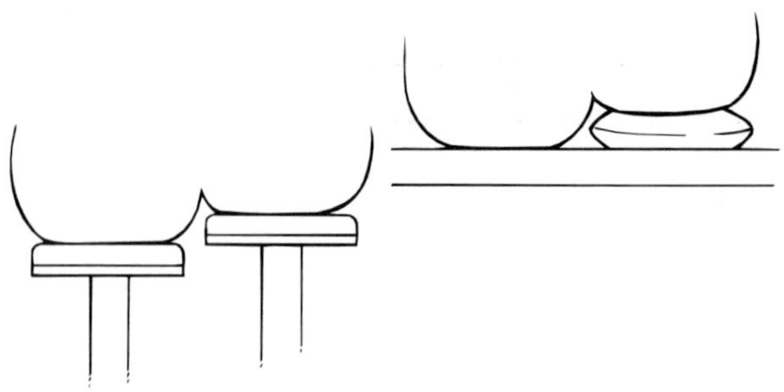

Fig. 8–10. Elevation of buttocks with use of the fracture table may aid the reduction of a subtrochanteric fracture.

(Fig. 8–11). Confirm its containment within the femur by means of AP and lateral fluoroscopic views. Ream the proximal fragment to a diameter of 10 mm in 0.5-mm increments with cannulated reamers. Reduce the proximal fragment to the distal fragment by means of the internal fracture alignment device (Fig. 8–12). Advance the guide rod into the center of the distal fragment until the tip reaches the old epiphyseal scar. Remove the internal fracture alignment device. Verify containment of the guide rod within the femur by image intensification.

Verification of the proper nail length may be determined by two separate methods, the guide rod method or the nail length gauge. In the guide rod method, place the distal end of the guide rod between the proximal pole of the patella and the distal femoral epiphyseal scar, overlap a second guide rod to the portion of the reduction guide rod extending proximally from the femoral entry portal. Subtract the length (XXX mm) of the overlapped guide rods from 900 mm to determine the nail length (Fig. 8–13). Alternatively, position the nail length gauge anterior to the femur (unaffected femur preoperatively; affected femur intraoperatively) with its distal end between the proximal pole of the patella and the distal femoral epiphyseal scar (Fig. 8–14). Move the C-arm to the proximal end of the femur and read from the image intensifier the correct nail length directly from the stamped measurements on the nail length gauge.

Ream the entire femur over the 3.2-mm guide rod in 0.5-mm increments until the desired diameter is achieved (Fig. 8–15). Usually, overream 1 mm larger than the selected nail diameter. In cases of excessive anterior bow of the femur detected on lateral radiographs or fracture extension into the distal one-fourth of the femur, overream 1.5 to 2 mm larger than the nail diameter. The final reamer diameter should be verified with the reamer template before nail selection and insertion. (Never insert a nail that has a larger diameter than the last reamer used.)

Introduce the medullary exchange tube over the guide rod to maintain fracture reduction. Replace the ball-tip guide rod with a 4-mm nail guide rod after the medullary exchange tube has entered the distal fragment in the distal metaphysis. Remove the medullary exchange tube. In cases of difficult alignment, one may choose not to remove the ball-tip reamer guide wire until the nail is seated in the distal metaphysis. In 12- to 14-mm Reconstruction nails, this is possible. In the 8- to 11-mm Reconstruction nails, however, a 3-mm driving guide wire is recommended.

Nail Insertion

Attach the selected nail to the proximal drill guide with the hexagonal bolt. When assembled properly, the nail will have an anterior bow and the keyed post of the proximal drill guide will point laterally.

Attach either the sliding hammer or supine driver to the bolt of the proximal drill guide and insert the nail over the guide rod. Use the keyed post as a handle to control rotation and aid insertion of the nail (Fig. 8–16). It is very important to never hit directly on the proximal drill guide; use the insertion instruments only. Striking the proximal drill guide may deform the alignment needed for proximal targeting. Retighten the bolt of the proximal drill guide assembly as needed and before final seating of the nail using the 11/16-inch open-end wrench or universal socket wrench.

Unlike most conventional interlocking femoral nails in which the nail is inserted until the proximal drill guide is flush with the tip of the greater trochanter, the Reconstruction nail must be inserted to the proper depth (with the aid of AP image intensification) to allow proximal screw placement in the femoral head. In obese patients, an offset Reconstruction/Delta Reconstruction driver may be attached to the proximal flat of the reconstruction proximal drill guide. This allows offset of the supine driver for easier insertion of the nail. In obese patients, a straight driver will tend to offset the

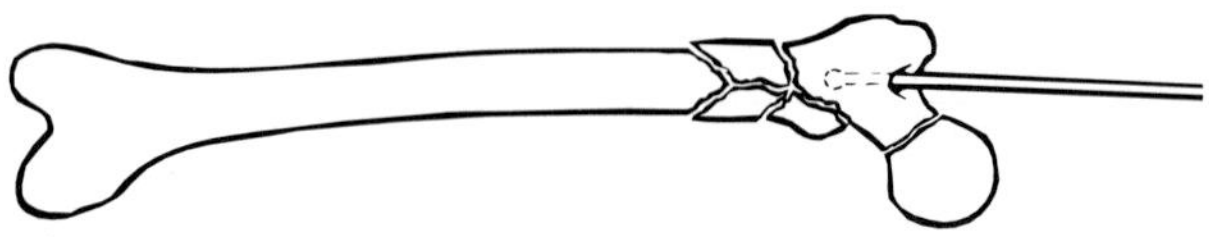

Fig. 8–11. Guide wire insertion for reduction of shaft fracture.

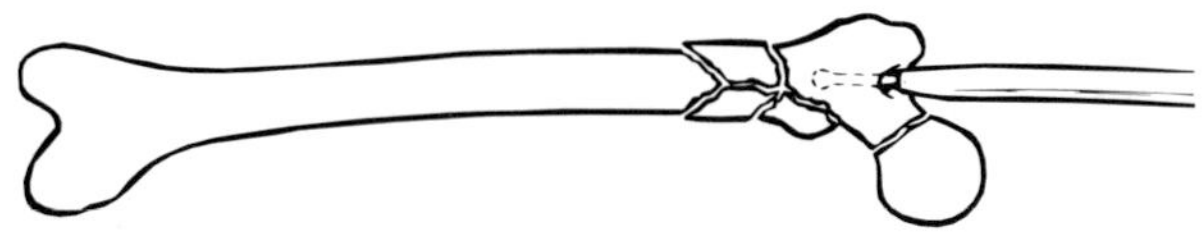

Fig. 8–12. Entry portal tool may be inserted over the guide wire to aid in reduction of the proximal fragment to the distal fragment.

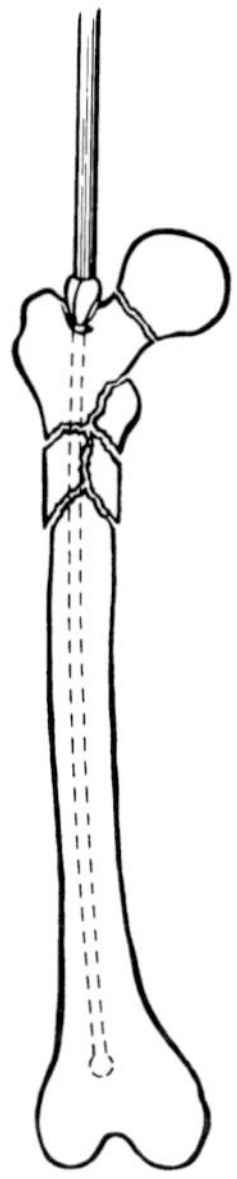

Fig. 8–15. Reaming of intramedullary canal in 0.5 mm increments when reaming cortical bone recommended. Usually reaming to 1 mm larger than the shaft diameter and 0.5 mm over the proximal expansion of the nail is recommended.

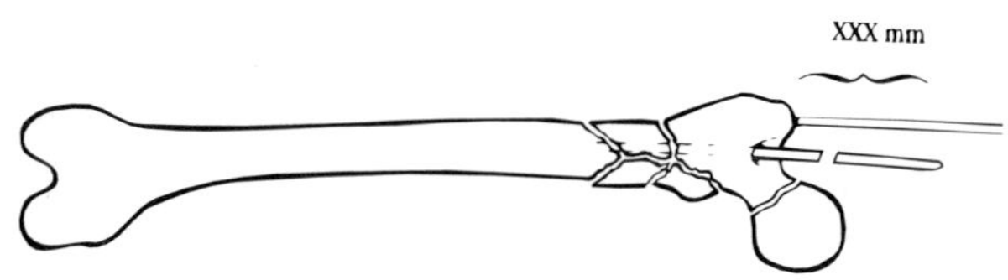

Fig. 8–13. Length measurement technique with the use of two equal length guide wires.

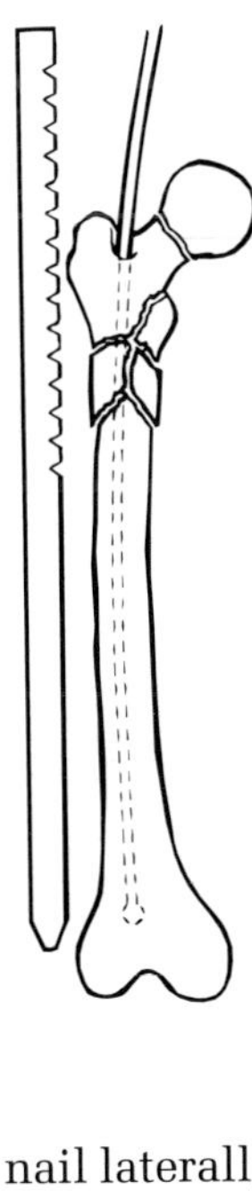

Fig. 8–14. Scanogram for estimation of leg length.

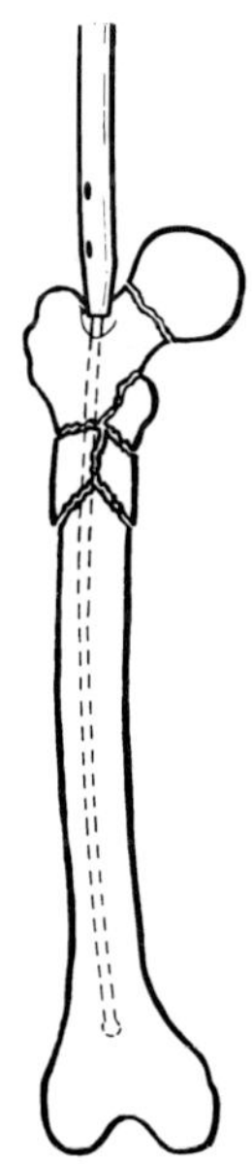

Fig. 8–16. During nail insertion, the nail may be used to reduce the proximal fragment to the distal fragment as the nail crosses the fracture site.

nail laterally and force the hip into varus if fracture extension or comminution is present medially. This occurs because of pressure of the driver on the lateral ilium. One may use the offset driver or remove the driving handle after nail seating to restore normal hip alignment.

To determine proper nail insertion depth, place the inferior drill sleeves (silver, green, blue, red) into the proximal drill guide to extrapolate the eventual location of the 8-mm inferior screw. If two screws are to be used, the nail should be inserted to a level allowing the 8-mm inferior screw to be placed just superior to the calcar, approximately 5 mm from the medial femoral neck cortex (Fig. 8–17). If only one screw is to be used, the nail should be inserted

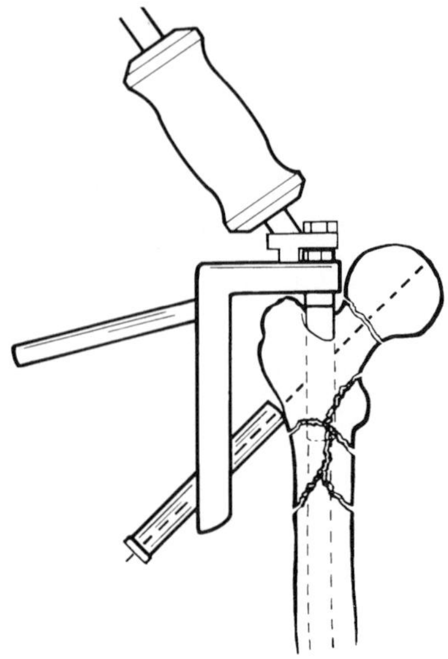

Fig. 8–17. Place the inferior proximal screw approximately 5 mm proximal to the medial femoral neck cortex to allow spacing for screw.

to a level allowing the 8-mm inferior screw to be centralized in the femoral head (Fig. 8–18).

Position the C-arm to obtain a true lateral view of the femoral head and neck. Align the keyed post to the axis of the C-arm by rotating the proximal drill guide in the transverse plane. The proximal targeting post is radiopaque to allow its' use for centralization of the proximal locking screws in the sagittal plane. A posterior and anterior portion of the femoral head must be seen in relation to the proximal drill guide (Fig. 8–19). Further verification of correct alignment may be obtained with an oblique C-arm view.

In most cases using the supine position, the femoral head is anterior to the shaft of the femur, thereby requiring the proximal drill guide to be rotated below horizontal to prevent proximal screw placement posteriorly to the femoral head. Notice that the anteversion in the nail is to compensate for the anterior offset of the femoral head and neck from the center of the medullary canal (the point known as the trochanteric or piriformis fossa). The proximal drill guide should point toward the femoral head and neck. The tendency during insertion is for retroversion of the proximal locking screws. Even though 8° of anteversion is built into the nail in relation to the distal locking holes, position the proximal drill guide slightly below the horizontal axis of the limb and then reconfirm rotational alignment and centralization of the guide by noting its bisection of the femoral head on the lateral radiographic view (Fig. 8–20).

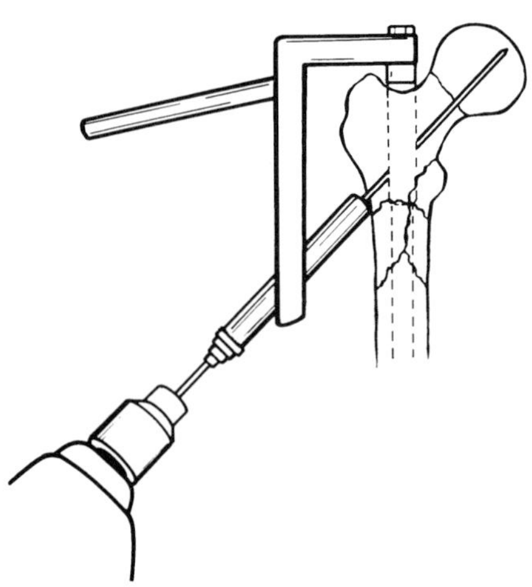

Fig. 8–18. If only one screw is used, center the inferior proximal locking screw in the center of the head.

Proximal Interlocking

Proximal interlocking involves the use of 6.4-mm and 8-mm lag screws with the 12- to 14-mm Reconstruction nails and two 6.4-mm screws with the Delta and Delta II Reconstruction nails. Therefore, the 3.2-mm-tip threaded guide pin, the red, blue, green, and silver drill sleeves, the femoral hexdriver and reconstruction/Delta reconstruction hex shaft, the large and small step drills, and quick release T-handle are required.

Stabilization of Neck Fracture

If only one screw is to be used for proximal interlocking, always use the 8 mm lag screw; however, the stronger mechanical construct is with both screws inserted. (To prevent rotation of the femoral head in femoral neck fractures, two screws are required.) Using the percutaneous knife, incise the skin and fascia through the inferior hole of the proximal drill guide. Insert the stacked drill sleeves with all four color-coded sheaths (9.5 mm silver, 8 mm green, 4.8 mm blue, 3.2 mm red) through the inferior hole. Push the drill sleeves to bone. Insert the 3.2-mm-tip threaded guide pin through the red drill sleeve and advance it into the femoral head at least 4 mm superior to the calcar to a level of approximately 5 mm beneath the subchondral

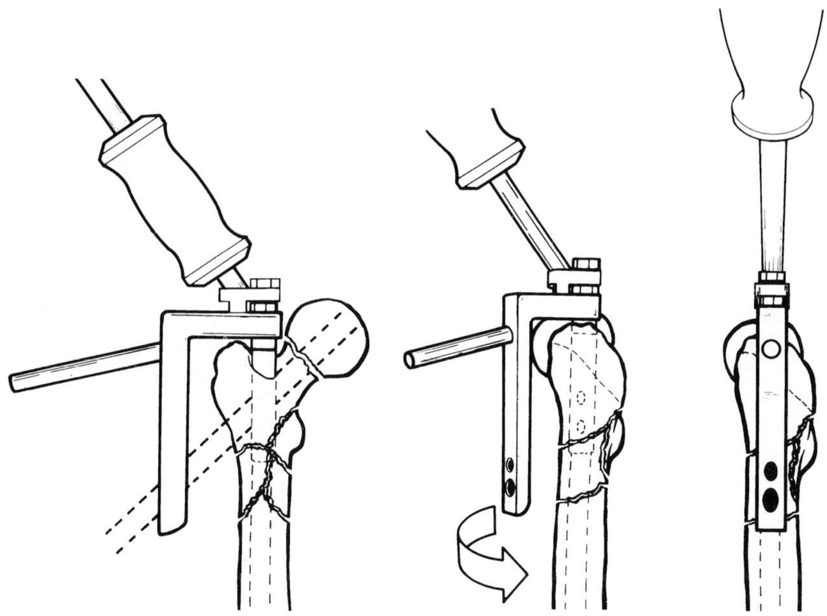

Fig. 8–19. Use the proximal targeting arm to aid in correct insertion in the femoral head. Rotate the proximal targeting arm until it bisects the femoral head on the true lateral view radiographically when femoral head can be seen anteriorly and posteriorly to the superimposed guide arm and nail. This screw will be centralized within the femoral head.

bone of the femoral head. Confirm the position of the guide pin within the head with AP and oblique lateral views with the C-arm.

If on the true lateral view the 3.2-mm-tip threaded guide pin is obstructed by the proximal drill guide but the femoral head anterior and posterior is visible, central placement of the pin can be inferred. For further confirmation, the C-arm may be obliqued anteriorly and posteriorly from the true lateral of the femoral head. If rotation of the femoral head is possible, another 3.2-mm-tip threaded guide pin in the superior hole should be used. Incise the skin and fascia through the superior hole of the proximal drill guide. Insert the stacked drill sleeves (8-mm green, 4.8-mm blue, 3.2-mm red) through the superior hole. Push the drill sleeves to bone. Insert the 3.2-mm-tip threaded guide pin through the red drill sleeve and advance the guide pin into the femoral head (Fig. 8–21).

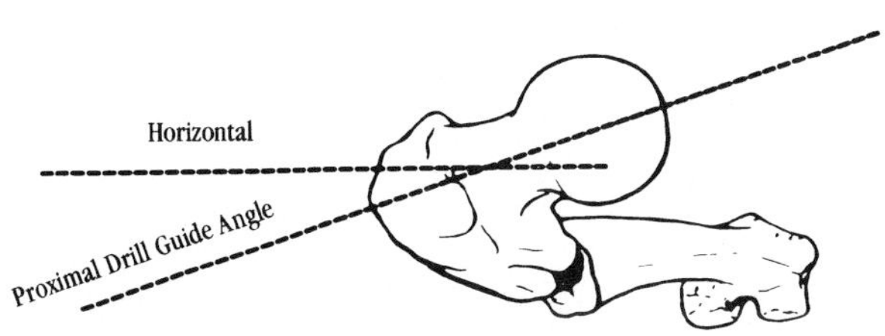

Fig. 8–20. Be aware of the extra anteversion that may be present with a subtrochanteric fracture.

Inferior Screw Placement

Remove the inferior 3.2-mm guide pin and blue and red drill sleeves. This will leave a pilot hole to center the large step drill. Insert the large step drill through the green drill sleeve into the femoral head to within 5 mm of subchondral bone; verify that the drill sleeves are against bone. Make the screw length measurement at this point using the drill calibrations and reading the depth against the top of the

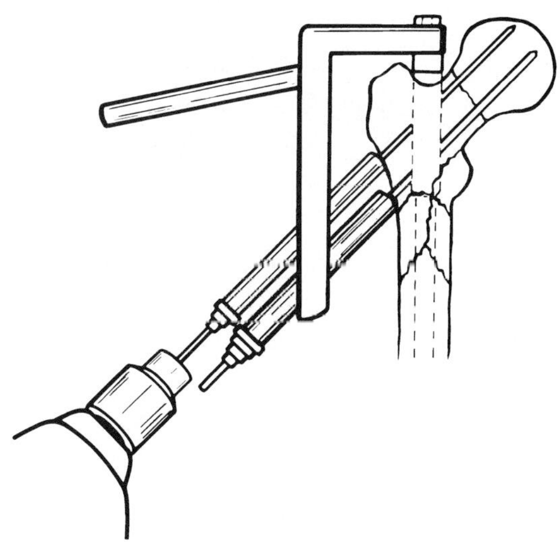

Fig. 8–21. Center both screws for maximum stabilization of a femoral neck component. The wire should be placed within 1 mm of the subchondral bone on AP and lateral views.

green drill sleeve (Fig. 8–22). In determining the length of the screw, consider potential impaction of the femoral head, if applicable. Remove the large step drill. The large and small step drill are designed to be semi-disposable, as the dense bone dulls the cutting flutes. Therefore, it is recommended to dispose of the step drills after five to ten uses.

Tapping for Proximal Screws

Tapping is usually recommended, but in very dense bone, tapping is required. The 8-mm tap shaft is attached to the quick release T-handle, and is used through the silver drill sleeve (Fig. 8–23). Return the green drill sleeve. Insert the selected 8 mm lag screw through the green drill sleeve by means of the Reconstruction/Delta reconstruction hex shaft, attached to the T-handle, into the femoral head (Fig. 8–24). Remove the green and silver drill sleeves.

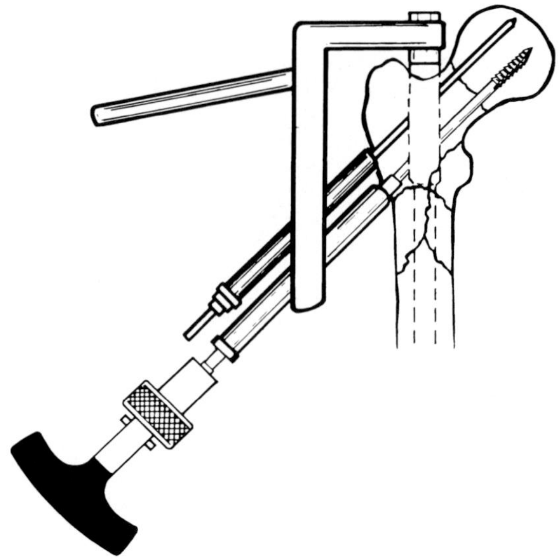

Fig. 8–23. Tapping is recommended for the screws to minimize femoral neck spinning and to facilitate screw insertion.

Superior Screw Placement

For two screw proximal fixation, insert the red, blue, and green drill sleeves through the superior hole of the proximal drill guide and advance the 3.2-mm-tip threaded guide pin, if not already in place, to within 5 mm of subchondral bone. The additional step of placing the 3.2-mm-tip threaded guide pin acts as a pilot hole for the drill. Remove the 3.2-mm-tip threaded guide pin and blue and red drill sleeve. Insert the small step drill through the green drill sleeve into the femoral head to within 5 mm of the subchondral bone. Verify that the drill sleeves are against bone. Make the screw length measurement at this point using the drill calibrations and reading the depth against the top of the green drill sleeve (Fig.

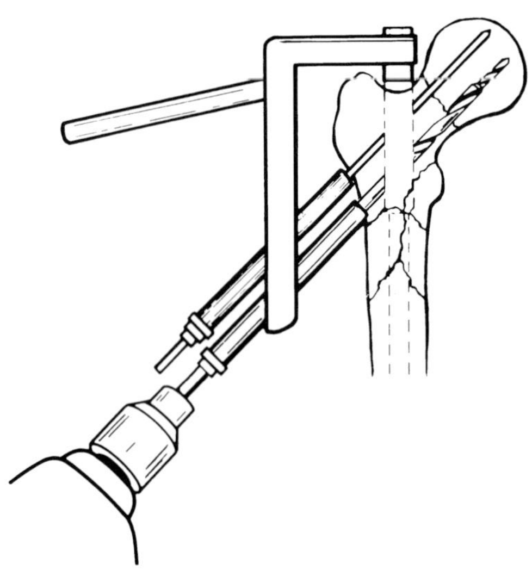

Fig. 8–22. Step drill for lag technique of inferior screw.

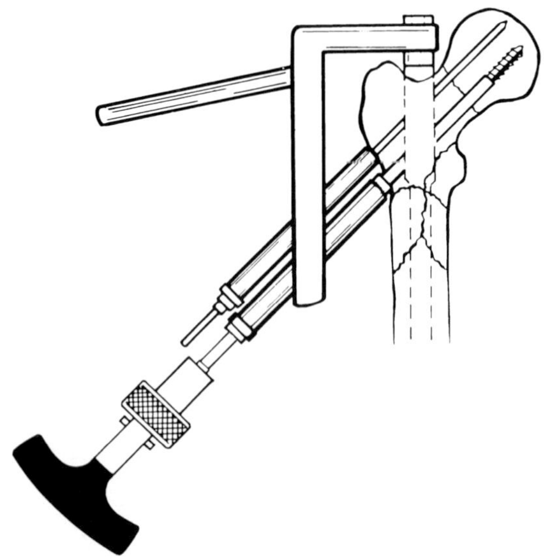

Fig. 8–24. The last screw should be inserted until threads are all contained within the femoral head and the screw head is on the lateral cortex.

8–25). Remove the small step drill. Tapping is usually recommended, but in very dense bone, tapping is required. The 6.4-mm tap shaft is attached to the quick release T-handle and is used through the green drill sleeve (Fig. 8–26). Insert the selected 6.4-mm lag screw by means of the Reconstruction/Delta reconstruction hex shaft, attached to the T-handle, into the femoral head (Fig. 8–27). Remove the green drill sleeve. Confirm containment of both screws in the femoral head with AP, lateral, and oblique views. For maximal stability, all threads of the proximal locking screws should be within the femoral head and the screw threads should pass across any fracture lines.

When femoral neck compression is not required and only one proximal screw is used, a set screw can be inserted to prevent the proximal screw from sliding. This technique is rarely used, but may be helpful if significant instability exists because of comminution of the femoral neck region. The screw is inserted through the proximal cannulation of the nail and engaged against the proximal screw by means of the femoral hexdriver. The long set screw secures the 8-mm proximal screw, whereas the short set screw secures the 6.4-mm proximal screw. If the 8-mm and 6.4-mm screws are both used and the short set screw is inserted, sliding is prevented for the 6.4-mm screw only. Proximal interlocking is now complete.

Distal locking is routinely advised with the Reconstruction nail techniques. A static construct is the most stable situation and least likely to result in malunion. Most commonly a freehand technique or radiolucent drill guide is used for distal interlocking screw placement.

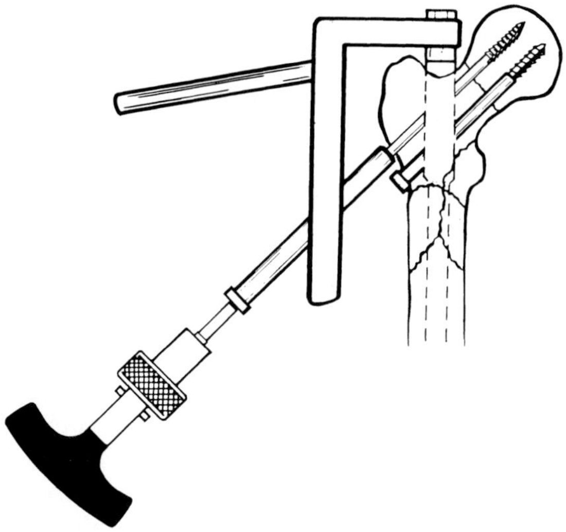

Fig. 8–26. Tapping of proximal locking screw.

TIPS AND TECHNIQUES

Entry portal selection for the reconstruction nail is significantly more difficult than a standard femoral nail insertion in two situations:

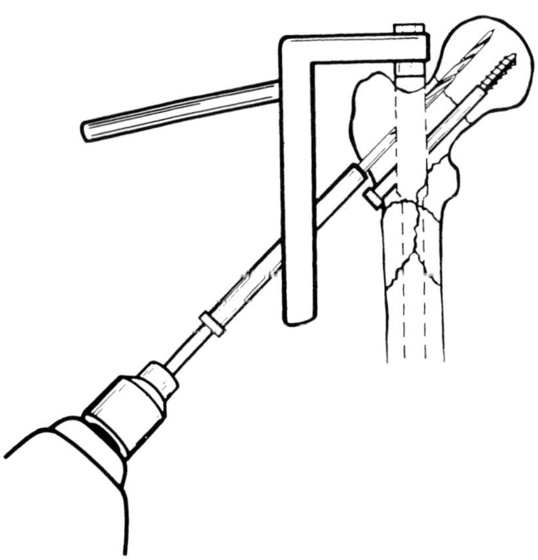

Fig. 8–25. Drilling of proximal locking screw with step drill.

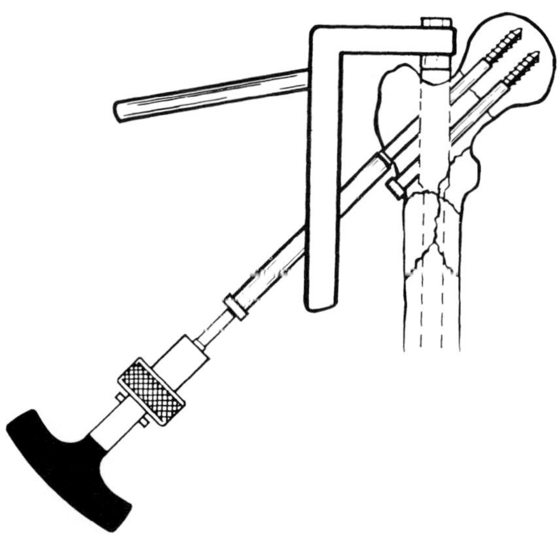

Fig. 8–27. Seating of proximal locking screw for maximum rotational ability of the proximal femur.

(1) subtrochanteric fractures with marked external rotation of the proximal fragment and (2) displaced femoral neck and shaft fractures. Subtrochanteric fractures by the nature of the deforming forces frequently rotate the proximal fragment externally and place the hip in varus. This makes it very difficult to visualize the entry portal on conventional views. This may be solved by either internally rotating the leg and attempting a closed reduction of the hip or by inserting a Schanz pin percutaneously into the trochanteric mass and using this as a joy stick to rotate the proximal femur into a more anatomically recognizable position.

We use a guide wire technique, the Day-Trafton technique, using a guide wire inserted in the piriformis fossa and over ream with an 8-mm cannulated reamer. The ipsilateral neck and shaft fracture presents the dilemma and concern of possible damage to the femoral neck fracture and femoral neck viability during nail insertion. This may be addressed by first performing an open reduction anteriorly of the femoral neck fracture and inserting provisional fixation. The use of a straight Charnley-type T-reamer inserted into the piriformis fossa can serve as a spacer during femoral neck provisional fixation. While provisional fixation is applied to the femoral head, it does not violate the medullary canal. It is frequently helpful to think of the provisional fixation of the femoral neck as being similar to pinning a slipped capital femoral epiphysis disruption, such that the pins need to be inserted from anterior on the greater trochanteric area posteriorly into the femoral head. Once the provisional fixation is in place, the T-handled reamer is removed from tho medullary canal and standard reduction and nailing of the shaft fracture can follow.

Proper selection of nail depth insertion in reference to the proximal femur and also rotation of the nail to maximize screw centralization of the femoral head are also problematic. Preoperative templating is very helpful in determining the diameter of the femoral neck and will aide in the selection of the proper implant. The standard Russell-Taylor Reconstruction nail has a spread of approximately 21 mm from screw to screw so it is recommended that the femoral neck width measure at least 25 mm for use of the standard Reconstruction nail. The Delta Reconstruction nail possesses an 18 mm spacing of these proximal locking screws which will be useful in smaller femurs.

Radiographic visualization of the proximal femur may be difficult and disorienting at first with Reconstruction nailing. Rotation of the C-arm until a true lateral of the femoral head neck is the key technique. This will be facilitated by rotating the proximal guide anteriorly. Once a true lateral of the femoral neck can be visualized and a reduction confirmed, rotate the handle posteriorly until the opaque guide bisects the femoral head. This will allow visualization of the femoral head anteriorly and posteriorly to the locking guide. This in effect is a cross-hair alignment by negative inference; if there is femoral head anterior and posterior to the proximal guide handle, the screws will be contained in the centered position of the femoral head. One should tend toward slightly anterior position of the screws into the femoral head. This rotation may be marked by an external skin marker to maintain correct anteversion during nail seating.

The next goal is to obtain proper depth insertion of the nail. This is facilitated again by preoperative planning and referencing the tip of the greater trochanter to the center of the femoral head. It is frequently helpful to outline the femoral head neck axis with a skin marker on the outside of the leg as a visual cue for proper depth insertion. The goal is to try to place the 8-mm lag screw just on the medial femoral cortex. If the nail is inserted too deep, it will be difficult to insert the screw. Allow 4 to 5 mm minimal spacing of the guide wire proximal to the medial femoral neck. The use of the 3.2-mm guide wire through the sheaths will help insure this is a correct portal. Lay the sheath and wire over the guide on the hip and obtain a radiograph to assist in confirmation. Alternatively, a Kirschner wire may be inserted percutaneously anteriorly over the femoral neck into the desired position and the proximal driving guide inserted to this point.

If during insertion the screw seems to go in a more inferior to superior tract into the femoral head or it is the surgeon's perspective that only one screw can be inserted, reevaluate the fracture for varus reduction. Because the screws are oriented in a 135° angle, it frequently is a clue that the hip may be reduced into varus when only one screw can be inserted.

Frequently during the proximal locking screw insertion, the surgeon will note that the proximal locking screw will seem to just spin. This is because of the fact that the partially threaded proximal screw is functionally a bolt. When all of the threads of the bolt become contained within the proximal nail, there are no threads to pull the nail into the bone. At this point, it is frequently helpful just to tap the bolt into the femoral head until threads can contact bone and start the threading process again.

The proximal screws must provide stable fixation in the operating room. In cases of severe osteoporosis or pathologic lesions where the screws do not have good fixation, augmentation of the proximal screw fixation with methylmethacrylate is advisable.

Postoperative Care

In the absence of other complicating injuries, patients with Reconstruction nails are mobilized the first postoperative day with bed to chair transfers and ambulation with walkers or crutches. Weight bearing is restricted to 10 to 15 kg on the affected extremity in comminuted cases. If bone to bone contact is achieved and good bone quality was present at the time of surgery, weight bearing is permitted as tolerated with crutches or walker. Range of motion exercises and straight leg lifts are started the first few days. The patients are usually discharged home per usual surgical guidelines (no fever, wound drainage, etc.) and when they demonstrate lower extremity control sufficient for household ambulation with ambulatory assist devices. Follow-up visits occur at 3-week intervals, with radiographs at that time. As callus is detected usually at 4 to 8 weeks, progressive weight bearing is allowed. Patients must demonstrate full weight bearing on the affected leg for 60 seconds, before crutches are discontinued. A progressive resistance exercise program is prescribed and swimming or stationary bicycling is recommended.

Implant removal is not considered until there is mature radiographic callus bridging the bone on both the AP and lateral radiographs. A general anesthetic is required and usually a 24-hour hospitalization. We place patients on crutches after implant removal until their gait returns to the preimplant removal status. After implant removal, contact sports are avoided for 3 months arbitrarily.

CLINICAL EXPERIENCE

Case Examples

Case One

A 49-year-old man experienced a chute malfunction while parachuting. On impact he sustained a closed unstable proximal femur fracture (Fig. 8–28). The patient underwent reamed

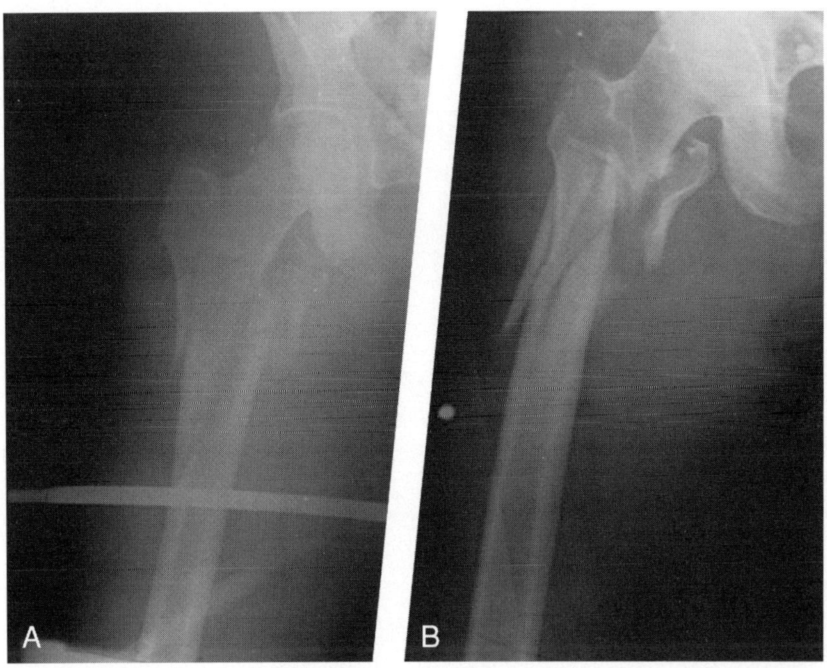

Fig. 8–28. AP and lateral radiograph of Russell-Taylor IB subtrochanteric femoral fracture. Subtrochanteric fracture with lesser trochanteric fracture. No involvement of fracture into the piriformis fossa.

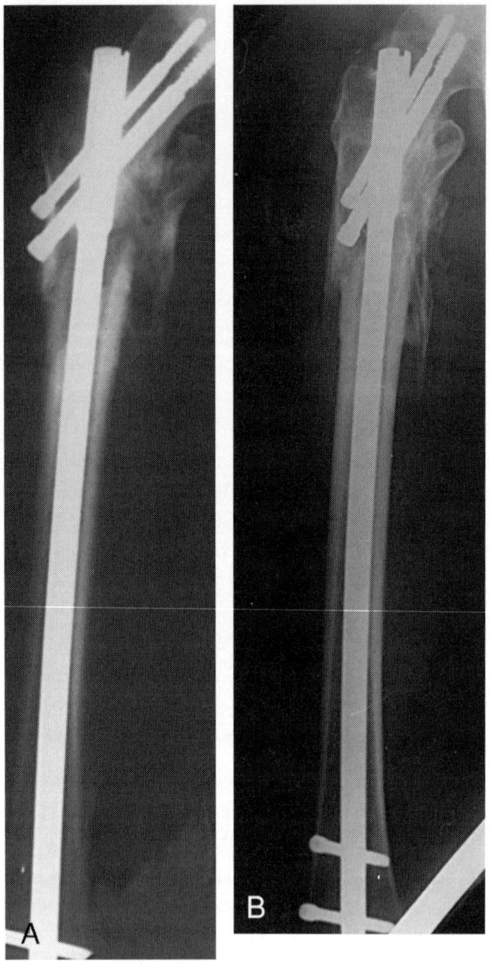

Fig. 8–29. Stabilization of subtrochanteric fracture Russell-Taylor IB with Reconstruction nail in static mode.

static Reconstruction nailing. His fracture united at 3 months and he returned to his former occupation without restrictions (Fig. 8–29). He demonstrates the subtrochanteric fracture for which the Reconstruction nail is best suited, that is, a subtrochanteric fracture with loss of the medial cortical stability with fracture of the lesser trochanter. The fracture does not extend into the piriformis fossa. (Russell-Taylor classification IA[5])

Case Two

A 26-year-old man sustained a gunshot injury to his proximal femur (Fig. 8–30). After initial irrigation and debridement, he underwent a statically-locked Reconstruction nailing. Delayed wound coverage was possible at 7 days. Union was documented at his 4-month follow-up visit (Fig. 8–31). The lesser trochanteric area was intact to the proximal femur and there was no comminution in the piriformis fossa. (Russell-Taylor classification IA)

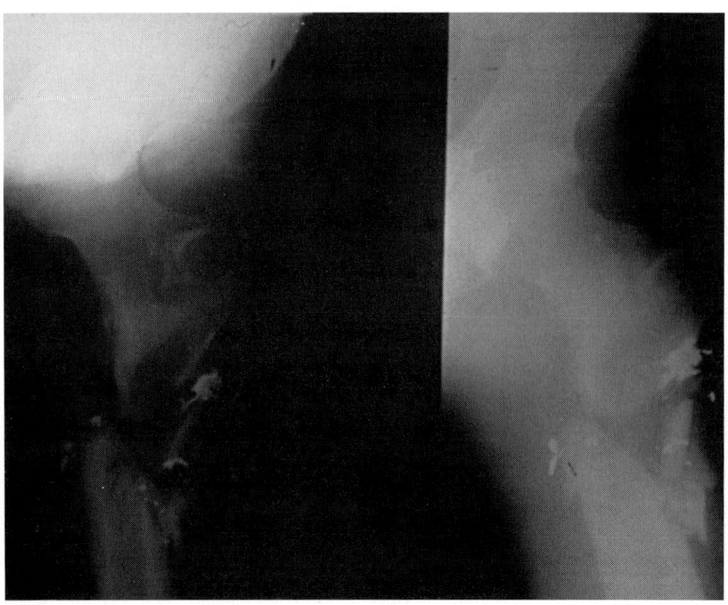

Fig. 8–30. AP and lateral radiograph of Russell-Taylor IA Fracture is secondary to a gunshot wound.

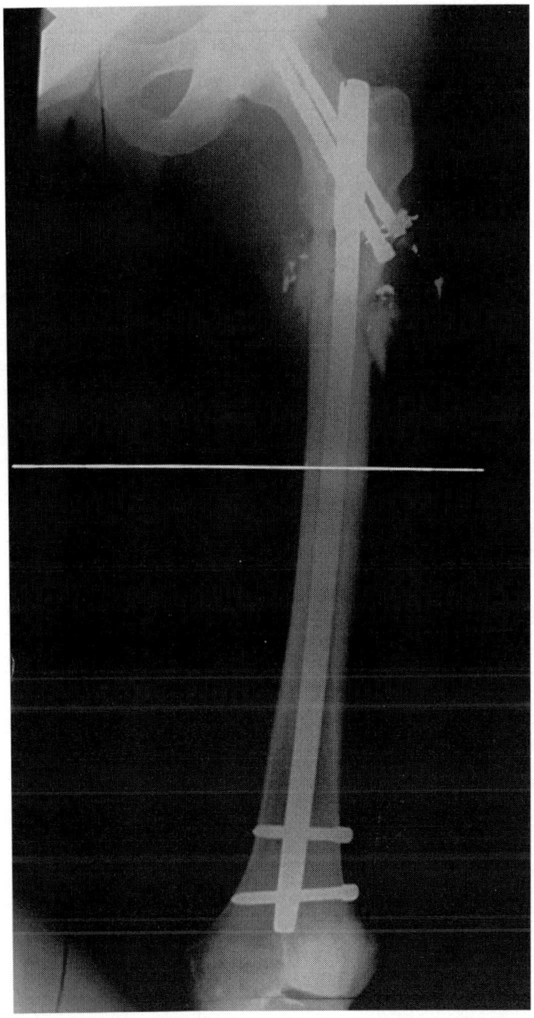

Fig. 8–31. Stabilization of an open fracture with Reconstruction nail.

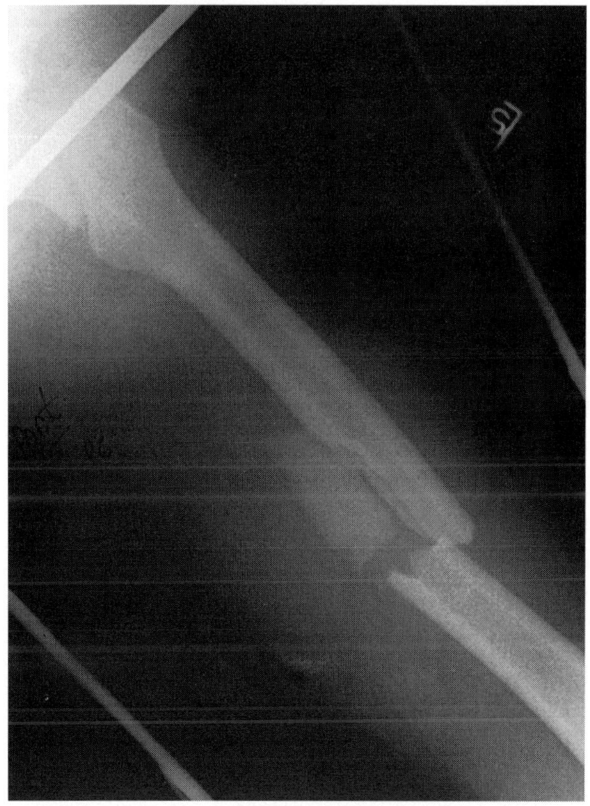

Fig. 8–32. Ipsilateral femoral neck and shaft fracture.

Case Three

A 22-year-old man involved in a motor vehicle accident sustained an ipsilateral femoral neck and open femoral shaft fracture (grade II Gustilo-Anderson) (Fig. 8–32). He underwent debridement and irrigation of the shaft fracture and closed reduction and internal fixation of both fractures with a static Reconstruction nail using a reamed technique. As the neck did not displace after traction was applied, open reduction was not required. At 6 months, all fractures were healed without infection (Fig. 8–33). At his 4-year follow-up, he was employed without limitations and there was no evidence of infection or avascular necrosis.

Case Four

A 29-year-old man with a history of polyostotic fibrous dysplasia developed increasing deformity of his leg after correction of a similar problem in childhood. Radiographs documented his severe maldevelopment and impairment (Fig. 8–34). Bone scans were consistent for stress failure at the apex of the deformity. The patient underwent Jewett nail removal, open segmental osteotomies with autogenous iliac grafting, and stabilization with the Reconstruction nail, initially in a static locked mode. He was dynamized at 6 months because of irritation from the distal screws. He was united and without deformity at 4-year follow-up (Fig. 8–35).

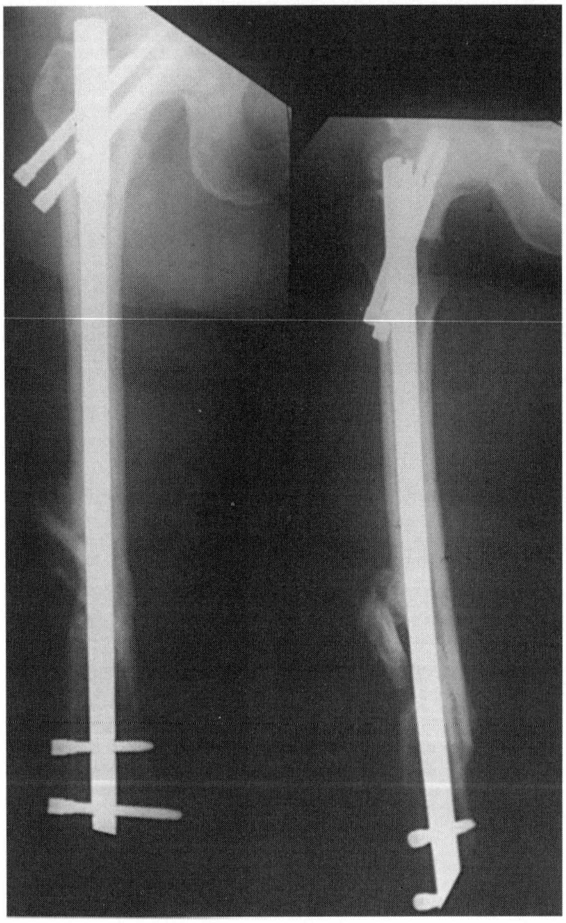

Fig. 8–33. Stabilization of ipsilateral femoral neck and shaft fracture in static mode.

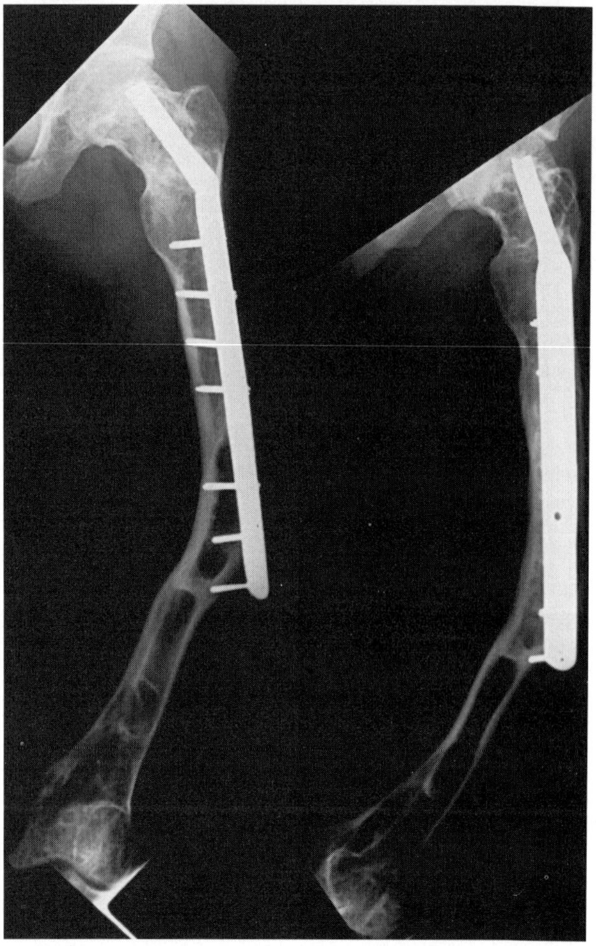

Fig. 8–34. Fibrous dysplasia with impending fracture. Previous Jewett plate fixation for fibrous dysplasia.

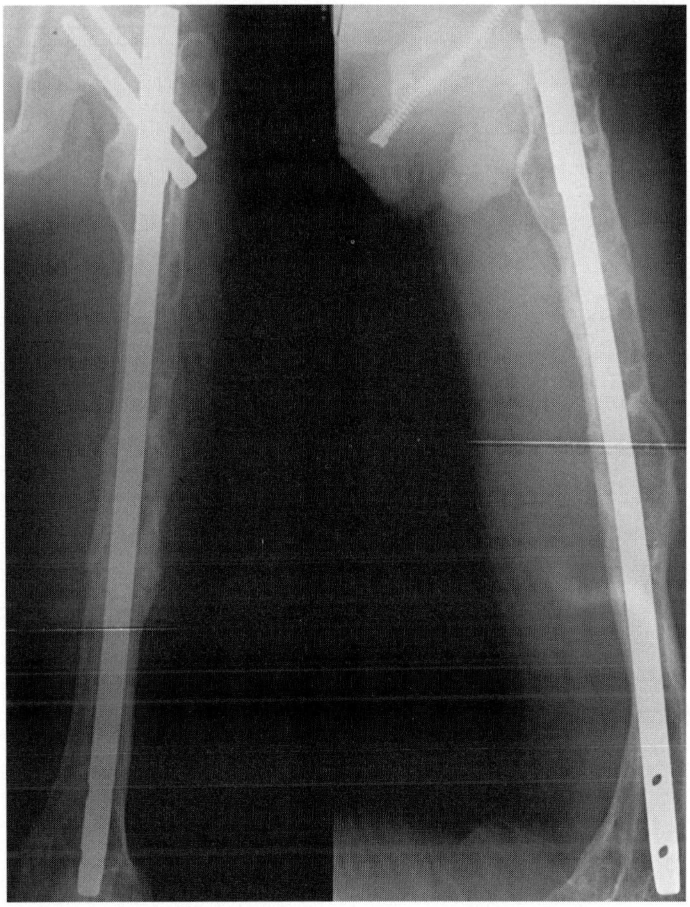

Fig. 8–35. Union of segmental osteotomies in fibrous dysplasia. Nail dynamized at 6 months. Plan retention of nail for prophylaxis.

CLINICAL RESULTS

Slater et al.[6] documented the results of 64 consecutive unstable subtrochanteric fractures treated with the Russell-Taylor Reconstruction nail. The majority were high-energy fractures with 56 closed and 8 open fractures. Fifty-nine percent of fractures involved loss of the medial femoral cortex or fracture of the lesser trochanter. Twenty-two percent involved extension into the trochanteric mass or piriformis fossa region. Seventy-four percent of the fractures were Winquist-Hansen type 3, Winquist-Hansen type 4, or segmental fractures. In the 12 cases with extension into the piriformis fossa, intraoperative difficulties were high, occasionally requiring open reduction for the entry portal. Of the 61 cases with follow-up at an average of 11 months, all fractures united without reoperation, bone grafting, or dynamization. There were no acute infections, but 2 patients developed late infections at 16 and 18 months postinjury because of sepsis from other new injuries. Both responded to implant removal and antibiotics. Seven nails have been removed without complication or refracture.

Azar and Russell[7] have presented a prospective study of 35 patients with ipsilateral femoral neck and shaft fractures. Thirty patients have a minimum follow-up of 2 years and an average of 3.3 years. There has been one femoral neck nonunion in a patient with preexisting varus deformity caused by old slipped capital epiphysis that subsequently united with internal fixation and autogenous iliac graft and one femoral neck malreduction that was reoperated within 5 days with valgus reduction obtained and fixation with the Reconstruction nail with accessory screw. There has been one deep infection that resolved after fracture union and nail removal with antibiotics. Only one case has developed avascular necrosis of the femoral head approximately 7 years postinjury from a completely displaced femoral neck fracture component treated at 2 weeks postinjury with open reduction and fixation with the Reconstruction nail. His bone scan at 2-year follow-up was normal. Pain and radiographic changes occurred after 7 years. Currently, he is managed with a cane and nonsteroidal anti-inflammatory medication. Eighty percent of patients have returned to their preinjury work and recreational activities.

OVERVIEW

Though technically more demanding than conventional interlocking femoral nails, the Reconstruction nail has achieved its design goals and has also ushered in a new era of implant design concepts. Continued efforts to improve instrumentation and implant design are ongoing. However, the Reconstruction nail has earned a place in the treatment of complex proximal femoral problems.

REFERENCES

1. Russell, T.A., Taylor, J.C., Lavelle, D.G., Beals, N.B., Brumfield, D.L, Durham, A.G.: Mechanical characterization of femoral interlocking intramedullary nailing systems. J. Ortho. Trauma *5*:332, 1991.
2. Bucholz, R.W., Ross, S.E., Lawrence, K.L.: Fatigue failure of the interlocking nail in the treatment of fractures of the distal part of the femoral shaft. J. Bone Joint Surg. *69*:1391, 1987.
3. Beals, H.B., Davidson, J.R.: Improved fatigue strength of interlocking nails. Second Annual Conference International Society for Fracture Repair, Minneapolis, MN, 1990 (abstract).
4. Surgical Technique Manual Smith & Nephew Richards Family of Reconstruction Interlocking Nails, T.A. Russell, J.C. Taylor, Lavelle, D.G., Smith & Nephew Richards, Memphis, TN.
5. Russell, T.A., Taylor, J,C.: Subtrochanteric fractures. *In* Skeletal Trauma. Edited by B. Browner.
6. Slater, J.C., Russell, T.A., Walker, B.J.: Intramedullary nailing of complex subtrochanteric fractures of the femur. submitted for publication. Presented at AAOS, Orthop. Transactions 1992.
7. Russell, T.A., Azar, F.M.: Ipsilateral femoral neck and shaft fracture treated with the Russell-Taylor Reconstruction Nail. submitted for publication. Presented at AAOS, Orthop. Transactions, Orlando, FL, 1995.

9

Closed Küntscher Nailing of Femoral Fractures

Robert G. Veith, Sigvard T. Hansen, Jr., and Robert A. Winquist

Closed intramedullary nailing of femoral shaft fractures was first reported by Küntscher in 1940.[1] Through a limited incision that exposed the greater trochanter, Küntscher stabilized femoral shaft fractures with a cloverleaf bullet-tipped nail after enlarging the medullary canal with graduated reamers. Despite Küntscher's success with this technique, his procedure did not gain widespread popularity in the United States until approximately one decade ago. General acceptance of the technique has been brought about by refinements in instrumentation and by the availability of the mobile image intensifier, which has reduced the radiation hazard to acceptable levels. Numerous published series describing femoral fractures treated with closed intramedullary nailing have demonstrated the superior results that can be achieved with this technique.[2–11] On this basis, many surgeons have adopted closed intramedullary nailing over nonoperative treatment.

The primary advantage that closed femoral nailing has over open fixation techniques, with either intramedullary nails or plates and screws, is that bony structure can be restored without exposure of the fracture hematoma or further compromise of local soft tissues and parosteal attachments. Blood loss is minimized, as are the risks of infection, delayed union, and nonunion.

The femur is well suited for intramedullary nailing because of its excellent soft-tissue coverage and the shape of its intramedullary canal. Although the intramedullary blood supply is temporarily compromised following the reaming process, this closed procedure does not interfere with the external blood supply near the fracture site. Clinical practice has shown that the femur tolerates the deleterious effects of reaming because it is surrounded by a richly vascular soft-tissue envelope.[12] The tibia, on the other hand, is less well suited for immediate intramedullary reaming and fixation because its vascular supply is limited. The Küntscher technique with reaming is not recommended for most open tibial fractures.

Closed femoral nailing has distinct medical and economic advantages over other techniques.[9,13] At Harborview Medical Center in Seattle, more than 750 acute femoral shaft fractures have been treated with closed intramedullary nailing since the technique was adopted in 1968. We feel that this procedure, modified as outlined in our AAOS Instructional Course Lecture,[14] offers the most physiologic treatment for femoral shaft fractures because bony structure is restored, the patient can be mobilized early, and the injured extremity can be rehabilitated more readily. However, closed femoral nailing is technically demanding, and fractures treated with this technique must be selected properly so that complications can be avoided. This chapter presents our approach to the management of patients with femoral shaft fractures and discusses means of minimizing the technical pitfalls of closed intramedullary nailing of the femur.

FRACTURE SELECTION

Not all femoral shaft fractures are amenable to the standard technique of closed intramedullary nailing following reaming. Stability of the fracture is a key element in determining the suitability of this technique for specific femoral shaft fractures. Unstable fractures generally are considered unsuitable for standard closed femoral nailing because an unacceptable amount of shortening, malrotation, or angulation may occur. Both the pattern and the location of the fracture in the femoral shaft are important in evaluating whether the fracture is stable, and both considerations must be assessed carefully by the surgeon when selecting the method of treatment.

In general, transverse fractures with less than 50% comminution can be considered stable. Short oblique fractures in the proximal shaft or midshaft also are stable, but some shortening can occur after standard nailing of short oblique fractures in the infraisthmal area. Long oblique, split segmental, and comminuted fractures with less than 50% cortical contact are regarded as unstable. In a segmental fracture, each fracture must be evaluated separately to determine its inherent stability.

The location of the fracture in the femoral shaft may render unstable an otherwise stable fracture. For example, a transverse fracture with less than 50% comminution usually is stable if it lies within the region 2.5 cm distal to the greater trochanter and 10 cm above the knee joint, provided that the intracondylar area is intact. Transverse fractures more proximal than 2.5 cm below the lesser trochanter are unstable, however, and may angulate or rotate if treated with standard closed nailing. Fortunately, the development of the interlocking femoral nail has extended the limits of closed nailing of femoral shaft fractures.[15] This chapter deals with the technique of interlocking femoral fixation only with respect to its role in the management of unstable fracture patterns.

The age of the patient is also an important consideration in the proper selection of fractures for closed intramedullary nailing of the femur. We do not favor nailing of femoral shaft fractures in children, but we do consider this technique to be the treatment of choice for adolescents.[16] Closed intramedullary nailing is particularly advantageous in the elderly patient because the procedure is well suited for osteoporotic bone. Elderly patients can bear weight without fear of failure of the fixation, and the worrisome stress-riser effect does not occur when a full-length nail is used.

SURGICAL TIMING

We recommend immediate fixation of femoral fractures in patients who are multiply injured, who have sustained ipsilateral fractures of the femur and tibia (floating knee), or who have open femoral fractures. Approximately one third of the patients with femoral shaft fractures also have sustained life-threatening injuries to the head, chest, or abdomen. In these patients, early femoral fixation reduces morbidity and mortality in the early postinjury phase. Multiply injured patients are at significant risk for pulmonary complications. Border et al. emphasized the value of the sitting or upright position for enhancing respiration;[17] consequently, traction should be avoided in these patients. With adequate femoral fixation, the patient can be mobilized, or at least enabled to sit upright, on the day after injury. In the patient with head injuries, femoral fixation should be provided. Immediate femoral fixation in patients with multiple injuries allows the health care team essentially to "ignore" the fracture after operation and to concentrate on important lifesaving measures. We believe that the period just after initial resuscitation of the patient is ideal for performing fracture fixation. If an emergency cranial or abdominal surgical procedure is performed, we follow that procedure with closed femoral nailing during sustained anesthesia.

Riska et al. have observed a reduction in the incidence of the fat embolism syndrome following early internal fixation of long bone fractures.[18] We also observed that early fracture fixation with intramedullary nailing decreased the risk of fat embolism in a retrospective series of 100 consecutive patients with femoral shaft fractures.[19] The incidence of fat embolism syndrome was 0% in the 57 patients whose fractures were treated with intramedullary nailing immediately and 11% in the 43 patients whose fractures were treated in a delayed manner. Regardless of whether immediate internal fixation diminishes the incidence of the ARDS, we believe that femoral fixation improves pulmonary management should patients develop this syndrome.

Patients with ipsilateral fractures of the femur and tibia tend to have a high incidence of additional life-threatening injuries. In patients with this combination of fractures, we recommend immediate internal fixation of both femoral and tibial fractures because such treatment simplifies nursing care in the postinjury period. Fixation of both fractures leads to improved functional end results.[20,21]

In the past, we treated open femoral fractures with immediate debridement and then placed the patient in traction. Closure of the wound was performed approximately 5 to 7 days after injury, and intramedullary nailing was performed an average of 14 days after injury. For the past 7 years, however, we have performed primary debridement and immediate internal fixation of all grade I and grade II open femoral fractures and have closed the wound after 5 to 7 days.[22] Administration of antibiotics is continued for 24 to 48 hours after the initial surgical procedure.

Immediate fracture fixation is less crucial in patients with isolated femoral shaft fractures than in patients with life-threatening injuries. In the past, we tended to place patients with isolated closed femoral shaft fractures in traction for 5 to 7 days prior to femoral fixation. Now we frequently perform immediate fixation in these patients because (1) the deleterious effects of immediate fixation are small, (2) our experience suggests that the risk of ARDS is reduced with immediate fixation,[19] and (3) the significantly shortened period of hospitalization associated with this treatment method has obvious economic and emotional benefits.

SURGICAL EQUIPMENT

Closed intramedullary nailing of the femur requires the use of expensive specialized equipment. An institution in which intramedullary nailing is performed on a regular basis must stock a full complement of prebent, bullet-tipped, or pathfinder cloverleaf femoral nails in addition to graduated flexible reamers and an appropriate power source with which to operate them. Further necessities are a mobile C-arm image intensifier and a suitable fracture table that allows traction during surgery. The table also should allow the unscrubbed surgeon easy access with the image intensifier and ease in manipulating the fractured extremity. We prefer a fracture table with a perineal post that can be offset distally. The image intensifier should be fully mobile and should have an image retention mechanism, which significantly decreases radiation exposure.

PREOPERATIVE MANAGEMENT

Upon admission to the emergency room, all patients receive treatment to stabilize vital functions; special attention is given to the cardiopulmonary, abdominal, and central nervous systems. The fractures usually have been splinted by paramedics in the field. The injured extremity is examined closely, the degree of soft-tissue injury is assessed, and the knee is examined for points of tenderness that may suggest a ligamentous injury.[23] Radiographs of the injured femur, as well as views of the ipsilateral knee, are taken. An anteroposterior view of the pelvis also is obtained to rule out an associated femoral neck fracture.

If an immediate surgical procedure is not performed, the patient is placed in skeletal traction in the emergency room; traction is applied through a proximal tibial Steinmann pin. Sufficient traction is applied to restore normal length or even to distract the fracture slightly. Traction averages 25 to 35 pounds (11 to 16 kg) in women and 30 to 45 pounds (14 to 20 kg) in men. For accurate radiographic assessment of the length of the fracture, radiographic beams must be directed perpendicular to the thigh. When the patient is in traction, the lateral radiograph provides the most reliable assessment of femoral length. Maintenance of proper length preoperatively greatly facilitates manipulation and reduction of the fracture during operation. This approach lessens the risk of sciatic nerve palsy, which can result from excessive and/or prolonged traction during operation.

If femoral nailing is not performed on the day of injury, a delay of approximately 5 to 7 days allows the swelling and the inflammatory response within the thigh to diminish, thus aiding manipulation of the femur during operation. During the interval before surgery, we observe the patient closely for complications, particularly ARDS. If any signs or symptoms suggest this syndrome, arterial blood-gas measurements are obtained immediately.

OPERATIVE PLANNING

Prior to surgical intervention, high-quality AP and lateral radiographs of the fractured extremity are obtained. The radiographs are scrutinized closely for undisplaced fractures, potential butterfly fragments, and undisplaced femoral neck fractures. Radiographs of the normal femur also are taken at a tube-to-plate distance of 1 meter, which produces a predictable 10% magnification of the femur. The width of the medullary canal and the length of the normal femur from the tip of the trochanter to the lateral joint line of the knee are measured. (The Küntscher ossimeter includes the 10% magnification on the green scale.[14]) These measurements allow the surgeon to select the nail of appropriate size. We then check the length of the nail by measuring the patient's uninjured extremity from the tip of the trochanter to the joint line. We recommend the use of a full-length nail that extends from the tip of the greater trochanter to the old distal femoral epiphyseal scar.

To determine the diameter of the nail, we measure the width of the canal on the radiograph of the uninjured femur both at the isthmus and at the level of the fracture site. Optimally, the nail should achieve at least 2 cm of cortical contact both proximal and distal to the fracture site. In proximal or infraisthmal fractures, however, excessive reaming to achieve this goal may lead to comminution when a nail with a larger diameter is inserted. Reaming the isthmus more than 2 to 3 mm, or more than half the thickness of the cortex, is excessive. Initially, we used larger nails, but currently the average nail diameter we use is 14 to 15 mm in men and 12 to 14 in women. Nails of 2 to 3 different diameters and 2 to 3 different lengths should be available in the operating room for each patient.

Before undergoing a standard closed femoral intramedullary nailing procedure, the patient is typed and cross-matched for 2 units of blood. A prophylactic antibiotic, usually a cephalosporin, is administered 1 hour before operation and is continued for 24 to 48 hours after the procedure.

OPERATIVE TECHNIQUE

The technical aspects of closed intramedullary femoral nailing are demanding and require experienced personnel, including a scrubbed surgeon and an unscrubbed surgeon, who participates actively throughout the operation. After a suitable regional or general anesthetic has been administered, particular attention is directed toward positioning the patient properly on the fracture table. We prefer to place the patient in a lateral decubitus position; the side that is not being operated on is down (Fig. 9–1). We have found that placing the patient in a lateral rather than a supine position facilitates insertion of the nail and manipulation of the fracture and improves rotational control. Occasionally, we use the supine position in patients with fractures of the spine or complex pelvic fractures for whom the lateral position might be hazardous. The supine position also allows retrograde intramedullary nailing of the femoral shaft when ipsilateral fractures of the femoral neck and shaft are managed.

With the patient in the lateral position, the use of an axillary pad prevents neurologic injury to the lower arm. The upper arm is placed in a padded armrest. The perineal post is rotated distally to allow visualization of the trochanter in both the anteroposterior and lateral planes. The fractured leg is placed over the perineal post; care is taken to prevent compression of the genitalia. The majority of the patient's weight must be supported under the opposite greater trochanter and thigh because excessive weight on the perineal post results in distal venous congestion and abduction of the proximal fragment of the femoral shaft. The uninjured leg is placed in gentle traction in line with the body. The injured extremity is placed on a straight traction, and the hip is flexed 20 to 30° and is slightly adducted. If a lengthy procedure or excessive traction is anticipated, the sciatic nerve must be protected by flexing the knee and inserting a femoral traction pin.

At this point, correct rotational alignment of the fractured femur must be obtained. Alignment is achieved by gently rotating the extremity internally and externally, while checking manually for proper relaxation of soft tissues and simultaneously studying skin folds to detect excessive tension from the rotation. Finally, one must remember that if the foot or patella is parallel to the floor, the fracture generally is rotated externally. To obtain proper alignment, one should place the leg in 20 to 30° of internal rotation.

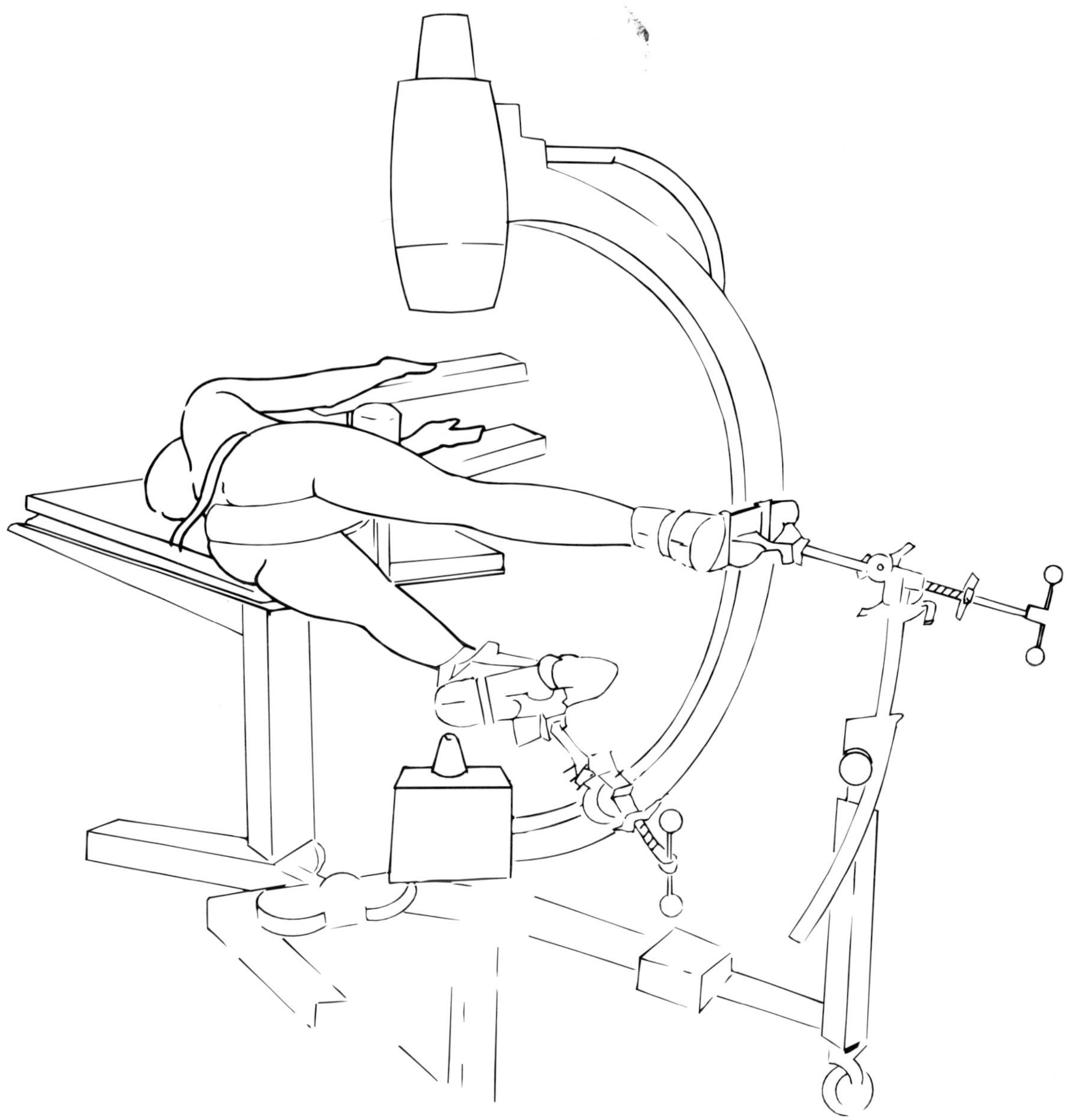

Fig. 9–1. Standard table position for intramedullary nailing of most femoral shaft fractures. Traction is applied to the injured extremity with the hip slightly flexed and the knee extended. Care is taken to obtain proper rotation of the extremity. (Note that the injured extremity is placed in apparent internal rotation of approximately 20 to 30° from the horizontal plane.) Gentle traction is applied through the contralateral extremity, which is aligned with the body.

When a distal femoral traction pin is used, the patient's knee is flexed and the foot and leg are placed on a padded Mayo stand that can be raised or lowered to provide proper rotation of the thigh (Fig. 9–2). After the patient is positioned, the C-arm image intensifier is used to visualize the fracture, the knee, and the prospective insertional point for the nail. We attempt a closed reduction of the fracture while still scrubbed. The radiographs of the injury then are reviewed again to determine where reductive forces should be directed. Traction is applied to obtain length, and the surgeons must realize that an increase in traction may make reduction more difficult by causing excessive soft tissue tension in the thigh.

The unscrubbed surgeon must think in three dimensions when the reduction maneuver is performed. With the use of leaded gloves or wooden rings, the surgeon applies localized

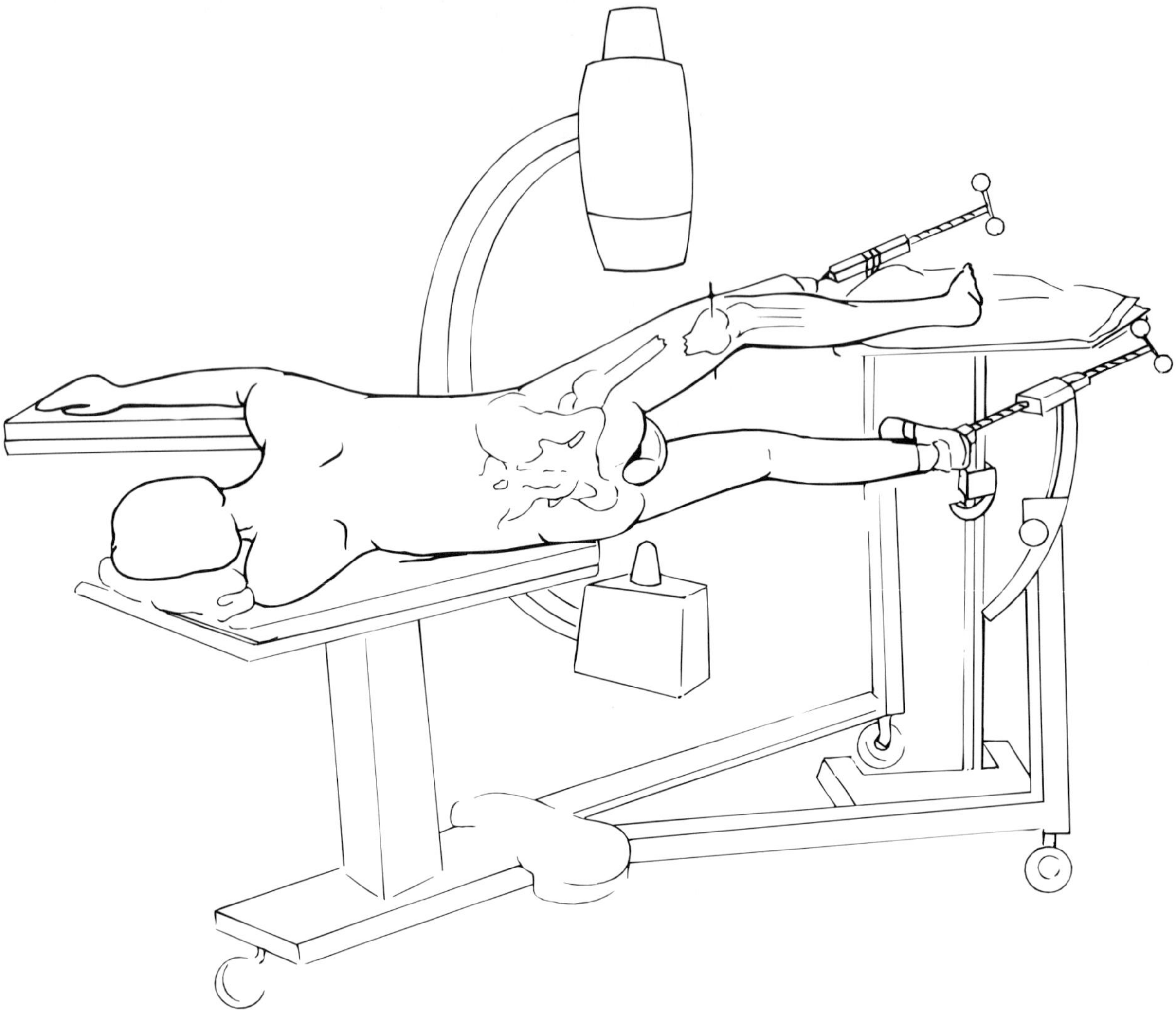

Fig. 9–2. The "flexed-knee table position" uses a distal femoral Kirschner wire. The foot rests on a padded stand, which can be raised or lowered to achieve proper rotation of the thigh. Flexing the knee relaxes the gastrocnemius muscle and the posterior knee capsule, aiding reduction of distal femoral shaft fractures. Knee flexion also relaxes the sciatic nerve.

pressure just proximal and distal to the fracture site. Before proceeding with the operation, the unscrubbed surgeon should be confident that reduction can be attained in both the anteroposterior and the lateral plane (Fig. 9–3). Certain fractures may require the use of rotatory force or increased angulation to recreate the deformity produced at the time of fracture before reduction can be achieved.

After reduction of the fracture is assured, the patient is prepared and draped for the surgical procedure. A sterile cover is applied to the C-arm image intensifier. A 5-cm incision, extending proximally from the tip of the greater trochanter, is made in line with the femur. The deep fascia is divided in line with the skin incision, and the fibers of the gluteus maximus are separated bluntly to allow palpation of the posterior tip of the greater trochanter.

An accurate insertional point for the nail is critical. Küntscher and others have advocated an insertional point lateral to the tip of the greater trochanter to avoid the risks of intracapsular infection, avascular necrosis of the femoral head, and iatrogenic femoral neck fracture. This lateral insertional point, however, may result in comminution of the medial femoral cortex of the proximal fragment, especially in more proximal fractures. Similarly, if the insertional point is too medial, the lateral

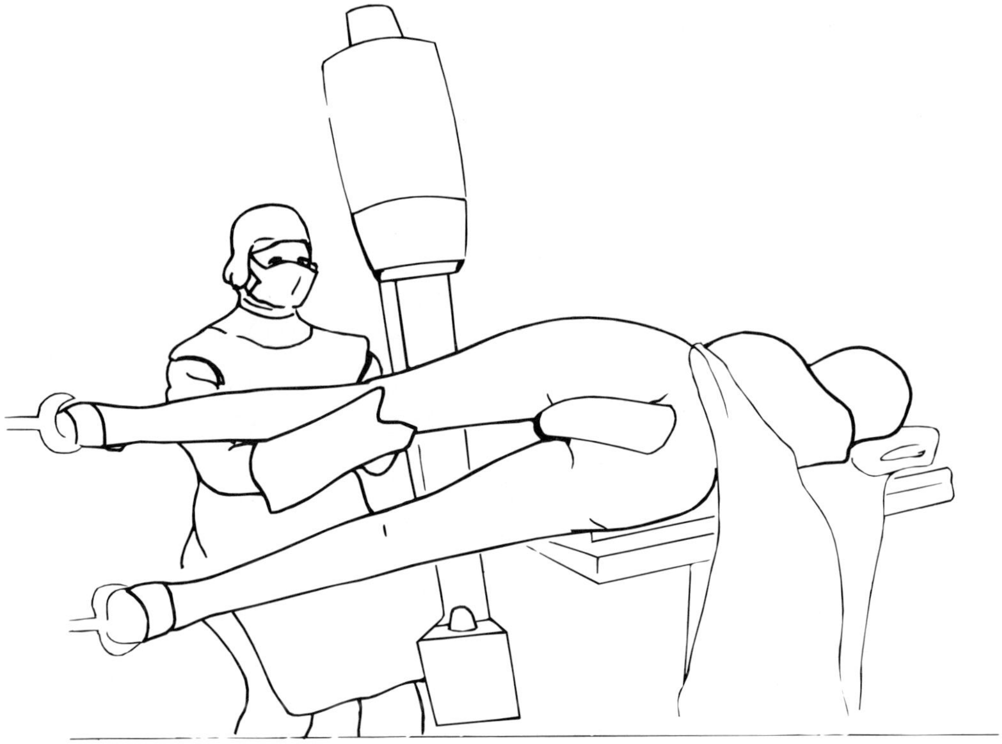

Fig. 9–3. Wearing protective gloves, the unscrubbed surgeon performs a reduction maneuver before preparing and draping the patient. This surgeon must determine whether fracture reduction is obtainable.

cortex of the proximal fragment may fracture. We believe that the ideal insertional point is in the piriform fossa just medial to the tip of the greater trochanter (Fig. 9–4).

The steps for standard closed intramedullary nailing of the femur are shown in Figure 9–5. The point of insertion is made with a sharp awl or T-handled drill. Before the cortex is penetrated, the prospective insertional point is checked carefully under fluoroscopy in both the anteroposterior and the lateral plane. The awl is directed centrally in line with the proximal medullary canal in both of these planes. The proximal metaphyseal bone is penetrated with the T-handled drill. A bulb-tipped guide with a slight bend at its end is advanced to the fracture site. The fracture is reduced by the unscrubbed surgeon, who checks the position of the fracture in both planes. The bulb-tipped guide then is advanced carefully across the fracture site into the distal segment. The unscrubbed surgeon again examines the fracture in both planes to ensure an intramedullary position of the guide. The guide is advanced centrally to the old epiphyseal scar, and its length

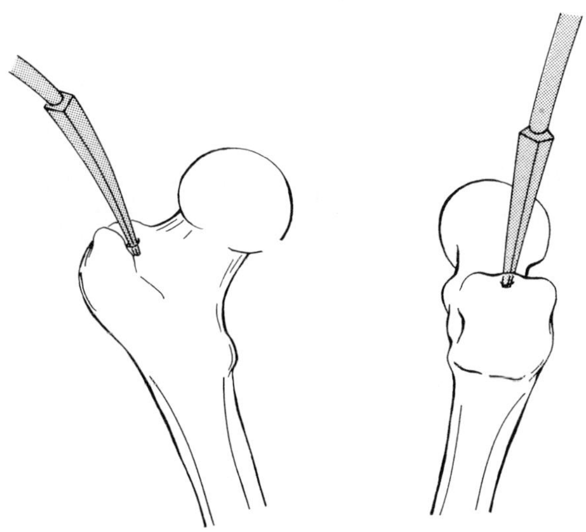

Fig. 9–4. The proper insertion point for the nail is located medial to the tip of the greater trochanter and slightly anterior to the trochanteric fossa. A sharp T-handled drill penetrates the proximal femur in line with the proximal femoral shaft in both anteroposterior and lateral planes.

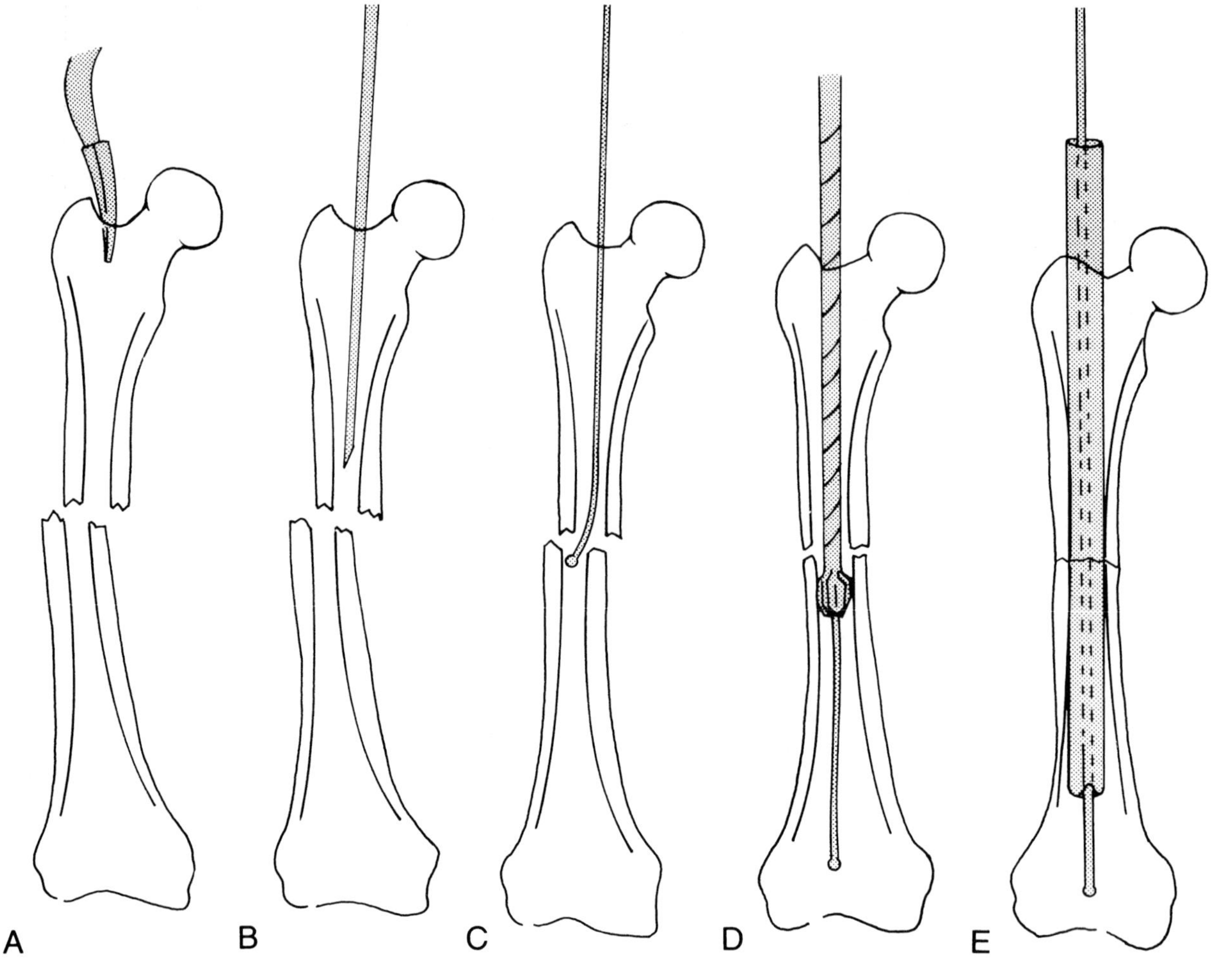

Fig. 9–5. Steps for standard closed intramedullary nailing. *A*, A sharp-tipped awl is used to make the insertion point. *B*, A T-handled drill perforates the bone and passes into the intramedullary canal. *C*, A bulb-tipped guide with a slight bend at the end traverses the fracture site. *D*, The femoral canal is enlarged with graduated flexible intramedullary reamers. *E*, The nail-driving guide is advanced past the bulb-tipped guide; the cloverleaf nail is then driven over the nail-driving guide.

then is measured to provide the final determination of the length of the nail.

We begin reaming the intramedullary canal with an 8-mm endbiting reamer used in conjunction with a skin protector. The size of the reamer then is increased by 1-mm increments until cortical resistance is encountered. The unscrubbed surgeon must maintain optimal alignment of the fracture to avoid eccentric cortical reaming. When resistance to reaming is encountered, the surgeon should increase the size of the reamer in increments of 0.5 mm until reaming is sufficient. During the reaming process, the bulb-tipped guide should be held so that it does not back out when the reamer is retracted. We generally overream the proximal fragment by 0.5 mm unless the fracture is proximal. We have determined that overreaming prevents binding of the nail in the isthmus during insertion and greatly lessens the risk of comminution of the proximal fragment while still providing excellent fixation of the fracture. If a reamer breaks, it can be retrieved by withdrawing the bulb-tipped guide. As previously mentioned, excessive cortical reaming requires the use of larger nails, which increases the risk of comminution during insertion of the nail and resultant loss of stability.

After ascertaining that the chosen nail will fit over the nail-driving guide, we insert the guide across the fracture site while the bulb-tipped guide is still in place. The position of the nail driving guide is checked in both planes before the bulb-tipped guide is removed. The surgeon inserts the prebent cloverleaf intramedullary nail proximally and makes sure that the anterior bow of the nail conforms to that of the femur. The nail is driven to the fracture site and then is driven carefully across the site while the unscrubbed surgeon maintains the reduction. After the nail has been driven a few millimeters across the fracture site, the nail-driving guide may be removed and traction may be decreased sufficiently to allow impaction of the fracture as the nail is inserted farther. The unscrubbed surgeon must support the fracture during the final driving of the nail, especially in distal fractures, which tend to sag into a valgus position. The unscrubbed surgeon also applies a counterpressure to the knee as the nail is driven distally. The tip of the nail should extend to the old epiphyseal scar. When insertion of the nail has been completed, the entire femur is scanned with the image intensifier, and the fracture is studied closely for comminution. The incision is irrigated well and closed without any drain.

After the patient is moved carefully from the operating table, the traction pin, if present, is removed. At this point, we check femoral rotation and closely examine the ligamentous stability of the knee. The leg then is placed in an antirotation splint, and the patient is taken to the recovery room. In the recovery room, permanent AP and lateral radiographs of the entire femur are obtained and are used to check position of the nail and to assess stability of the fracture.

This operative procedure represents our standard nailing of stable transverse or short oblique fractures in the middle third of the femur (Fig. 9–6). This procedure must be modified under certain conditions. Modifications must be made for open fractures, for fractures

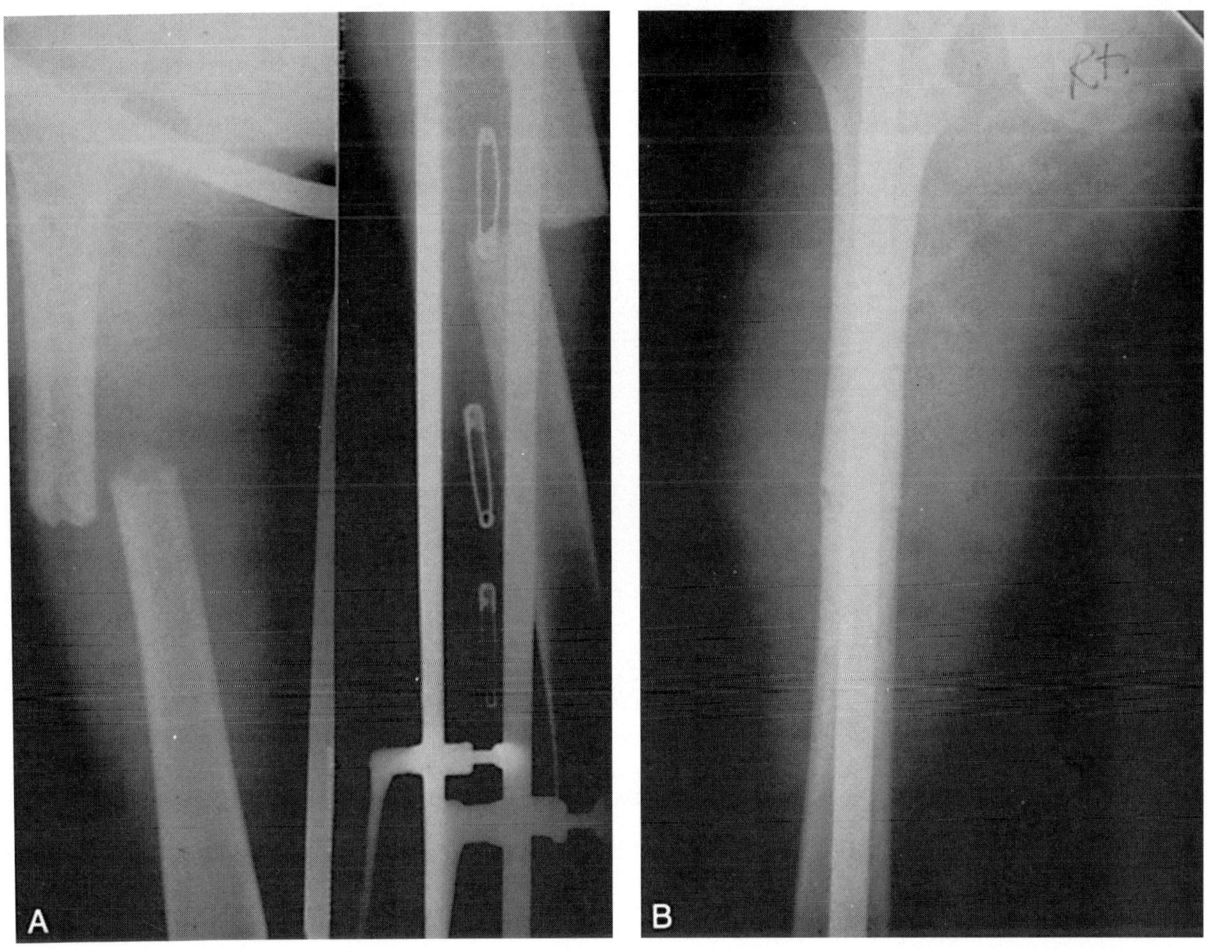

Fig. 9–6. *A,* Anteroposterior and lateral radiographs of a closed transverse fracture of the midshaft of the femur sustained by a 26-year-old man in a motorcycle accident. *B,* Postoperative radiographs demonstrate anatomic reduction with stable nail placement.

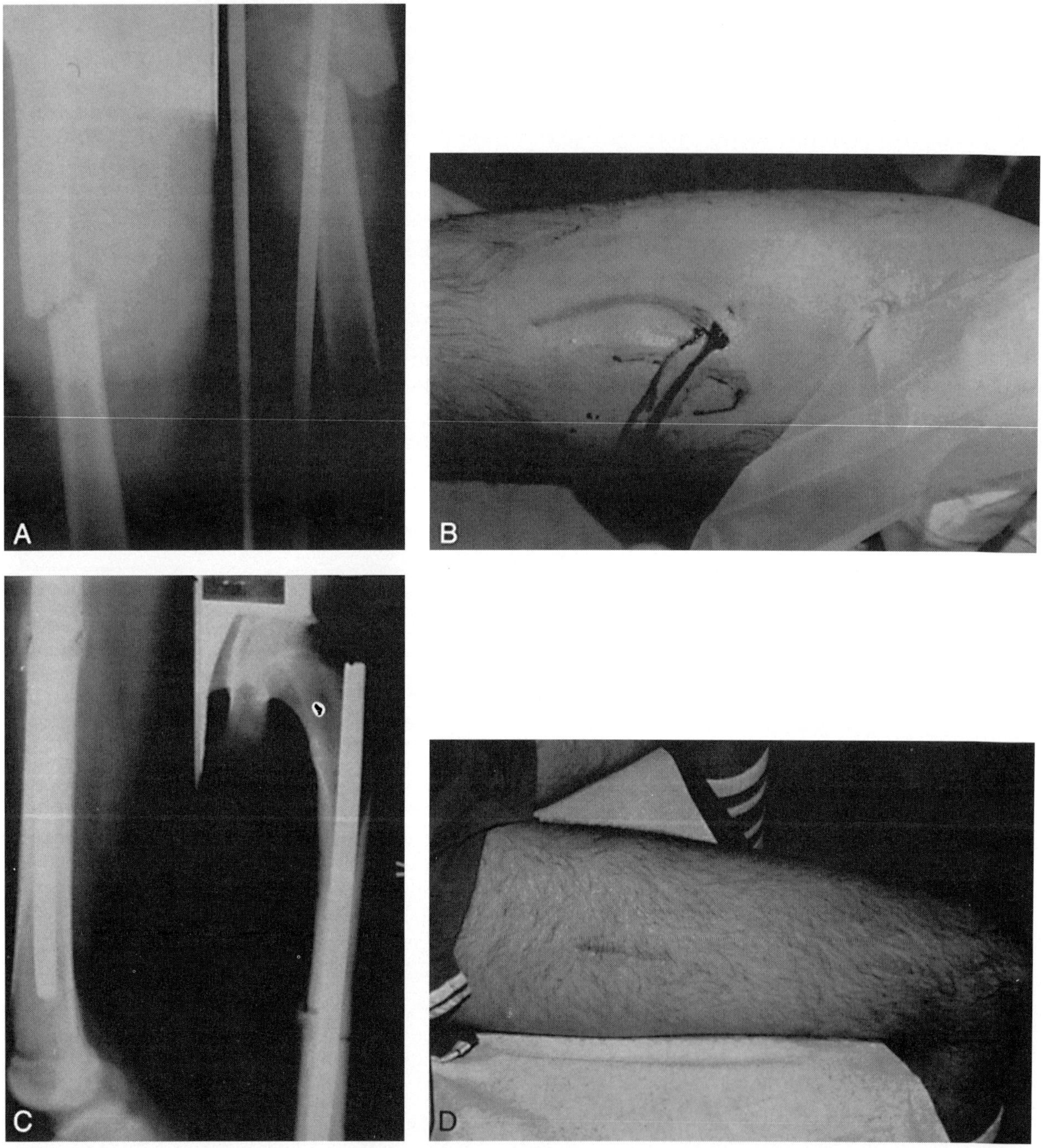

Fig. 9–7. *A,* Anteroposterior and lateral radiographs of a grade I open femoral fracture in a 28-year-old man involved in a motorcycle accident. *B,* The patient is positioned on the table for debridement of the open wound followed by immediate intramedullary nailing of the fracture. The traumatic wound is not closed primarily. *C,* Anteroposterior and lateral radiographs of the femur obtained 2 months after injury show anatomic position with excellent healing of the fracture. *D,* Two months after injury, the open wound has healed cosmetically and the patient has gained full range of motion of the knee.

that are very distal or proximal; and for segmental, comminuted, or long oblique fractures.

Open Fractures

We regard an open femoral shaft fracture as an indication for immediate operative stabilization, particularly in the multiply injured patient (Fig. 9–7). The technique previously described is altered in only two major respects. First, a thorough and meticulous debridement of the open fracture is performed before nailing. Second, the traumatic wound always is left open and is closed secondarily in 4 to 6 days. During our early experience with intramedullary nailing at Harborview Medical Center, all open femoral fractures were debrided primarily, and nailing was delayed for approximately 2 weeks after injury. As we became aware of the benefits of immediate internal fixation, however, our approach changed to the performance of immediate intramedullary nailing of open fractures. In this case, the traumatic wound must be left open initially. We do not advocate the use of antibiotics for longer than 48 hours after injury.

Proximal Fractures

Closed intramedullary nailing of proximal fractures can pose significant technical difficulties. Our limit for the use of standard intramedullary nailing for proximal fractures has been 2.5 cm below the lesser trochanter. The interlocking femoral nail, however, allows nailing of even more proximal subtrochanteric fractures, provided that the lesser trochanter is intact. Proper intramedullary nailing of very proximal fractures requires an accurate insertional point for the nail and an excellent reduction of the fracture. Both conditions are difficult to achieve because the short proximal fragment usually is pulled into flexion at the hip and generally also into abduction and external rotation. The insertion of the sharp-tipped awl into the proximal fragment too far anterior to the correct insertional point is a common pitfall. With subsequent reaming and insertion of the nail, posterior comminution of the proximal fragment may result. This error can be avoided when the flexed position of the proximal fragment is kept in mind while using the sharp-tipped awl. Fracture reduction must be obtained by the scrubbed surgeon, who accomplishes the reduction by inserting the bulb-tipped guide into the proximal fragment and reaming this fragment to 11 mm in diameter. The scrubbed surgeon then places a 10-mm nail over the bulb-tipped guide and uses it to manipulate the proximal fragment while the unscrubbed surgeon manipulates the distal fragment (Fig. 9–8).

Distal Fractures

Distal femoral fractures within 10 cm of the joint line often can be treated successfully with standard intramedullary nailing (Fig. 9–9). This technique is often safer and simpler to use than other methods of internal fixation. In more un-

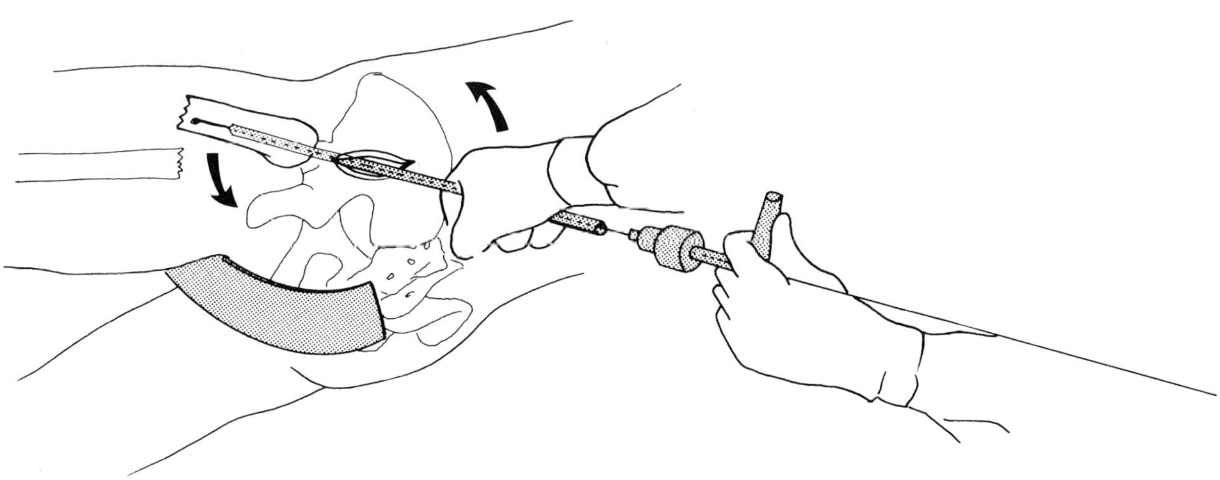

Fig. 9–8. In fractures of the proximal femoral shaft, a 10-mm nail inserted over the bulb-tipped guide aids in manipulating the flexed proximal fragment.

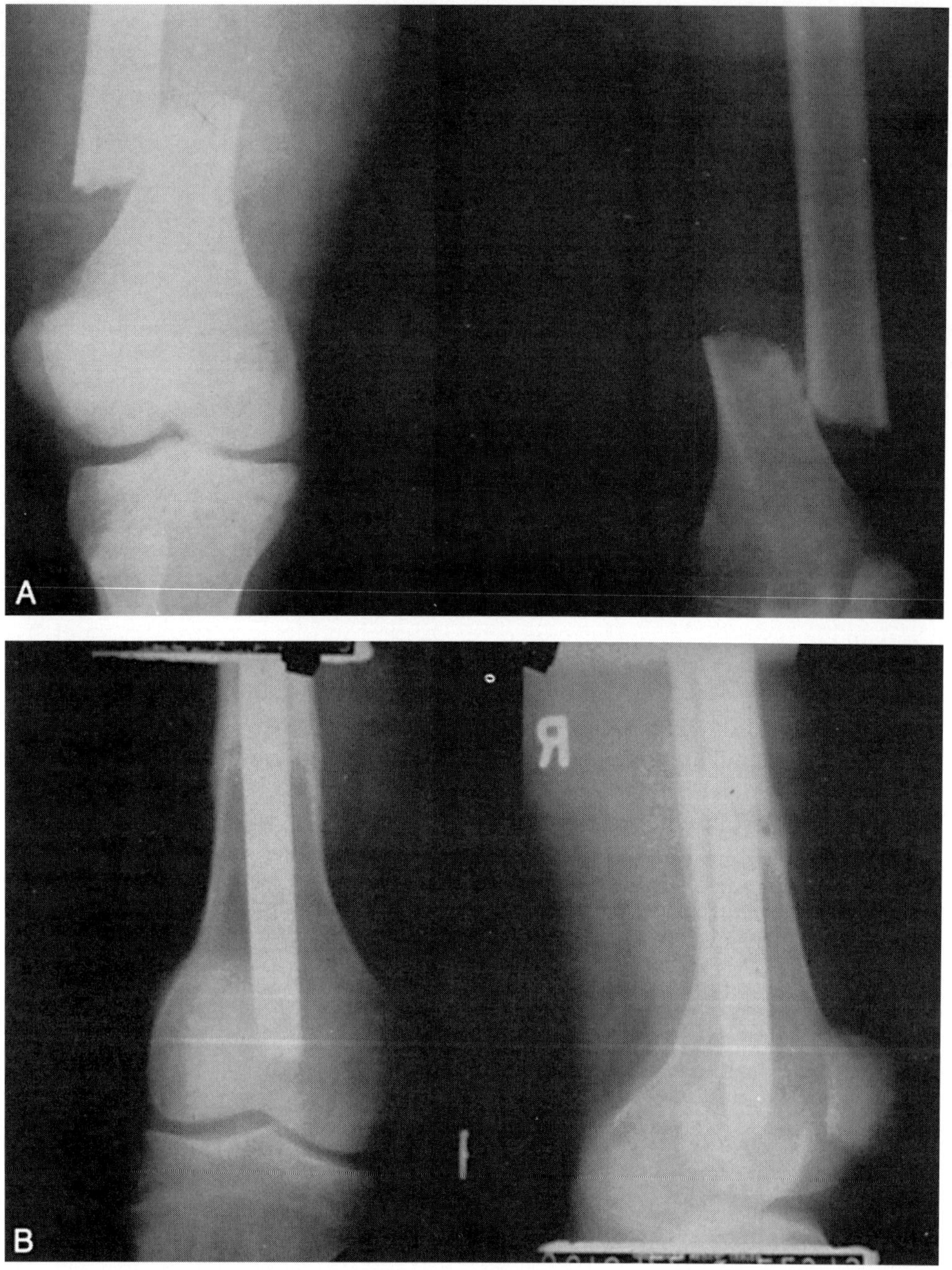

Fig. 9–9. *A,* Anteroposterior and lateral radiographs of a distal femoral shaft fracture in a 22-year-old man injured in a motor vehicle accident. Note the posterior displacement of the distal shaft with anterior angulation of the distal fragment. Traction placed through the foot will accentuate the deformity, preventing fracture reduction. Thus, the "flexed-knee table position" with a distal femoral traction pin is required. *B,* Postoperative anteroposterior and lateral radiographs of the femur show anatomic reduction with stable fixation.

stable distal fractures, we now tend to improve fixation of the distal fragment with the use of the interlocking nail. When treating distal fractures, the knee must be flexed and a distal femoral traction pin must be inserted. The flexed-knee position relaxes the posterior knee capsule and the gastrocnemius muscle, thereby avoiding a hyperextension deformity at the fracture, which can prevent fracture reduction. The femoral traction pin is inserted anteriorly just proximal to the adductor tubercle, and it is placed from the inframedial to the superolateral side to pull the fracture out of valgus angulation. The foot and leg then are placed on a Mayo stand that is raised or lowered to control rotation. With the patient in the lateral decubitus position, the weight of the leg produces valgus angulation at the fracture site. If the deformity is not corrected during the insertion of the nail, the nail will be driven into the medial femoral condyle, and a valgus deformity will result (Fig. 9–10). The unscrubbed surgeon must prevent this deformity by supporting the leg during insertion of the nail. Distal purchase of the nail is critical for the stability; thus, the cancellous bone is not reamed, and the nail is driven through the old epiphyseal scar to the level of the intercondylar notch. The use of a full-length nail, important in all femoral fractures, is essential in the more distal fractures.

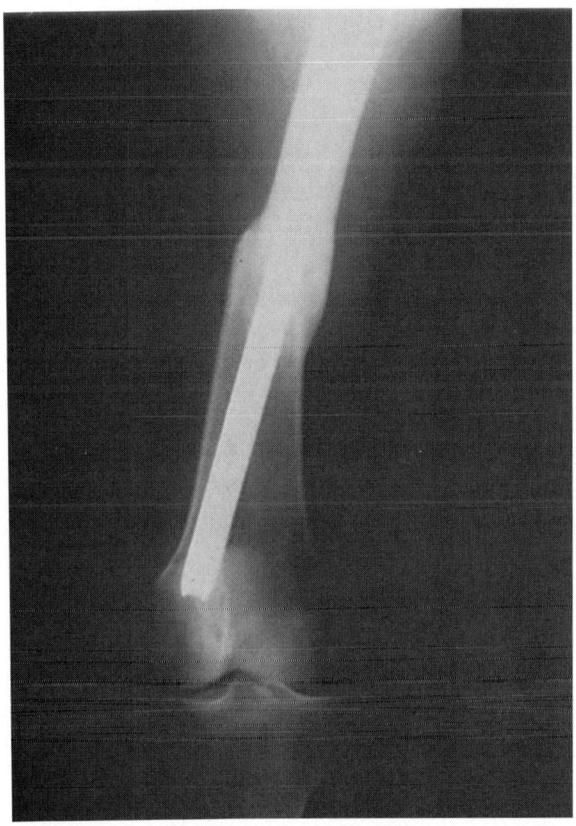

Fig. 9–10. Anteroposterior radiograph of a femoral fracture demonstrates a valgus malunion in a patient referred 12 months after injury. During the nailing process the fracture was allowed to sag into valgus alignment while the patient was in the lateral decubitus position on the fracture table. Note the improper placement of the distal tip of the nail in the medial femoral condyle.

Segmental Fractures

Segmental fractures may be managed effectively with closed intramedullary nailing.[10] There is a theoretic risk that the segmental fragment may spin during reaming if its fascial attachments have been disrupted by the injury. Preoperatively, both fractures are evaluated for their inherent stability, and the segmental fragment is examined for fracture comminution. If either fracture is deemed unstable, or if a segmental fragment is split, a static interlocking nail should be used. Each fracture should be reduced separately and externally while the bulb-tipped guide is passed carefully. Because external manipulation is not always successful in reducing these fractures, a rigid, sharp-tipped, curved guide may be necessary for internal manipulation. Reaming and nailing are carried out exactly as in the standard nailing procedure. The proximal and middle fragments are over-reamed by 0.5 mm to prevent difficulty when inserting the nail. The distal fragment may be quite short, and valgus sag must be prevented during nailing (see the previous section on distal fractures).

In segmental fractures, linear traction may fail to distract one of the two fractures, thereby making reduction difficult. If simple internal measures with sharp or bulb-tipped angled guides are not sufficient to produce alignment, a percutaneous hook can be inserted quickly from a direct anterior approach, and alignment can be achieved easily (Fig. 9–11). The hook is kept aligned with the muscle fibers to avoid damage to the muscle. The reamer guide is passed across the fracture site, and then the hook is removed.

Comminuted Fractures

Excellent results may be obtained with the use of standard intramedullary nailing in selected patients with comminuted fractures.[24] Fortunately, the interlocking nail has extended significantly the limits of intramedullary nailing, thereby allowing treatment of more severe degrees of comminution and, thus, has minimized the problems associated with postoperative instability, malrotation, and/or shortening of the fracture. Because these fractures appear to be unstable, the inexperienced surgeon tends to use a large nail. Unfortunately, the use of

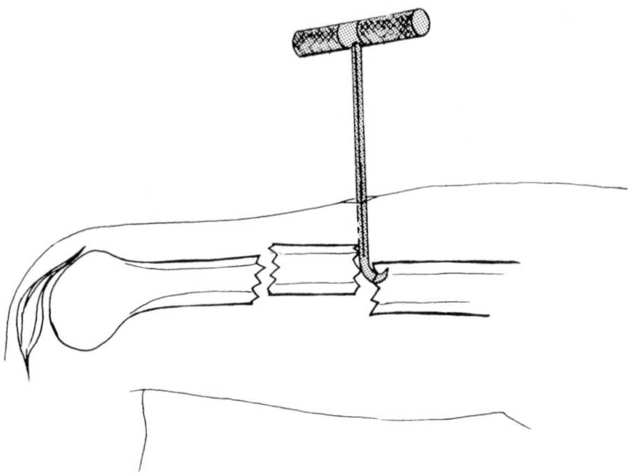

Fig. 9–11. In segmental fractures wherein simple measures have not proved sufficient to produce alignment, minimal open reduction may be achieved with the use of a percutaneous hook inserted quickly through a directly anterior approach. Care is taken to align the hook with the muscle fibers to avoid muscle damage. After the reamer guide has been passed across the fracture site, the hook is removed.

such a nail leads to further comminution and greater instability.

Preoperatively, the degree of fracture comminution must be determined according to a system of classification from grade I to grade IV.[24] In a grade I comminuted fracture, only a small piece of bone has broken off, and the effect of this fragment on the stability of the fracture is negligible. In a grade II comminuted fracture, the fragment is larger than that of the grade I fracture, but there is still at least 50% contact of the abutting cortices, which prevents shortening and helps to control rotation. A grade III comminuted fracture has less than 50% cortical contact of the proximal or distal fragments; thus, rotation, translation, and shortening of the fracture may occur. Grade IV comminuted fractures have segmental comminution and have lost the circumferential buttress of the bone; thus, there is no length or rotational stability.

In general, we treat grade III and grade IV comminuted femoral fractures with static interlocking intramedullary fixation. Grade I and grade II comminuted fractures may be treated with standard femoral nailing. As in transverse fractures, progressive, circumferential contact reaming is desirable to avoid further comminution. By directing the bulb-tipped guide away from a potential fragment, one may be able to prevent further comminution, especially when the fragment could be a large butterfly fragment. The cortex opposite a displaced oblique or butterfly fragment is not reamed because there is no cortical counter-resistance to the reamer. As the nail is driven through this area, the cortex can be fractured away (Fig. 9–12). The use of a larger nail increases the likelihood of such intraoperative comminution.

Long Oblique (Spiral) Fractures

Long oblique fractures represent an unstable pattern in regard to potential shortening. These fractures, which occur most commonly in the elderly patient, are caused by a low-velocity twisting injury that produces a long spiral pattern. When a long oblique fracture occurs in the midshaft, excellent nail fixation may be achieved with only slight subsequent shortening. Because the medullary canal of the femur widens proximally and distally, however, long oblique fractures in these areas cannot be stabilized rigidly with a standard intramedullary nail. Thus, proximal or distal long oblique fractures are best treated with static interlocking nail fixation or with standard nailing and supplemental cerclage fixation (Fig. 9–13).

Supplemental Cerclage Wiring of Unstable Shaft Fractures

The use of supplemental cerclage wiring for long oblique fractures carries the inherent risks of excessive blood loss, infection, and delayed union. Sciatic nerve palsy also may result from prolonged traction if the knee is in the extended position during operation. In years past, we used intramedullary nailing with supplemental cerclage wiring to treat selected grade III and grade IV comminuted fractures and long oblique fractures.[25] These fractures now are managed more safely and easily with static interlocking femoral fixation. We reserve supplemental cerclage wiring for use in proximal or distal long oblique fractures without comminution and, at times, for reduction of large comminution fragments in open fractures at the time of fracture debridement.

If cerclage wires are used, blood loss can be minimized by positioning the patient on the fracture table in such a way that as much weight as possible is placed on the trochanteric rest rather than on the perineal post. Risks of infection and delayed healing are minimized by avoiding excessive stripping of the fracture

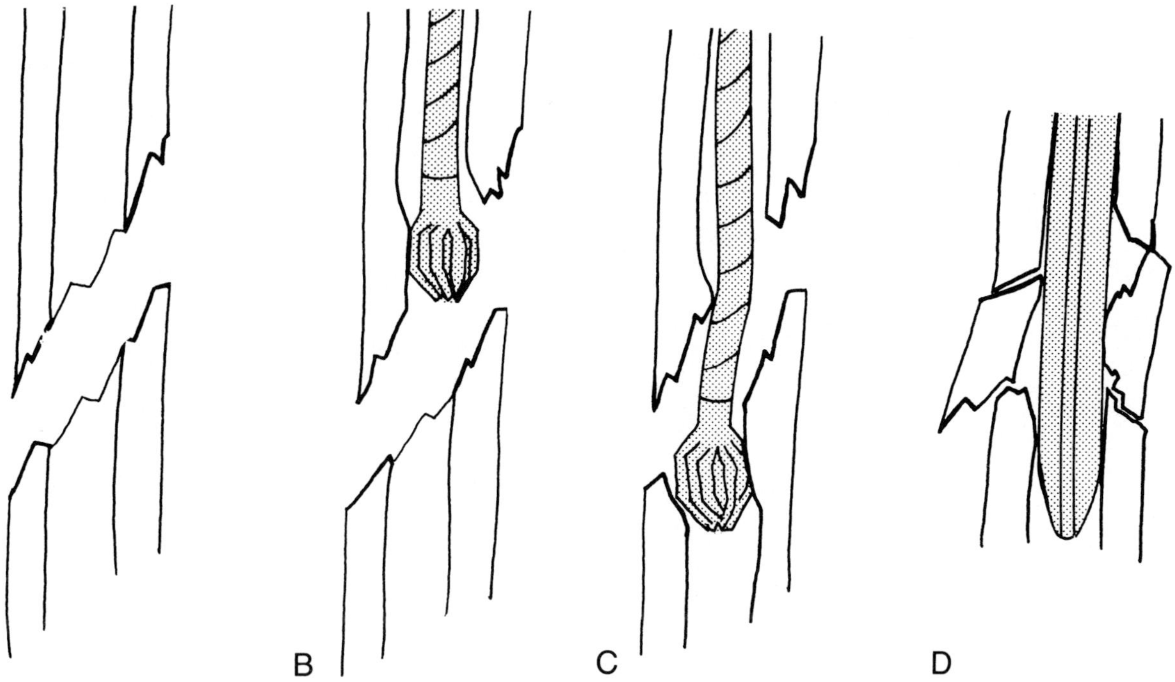

Fig. 9–12. *A,* Comminution of a fracture with a displaced oblique or butterfly fragment may occur intraoperatively. *B,* As the flexible reamer is moved toward the fracture site, it angles away from the longer side of the proximal bone fragment when it no longer encounters pressure from the opposite side. *C,* Eccentric reaming also occurs when the reamer enters the distal fragment. *D,* If several millimeters of the cortex are reamed, these angular projections of bone can be broken off when the nail is passed. Such comminution is more likely to occur if a larger nail is used. Intraoperative comminution may significantly reduce fracture stability, with resultant shortening and/or rotation of the fracture.

fragments. Also, Parham bands should not be used; Rhinelander has shown that they interfere with local vascularity of the bone and impede the healing process.[12] We prefer No. 18 gauge cerclage wires spaced 1 to 2 cm apart, depending on the fracture pattern. The risk of sciatic nerve palsy is essentially eliminated by flexing the knee and applying traction through a distal femoral pin. After the fracture has been reduced and cerclage wiring has been applied, standard nailing is performed as previously outlined. In general, reaming is minimized so that a nail with a slightly smaller diameter can be used,thereby reducing the risks of comminution and distraction during insertion of the nail.

Femoral Fractures in Adolescents

The standard nailing technique is changed slightly for femoral fractures in adolescents.[16] Special care is taken to avoid injury to the trochanteric apophysis when the insertional point is made. Selection of a nail with the correct length is important to avoid penetration of the nail into the distal femoral epiphysis. Excessive reaming should be avoided when treating femoral fractures in adolescents (Fig. 9–14).

POSTOPERATIVE CARE

After operation, the leg is placed in a special splint that adds rotational stability. In the majority of patients, physical therapy is initiated on the first postoperative day. Quadriceps muscle sets and straight-leg lifts are begun, and if possible, the patient is placed in a bedside chair. From the perspective of pulmonary care, one must take advantage of the benefits of femoral fixation by minimizing recumbency.

Protected crutch-assisted ambulation can begin when the patient can perform a straight-leg lift and can demonstrate control of the injured extremity. The degree of weight bearing allowed is determined by the stability of the fracture pattern. The patient is discharged from the hospital when fully independent. An active

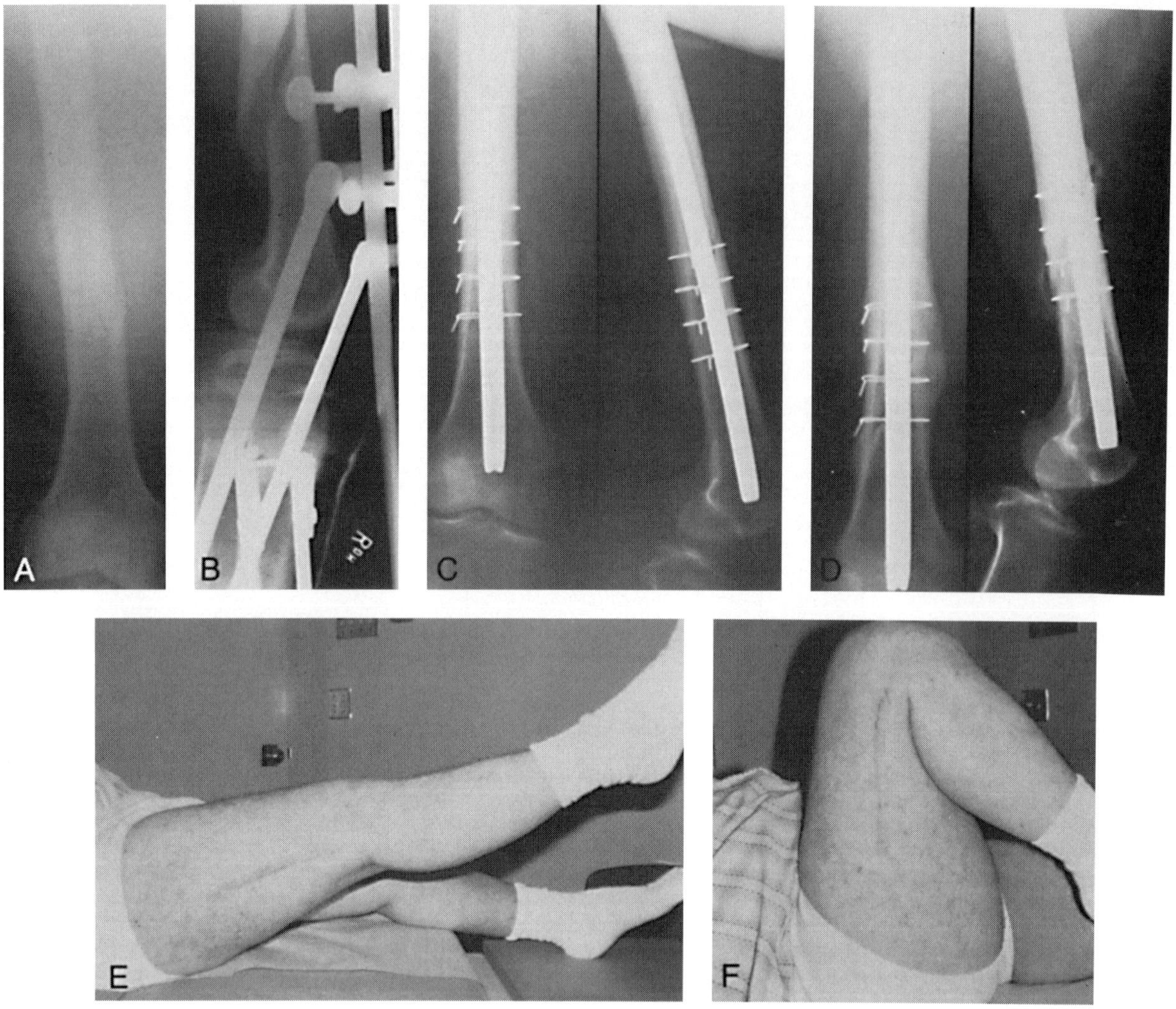

Fig. 9–13. Anteroposterior *(A)* and lateral *(B)* radiographs of a long oblique (spiral) fracture in the distal femoral shaft in a 50-year-old man injured in a 3-m fall. *C,* Radiographs following open reduction, cerclage wiring, and intramedullary nailing show anatomic reduction. *D,E,F,* Three months after injury, the fracture has healed and the patient has achieved an excellent functional end result with full range of knee motion.

quadriceps rehabilitation program and range-of-motion knee exercises are emphasized after discharge. Outpatient physical therapy supervision is encouraged and hastens functional recovery. The patient continues to use crutches to support ambulation until sufficient strength for independent ambulation and 90° of knee flexion have been achieved. For stable fractures, a 4- to 6-week recovery period is required before the patient can walk.

The patient returns for postoperative radiographic and physical examinations at 1, 3, 6, and 12 months. If postoperative radiographs indicate insufficient fracture stability to allow full weight-bearing ambulation, the patient's postoperative regimen is modified accordingly to include partial or toe-touch weight-bearing ambulation or, infrequently, postoperative traction or a spica cast. In most patients, removal of the nail is encouraged in patients younger than 50 years of age after 12 to 18 months, provided that a solid union has been achieved. The nails should not be removed in elderly patients or in patients who have sustained a pathologic fracture. Nail extractors are required and may necessitate a 1- or 2-day hospital stay. Patients are allowed unlimited weight bearing without crutches after removal of the nail.

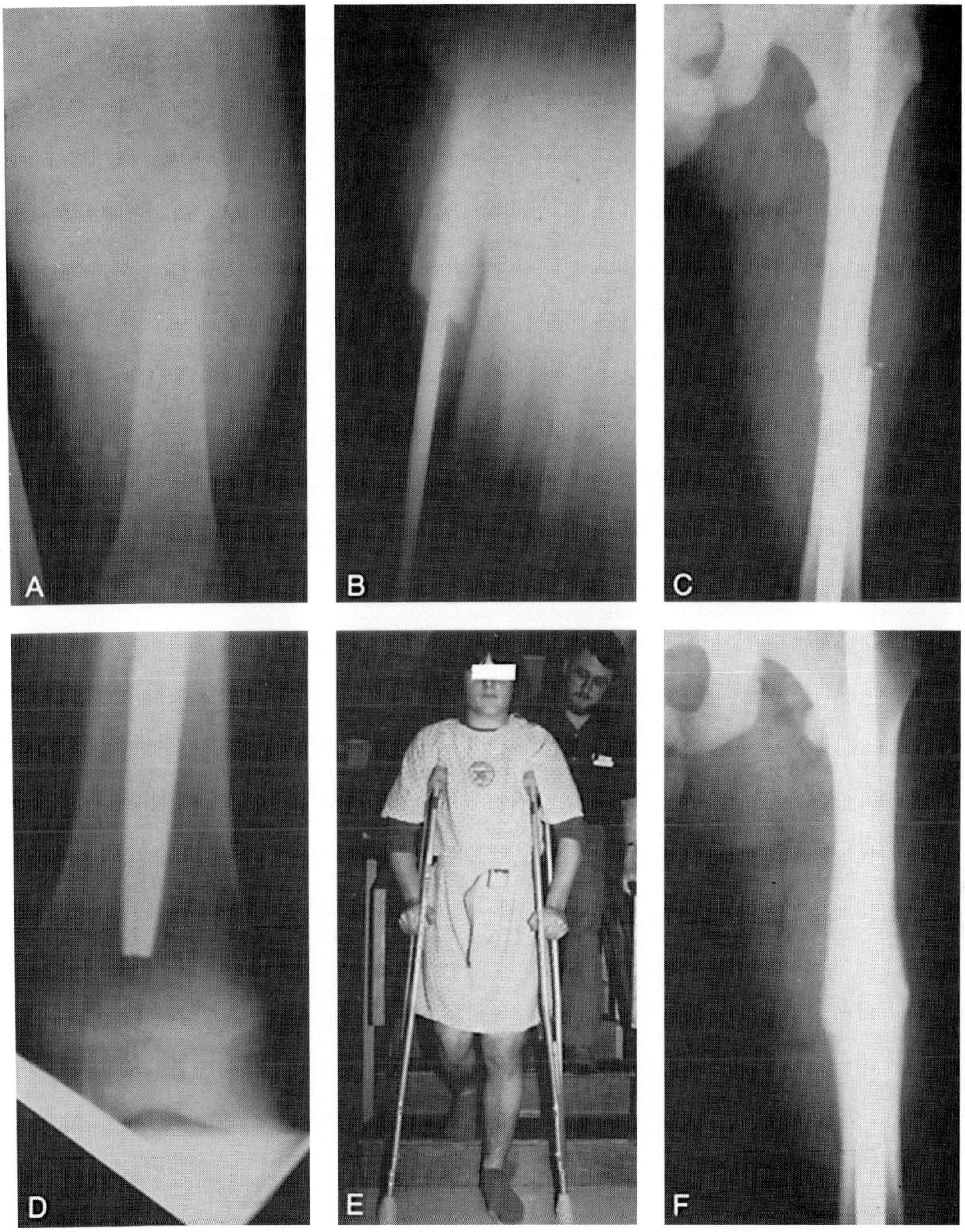

Fig. 9–14. *A,B,* Anteroposterior and lateral radiographs of a short oblique fracture of the midshaft of the femur sustained by a 14-year-old adolescent male during a motocross competition. *C, D,* Postoperative radiographs show anatomic reduction. Note that the nail does not violate the distal femoral epiphysis. *E,* On the second postoperative day, the patient was able to ambulate independently with crutches and was discharged from the hospital. *F,* Radiograph 9 months after injury shows solid union with both femora equal in length.

RESULTS

Since the introduction of closed intramedullary nailing into the University of Washington teaching program in 1968, the technique has been modified and refined with experience. We (Winquist and Hansen) reviewed the first 520 consecutive femoral shaft fractures treated between 1968 and 1979.[11] The average age of the 347 men and 153 women was 29.5 years (range 10 years, 10 months to 92 years). The majority of injuries were caused by motor vehicle accidents, and associated injuries commonly resulted from these high-energy accidents. Of the 500 patients, 143 sustained serious injuries to the head, chest, or abdomen; 27 patients had bilateral femoral shaft fractures; 54 patients had ipsilateral femoral and tibial fractures; and 27 had ipsilateral fractures of the hip, including femoral neck and intertrochanteric fractures. Also, 86 fractures were open.

The fracture was located in the proximal one third of the femur in 85 patients, in the middle one third in 325 patients, and in the distal one third in 110 patients. The series included 124 transverse fractures, 101 short oblique fractures, 30 spiral or long oblique fractures, and 261 comminuted fractures, including 26 segmental fractures.

The average time from injury to nailing was 7 days. In patients with isolated femoral fractures, the average length of the hospital stay was 13.3 days and the time on crutches averaged 5.8 weeks. For multiply injured patients, total length of hospital stay averaged 26.9 days. Of all the fractures, 87% appeared to be solidly united at 3 months. Postoperative range of motion of the knee averaged 132°. Only 8 patients experienced knee flexion of less than 125°, which was often related to additional injuries to the ipsilateral extremity. The incidence of significant ligamentous injuries to the knee was 9%.

Complications included 4 infections (0.9%), of which 2 occurred in open fractures and 2 in closed fractures. All 4 fractures ultimately healed without residual infection after aggressive management. Only 4 cases of nonunion were reported (0.9%). Shortening of more than 2 cm occurred in 2% of patients, and shortening of 1 or 2 cm occurred in 7.1%. External rotation malunion of 10° or more occurred in 43 patients; such malunion of more than 20° was seen in 12 patients. Closed intramedullary derotational osteotomies were required by 3 patients. Valgus angulation occurred in 8 patients in the series and ranged from 5 to 11°. Most cases of angulation were caused by technical complications of the nailing; valgus sag at the fracture site was not corrected by supporting the thigh during the nailing. In all patients, the angulation was asymptomatic and did not require correction. Varus angulation did not exceed 5° in 4 patients.

Medical complications included ARDS in 55 patients, which was related to the severity of initial injury and accompanying shock. All patients were managed with supportive respiratory measures, and all recovered completely. Pulmonary embolism occurred in 9 patients and led to death in 1 patient. Of the 500 patients, 11 died within a year of injury. One patient died 2 months after injury from complications of severe brain trauma, and 5 other patients died from associated multiple injuries. None of the deaths was related directly to the femoral fracture.

SUMMARY

Closed intramedullary nailing following reaming is a safe and effective means of treating most patients with femoral shaft fractures. The procedure is technically demanding and requires properly trained personnel and expensive equipment. Selection of the proper fracture pattern for standard nailing is important. Fortunately, the closed interlocking femoral nail has extended the limits of closed femoral nailing for fractures that would be unstable with regard to length and rotation after standard femoral nailing.

REFERENCES

1. Küntscher, G.: Die Marknagelung von Knochenbruchen. Arch. Klin. Chir. *200*:443, 1940.
2. Bohler, J.: Closed intramedullary nailing of the femur. Clin. Orthop. *60*:51, 1968.
3. Christensen, N.O.: Techniques, errors, and safeguards in modern Küntscher nailing. Clin. Orthop. *115*:182, 1976.
4. Clawson, D.K., Smith, R.F., Hansen, S.T.: Closed intramedullary nailing of the femur. J. Bone Joint Surg. *53A*:681, 1971.
5. Gherlinzoni, G., Vasciaveo, F., Murena, P.F.: Closed reduction reaming and nailing in fractures of the femoral shaft. Ital. J. Orthop. Traumatol. *1*:117, 1975.
6. Hansen, S.T., Winquist, R.A.: Closed intramedullary nailing of the femur. Clin. Orthop. *138*:56, 1979.
7. Kootstra, G.: Femoral Shaft Fractures in Adults. A Study of 329 Consecutive Cases with a Statistical Anal-

ysis of Different Methods of Treatment. Assen, The Netherlands, Van Gorcum, 1973.

8. Rascher, J.J., Nahigian, S.H., Macys, J.R., Brown, J,E.: Closed nailing of femoral-shaft fractures. J. Bone Joint Surg. *54A*:534, 1972.
9. Rokkanen, P., Slatis, P., Vankka, E.: Closed or open intramedullary nailing of femoral shaft fractures? A comparison with conservatively treated cases. J. Bone Joint Surg. *51B*:313, 1969.
10. Winquist, R.A., Hansen, S.T.: Segmental fractures of the femur treated by closed intramedullary nailing. J. Bone Joint Surg. *60A*:934, 1978.
11. Winquist, R.A., Hansen, S.T., Clawson, D.K.: Closed intramedullary nailing of femoral fractures. A report of five hundred and twenty cases. J. Bone Joint Surg. *66A*: 529, 1984.
12. Rhinelander, F.W.: Tibial blood supply in relation to fracture healing. Clin. Orthop. *105*:34, 1974.
13. Carr, C.R., Wingo, C.H.: Fractures of the femoral diaphysis. J. Bone Joint Surg. *55A*:690, 1973.
14. Hansen, S.T., Winquist, R.A.: Closed intramedullary nailing of fractures of the femoral shaft. Part II: Technical considerations. In The American Academy of Orthopaedic Surgeons Instructional Course Lecture. Vol. 27. St. Louis, C.V. Mosby Co., 1978.
15. Kempt, I., Grosse, A., Lafforgue, D.: L'apport du verrouillage dans l'enclouage centro-medullaire des os longs. Rev. Chir. Orthop. *64*:635, 1978.
16. Kirby, R,M., Winquist, R.A., Hansen, S.T.: Femoral shaft fractures in adolescents: A comparison between traction plus cast treatment and closed intramedullary nailing. J. Pediatr. Orthop. *1*:193, 1981.
17. Border, J.R., LaDuca, J., Seibel, R.: Priorities in the management of the patient with polytrauma. Prog. Surg. *14*: 84, 1975.
18. Riska, E.B., et al.: Prevention of fat embolism by early internal fixation of fractures in patients with multiple injuries. Injury *8*:110, 1976.
19. Talucci, R.C., et al.: Early intramedullary nailing of femoral shaft fractures: A cause of fat embolism syndrome. Am. J. Surg. *146*:107, 1983.
20. Karlstrom, G., Olerud, S.: Ipsilateral fractures of the femur and tibia. J. Bone Joint Surg. *59A*:240, 1977.
21. Veith, R.G., Winquist, R.A., Hansen, S.T.: Ipsilateral fractures of the femur and tibia: A report of 57 consecutive cases. J. Bone Joint Surg. in press.
22. Gustilo, R.B.: Management of Open Fractures and Their Complications. Philadelphia, W.B. Saunders Co., 1982.
23. Pedersen, H.E., Serra, J.B.: Injury to the collateral ligaments of the knee associated with femoral shaft fractures. Clin. Orthop., *60*:119, 1968.
24. Winquist, R.A., Hansen, S.T.: Comminuted fractures of the femoral shaft treated by intramedullary nailing. Orthop. Clin. North Am., *11*:633, 1980.
25. Morris, M.E., Veith, R.G., Winquist, R.A.: Unpublished data.

10

Locked Nailing of Femoral Fractures

Charles M. Court-Brown and Bruce D. Browner

NAILING OF THE FEMUR

The use of intramedullary nails in the treatment of femoral fractures has a long history. Hey Groves in Bristol, England, used both fenestrated and solid metal nails to treat the femoral fractures referred to him during and after World War I. He found the use of metal nails to be a great improvement over the bone and ivory pegs that he had used before the war.[1]

The next major contribution to intramedullary nailing was provided by the Rush family in the United States[2] and Gerhard Küntscher in Germany.[3] The Rush family introduced the concept of unreamed narrow nails, which could be used to treat femoral diaphyseal fractures by bending them to provide three-point fixation. These nails were the forerunners of the Hackethal and Ender's nails. The use of these devices is described elsewhere in the book.

Küntscher is unquestionably the father of reamed intramedullary nailing. Together with the engineer Pohl he designed a series of nails that culminated in the famous cloverleaf shape. Küntscher maintained that reaming was important. He felt that reamed nailing was advantageous for three reasons. First, it permitted the insertion of a nail of sufficient thickness to take over the function of the bone and therefore allowed early mobility. Second, reaming increased the area of endosteal contact made by the nail. Finally, reaming allowed for an accurate fit between the nail and the reamed part of the endosteal cortex. In addition to stating these basic concepts, Küntscher also believed that the surgical incision should be as far from the fracture as possible. Thus, unlike Hey Groves who practiced retrograde open nailing, Küntscher advocated closed nailing techniques. To facilitate these he also helped to pioneer the use of image intensification and, lastly, he developed the "Detensor" nail that allowed for interlocking fixation using transfixion bolts.

Küntscher presented his early work at a meeting of the German Surgical Society in 1968 shortly after his retirement, and he obviously influenced Klaus Klemm. Both Klemm and his coworker Schellman and later Grosse and Kempf from Strasbourg developed locking intramedullary femoral nails that were contoured to allow for the normal femoral recurvatum and had both distal and proximal cross screws through which screws or bolts could be inserted. This basic design, perfected in the late 1970s, has not been significantly altered over the last 15 years and virtually all modern femoral nails now have a similar design. Commercial constraints have altered the location and angle of the cross screws and the shape and diameter of the nail, but essentially the original design of Klemm and Schellman and Grosse and Kempf remains. Modifications such as the distal fins of the Brooker Wills nail have come and gone, but thus far, no one has devised an adequate replacement for locking screws or bolts.

The basic concept in interlocking nailing of the femur is straightforward. The locking screws are passed from lateral to medial femoral cortices through the holes in the nail. There are two basic modes of fracture fixation, static and dynamic. The term static locking

(Fig. 10–1) refers to the practice of inserting proximal and distal locking screws. This mode is used to treat fractures that are inherently unstable, particularly if there is cortical comminution or bone loss. Essentially, the femoral diaphysis is suspended between the proximal and distal cross screws. The dynamic mode of fixation (Fig. 10–2) refers to the practice of inserting cross screws either proximally or distally. This is used mainly for stable femoral fractures that are either proximal or distal to the isthmus. These fractures will not shorten but will remain rotationally unstable and require screw fixation in the shorter segment. Stable isthmic fractures are the fractures that are best treated by the classical Küntscher nail, and this type of fracture can easily be treated by an unlocked nail if the surgeon is confident about fracture stability.

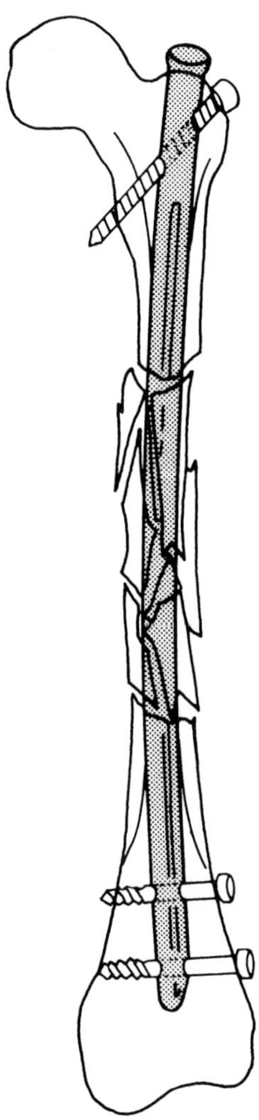

Fig. 10–1. Statically locked Grosse-Kempf intramedullary nail.

Surgical Technique

Unlike tibial nailing, in which there has been some evolution of surgical technique in the last few years, the technique of femoral nailing has not changed significantly over the last 15 to 20 years. There will be slight variations in the technique of femoral nailing and cross screw insertion depending on the type of nail used, but the basic operation is similar for all nails. In this chapter it will be described using the Grosse-Kempf intramedullary nail.

Preoperative Planning

Prior to commencing closed nailing of a femoral fracture, it is important to have adequate radiographs of the complete length of the femur. Not only should the fracture morphology be appreciated, but failure to visualize the whole length of the bone may result in the surgeon missing a proximal or distal fracture. This is particularly important if the surgeon is nailing a pathological fracture in the subtrochanteric area. Inadequate radiographs may prevent the demonstration of distal metaphy-

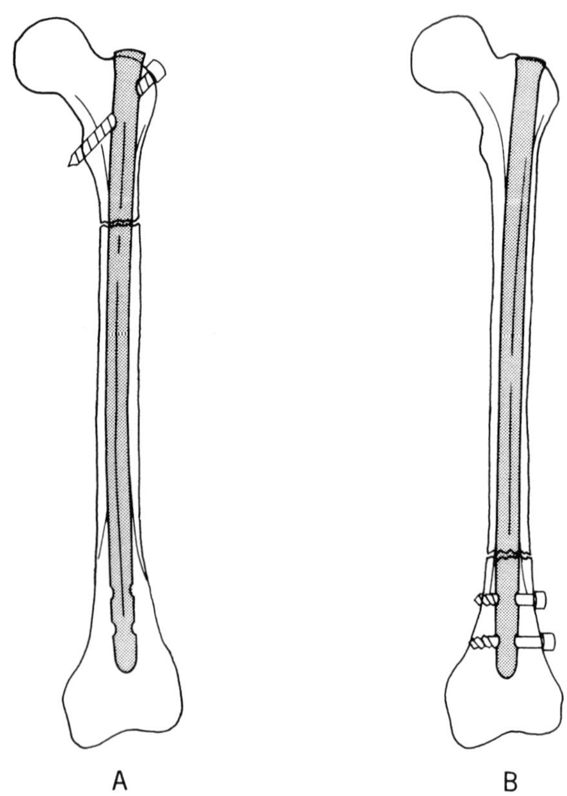

Fig. 10–2. Dynamically locked nail.

ses, which may preclude nailing or interfere with distal cross screw insertion.

The surgeon should study the preoperative radiographs very carefully, bearing in mind that he or she might cause a femoral neck fracture, proximal diaphyseal comminution, or increased comminution of the fracture, merely by the insertion of the femoral nail. It is therefore essential to know if these problems existed before surgery, as nailing may cause displacement of undisplaced fracture lines around the main fracture. If undisplaced fractures subsequently are displaced, a fracture that might have been treatable with a dynamic lock will require a static lock.

A surgeon should also be aware of the presence of osteoarthritis of the hip, which may interfere with movement of the hip during nailing. In severe cases of hip osteoarthritis, the hip may be so stiff that conventional supine nailing is impossible. It is obvious that the surgeon must look for the presence of a hip or knee arthroplasty. The former will clearly preclude femoral nailing. Although the latter does not, care must be taken not to damage or loosen a knee prosthesis during the operation.

The surgeon must also be careful not to start a femoral nailing procedure without the correct equipment. He or she should check that the operating room is equipped with a full set of nails of appropriate sizes and the complete nailing and reaming instrumentation. In addition, the correct nail extraction equipment should be on hand should the surgeon run into difficulties. The fracture table should be modified for nailing and the image intensifier should always have a memory to minimize the amount of radiation to which the surgeon is exposed.

Patient Positioning

There are two basic positions for femoral nailing, the lateral decubitus position (Fig. 10–3) and the supine position (Fig. 10–4). Each has its merits and the surgeon will usually select the patient position based on personal preference, although there are some specific indications for each position.

The lateral position provides easy access to the greater trochanter and with appropriate positioning of the image intensifier good visualization of the complete femoral shaft can be obtained. However, it is more difficult to accurately place the patient in the lateral position, particularly if the operating room staff are inexperienced in the use of this position. Other disadvantages include respiratory compromise because of the compression of the dependent lung, a valgus malposition at the fracture site secondary to the action of gravity, and increased difficulty in assessing the degree of any rotational malalignment. Distal screws are a little more difficult to insert and the use of a plastic isolation drape is virtually impossible.

However, the fact that the hip joint is flexed during nailing in the lateral position may make nailing of a patient with an osteoarthritic hip

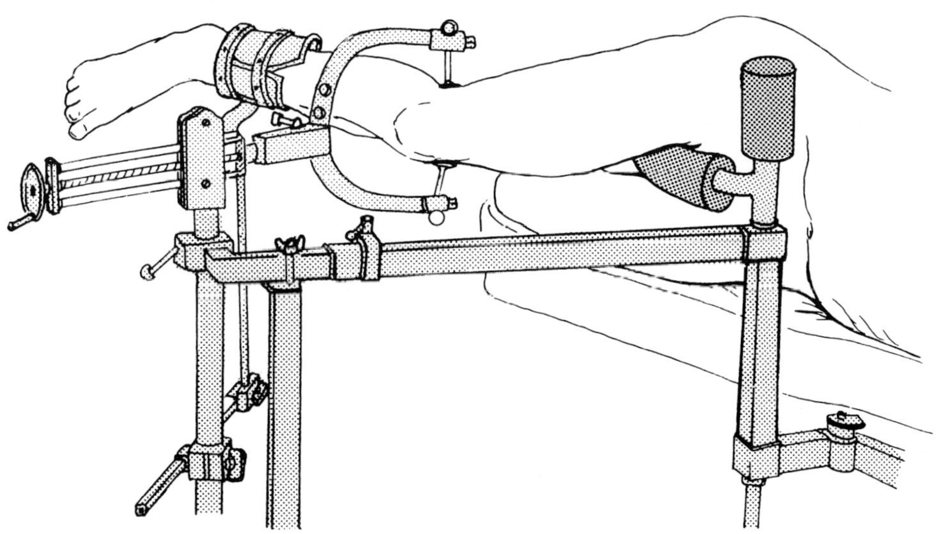

Fig. 10–3. The lateral decubitus position for nailing.

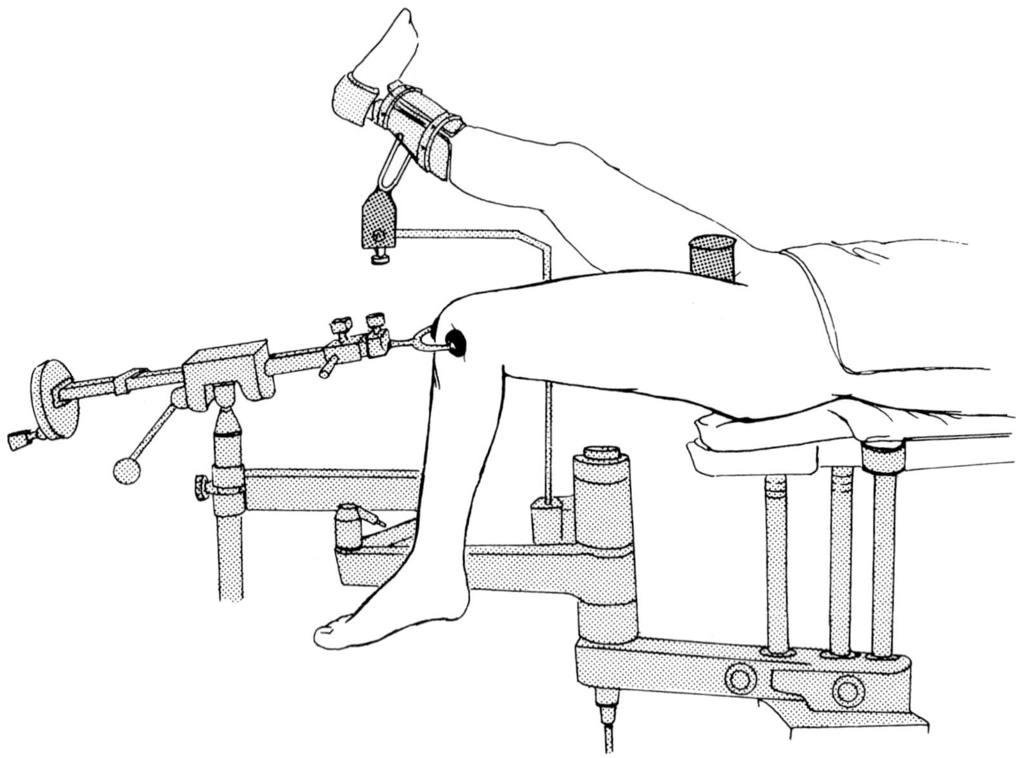

Fig. 10–4. The supine position for nailing.

somewhat easier, because allowance is made for the fixed flexion deformity that may be present in the hip joint. Some surgeons also prefer the lateral position when nailing proximal femoral fractures, because in these fractures the proximal femoral fragment tends to assume a flexed position.

In the supine position the patient is placed supine on the orthopaedic table. The contralateral limb is flexed at the hip and knee and placed on a well-padded support. This position allows for easy use of an image intensifier to visualize the femur. Access to the proximal femur is facilitated by adducting the leg, and if the patient is overweight, a pad placed in the flank will facilitate access. There are few disadvantages to the supine position, although proximal femoral fractures and fractures adjacent to an osteoarthritic hip may provide a problem, and the surgeon should be aware of this. Moran et al.[4] described using the supine position for nailing femoral fractures in patients with fixed flexion deformities in osteoarthritic hips. They approached the proximal femur from below. However, this is an awkward technique and surgeons may well elect to use the lateral approach.

Entry Point

Surgeons often describe the insertion of the distal cross screws as being the most difficult aspect of femoral nailing. However, the most critical maneuver in femoral nailing is, in fact, the selection of the correct nail entry point. There is some debate concerning the optimal entry point. Küntscher and, subsequently, the AO group advocated the tip of the greater trochanter (Fig. 10–5). It was argued that a more medial entry point would compromise the blood supply to the femoral head and possibly cause a femoral neck fracture. However, if this point is chosen, the nail will be forced to travel medially and therefore strike the medial cortex of the upper femur. This may well result in femoral comminution and in varus malalignment of proximal fractures. It also frequently results in the nail twisting as it passes down the femur. This may make the nail difficult to insert, cause deformity at the fracture site, and result in the insertion of the distal cross screws being awkward.

The alternative starting point is the piriform fossa just medial to the greater trochanter. This tends to be situated in the axis of the femur above the intramedullary canal and its use results in the nail passing directly down the intramedullary canal. The use of the piriform fossa is not associated with the same risk of comminution or nail twisting. Care must be taken not to attempt nail insertion medial to the piriform fossa, because there is a significant risk of femoral neck fracture.

It is recommended that the image intensifier be used to locate the correct entry point. Digital examination will indicate the position of the piriform fossa, but the intensifier will show the surgeon if the selected entry point is above the medullary canal of the femur. Once the correct position is selected, a bone awl can be used to make an initial defect in the bone. Alternatively, a standard hip fracture guide wire may be inserted into the bone in the piriform fossa and an overdrill can be used to establish the nail entry point.

Closed Reduction and Reaming

Reduction is achieved by a combination of traction, external manipulation of the fracture by the surgeon or a scrubbed assistant and occasionally by using a small hollow nail in the proximal fragment to allow manipulation of this fragment. Closed reduction may be difficult to achieve, and the surgeon must under no circumstances attempt closed nailing of the femur until it has been demonstrated that the fracture is reducible by closed means and that he or she is aware of what maneuver is required to reduce the fracture. If the fracture cannot be reduced by closed means, closed nailing should not be attempted and another treatment method should be selected.

Traction can be applied through a skeletal pin or an orthopaedic boot. If there has been little delay before surgery and the patient is not overweight or extremely muscular, the use of an orthopaedic boot, as used commonly in hip fracture surgery, will be adequate. However, if surgery has been delayed or if the patient is extremely muscular, it is always safer to apply traction through a skeletal pin. The pin can be inserted through the distal femur or the proximal tibia. A distal femoral pin provides for a more direct pull on the fracture but may obstruct the passage of the nail in a distal fracture. However, in reality either pin location can be used fairly easily.

Once the patient has been prepared and draped, the surgeon should make the skin incision. The most common error made by surgeons in femoral nailing is to center the proximal skin incision on the greater trochanter. In fact, the skin incision should start at the level of the greater trochanter and be carried proximally for about 10 cm. This will allow the instrumentation required in closed nailing to be contained within the wound.

Once the surgeon has dissected down to the level of the proximal femur, the entry point has been determined, and a defect has been made in the proximal femoral cortex, a hand reamer can be used to make a track between the proximal femoral defect and the intramedullary canal. The metaphyseal bone in the trochanteric area may be hard in young people, and it is important to make a tract between the entry point and the canal before reaming is undertaken to facilitate the passage of a guide wire.

Once the tract exists between the entry point and the intramedullary canal, an olive-tipped guide wire can be passed into the femur. If the fracture is well aligned, a straight guide wire can be employed, but usually it is necessary to "feel for" the distal fracture with the guide wire. To facilitate this, the end of the guide wire should be bent by approximately 20°, about 2 cm from the tip. If the femur is to be reamed, the surgeon must ensure that there is an olive-tip on the wire in case the reamer becomes stuck. If this occurs, the presence of the olive facilitates reamer removal.

Once the guide wire has crossed over the fracture site, it should be passed distally into the center of the distal fragment as visualized on the anteroposterior intensifier view. It is important that the guide wire is not passed down the medial or lateral femoral cortices, as the subsequent introduction of a nail into these locations will cause a valgus or varus deformity. The guide wire should be placed into the distal metaphyseal bone to minimize the risk of it backing out later.

The reamers are introduced over the olive-tipped guide wire. In most reaming sets, the initial reamer is end-cutting and enlarges the tract to about 9 mm. Subsequent side-cutting reamers are used to expand the tract in 0.5-mm in-

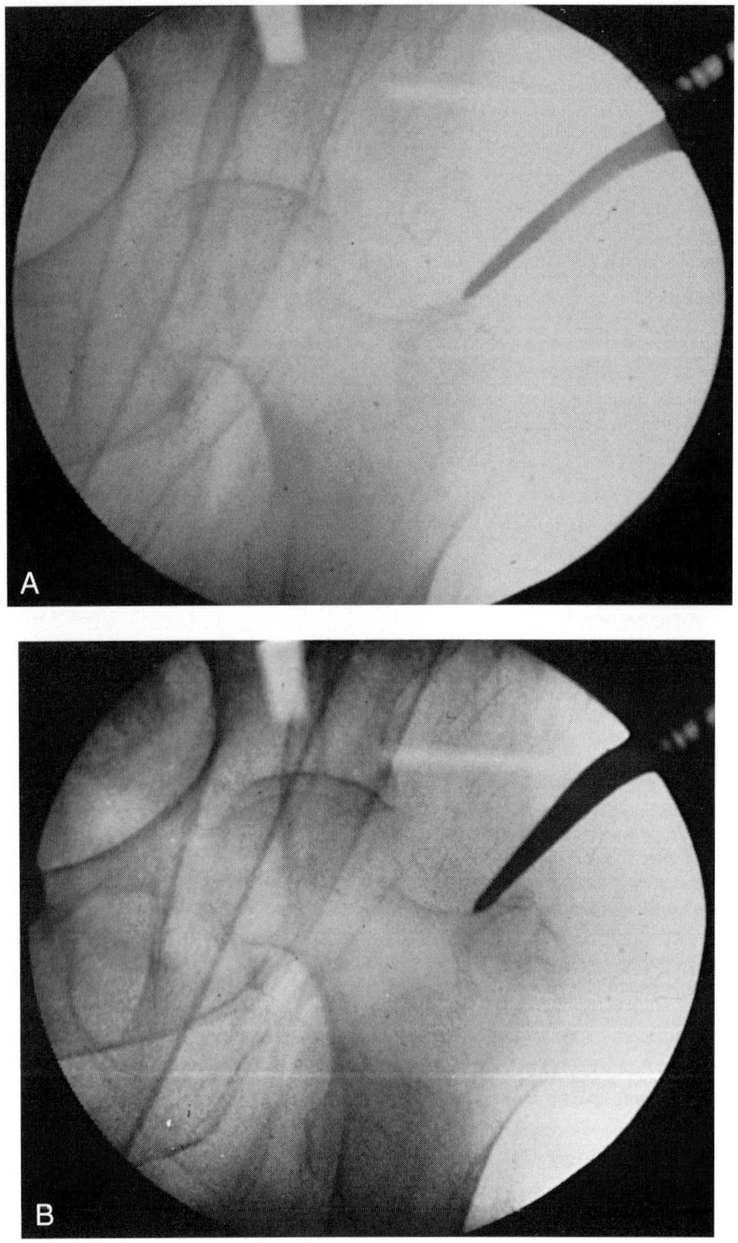

Fig. 10–5. *A,* An image intensifier view showing a bone awl place on the tip of the greater trochanter. It is clear that this location is lateral to the axis of the femur and if the nail is introduced from this site, it will bend as it is advanced down the intramedullary canal. *B,* The bone awl has been placed in the piriformis fossa. This is medial to the tip of the trochanter and is a more appropriate site for the insertion of the intramedullary nail. (continued)

crements. It is important that the surgeon resists the temptation to progress in larger increments, as the reamers may well become stuck within the canal. Care should be taken to ream the whole length of the femur. Failure to do this may result in cortical damage as the nail is hammered into unreamed bone.

Reaming should be carried out until the resultant track in the medullary canal is 1 mm wider than the intramedullary canal that the surgeon proposes to use. Unslotted nails tend to be stiffer than slotted nails, and it is suggested that if an unslotted reamed femoral nail is used, the surgeon should ream the canal 2 mm larger than the size of the proposed nail. In adult femora, it is adequate to use a 12- or 13-mm

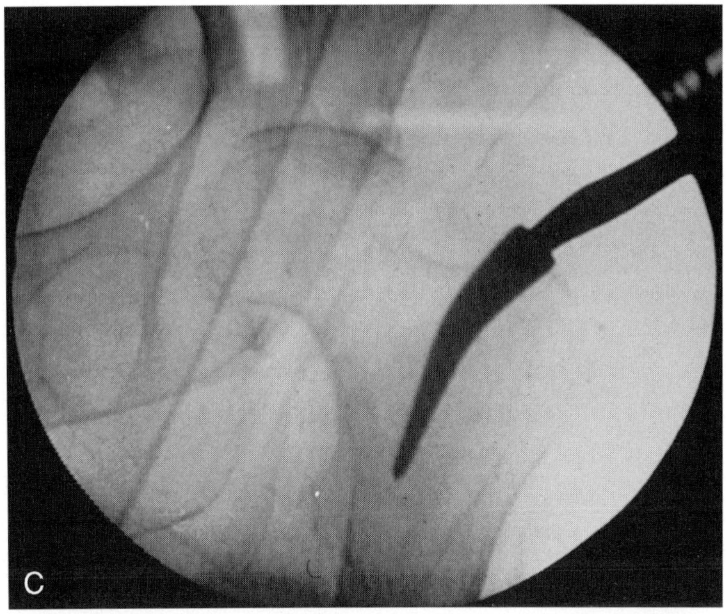

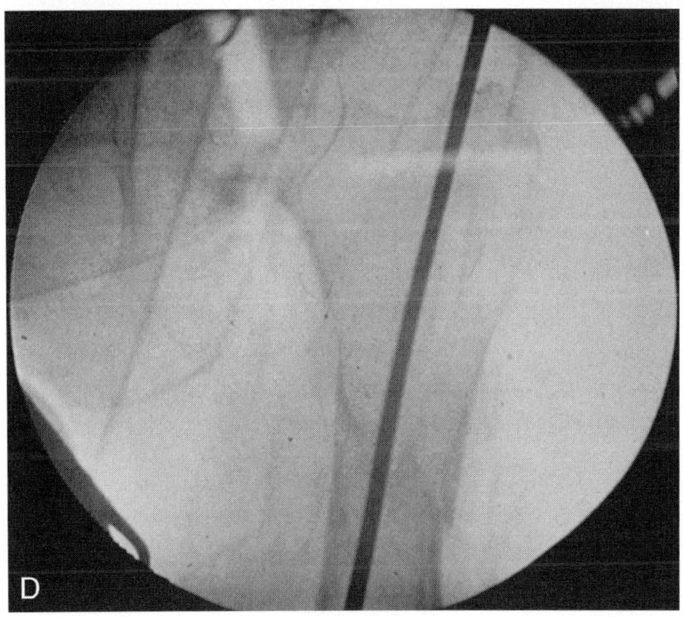

Fig. 10–5. (continued) *C,* The bone awl has been placed into the piriformis fossa and a channel has been made into the intramedullary canal. This maneuver is essential before a guide wire can be passed into the femur. *D,* A guide wire has been passed down the femoral canal.

nail. In older patients, the medullary canal may be wider and nails of 15 or 16 mm may be employed. Once the femoral canal has been reamed, a nail of the appropriate length is selected. Femoral length can be assessed by using a ossimeter, by preoperative measurement of the length of the contralateral femur (if this is intact), or by measuring the guide wire. Thus, the olive-tipped guide wire should be replaced by a graduated straight guide wire over which the nail can be inserted. Changing the guide wires is facilitated by placing a plastic sleeve over the olive-tip guide wire prior to removal to allow for maintenance of fracture position.

Once the correct length and diameter have been calculated, the nail should be mounted on the appropriate introducer and passed down the femoral canal (Fig. 10–6). Care should be

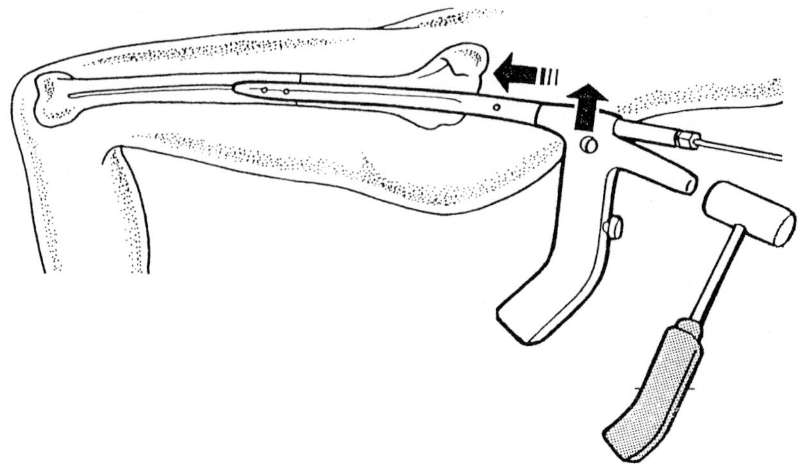

Fig. 10–6. Once the intramedullary canal has been reamed, a straight nontipped guide wire is inserted to the distal end of the femur and the nail is passed over it into the intramedullary canal.

taken so that the nail does not damage the bone at the fracture site as it is hammered across this area. Excessive hammering will cause bone damage and should never take place. If this is required, there probably has not been adequate reaming or the end of the nail is abutting against cortical bone. The nail should be fully inserted so that the top of the nail is flush with the proximal femur and the distal end of the nail is embedded into the distal femoral metaphysis.

Proximal cross screw insertion is usually straightforward. All of the nails have adequate jigs that allow the surgeon to insert a proximal cross screw. Most nails now use a diagonal cross screw, running from the greater trochanter downwards and medially into the lesser trochanter. Only one proximal cross screw is required. The surgeon should be careful that the cross screw is not placed above the lesser trochanter into the base of the femoral

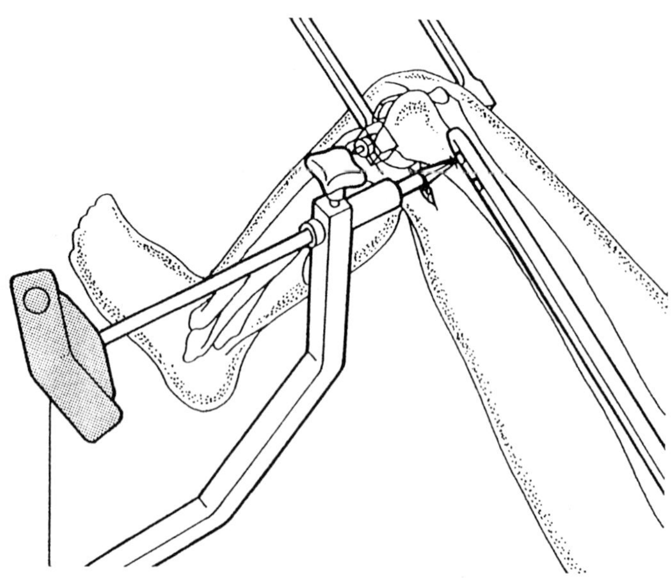

Fig. 10–7. The use of an intensifier-mounted jig to insert a distal cross screw. Once the jig has been aligned so that the distal nail hole can be visualized in the beam of the C-arm, a mark is placed on the skin and subsequently on the bone to facilitate drill and screw placement.

neck, because this may well weaken the femoral neck and cause a fracture.

Distal Locking

Three methods of distal locking are available to guide drilling and insertion of the screws through the distal holes in the nail.

Image Intensifier Mounted Target Device

With this technique, a metal gantry is attached to the image intensifier so that the intensifier beam passes through an alignment hole and then through the holes in the nail. A pointer is placed in the alignment hole and pressed against the skin. A small skin incision is then made, and the pointer advanced to mark the bone (Fig. 10–7). A drill sleeve is then mounted instead of the pointer. Once the intensifier beam is perfectly aligned with the drill sleeve and the holes in the nail, a drill bit can be placed through the drill sleeve and into an appropriately placed skin incision and then used to create a hole in the distal femur to allow the passage of a cross screw (Fig. 10–8). Once the hole has been drilled, the image intensifier mounted device is removed and a depth gauge is used to select the appropriate size of distal screw or bolt, which is then inserted.

Nail Mounted Target Device

In the mid-1980s there was a vogue for using a nail-mounted target device. The rationale behind the use of these devices was straightforward. A siting device was screwed onto the end of the nail such that poles in the distal part of the siting device were aligned with the holes in the distal part of the nail. Once the nail had been passed into the femur, it was theorized that it would be straightforward to then insert a drill sleeve into the distal holes of the nail-mounted jig and consequently insert distal screws or bolts.

Unfortunately, it soon became clear that femoral nails twist and deform as they are passed into the intramedullary canal. This is particularly true of the slotted nails like the Grosse-Kempf nail, but even solid section nails such as the Russell-Taylor nail also deform, rendering nail-mounted devices useless. Few people now use these devices and most surgeons have turned to the use of a freehand technique to facilitate the insertion of distal cross screws.

A

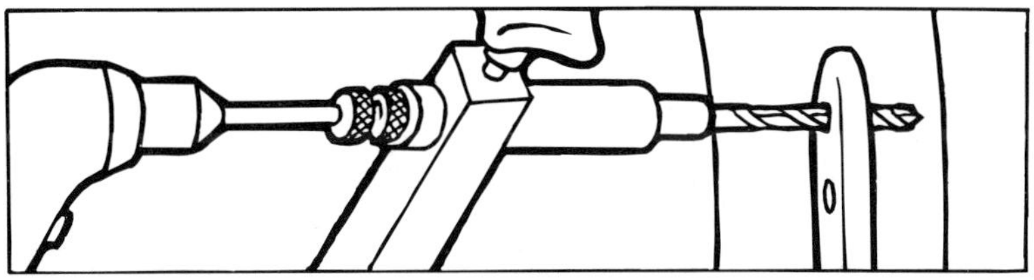

B

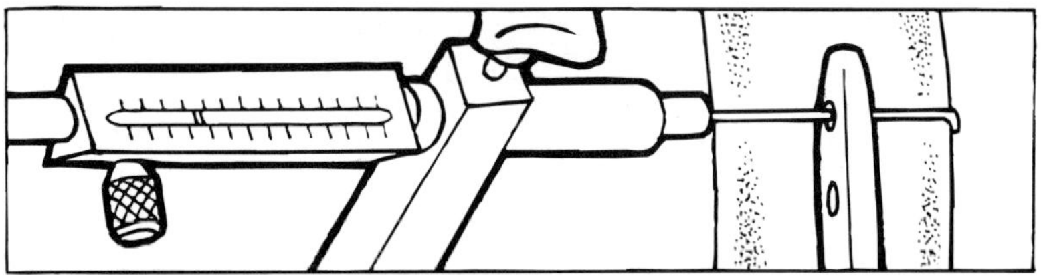

C

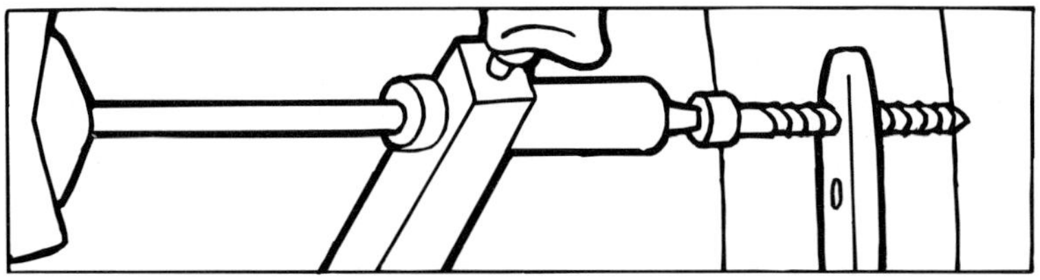

Fig. 10–8. *A,* The drill bit is advanced through the sleeve in the jib and through the distal screw hole. *B,* A depth gauge is used to assess the correct length of screw. *C,* A screw is then advanced into the nail.

Freehand Technique

To prepare for distal cross screw insertion using a freehand technique, the C-arm of the image intensifier is placed in a lateral position with the beam exactly at right angles to the bone (Fig. 10–9). The surgeon should never start drilling for distal screw placement until one of the distal screw holes appears as a perfect circle on the image intensifier screen. Because the nail frequently rotates during insertion, it is helpful to have an orthopaedic table which will rotate to regain alignment of the nail within the intensifier beam.

If the holes in the distal part of the nail appear elliptical, they are not correctly lined up in the intensifier beam. If the nail is correctly rotated and the intensifier beam is not at right angles to the nail, then the hole will appear to be elliptical in the longitudinal plane. If the rotation of the nail is incorrect but the image intensifier is correctly placed, the ellipse appears in the transverse plane. By altering the rotation of the patient and the angle that the C-arm makes with the distal femur, it is possible to get an exact circle.

When a perfect circle is achieved, the surgeon should use a long pointer to delineate the exact center of the pole in the intensifier beam. Once this is done, an appropriate skin incision can be made. The sharp pointer can then be inserted through the soft tissues onto the lateral cortex of the femur and once again aligned to appear in the center of the hole. Once this is

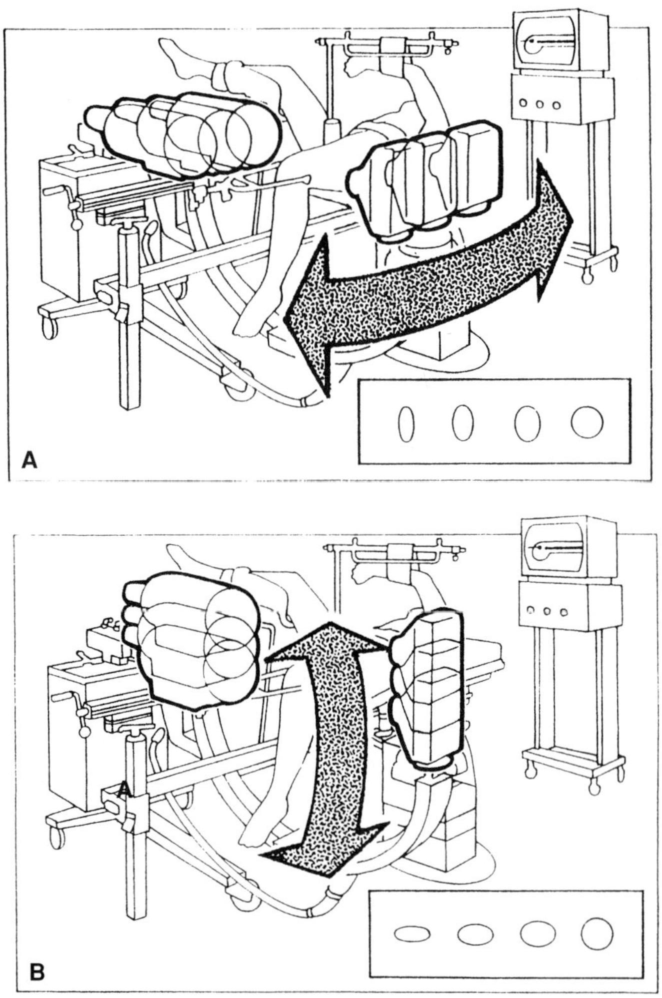

Fig. 10–9. *A,* This demonstrates the appearance of the distal hole where the C-arm of the image intensifier is incorrectly aligned but the nail rotation is correct. The C-arm should be exactly at right angles to the femur to get a perfect circle. Distal cross screw insertion should not commence until a perfect circle is seen. *B,* A transverse ellipse is seen where the rotation of the nail is incorrect with respect to the C-arm of the intensifier. This must be corrected to get a perfect circle.

done, the pointer or awl can be used to make a defect on the lateral cortex of the femur and an appropriate drill bit can then be inserted into the femoral defect and a hole placed between the cortices of the femur through the distal hole of the nail. A depth gauge can then be used to estimate the correct screw or bolt size, and an appropriate screw or bolt is then inserted.

There are a number of tips which are useful to facilitate the insertion of distal cross screws. The radiographer can be allowed to drop the C-arm to allow the surgeon access to the lateral femur but should not be allowed to remove the C-arm in any other way. It is relatively simple to drop and subsequently raise the C-arm of the intensifier, but if the intensifier is moved in any other way from its original position, it is frequently difficult to reposition it properly.

It is also suggested that the surgeon checks that the drill bit is within the hole in the nail once it has been inserted through the femur. This maneuver should be repeated when the screw has been inserted through the lateral cortex of the femur and the nail to ensure that an adequate position has been achieved.

A number of devices have been invented to facilitate freehand distal cross screw placement. The best known of these is the offset radiolucent drill. It permits a drill bit to be driven at 90° to a power drill in a device that is radiolucent. By aligning the siting rings with the distal hole in the nail, it is relatively easy to insert a distal cross screw. A number of manufacturers produce such devices. Other techniques have been suggested. Kirschner wires have been used to drill a siting hole through the femoral cortices and surgeons have experimented with the use of lasers and ultrasound, but none of these techniques have been proven in clinical practice. The freehand technique remains the technique of choice for distal cross screw insertion, although the offset radiolucent drills do provide a useful alternative method.

The question always arises concerning whether the surgeon should use one or two distal cross screws in the treatment of femoral diaphyseal fractures. It has been suggested that if the proximal of the two distal screw holes remains empty, this acts as a point of fatigue failure facilitating nail breakage.[5] Review of the clinical results of the use of reamed nails in the management of femoral diaphyseal fractures has not supported the contention that nail breakage is a major problem. This was confirmed by Hajek et al.[6] who performed a biomechanical and clinical analysis of the use of one or two distal cross screws in the treatment of diaphyseal femoral fractures and concluded that one distal screw provided adequate distal fixation. The investigators emphasized that this applied solely to diaphyseal fractures. The indications for the use of two distal cross screws are distal diaphyseal or metaphyseal fractures and if the bone is osteoporotic. In elderly osteoporotic bone maximal purchase is required and two screws should be used.

Nailing of Proximal Femoral Fractures

Nailing of proximal femoral fractures often provides the surgeon with the additional challenge of reducing the fracture fragments. Because of the unopposed actions of the hip flexors, the proximal femoral fragment may be pulled into a considerable degree of flexion. If the surgeon elects to use the supine position, it may prove difficult to bring down the proximal femoral fragment to a position that allows a guide wire to be passed successfully into the distal fragment.

The best method for reducing a proximal femoral fracture is to insert a cannulated metal rod into the proximal fragment, lever the fragment downwards, and pass the guide wire through the metal rod and across the fracture. A short Küntscher nail can be useful, but a number of the nailing sets now provide a instrument specifically for this maneuver. This is illustrated in Figure 10–10, with reference to the Grosse-Kempf instrumentation. Once the guide wire is successfully across the fracture, reaming and nailing can be undertaken in the usual way.

Postoperative Care

Postoperative management varies according to the type of fracture, the age of the patient, and the preoperative mobility of the patient and the extent of any coexisting injuries. Clearly, in multiply-injured patients the rehabilitation program may be dictated by the nature of other injuries. In isolated femoral fractures in physically-fit people, the use of reamed intramedullary nails permits early weight bearing. Surgeons tend to dictate a time scale to the patient based on their perception of the fracture, but in reality, patients will only weight bear when pain permits. Thus, in nailed mid-

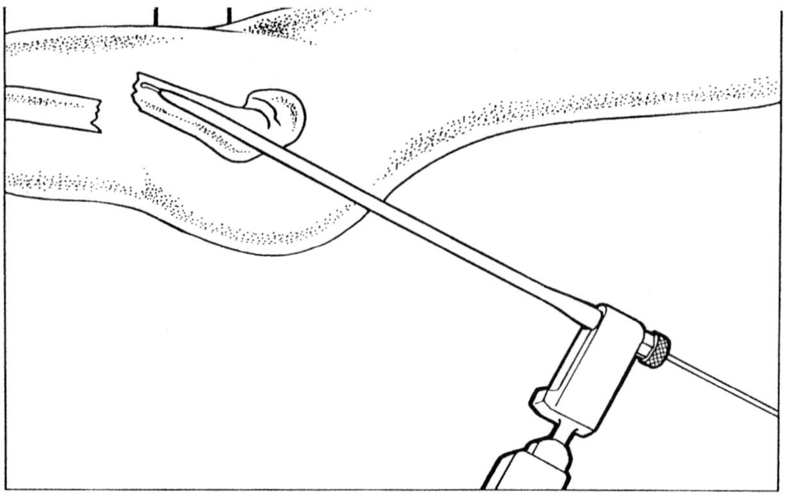

Fig. 10–10. The use of a cannulated long metal rod to adjust the position of the proximal femoral fragment in a high femoral diaphyseal fracture. In this fracture the proximal fragment flexes and it can be difficult to reduce the fracture before passing a guide wire and nail across it.

shaft transverse femoral fractures, weight bearing is early, but in comminuted fractures extending over large areas of the femur, weight bearing is often delayed for 2 to 3 months.

Dynamization is still practiced by many surgeons, but there is no evidence that it is useful in terms of securing union. Dynamization tends to be undertaken 6 to 8 weeks after nailing, if there is little sign of fracture union. Surgeons forget that in more severe fractures there may be no sign of fracture at this time, and they attribute the natural later evolution of callus to their dynamization, rather than to the natural history of fracture healing. Dynamization is, however, useful if the surgeon inadvertently lengthens the fracture during nailing. This will undoubtedly cause delayed union or nonunion, and fracture reduction is facilitated by removal of the distal screw or screws 4 to 6 weeks after nailing.

RESULTS

After its introduction, interlocking intramedullary nailing quickly became the treatment of choice for closed femoral fractures and for all but the most severe open femoral fractures (Fig. 10–11). Kempf et al.[7] documented the treatment of 52 comminuted femoral fractures and showed good results. Four patients had nonunions, all of which healed after further nailing. Three patients with bone loss were successfully treated by grafting and only 1 of their patients developed infection. They compared their results with the results of traction, femoral plating, and narrow-diameter nails, and intramedullary nailing showed considerable improvement in mobility and length of hospital stay. The investigators advocated the technique based on their improved patient mobility and the reduced requirement for bone grafting. Their results and complications are summarized in Table 10–1, which lists data taken from reports dealing with unselected series of femoral fractures treated by interlocking nailing.

Similar results were gained by Wiss et al.[8] They analyzed 112 patients with open and closed femoral diaphyseal fractures. Their patient population tended to be more severely injured, with 58% having other injuries and 15% having sustained their femoral fracture as a result of a gunshot injury. They had a higher rate of complications, but these were mainly minor malunion problems. Seven patients were lengthened by 1 cm or more and 14 had varus or valgus of more than 5°. However, it is clear that most complications were secondary to surgical inexperience and there were no cases of wound infection or osteomyelitis. There were only 2 nonunions. The investigators recorded that there were technical complications in 18% of the patients. They had minor problems inserting the distal cross screws in 8 patients, but their major problems were that 1 patient had a subcapital fracture preoperatively and another

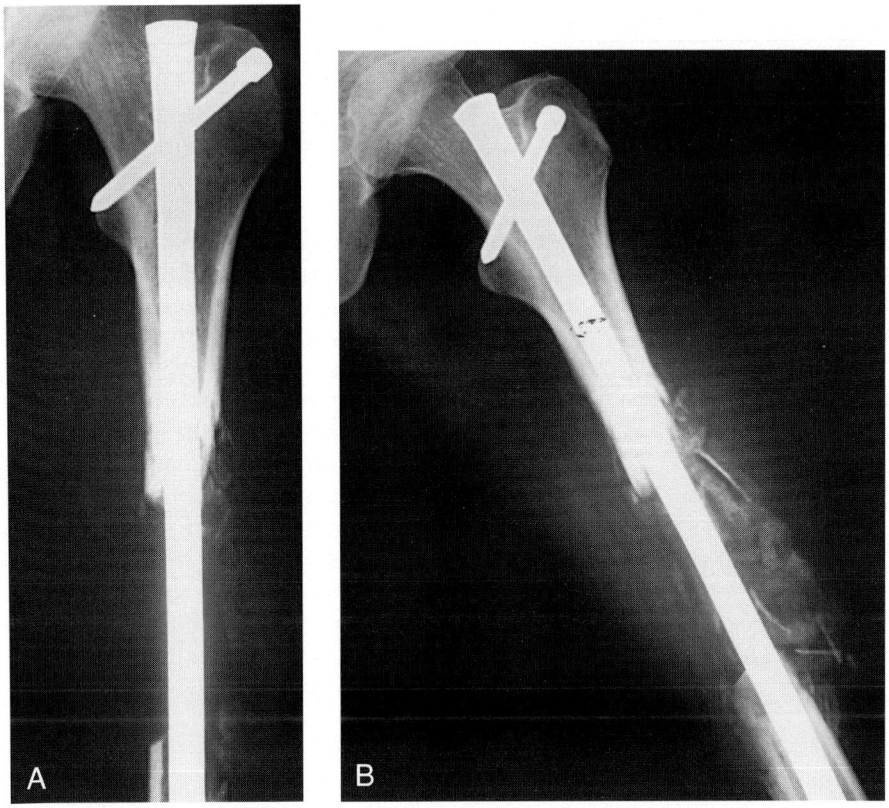

Fig. 10–11. A Gustilo IIIb femoral fracture that required bone excision and subsequent corticocancellous grafting to secure union. This difficult problem illustrates the use of a statically locked intramedullary nail.

showed displacement of a previously undisplaced intertrochanteric fracture. Two patients developed fat embolism syndrome.

Klemm and Borner[9] described the use of interlocking femoral nailing in 266 femoral fractures, 84% of which were closed. Unlike the other investigators, they carefully assessed their functional results. They produced a simple classification of function following femoral nailing that is shown in Table 10–2. They defined an excellent result as consisting of full hip and knee motion, no muscle atrophy, and normal radiographic alignment. A good result had slight loss of hip or knee movement, less than 2 cm of muscle atrophy, and an angular deformity of less than 5°. Fair results were defined as having 25% loss of hip or knee motion and less than 2 cm of muscle atrophy or less than 5° of angular deformity. Using these relatively straightforward criteria, they had 97 good or excellent results with 79.3% of the results being excellent. Fourteen patients developed compli-

Table 10–1. Results and complications of trials documenting unselected series of femoral fractures treated by reamed interlocking nailing

Author	*Number*	*Malunion*	*Infection*	*Comminution*	*Neck Fracture*	*Nonunion*	*Nerve Palsy*
Kempf et al. (1985)	52	21.1%	2.1%	3.8%	—	7.6%	—
Wiss et al. (1986)	112	14%	0%	—	0.9%	1.8%	—
Klemm and Borner (1986)	266	3.0%	2.6%	—	—	1.5%	0.3%
Christie et al. (1988)	120	2.5%	0%	5%	2.5%	1.6%	2.5%
Sjojberg et al. (1990)	40	22.5%	0%	—	—	0%	—

Table 10–2. Simple functional outcome measures following femoral nailing proposed by Klemm and Borner (1986). Their results in terms of their outcome measures are shown

Results	*Functional Outcome*	*Number*	*%*
Excellent	Full hip and knee motion No muscle atrophy Normal radiographic alignment	211	79.3
Good	Slight loss of hip or knee motion Less than 2 cm muscle atrophy Angular deformity less than 5°	47	17.7
Fair	Moderate (25%) loss of hip or knee motion More than 2 cm muscle atrophy Angular deformity 5 to 10°	8	3.0

cations. Four patients had a nonunion, 2 of which required bone grafting. Seven patients had deep infection, although 6 of them were successfully treated with appropriate therapy. One patient developed a peroneal nerve palsy.

Christie et al.[10] reviewed 120 femoral shaft fractures treated with the Grosse-Kempf nail. Twenty fractures were open and 13 were pathological. The mean time to union was 17 weeks, with a range of 10 to 28 weeks. Knee flexion was excellent, although the investigators noted that it took several months for knee flexion to return after distal femoral diaphyseal fractures. There were no bone infections, but 5 patients had positive culture from either the skin wound or drain sites. There were 2 nonunions and 2 implant failures. The major problems encountered were proximal comminution in 6 cases, caused by too lateral a starting position, and femoral neck fracture in 3 patients. They also had 3 cases of pudendal neuropraxia. As earlier workers had done, they emphasized the advantages of femoral nailing in facilitating patient mobilization.

Later reports dealing with femoral nailing detailed similar results. Sojbjerg et al.[11] examined the usefulness of nailing in 80 comminuted and unstable femoral fractures. There were no nonunions but 3 patients had lateral rotation deformities of between 5° and 10°. Three further patients had shortening of between 1 and 2 cm and 2 had lengthening of 1 cm. They did not use dynamization and noted that despite this they had 100% union. They also had no infections and excellent patient mobilization with good knee movement being preserved. They emphasized the need for attention to detail in femoral nailing and they reinforced Browner's[12] belief that experience was necessary to carry out the technique successfully.

The literature dealing with nailing of diaphyseal femoral fractures indicates that, with increasing familiarity, surgeons have operated earlier and allowed earlier weight bearing. There has, if anything, been a decrease in morbidity and complications and now there is no doubt that the literature supports early closed femoral nailing with weight bearing being encouraged when the local symptoms and other injuries permit.

More recently, surgeons have begun to analyze specific types of fracture and assess their suitability for nailing. However, Brumback et al.[13,14] have continued to analyze the use of femoral nailing in the general population. In a trilogy of articles, this group has assessed the complications and errors associated with femoral nailing, as well as the influence of static fixation on fracture healing and femoral osteopenia. The investigators analyzed the use of dynamic femoral nailing in 133 fractures. Fourteen (10.5%) fractures were complicated by loss of fixation and reduction, with 13 fractures shortening by 2 cm on average. Eight fractures required secondary surgery. The reasons for the loss of reduction were identical to those illustrated in previous articles. The surgeons had usually failed to appreciate the fracture pattern preoperatively or had caused increased fracture comminution by the action of nailing. They reasonably advocated high quality preoperative radiographs, with the surgeon being prepared to statically nail the femur if there was any indication of fracture instability.

In their second report, Brumback et al.[15] analyzed the use of static interlocking fixation with a view to examining the need for dynamization. They examined 100 patients who had fresh diaphyseal fractures treated by static nailing. All but 2 patients healed without dynamization, and they concluded that this procedure should not be performed routinely. In the third report in the series Brumback et al.[16] again examined static interlocking nailing, but this time with a view to checking the stress shielding effect of the nail or whether any stress risers were created. The investigators divided 214 fractures into two groups. In group 1 (111 fractures) the static interlock was retained and in group 2 (103 fractures) the interlocking nail and cross screws were removed at an average of 14 months after the initial surgery. They encountered no femoral fracture in group 1 and only diaphyseal fractures in group 2. Their conclusions were that any problems associated with stress shielding and stress risers were not clinically relevant and that the conversion to dynamic intramedullary fixation for a period of time before nail removal was unnecessary. They did advocate that circumferential healing of the femoral cortex should be evident before the intramedullary nail was removed.

As surgeons have become more accustomed to femoral nailing, they have examined its usefulness in specific fracture types. Wiss and Brien[17] reviewed their experience in subtrochanteric fractures. They treated 95 such fractures with the Grosse-Kempf nail of which 26 were open fractures. The fact that 77% of these fractures were high energy is reflected by the fact that their mean union time was 25 weeks. However, there was only one nonunion that required cancellous bone grafting. Hip and knee flexion was reasonable and malunion rates were less than in the early series summarized in Table 10–1. They did encounter a number of nerve palsies involving the sciatic, peroneal, and pudendal nerves. Despite this, they felt that the technique was very useful in these fractures and could be used in all subtrochanteric fractures regardless of the fracture pattern or the degree of comminution, provided the lesser trochanter was intact.

Distal diaphyseal femoral fractures can also be nailed successfully. Leung et al.[18] examined the treatment of 37 supracondylar and intercondylar femoral fractures using the Grosse-Kempf nail. The investigators combined the use of interfragmentary screws with intramedullary nailing for intercondylar fractures and used a modified knee rating system based on that of the Hospital for Special Surgery. They found that 35% of their patients had an excellent result, 59% had a good result, and 5% had a fair result. They had no infection or wound problems. Their main problem was irritation from the distal screws during the early postoperative period. The investigators suggest that the distal screws should routinely be removed after fracture union in these patients. Again, they emphasize the close attention to detail that is required to successfully nail these somewhat difficult fractures.

The use of intramedullary nailing to stabilize segmental fractures has been discussed in a number of reports.[19–21] Wiss and his coworkers treated 33 segmental fractures with the Grosse-Kempf nail. As expected, their union time was prolonged with an average of 32 weeks. There was only one nonunion and two malunions. Dynamization was not routinely employed and they encountered little difficulty in the technique of reaming or nail insertion with these fractures. Complications were few involving two nerve palsies and two nonunions.

Butler et al.[20] examined a less common group of segmental fractures. They looked at 23 patients who had a diaphyseal fracture and an ipsilateral fracture of the distal femur. Twelve patients had an ipsilateral supracondylar fracture, with the remaining 11 having an intercondylar fracture. The mean time to union was 19 weeks. In group 1, patients with a supracondylar fracture achieved good fracture alignment. In group 2, patients who had the intercondylar fractures exhibited impressive results, with 3 fractures healing with slight displacement. Function was good and complications were few.

Wu et al.[21] compared closed and open nailing in the management of segmental femoral fractures and showed that closed nailing was the better technique. The nonunion rate was 11.8%. This was higher than the results of Wiss et al.[19] and Butler et al.,[20] but their nonunion rate in closed nailing was half of the rate of nonunion in open nailing. Interestingly, they had a high rate of iatrogenic femoral neck fracture at 5.9%. All these investigators advocate interlocking nailing in preference to other techniques for the management of segmental femoral fractures.

As surgeons have become more confident about the use of interlocking femoral nailing, they have turned to the technique for the management of open femoral fractures (Fig. 10–12). The series listed in Table 10–1 contain open fractures, but a number of authors have selectively looked at the use of intramedullary femoral nailing for open fractures. Lhowe and Hansen[22] analyzed 42 patients who presented with open fractures. They used both unlocked and locked reamed intramedullary nails. Using the Gustilo grading system, 36% were grade I,

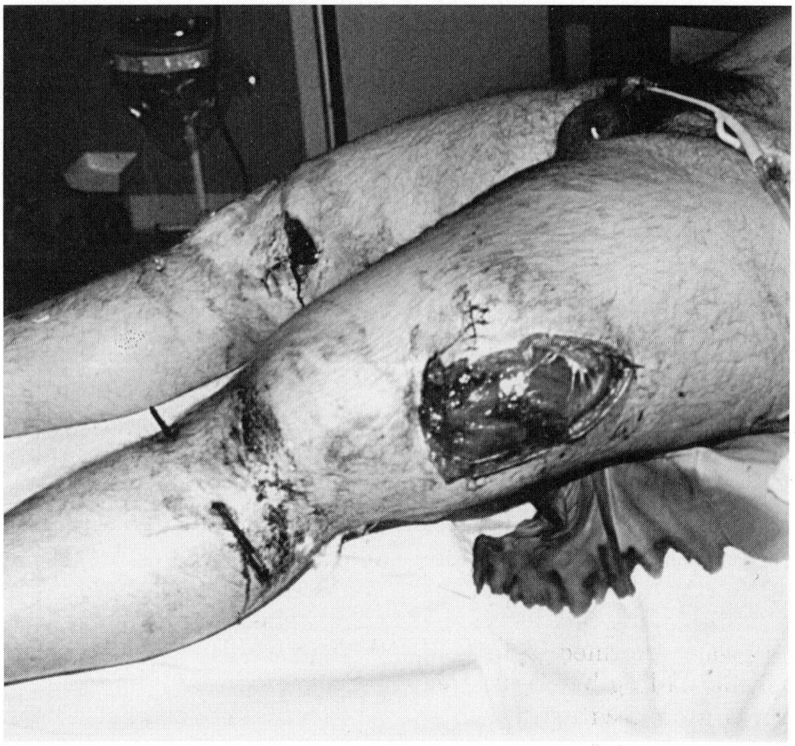

Fig. 10–12. The clinical appearance of a Gustilo IIIb femoral fracture in a multiply injured patient. Nailing has now become the treatment of choice for this difficult clinical problem.

45% were grade II, and there were only 19% grade III injuries. All fractures healed within 4 months and excellent knee and hip movement was achieved. Complications were relatively few. They experienced a 16% incidence of malunion, but this is almost certainly because in the early days of their trial they were using unlocked nails. They had a low incidence of infection, nonunion, and nerve palsy. The investigators concluded that the procedure was safe, but emphasized the need for proper soft-tissue debridement and surgical expertise.

Brumback et al.[16] were a little more circumspect in their recommendations. They analyzed 89 open femoral fractures of which 46 were grade III in severity. They only practiced immediate femoral nailing in fractures in which irrigation and debridement could be undertaken within 8 hours of the injury. In other cases, nailing was delayed for about 10 days. They had no infection in Gustilo grade I, II, or IIIa fractures, but they had 3 infections in grade IIIb fractures. However, two of these infections were in delayed nailings. Complications were few, and they concluded that the technique was reasonable for all fractures except for those grade III fractures that were unsuitable for immediate nailing. The decision as to suitability for immediate nailing was based on the extent of any associated injury, the extent of soft-tissue damage, and the degree of soft-tissue contamination.

O'Brien et al.[23] treated 63 open femoral fractures by primary reamed intramedullary nailing. Twenty-two were grade I fractures, 26 were grade II fractures, and the remaining 15 were grade III fractures. The infection rate was slightly higher than in other series with 5 early soft-tissue infections and 3 later bone infections. They concluded that it was a useful technique, especially in multiply-injured patients. However, they did note a number of serious respiratory complications, although none were fatal.

Grosse et al.[24] published the combined open fracture series of Strasbourg, France and Edinburgh, Scotland. This report totalled 115 consecutive open femoral fractures treated by the Grosse-Kempf interlocking nail. There were only 3 fractures that required bone grafting, with the rest uniting uneventfully. Joint stiffness was not a problem, but 3 patients did develop infection. There were also 2 sciatic nerve palsies and 1 femoral neck fracture. The investigators concluded that if an adequate debridement was performed, all grades of open femoral fractures could be nailed.

The relative frequency of gunshot femoral fractures in the United States has prompted a number of authors to investigate the use of nailing in these injuries. Wiss et al.[25] examined 56 patients who had a low velocity gunshot injury treated by interlocking nailing using the Grosse-Kempf system. The investigators did not routinely perform wound irrigation and debridement but used a first generation cephalosporin and an aminoglycoside for 72 hours. Nailing was delayed for 10 to 14 days, except in those patients who had life-threatening or limb-threatening injuries. Closed intramedullary nailing was performed in 89% of the patients with static nailing being used in 93%. All 50 fractures united without further surgical intervention other than occasional dynamization. Five vascular repairs were performed prior to nailing; all were successful. The investigators recorded 5 peripheral nerve injuries. There were 3 sciatic palsies and 2 peroneal palsies.

More recently Nowotarski and Brumback[26] have investigated immediate nailing for femoral fractures caused by low-velocity and mid-velocity gunshot injuries. In a retrospective review of 39 fractures nailed within 18 hours of injury, only 2 nonunions and no malunions were recorded. One infection did occur, which was successfully treated, and they concluded that not only was immediate nailing clinically reasonable, but it was cheaper, saving approximately $7,000 per patient compared with delayed nailing.

COMPLICATIONS

The literature clearly points to a reduction in the complications associated with femoral nailing over the last decade. Formally there was a relatively high incidence of malunion, but improved surgical technique and the importance of avoiding complications if clinical outcome is to be satisfactory has reduced the complication rate. However, all surgical techniques have problems, and surgeons should be aware of the complications associated with femoral nailing and how they might best be reduced or avoided altogether.

Malunion

Malunion rates have dropped principally because surgeons have recognized the importance of statically locking any femoral fracture that is potentially unstable. Brumback and colleagues[13,15] have shown that static locking is not associated with nonunion and does not increase union time. Thus, the use of static locking is to be encouraged, unless the surgeon is completely confident that the fracture is stable after dynamic nailing. Rotational malalignment has decreased, because surgeons have become aware of the problem and are now more careful in aligning the femur prior to nailing.

Infection

Infection rates following femoral nailing are very low (Table 10–3; see also Table 10–1). Not surprisingly they are higher in open fractures than in closed fractures, but as with other open fractures, the incidence of infection is associated more with the surgeon's skill in debridement and soft-tissue closure than with the type

Table 10 3. Results and incidence of complications of open fractures treated by reamed intramedullary nailing. The papers designated by an asterisk* refer exclusively to gunshot wounds

Author	*Number*	*Malunion*	*Infection*	*Comminution*	*Neck Fracture*	*Nonunion*	*Nerve Palsy*
Lhowe and Hansen (1988)	42	16%	5%	—	—	7%	2%
Brumback et al. (1989)	89	2.2%	3.4%	2.2%	—	0%	—
O'Brien et al. (1991)	63	12.7%	4.8%	—	—	4.8%	—
Grosse et al. (1993)	115	1.7%	2.6%	—	0.8%	3.5%	1.7%
*Wisse et al. (1991)	56	10.7%	0	—	—	3.6%	8.9%
Nowotarski and Brumback *(1994)	39	0	2.5%	—	—	5.1%	5.1%

of implant involved. Infection is usually easy to treat if it is detected early. Treatment involves adequate bone and soft-tissue debridement, rereaming to remove the endosteal membrane, and exchange nailing with a larger nail. This technique has been described in detail for the tibia[27] but the same protocol applies to the femur. If it is employed, complications associated with infection in nailed femoral fractures should be low.

Nonunion

As with bone infection, the incidence of nonunion is low and is related mainly to the force of the injury. The usefulness of reaming the femur is as yet unknown, but it is likely that reaming does have an osteoinductive effect and that this, in part, explains the low incidence of nonunions. Aseptic nonunion should be treated by exchange nailing, unless there is a large bony defect in which case corticocancellous bone grafting, vascularized bone grafting, or segmental transport can be used. Dynamization seems to have no particular purpose except to close an over-distracted fracture. There are no reports in the literature proving the usefulness of dynamization for any other reason, and it is suggested that surgeons abandon the practice of dynamization if it is being used to stimulate union.

Femoral Neck Fracture

Femoral neck fracture (Fig. 10–13) is referred to sporadically as a complication of nailing. It is often difficult to know whether nailing has caused a femoral neck fracture or merely displaced a fracture that was caused by the injury. There is, however, no doubt that the former situation occurs and the surgeon should be aware of the possibility of femoral neck fractures. Harper and Henstorf[28] documented 2 femoral neck fractures after femoral intramedullary nailing, and suggested that they were caused by too medial a starting point for the femoral nail.

Christie and Court-Brown[29] reported on an additional 4 fractures, 3 of which occurred in slightly built female patients with small intramedullary canals. All 4 fractures were vertical extracapsular fractures with little or no displacement. Three were treated with the use of compression screws placed around the proximal end. One was treated nonoperatively. The authors also felt that the entry point for femoral nailing was crucial and failure to select the entry point properly accounted for this complication.

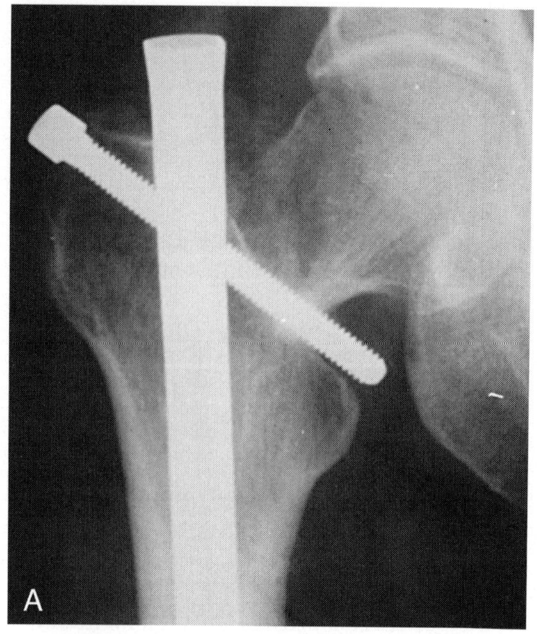

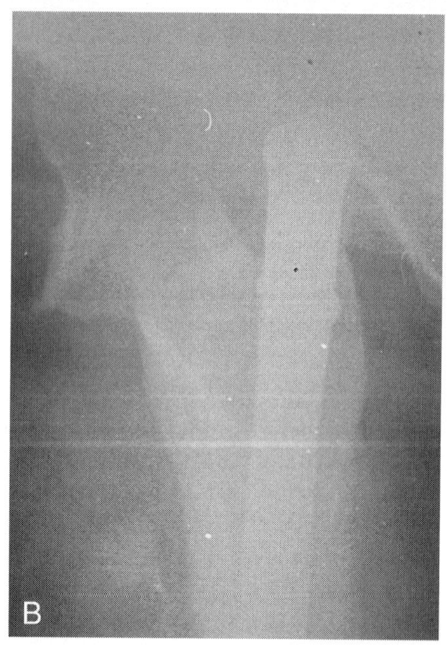

Fig. 10–13. An iatrogenic femoral neck fracture. The femoral neck was intact prior to nailing and it can be seen that in this case the nail has not been sufficiently advanced into the femur. The result of this is that the proximal screw has been placed in too proximal a location and has caused a femoral neck fracture. The fracture was treated by the insertion of cancellous screws around the nail and it healed uneventfully.

Proximal Femoral Comminution

Promixal femoral comminution can occur under three circumstances. If the proximal femur is inadequately reamed and the nail is wider than the medullary canal, a fracture of the proximal femur may occur. However, it is more common for proximal comminution to occur following the use of an incorrect starting point. If the initial bone defect is placed too laterally in the greater trochanter, the nail may pass medially and impinge on the proximal femoral cortex causing a fracture, particularly if it has been used to treat a fracture in an elderly patient where the bone is osteoporotic.

The third cause of proximal femoral comminution is if the entry point is too anterior or posterior. The resulting damage from hammering a nail into an anterior or posterior entry point may be considerable. Court-Brown[30] estimated that the incidence of proximal comminution was 5% over the first 3 years of femoral nailing in his center, but he noted that the incidence fell markedly as the surgeons gained experience in the technique.

Nerve Palsy

Tables 10–1 and 10–3 illustrate that nerve palsies are a complication of femoral nailing. The three nerves involved are the sciatic nerve, the common peroneal nerve, and the pudendal nerve. The problem of nerve palsies is associated with traction causing a neuropraxia of the nerve; the condition is usually self-limiting. Pudendal nerve palsy is a complication that is virtually specific to femoral nailing. It presents with alteration in labial sensation in females and alteration in scrotal and penile sensation and erectile dysfunction in males. In the series by Christie et al.,[10] shown in Table 10–1, the three pudendal neuropraxias resolved within 3 months. It is theorized that the condition is caused by excessive traction on the orthopaedic table with the groin being forced against the traction post.

The condition was investigated in some detail by Brumback et al.[31] They undertook a prospective study of 106 patients who had static interlocking nailing of a femoral diaphyseal fracture. The investigators measured the magnitude of the perineal pressure with a strain gauge mounted in the traction post. They also documented the time over which the perineal pressure was applied.

Ten (9.4%) patients had a pudendal nerve palsy. Nine only had sensory changes and 1 male complained of erectile dysfunction. The investigators showed that the duration for which traction was applied did not affect the incidence of pudendal nerve palsy but the magnitude of the total traction force did. They demonstrated that hip adduction in addition to fracture manipulation increased the magnitude of the traction force. The pudendal nerve palsy occurred more frequently in patients who had reconstruction femoral nailing than in those who had undergone standard interlocking femoral nailing. The surgeon should be aware of this important problem. Pudendal nerve palsy can be minimized or avoided by decreasing the traction pressure, and it is recommended that the traction post is placed in the contralateral groin.

Heterotopic Ossification

The fact that heterotopic ossification occurs in the soft tissues around the proximal femur after femoral nailing has been known for many years (Fig. 10–14). It is not uncommon to see heterotopic bone related to the proximal part of the nail and to have to remove this bone before the nail can be removed from the femur. The amount of bone can be considerable and Court-Brown[30] described a piece of bone measuring 9 cm (by 6 cm in diameter) associated with protruding Küntscher nail.

The incidence of heterotopic ossification about the hip after intramedullary nailing has been investigated by Brumback et al.[32] They prospectively studied 100 consecutive unilateral femoral fractures to assess the incidence of heterotopic ossification and to examine whether lavaging the bone debris from the soft tissues after nailing decreased its incidence. They found that 26% of patients had moderate or severe heterotopic ossification about the hip after intramedullary nailing. Forty percent had no heterotopic bone and the remaining 34% showed minor ossification. There was no correlation between the degree of heterotopic ossification and the age or sex of the patient, the severity of the injury, the presence or absence of a closed intracranial injury, the level or type of comminution of the fracture, the timing of the nailing, or the type of intramedullary fixation. They also showed no statistical difference between those fractures that had saline lavage

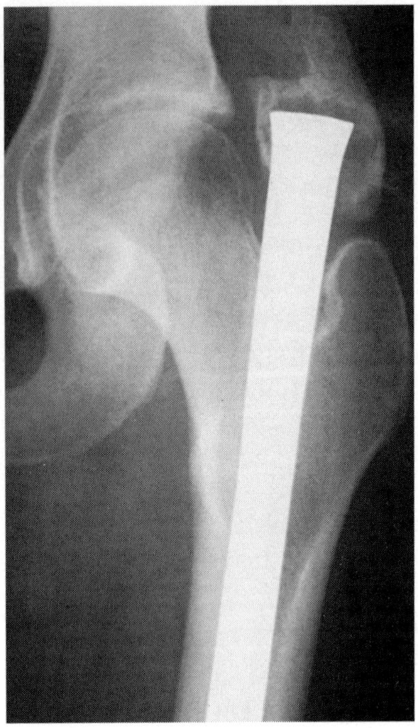

Fig. 10–14. Heterotopic bone around the end of an intramedullary nail. It is not unusual to see heterotopic bone in this location.

to remove the bone reamings and those that had not.

Heterotopic ossification is therefore usually a fairly minor problem that may manifest with some gluteal pain but rarely restricts hip movement or is serious enough to warrant surgical intervention.

Radiation Dosage

Surgeons are understandably concerned about the radiation that they might absorb during femoral nailing. This is particularly true of surgeons in training who may take some time to nail a femur. Obviously radiation can be minimized by adherence to good surgical technique and by the use of modern image intensification equipment. However, despite these precautions surgeons will absorb radiation, and it is important to know whether the degree of radiation associated with femoral nailing is in any way hazardous. Kempf et al. [7] had a total screening time of 3.43 minutes for their femoral nailing procedures. More recently, however, published screening times have been longer, with Levin et al.[33] having a total screening time of 12.6 minutes and Sugarman et al.[34] publishing an average screening time of 12.08 minutes. It is possible that the longer screening times represent surgical inexperience. Even despite these relatively long screening times, Sugarman and his coworkers showed quite clearly that a surgeon would have to nail about 700 femora a year before the acceptable radiation dose was exceeded.

Sanders et al.[35] undertook a similar study of 65 orthopaedic procedures performed with fluoroscopic assistance. They found that the average fluoroscopic time for statically nailing a femoral fracture was 6.26 minutes and they also estimated that the surgeon could perform about 750 such operations per year safely. Therefore, there is no evidence to demonstrate that the level of radiation absorbed by the surgeon or the patient is in any way hazardous.

Pulmonary Complications

It is accepted that femoral stabilization is imperative in the treatment of multiply injured patients. As intramedullary nailing provides the best method of stabilizing the femur, it was quickly adopted as the method of choice for stabilizing femora in multiply injured patients. However, recent experience with echocardiography has shown that reaming produces cascades of material that pass through the right side of the heart and if there is a patent foramen ovale they can enter the left side of the heart and therefore the systemic circulation. It would appear that if the lungs are normal, they will successfully absorb all of the material passing into them from the right side of the heart. Yet, there is concern about their ability to absorb any fat and other debris if there has been significant pulmonary trauma. The level of concern is such that a number of surgeons have opted not to use femoral nailing if there is significant lung damage in the multiply injured patient.

What little research there is into this problem is confusing. Wolinsky et al.[36] developed an open-chested sheep model to study the effects of major orthopaedic procedures on pulmonary physiology. They concluded that reamed intramedullary femoral nailing was not detrimental to sheep with otherwise normal lungs. Wozasek et al.[37] also used a sheep model and compared reamed femoral nailing, unreamed femoral nailing, and femoral plating. They showed that reamed intramedullary nailing caused more fat embolization in comparison to unreamed nailing and plating, but there was no difference in the arterial pressure response of the lung even in the presence of blunt thoracic trauma.

Using a similar model, Duwelius et al.[38] showed that pulmonary dysfunction following femoral fracture alone was minimal. They indicated that reaming had a modest effect on pulmonary vascular resistance which was not observed in their nonreamed group. However, they did find fat in the pulmonary circulation following both reamed and unreamed femoral nailing.

Further investigation is needed in this area, but it is important that surgeons do consider the possibility of embolization in the multiply injured patient with thoracic trauma. At the moment, it would be inappropriate to advise against reamed intramedullary nailing, but this area of research is advancing rapidly and it may be that another method of femoral stabilization may be shown to be appropriate for this small subgroup of patients.

CONCLUSIONS AND RECOMMENDATIONS

1. Femoral nailing is the best method of managing femoral diaphyseal fractures.
2. It is an appropriate technique for all fractures below the lesser trochanter and 5 cm above the knee joint.
3. It can be combined with interfragmentary screw fixations to successfully treat shaft fractures associated with intercondylar femoral fractures.
4. Open femoral fractures of all grades of severity can be treated by primary reamed intramedullary nails.
5. The principal complications are malunion and pudendal nerve neuropraxia.
6. The incidence of infection and nonunion is low.
7. The incidence of all complications can be minimized by adherence to correct surgical technique.
8. Radiation dosage does not constitute a significant problem for the surgeon or the patient.
9. In multiply injured patients with thoracic trauma, the surgeon should be aware of the theoretical possibility that reaming will cause pulmonary compromise and should be prepared to use another fixation method if this is considered appropriate.

REFERENCES

1. Hey Groves, E.W.: Some clinical and experimental observations on the operative treatment of fractures with especial reference to the use of intramedullary pegs. Br. Med. J. *2*: 1102–1105, 1912.
2. Rush, L.V., Rush, H.L.: A technique for longitudinal pin fixation of certain fractures of the ulna and of the femur. J. Bone Joint Surg. *21A*:619–628, 1939.
3. Küntscher, G.: Die marknagelong von knochenbruchen. Langenbecks Arch. Chir. 200:443–455, 1940.
4. Moran, C.G., Gibson, M.J., Cross, A.T.: Intramedullary locking nails for femoral shaft fractures in elderly patients. J. Bone Joint Surg. *72B*:19–22, 1990.
5. Bucholz, R.W., Ross, S.E., Lawrence, K.L.: Fatigue fracture of the interlocking nail in the treatment of fractures of the femoral shaft. J. Bone Joint Surg. *69A*: 1391–1399, 1987.
6. Hajek, P.D., Bicknell, H.R., Bronson, W.E., Albright, J.A., Saha, S.: The use of one compared with two distal screws in the treatment of femoral shaft fractures with interlocking intramedullary nailing. J. Bone Joint Surg. *75A*:519–525, 1993.
7. Kempf, I., Grosse, A., Beck, J.: Closed locked intramedullary nailing. Its application to comminuted fractures of the femur. J. Bone Joint Surg. *67A*:709–720, 1985.
8. Wiss, D.A., Fleming, C.H., Mata, J.M., Clark, D.: Comminuted and rotationally unstable fractures of the femur treated with an interlocking nail. Clin. Orthop. *212*:35–47, 1986.
9. Klemm, K., Borner, M.: Interlocking nailing of complex fractures of the femur and tibia. Clin. Orthop. *212*: 89–100, 1986.
10. Christie, J., Court-Brown, C., Kinninmonth, A.W.G., Howie, C.R.: Intramedullary locking nails in the management of femoral shaft fractures. J. Bone Joint Surg. *70B*:206–210, 1988.
11. Sojbjerg, J.O., Eiskjaer, S., Moller-Larsen, S.: Locked nailing of comminuted and unstable fractures of the femur. J. Bone Joint Surg. *72B*:23–25, 1990.
12. Browner, B.D.: Pitfalls, errors, and complications in the use of locking Küntscher nails. Clin. Orthop. *212*: 192–208, 1986.
13. Brumback, R.J., Reilly, J.P., Poka, A., Lakatos, R.P., Bathon, G.H., Burgess, A.R.: Intramedullary nailing of femoral shaft fractures. Part I: Decision making errors with interlocking fixation. J. Bone Joint Surg. *70A*: 1441–1452, 1988.
14. Brumback, R.J., Ellison, T.S., Poka, A., Bathon, G.H., Burgess, A.R.: Intramedullary nailing of femoral shaft fractures. Part III: Long term effects of static interlocking fixation. J. Bone Joint Surg. *74A*:106–112, 1992.
15. Brumback, R.J., Uwagie-Ero, S., Lakatos, R.P., Poka, A., Bathon, G.H., Burgess, A.R.: Intramedullary nailing of femoral shaft fractures. Part II: Fracture healing with static interlocking fixation. J. Bone Joint Surg. *70A*: 1453–1462, 1988.
16. Brumback, R.J., Stribling, E.P., Poka, A., Lakatos, R., Bathon, G.H, Burgess, A.R.: Intramedullary nailing of open fractures of the femoral shaft. J. Bone Joint Surg. *71A*:1324–1330, 1989.
17. Wiss, D.A., Brien, W.W.: Sub-trochanteric fractures of the femur. Results of treatment by interlocking nailing. Clin. Orthop. *283*:231–236, 1992.
18. Leung, K.S., Shen, W.Y., So, W.S., Mui, L.T., Grosse, A.: Interlocking intramedullary nailing for supracondylar and intercondylar fractures of the distal part of the femur. J. Bone Joint Surg. *73A*:332–340, 1991.
19. Wiss, D.A., Brien, W.W., Stetson, W.B.: Interlocked nailing for treatment of segmental fractures of the femur. J. Bone Joint Surg. *72A*:724–728, 1990.

20. Butler, M.S., Brumback, R.J., Ellison, T.S., Poka, A., Bathon, G.H., Burgess, A.R.: Interlocking intramedullary nailing for ipsilateral fractures of the femoral shaft and distal part of the femur. J. Bone Joint Surg. *73A*: 1492–1502, 1991.
21. Wu, C.C., Shih, C.H., Yuang, W.N., Chen, Y.J.: Treatment of segmental femoral shaft fractures. Clin. Orthop. *287*:224–230, 1993.
22. Lhowe, D.W., Hansen, S.T.: Immediate nailing of open fractures of the femoral shaft. J. Bone Joint Surg. *70B*: 812–820, 1988.
23. O'Brien, P.J., Meek, R.N., Powell, J.N., Blachat, P.A.: Primary intramedullary nailing of open femoral shaft fractures. J. Trauma *31*:113–116, 1991.
24. Grosse, A., Christie, J., Taglang, G., Court-Brown, C., McQueen, M.: Open adult femoral shaft fracture treated by early intramedullary nailing. J. Bone Joint Surg. *75B*:562–565, 1993.
25. Wiss, D.A., Brien, W.W., Becker, V.: Interlocking nailing for the treatment of femoral fractures due to gunshot wounds. J. Bone Joint Surg. *73A*:598–606, 1991.
26. Nowotarski, P., Brumback, R.J.: Immediate interlocking nailing of fractures of the femur caused by low- to mid-velocity gunshots. J. Orthop. Trauma *8*:134–141, 1994.
27. Court-Brown, C.M., Keating, J.P., McQueen, M.M.: Infection after intramedullary nailing of the tibia. J. Bone Joint Surg. *74B*:770–774, 1992.
28. Harper, M.C., Henstorf, J.: Fractures of the femoral neck associated with technical errors in closed intramedullary nailing of the femur. J. Bone Joint Surg. *68A*:624–626, 1986.
29. Christie, J., Court-Brown, C.: Femoral neck fracture during closed medullary nailing: Brief report. J. Bone Joint Surg. *74B*:6, 1988.
30. Court-Brown, C.M.: An atlas of closed nailing of the tibia and femur. Martin Dunitz, London, 1990.
31. Brumback, R.J., Ellison, T.S., Molligan, H., Molligan, D.J., Mahaffey, S., Schmidhauser, C.: Pudendal nerve palsy complicating intramedullary nailing of the femur. J. Bone Joint Surg. *74A*:1450–1455, 1992.
32. Brumback, R.J., Wells, J.D., Lakatos, R., Poka, A., Bathon, G.H., Burgess, A.R.: Heterotopic ossification about the hip after intramedullary nailing for fractures of the femur. J. Bone Joint Surg. *72A*:1067–1073, 1990.
33. Levin, P.E., Schoen, R.W., Browner, B.D.: Radiation exposure to the surgeon during closed interlocking intramedullary nailing. J. Bone Joint Surg. *69A*:761–765, 1986.
34. Sugarman, I.D., Adam, I., Bunker, T.D.: Radiation dosage during AO locking femoral nailing. Injury *19*: 336–338, 1988.
35. Sanders, R., Koval, K.J., Dipasquale, T., Schmelling, G., Stenzler, S., Ross, E.: Exposure of the orthopaedic surgeon to radiation. J. Bone Joint Surg. *75A*:326–330, 1993.
36. Wolinsky, P.R., Sciadini, M.S., Parker, R.E., et al.: Effects on pulmonary physiology of reamed intramedullary nailing in an open chested sheep model. Orthopaedic Trauma Unit, Los Angeles, 1994.
37. Wozasek, J.E., Neudeck, F., Obertacke, U., Redl, H., Schlag, G.: Intra- versus extra-medullary femoral fracture fixation in thoracic trauma. Orthopaedic Trauma Association, Los Angeles, 1994.
38. Duwelius, P.J., Mullins, R.J., Woll, T.S., et al.: The effects of femoral intramedullary reaming in a sheep lung model: A pilot study. Orthopaedic Trauma Association, Los Angeles, 1994.

11

The GSH Supracondylar Nail

William G. DeLong, Jr. and Frederick S. Bennett

The GSH supracondylar intramedullary nail developed by Green, Seligson, and Henry[1] and manufactured by Smith & Nephew Richards since 1990, is a cannulated closed-section stainless steel intramedullary device designed specifically to provide fixation of supracondylar fractures of the distal femur including those with intraarticular extension. It has an 8° apex-anterior bend near the distal end to accommodate the geometry of the femoral condyles, and there are transverse holes along its entire length to allow interlocking with 5-mm diameter screws (Fig. 11–1). The nail is currently available in 11-, 12-, and 13-mm diameters and lengths of 150, 200, and 250 mm. Interlocking is accomplished with a targeting device connected by means of a driving attachment to the distal end of the nail. The device was initially designed for use in elderly patients with osteoporotic bone; its use was subsequently extended to the younger population with particular advantage in cases of polytrauma.

The most unique feature of the GSH supracondylar nail is its intraarticular starting point, which allows it to be used for very distal fractures. The ability to lock the nail proximally enables more rigid fixation than any other available intramedullary device inserted at the level of the knee, including Ender's nails and the Zickel supracondylar device. The Huckstep nail (Fig. 11–2) was nearly identical in design and technical details of insertion but had a square cross section and was inserted antegrade from a starting point at the hip.[2] The Modny nail (Fig. 11–3), although designed for use in supracondylar fractures and capable of being interlocked both proximally and distally, had an X-shaped cross section and was inserted through the fracture site into the proximal fragment then advanced distally with a bone tamp using the holes in the nail.[3]

The GSH supracondylar nail was designed to extend the practical and theoretical advantages of intramedullary nailing to very distal fractures of the femur. Closed placement with indirect reduction of the fracture minimizes soft-tissue and periosteal damage, thus preserving vascularity of the fracture site. This optimizes the probability of bony union. The intramedullary position of implant places it closer to the line of muscle-generated forces than side-plate devices providing for a biomechanically sound construct (Fig. 11–4). Less surgical dissection is required in comparison to that required to insert screw and side-plate devices, resulting in less blood loss, less muscle damage, and less postoperative discomfort.

At the present time, the design of the nail remains in its evolutionary stages. When originally released on the market it was available in 11- and 12-mm diameters for use with 6.4-mm diameter interlocking screws. An unacceptably high (15%) rate of fatigue failure, which always occurred through unused screw holes near the middle of the nail, led to the current design with larger 12-mm and 13-mm diameter nails, increased wall thickness, and smaller 5-mm diameter interlocking screws. The resultant reduction of stress concentration within the nail increased the fatigue life by a factor of five in laboratory bench tests.[4] Only one fatigue fracture has occurred subsequent to these design changes, but this has prompted developers to consider further design modifications, such as

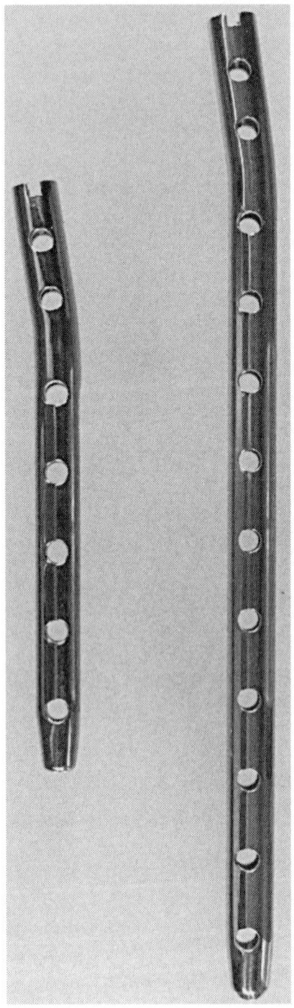

Fig. 11–1. Supracondylar nails in 250 mm and 150 mm lengths. Note 8° apex-anterior bend near the distal end.

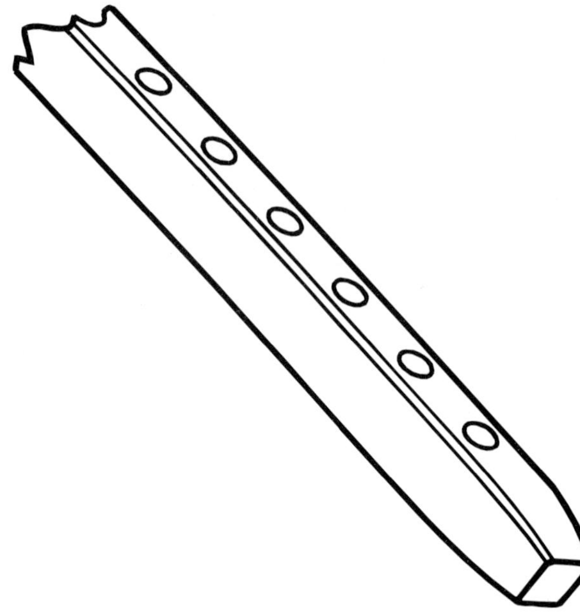

Fig. 11–2. Representative section of the Huckstep nail showing square cross section and holes for interlocking screw placement. The Huckstep nail is inserted in an antegrade direction from a starting point at the hip.

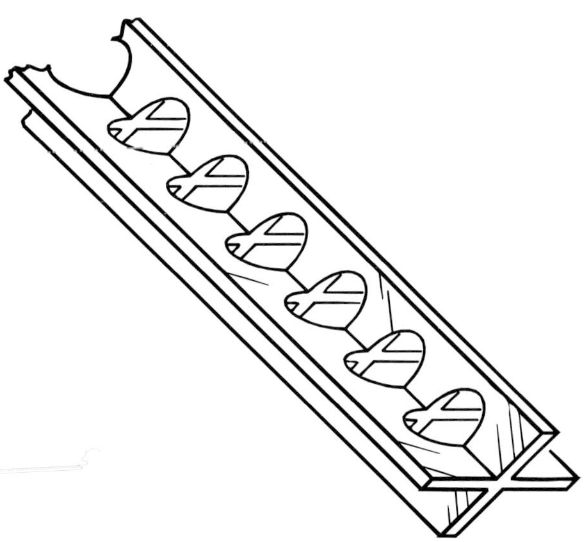

Fig. 11–3. Representative section of the Modny nail showing X-shaped cross section and holes for interlocking; it was designed for insertion at the supracondylar fracture site.

eliminating the intermediate screw holes near the central portion of the nail where the effects of working length at the fracture nail construct are focused. These modified nails demonstrate a significant increase in strength and recently have become available for clinical use. Figure 11–14 demonstrates this new design having three holes distally and just two proximally.

The targeting device for interlocking screw insertion is of paramount importance to expeditious insertion of the supracondylar nail. Its design has evolved to progressively eliminate all degrees of freedom and to maximize the probability of accurately targeting the proximal screws. The first generation targeting device allowed relative rotation about an axis orthogonal to the nail axis. The second generation device achieves an absolute lock-in of alignment with the undistorted nail, but may impinge on the soft tissues when the thigh is large (Fig. 11–5). A wider driving attachment with greater distance between the nail and targeting device is now available. It provides two positions to accommodate most patients as demonstrated in Figure 11–15.

The supracondylar nail was originally intended as an alternative to side plate devices

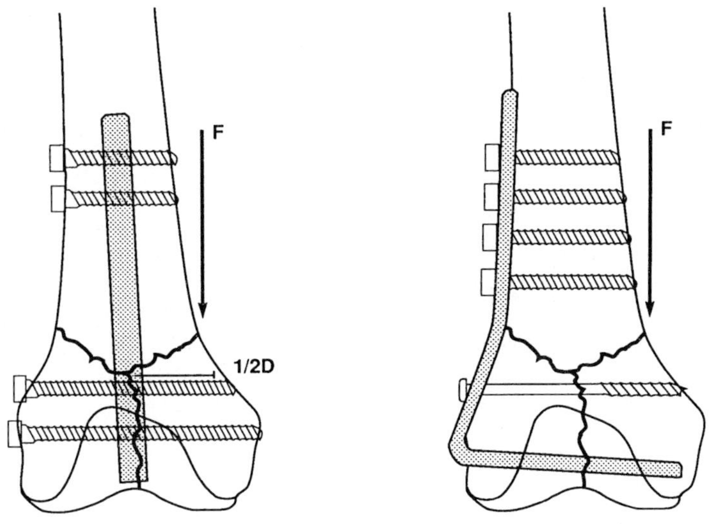

Fig. 11–4. The supracondylar nail is positioned closer to the line of force transmission across the distal femur than are side-plate devices. This reduces the moment arm through which these forces act upon the implant.

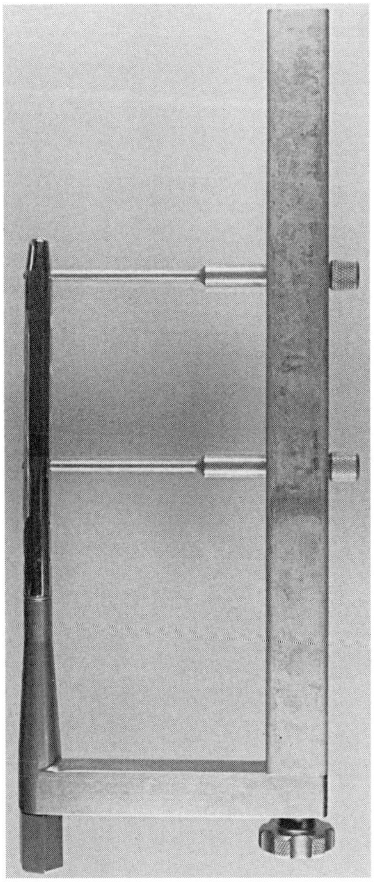

Fig. 11–5. Supracondylar nail ready for insertion attached to targeting device. Cross-pins are for alignment of nail to insure accurate targeting and are removed prior to insertion of the nail.

primarily for use in fractures that were located too far distally in the femur for use of standard antegrade nails, particularly those where osteopenia would be expected to also make screw fixation and side-plate fixation tenuous. However, experience with the device at a Level I trauma center has revealed additional clinical situations in which the supracondylar nail provides distinct advantages over all other currently available implants, including standard antegrade nails. Ipsilateral diaphyseal femoral and tibial fractures for example, when the femoral fracture is located within 20 cm of the knee joint, can be rapidly stabilized under tourniquet control on a standard operating room table through the same small incision which would normally be used for a closed tibial nailing (Fig. 11–6). The ability to use a tourniquet minimizes blood loss and the reliability of the targeting device reduces operative time. Further time is saved by avoiding the use of a fracture table. Clearly the potential reduction in blood loss and operative time are crucial advantages for multiple-trauma patients with life threatening injuries to the head, chest, and abdomen (Fig. 11–7).

Furthermore, the rigidity of fixation and length and rotational stability are superior to that obtained with any other variety of retrograde device. This enables the patient to be out of traction and receiving optimal pulmonary care and nursing care without concern of losing

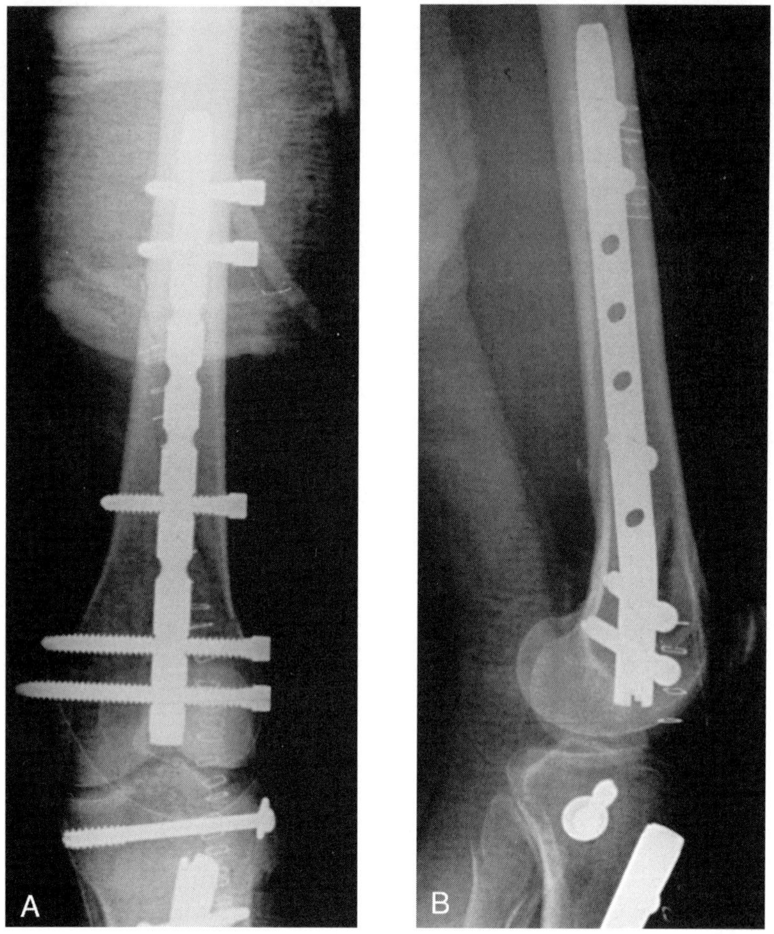

Fig. 11–6. Floating knee injury in 29-year-old female with a closed head injury, pneumothorax, and ruptured spleen has been stabilized rapidly on a standard operating room table under tourniquet control with minimal blood loss. A single incision at the knee provided access to drive a supracondylar nail proximally and a tibial nail distally. *A,* AP view. *B,* Lateral view.

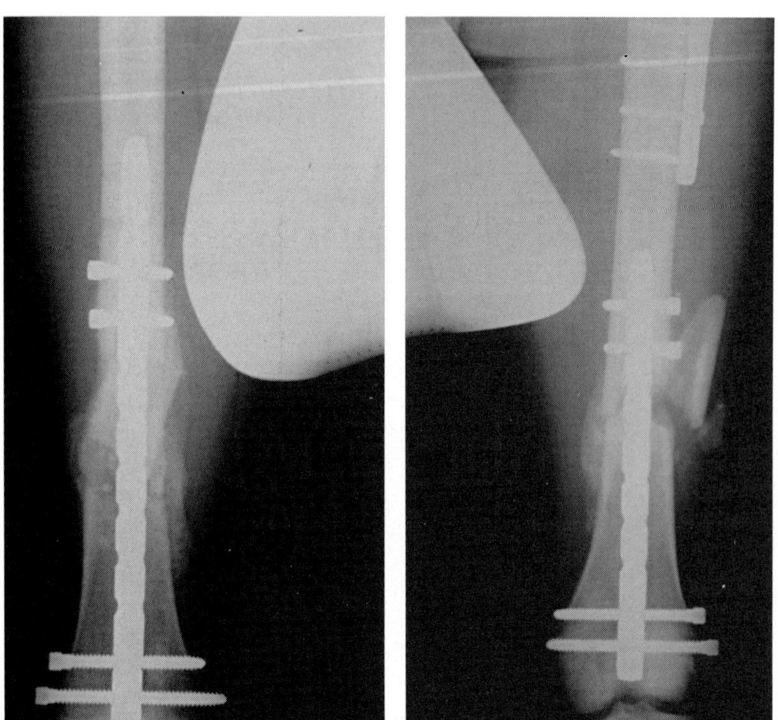

Fig. 11–7. Bilateral supracondylar nails inserted in 32-year-old male with life-threatening multi-systems trauma including head, chest, and abdominal injuries. The ability to use a standard operating table and tourniquet control and the ability to approach both extremities simultaneously using two operating teams, minimized orthopaedic operative time and blood loss and thus contributed to the survival of the patient. The presence of the left supracondylar nail did not interfere with subsequent fixation of nondisplaced ipsilateral left femoral neck fracture with compression hip screw and side-plate, which was carried out in a delayed fashion after resuscitation was completed.

fixation. In addition to the floating knee injury, other clinical situations in which we have found the supracondylar nail to be ideally suited for fixation of diaphyseal femoral fractures potentially treatable with standard femoral nailing include the following:

1. The critical multi-trauma patient with bilateral femoral fractures, so that both sides can be approached simultaneously by two operative teams.
2. The morbidly obese patient, so that the difficulty establishing a suitable entry portal in the piriformis fossa is eliminated.
3. Patients with distorted proximal femoral anatomy from previous injury, neoplasm, arthroplasty, or metabolic bone disease.
4. Ipsilateral femoral neck and shaft fractures, so that the femoral neck can be stabilized first without compromising the stability that can be achieved for the diaphyseal fracture component.
5. Delayed definitive fixation of the femur after external fixation and vascular repair for grade III open injuries, where reduction forces can be more carefully controlled than with the fracture table thus reducing the risk of disrupting the repair.
6. Pregnant patients, because no direct radiation of the pelvic region is necessary.
7. Patients with poor quality skin in the buttock and trochanteric region, where an incision for standard antegrade nailing would normally be made.

SELECTION OF FRACTURES

The supracondylar nail can be used for virtually any intraarticular or extraarticular distal femoral fracture (closed or open) that extends no further proximally than approximately 20 cm from the knee joint, provided that comminution of the medial or lateral epicondylar cortices does not prevent secure bicortical purchase of at least two distal interlocking screws (Fig. 11–8). Under such circumstances a condy-

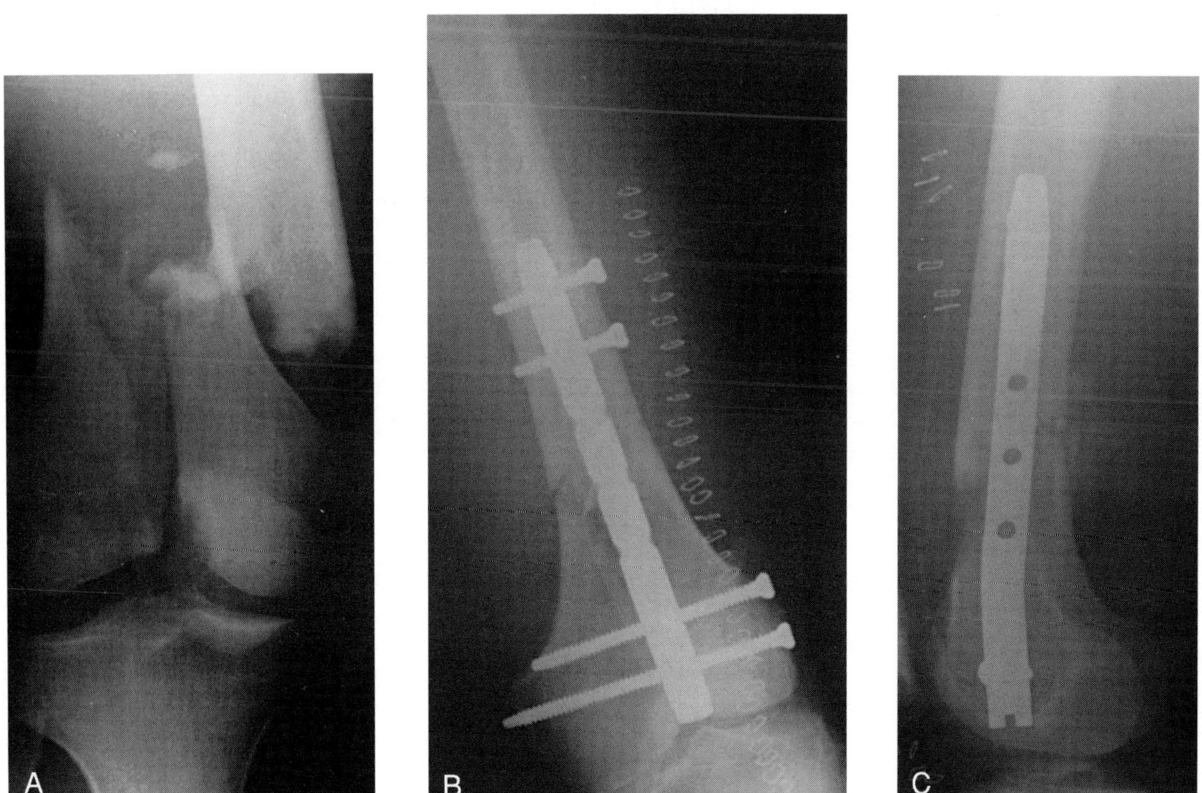

Fig. 11–8. AO type C2 distal femur fracture. *A,* Preoperative AP view. *B,* Postoperative AP view after insertion of 12 mm × 150 mm supracondylar intramedullary nail. Note the presence of sufficient intact cortex both medially and laterally to allow secure bicortical purchase of two screws distal to the metaphyseal/diaphyseal component of the fracture. *C,* Postoperative lateral view.

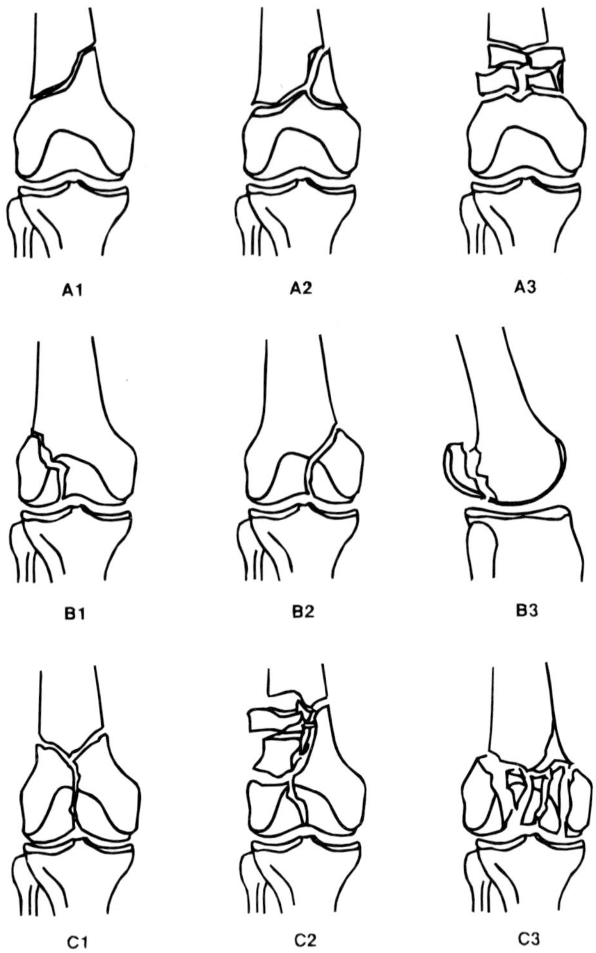

Fig. 11–9. AO classification of distal femoral fractures. Types amenable for use of the GSH supracondylar nail include A1, A2, A3, C1, C2, and some type C3 fractures.

lar buttress plate would be a better choice. Using the AO classification suitable fracture types include A1, A2, A3, C1, C2, and C3 (Fig. 11–9),[5] although most C3 fractures are managed equally or better with condylar buttress plates.

Extraarticular diaphyseal fractures with at least 7 to 9 cm of intact distal femur are better treated with standard antegrade femoral nailing except under the circumstances mentioned previously, because the knee joint is not violated making it less prone to stiffness. However, the intraarticular entrance point is a worthwhile compromise when the poor overall condition of the patient mandates immediate femoral stabilization with minimal surgical insult and blood loss and reduced operative time. In addition to acute fractures, we have used the supracondylar nail successfully in the treatment of distal diaphyseal nonunions, pathologic fractures, and corrective osteotomies for malunion.

PREOPERATIVE PLANNING

Preoperative planning is essential to gain a thorough understanding of the fracture pattern. This will confirm the applicability of the supracondylar nail and determine the minimum possible surgical exposure necessary for its insertion. Preoperative radiographs must be adequate to determine whether or not a formal arthrotomy is necessary to reduce and stabilize displacement of the articular surface. Traction radiographs may help determine whether or not there is intraarticular extension. When the joint surface is intact (AO type A fractures) percutaneous or arthroscopically assisted nail insertion can substantially reduce the invasiveness of the procedure. Fractures with articular or intercondylar displacement (AO type C fractures) are best approached though formal medial parapatellar arthrotomy, which provides adequate exposure for open reduction of the articular surface.

The geometry of the distal canal must be relatively normal without deformity from old fracture or metabolic bone disease. Although it may be possible to eliminate reaming when the canal diameter is more than 14 mm throughout the region of anticipated instrumentation, we recommend overreaming by at least 1 mm in the vast majority of cases. Overreaming by 1.5 or 2 mm facilitates locking when the 250 mm length nail is used by minimizing distortion of the nail within the intramedullary canal. Static locking is recommended for all fractures. The distal screws prevent the nail from protruding into the knee joint. Addition of proximal locking provides length and rotational stability.

Selection of optimal nail length involves compromise. The longest available nail (250 mm) provides the maximum possible stability but may complicate proximal interlocking. This is because the same problems encountered with guided distal interlocking of standard antegrade nails are encountered during proximal interlocking of the 250 mm supracondylar nail. Namely, distortion of the nail by the shape mismatch within the canal alters the alignment of the nail holes with the interlocking guide. Furthermore, freehand targeting methods are more difficult to apply proximally in the thigh, although it can be accomplished with appropriate

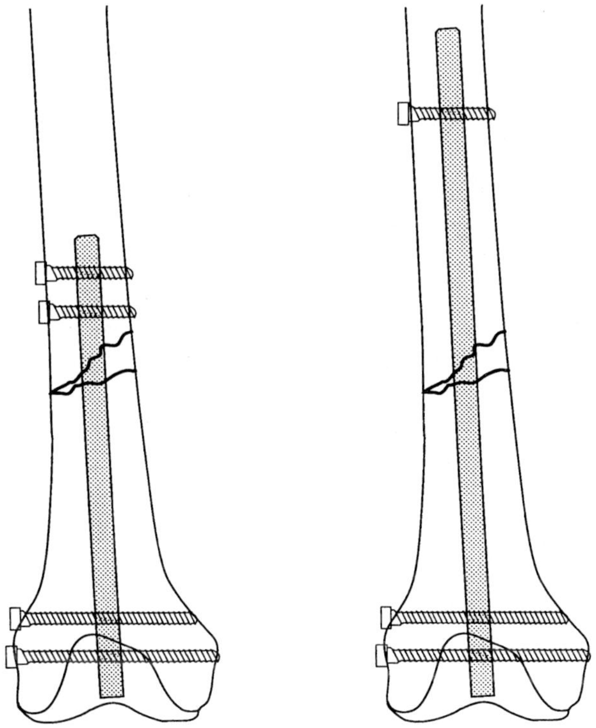

A. B.

Fig. 11–10. Two acceptable configurations for fixation of supracondylar femur fracture using the supracondylar nail. Illustration A on the left depicts use of a shorter, more reliably interlocked nail with two proximal screws, while illustration B on the right depicts use of a longer nail to gain a longer span of intramedullary purchase thus making placement of a single proximal interlocking screw sufficient.

positioning by surgeons skilled in the technique. For these reasons, we occasionally use shorter nails when appropriate; that is, when the nail will engage at least 5 cm of intact proximal femur so that at least two proximal screws will achieve secure bicortical purchase. Alternatively, the risk of potentially difficult proximal interlocking can be accepted and a relatively long nail selected to achieve a longer span of intramedullary purchase (Fig. 11–10).

Comminution that extends more than 20 cm proximally from the knee joint precludes effective stabilization with even the longest available supracondylar nail. Comminution of either the medial or lateral condylar cortex that extends to within approximately 5 cm of the roof of the intercondylar notch prevents adequate bicortical purchase of two distal interlocking screws.

OPERATIVE TECHNIQUE

There is no single technique for supracondylar nail insertion. Any of a variety of methods can be used depending upon the fracture pattern, the medical condition of the patient, the equipment available, and the preferences and the familiarity of the operating surgeon. Immediate nailing is optimal except for the most severely contaminated open farm equivalent injuries, and those where arterial reanastomosis must be performed at once because of prior delays in treatment. Under these conditions interim external fixation is useful to maintain length and gross alignment at the fracture site until nailing can be performed. The exchange is preferably made within 7 to 10 days while the pin tracts are still relatively free of contamination. Immediate nailing of open fractures, however, is contingent upon observing the established principles of thorough debridement of all devitalized bone and soft tissues.

Supracondylar nailing is performed in the supine position on a regular operating table equipped with a radiolucent foot extension long enough to allow imaging of the distal two-thirds of the thigh. Standard prophylactic antibiotics are administered preoperatively. The limb is draped free. A sterile tourniquet can be used unless there are specific contraindications, such as vascular injury, previous arterial anastomosis, or graft placement or noncompliant calcified vessels with risk of plaque dislodgement. Several sterile sheets are placed beneath the distal thigh to flex the knee, this moves the proximal tibia out of the way allowing access to the intracondylar notch and relaxes the gastrocnemius muscle avoiding recurvatum deformity.

Extraarticular fractures can be approached through a limited incision using a variety of techniques. An infrapatellar incision 4 to 5 cm long is made either directly over the patellar tendon or at its medial edge (Fig. 11–11). The patellar tendon is correspondingly then either split longitudinally or retracted laterally (as for tibial nailing, hence the ability to fix a floating knee with minimal dissection). Direct visualization of the entry site in the intercondylar notch (Fig. 11–12) can be accomplished by excision of the fat pad. Alternatively, it can be viewed arthroscopically through a standard anterolateral or anteromedial portal. One further option is to use the C-arm to confirm that the entry site is along the axis of the distal fragment in

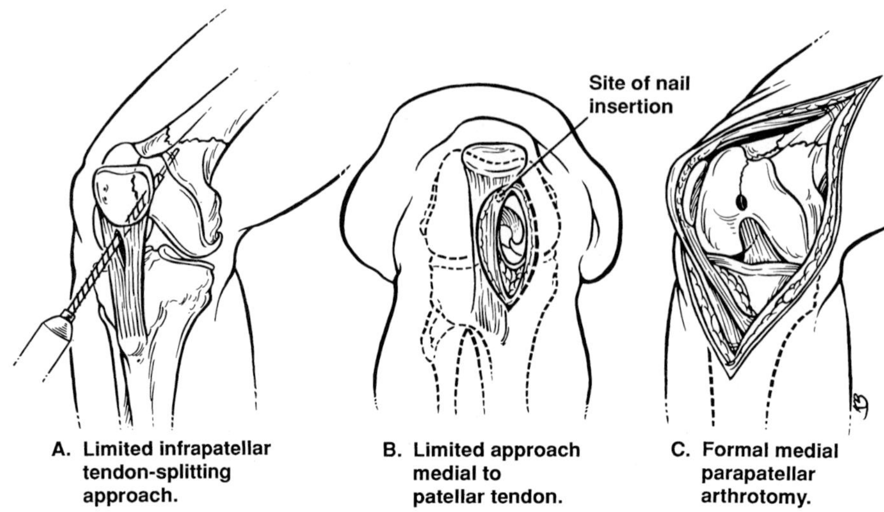

Fig. 11–11. Potential incisions and approaches for supracondylar nail insertion. *A*, Limited infrapatellar tendon-splitting approach. The entry site for supracondylar nail insertion can be viewed arthroscopically or located percutaneously using the C-arm. *B*, Approach medial to the patellar tendon. Excision of the fat pad allows direct visualization of the notch for nail insertion. *C*, Formal medial parapatellar arthrotomy, which allows direct visualization and reduction of displaced articular fracture lines and facilitates reduction of the extraarticular metaphyseal/diaphyseal fracture component.

both the AP and lateral planes. Either of the two infrapatellar incisions is easily extended to a formal medial parapatellar arthrotomy if necessary. A ¼-inch twist drill or Steinman pin is used to perforate the subchondral cortex. The subsequent path created in the distal fragment by either deepening the drill hole or by passage of hand-held reamers is the most crucial reduction maneuver of the entire procedure. Intraoperative imaging must confirm that the path taken is in perfect alignment along the longitudinal axis of the distal fragment, because the final varus/valgus and sagittal alignment of the fracture will be determined at this time.

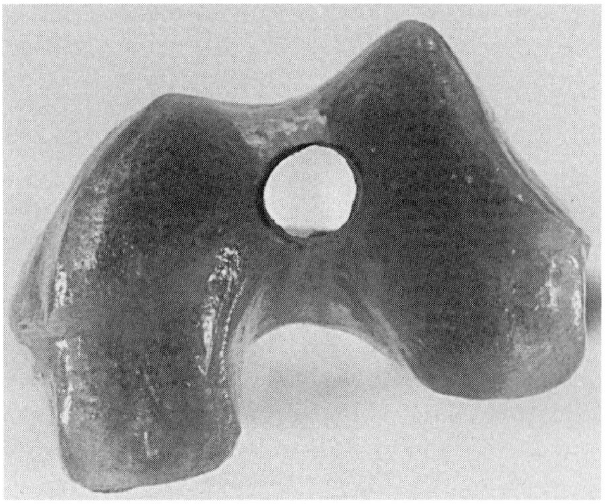

Fig. 11–12. Insertion site for the supracondylar nail within the notch, approximately 1 cm anterior to the femoral origin of the posterior cruciate ligament in line with the intramedullary canal in both the AP and lateral planes.

A guide wire compatible with available flexible intramedullary reaming equipment is then passed into the axial path created in the distal fragment. The fracture is reduced by manual traction and application of corrective translational forces to the thigh, allowing the guide wire to be passed into the proximal canal. If difficulty is encountered, as occasionally occurs with delayed nailings, one of the drill sleeves included in the instrument set can be passed over the guide wire to serve as a short rod for application of leverage on the distal fragment. Alternatively, a femoral distractor can be applied to achieve reduction, but it must be positioned where it will not interfere with either the nail or its lateral targeting device. Length and alignment are maintained manually or with a femoral distractor while the canal is reamed incrementally to at least 1 mm greater than the anticipated nail diameter. Overreaming by up to 2 mm may be necessary when the 250-mm length nail is used to minimize the distortion within the canal, which can complicate proximal interlocking. The reamers must be passed far enough proximally to accommodate the length of the nail being used. The nail is driven over the guide wire with the targeting device on the lateral side. The distal end of the nail should be seated at least 1 mm deep to the subchondral bone. Length and alignment are confirmed on the image intensifier prior to interlocking. The nail should be statically locked in all cases. At least two screws should achieve secure bicortical purchase in the distal fragment. The same is true proximally unless using a nail long enough to gain at least approximately 10 cm of secure circumferential intramedullary purchase in which case a single proximal interlocking screw may suffice.

It is best to drill the most proximal interlocking screw hole first, leaving the drill and drill sleeves in place. This will further fine-tune and secure the alignment of the targeting device with the remaining holes in the nail. At this point in the procedure, there are several technical fine points that are crucial. The stab wounds must be generous enough to easily accommodate the drill sleeves so that there is no tendency for the skin to redirect their path. Likewise, and for similar reasons, the fascia lata should be adequately divided, either sharply or by blunt spreading. The drill sleeves must be passed through the vastus lateralis all the way down to bone to minimize the tendency for the drill to ramp off course along the incline of the convex lateral cortical surface. The surgeon must hold the drill in precise alignment with the drill sleeves during drilling and get the drill started into bone before pushing with significant force. Only sharp new drill bits should be used because dull drill bits will tend to slide off course instead of cutting the desired path.

One helpful, time-conserving method during placement of interlocking screws is to drill up to, but not through, the far (medial) cortex and to measure the depth of penetration of the calibrated drill bit using the drill sleeve. Adding 5 mm to the measurement gives the necessary screw length. This will avoid the time necessary to move the C-arm to the AP view. Distally, however, the cortex is often too thin to feel with the drill. In this case palpation medially or direct visualization is more accurate than AP imaging because of the trapezoidal shape of the distal femur; this method serves equally well to conserve time by obviating the need for an AP view. Precise fracture length and depth of nail seating must be finalized prior to drilling for the proximal screws or else the distal end of the nail will either protrude and impinge upon the patella or be buried too deeply in the distal fragment, compromising distal purchase and making nail removal more difficult. After drilling the most proximal hole and leaving the drill and guide sleeves in place, the distal screws are inserted through stab incisions using a second set of drill sleeves. Proximal screw insertion is then completed. Intermediate fragments can be captured with additional interlocking screws in the central region of the nail. Structural bone grafts used to replace bone loss can also be stabilized with interlocking screws. Maximizing the distance between the two proximal screws by selecting nonadjacent holes in the nail should improve proximal fixation. When the distal fragment can accommodate three interlocking screws, this also enhances the overall stability of fixation. A suction drain is inserted and the knee joint is closed in a routine fashion after thorough irrigation to remove debris from reaming.

Fractures with intraarticular extension are best addressed with a formal medial parapatellar arthrotomy. This allows anatomic reduction and interfragmentary screw stabilization of the articular fragments. Simple intercondylar split patterns (AO type C1 and C2) are stabilized by passing 6.5-mm cancellous lag screws anterior and/or posterior to the anticipated path of the nail. Additional support is obtained during entry hole preparation, reaming and nail insertion with a large pointed reduction tenaculum applied across the condyles. Coronal splits in type C3 fractures are stabilized with screws passed from anterior to posterior. The screw heads are counter sunk when the screws pass through articular cartilage. Once anatomic reconstruction of the articular segment has been accomplished, reaming, nail insertion, and interlocking proceeds as described above for extraarticular fractures, provided that care has been taken not to insert medial-lateral interfragmentary screws along the path of the nail or AP screws where the interlocking screws must pass.

The exposure provided by a formal arthrotomy confers certain advantages during fracture reduction not afforded by the more limited infrapatellar exposures previously described. Following arthrotomy, the metaphyseal/diaphyseal fracture extension will essentially be exposed, converting the procedure to a limited open rodding with opportunity to clamp the fracture in a reduced position. Therefore, full arthrotomy may be worthwhile for critical patients with extraarticular fractures that must be stabilized in the shortest possible time. Additional subperiosteal dissection should be avoided, however. Pointed forceps are preferable when they will suffice because they interfere less with periosteal blood supply.

POTENTIAL PITFALLS AND POSTOPERATIVE COMPLICATIONS

As with any intramedullary nailing procedure, the potential pitfalls and complications of supracondylar nailing are numerous. Those potentially pertinent to supracondylar nailing include (1) errant interlocking screw placement, (2) limb length discrepancy, (3) rotational malalignment, (4) knee stiffness, (5) infection, (6) patello-femoral degeneration, (7) nonunion, (8) implant failure, and (9) loss of fixation. Accurate interlocking screw placement depends upon meticulous adherence to the technical fine points previously discussed and should always be confirmed at the end of the procedure by lateral views with the image intensifier. When difficulty is encountered, we readily resort to the freehand technique using the drill sleeves and holes in the targeting device to site in on the holes in the nail. Correct length is usually achieved in fresh fractures by simply pulling on the leg with near maximal force. Significant over distraction at the fracture site is unlikely to occur because traction is applied manually during reduction, not by means of a fracture table. Shortening of the limb, however, is a distinct possibility with oblique or comminuted fracture patterns. If the nail has already been locked proximally or a drill bit inserted with the fracture out to length, subsequent shortening will cause the nail to protrude into the knee joint interfering with the patella during knee flexion. Additional traction must be applied either manually or with a femoral distractor prior to setting the position of distal fragment by distal locking. Use of the femoral distractor, however, reintroduces the possibility of over distraction. Although use of a formal arthrotomy may afford enough exposure to gain some clues with regard to length and to clamp some fracture patterns in a reduced position, establishment of correct limb length during supracondylar nailing more closely resembles the process used for standard closed antegrade nailing of diaphyseal femoral fractures. The same is true regarding rotational alignment.

One could postulate that the hollow nail might act as a conduit for infection to pass into the knee joint from an infected fracture site, yet infection has not occurred in any of our patients, perhaps because an aggressive approach was taken towards debridement of open fractures. All patients were returned to the operating room every 2 days for repeat debridement until the wounds remained clean and cultures negative.

Impaired knee motion is common after supracondylar fractures because of associated injury to the quadriceps muscle and other surrounding soft tissues regardless of whether or not an arthrotomy is performed. Stiffness of the knee is minimized by use of continuous passive motion machines, by aggressive physical therapy, and by positioning the nail and interlocking screws appropriately. Any patient who does not readily achieve an arc of knee flexion of at least 0 to 90° within 1 week after surgery is treated with manipulation under anesthesia. If motion is found to be decreased at follow-up, arthroscopic or open lysis of adhesions is performed. Care is taken to avoid inserting interlocking screws which are too long since pain secondary to impingement on the soft tissues can result in difficulty when moving the knee. The nail is always seated at least 1 mm deep to the subchondral bone of the intercondylar notch to prevent impingement upon the patella during knee flexion.

Fatigue fracture of the supracondylar nail was a significant problem prior to design changes which increased available nail diameters to 12 and 13 mm, increased the wall thickness, and decreased interlocking screw diameter to 5 mm. Fatigue failure occurred at a rate of 15% (4 of 27) with both the 11- and 12-mm diameter nails when 6.4-mm interlocking screws were used. Only one of 14 nails with the new design (5-mm diameter interlocking screws) have failed. Fatigue testing has demonstrated a fivefold increase in the number of cycles to failure with reduction in interlocking screw size from 6.4 mm to 5 mm.[4] It is recommended that patients remain strictly non-weight bearing for at least 6 weeks until adequate bridging callus has formed. When severe comminution, segmental bone loss or large metaphyseal/diaphyseal bone defects are present, early bone grafting should be performed to promote healing.

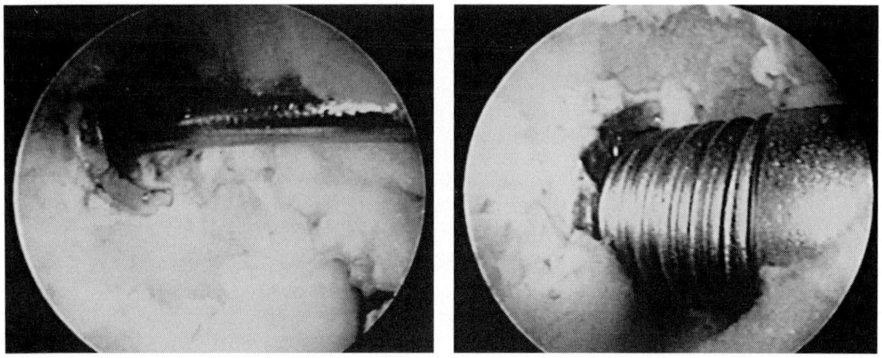

Fig. 11–13. Arthroscopic-assisted supracondylar nail removal. Once the distal end of the nail has been exposed in the notch using shavers and curettes, a guide wire (left) is inserted into the nail to guide placement of the threaded extraction device (right). Interlocking screws are removed through stab incisions prior to extraction of the nail.

POSTOPERATIVE TREATMENT

When stable fixation is achieved and a stable soft-tissue envelope is present, continuous passive motion of the knee can be initiated immediately. Straight leg lifts are begun soon thereafter. A hinged knee, long leg fracture brace is used when severe comminution precludes optimal fixation. An arc of at least 0 to 90° degrees of knee motion must be achieved prior to discharge. If the patient is judged to be delayed in progression towards this goal, the knee is manipulated under anesthesia. Motion lost at follow-up is aggressively regained with manipulation under anesthesia or open or arthroscopic lysis of adhesions as necessary. All patients are instructed to remain non-weight bearing for at least 6 to 8 weeks until substantial early fracture callus is visualized on follow-up radiographs. A gradual progression to full weight bearing is then allowed along with continuation of active and passive range of motion exercises for the knee. Late rehabilitation focuses on regaining the strength and bulk of the quadriceps muscle through progressive resistance exercises. Nail removal is delayed until at least 1 year after the initial surgery. This is usually accomplished percutaneously through a small infrapatellar tendon-splitting incision with arthroscopic assistance (Fig. 11–13).

CLINICAL EXPERIENCE

Forty patients with 43 fractures of the distal femur were treated with the supracondylar nail device between March 1990 and August 1992.[6] One patient died from a severe head injury in the early postoperative period. Another patient, whose grade IIIc open fracture was stabilized uneventfully by immediate supracondylar nailing prior to vascular repair, required an above knee amputation in the early postoperative period because of failure of the vascular repair. The remaining 38 patients with 41 distal femoral injuries are described here. There were 20 males and 18 females aged 16 to 90 years. Twenty-two fractures were open. Nineteen were closed injuries. Among the 22 open fractures, there was 1 grade I, 6 grade II, 7 grade IIIa, 7 grade IIIb, and 1 grade IIIc injury.[7] According to the AO classification system, there were 3 type A2, 16 type A3, 6 type C1, 6 type C2 and 10 type C3 supracondylar fractures.[5] The length of follow-up ranged from 4 to 26 months, averaging greater than 1 year. Each patient was followed at least until the time of radiographic union. This was defined as the presence of bridging callus in all four quadrants on routine AP and lateral radiographs of the distal femur. Knee range of motion and any evidence of angulation were recorded.

Level of activity and function were also noted, but they did not always directly reflect the outcome of the distal femoral injury because of other associated severe musculoskeletal and neurologic injuries. There were 7 patients with fractures of the ipsilateral tibia (floating knee injury). Four of the 7 patients were treated with intramedullary nailing of the tibia through the same incision used for insertion of the supracondylar intramedullary nail. Twenty-eight of the 38 patients in this series sustained multiple injuries, while the remaining 10 patients had isolated distal femoral fractures. Thirty-two of the 41 fractures healed within 4 months after the original nailing procedure. Four patients with bone loss at the fracture site after severe open injuries underwent early iliac crest bone grafting to prevent anticipated delays in healing. There were 5 delayed unions and 4 nonunions. One of the delayed unions healed by 7 months without additional intervention. Two required dynamization by removal of the distal interlocking screws. (When dynamizing, we prefer to remove the proximal screws to avoid rod protrusion into the notch unless the distal screws are significantly symptomatic). One patient was treated by revision with an antegrade femoral nail and application of iliac crest bone graft 4 months after the index procedure. The fifth patient, whose fracture developed progressive valgus angulation because of inadequate distal fixation with only a single interlocking screw was successfully revised with a lateral plate and bone graft 10 weeks after the initial nailing procedure. All 4 nonunions were associated with fatigue fracture of the supracondylar nail. These 4 fatigue failures all occurred among the 27 femurs treated with 11 mm diameter nails in conjunction with 6.4-mm diameter interlocking screws. All four nails failed through empty screw holes near the middle of the nail at the level of the fracture. Three of the 4 patients were noncompliant postoperatively with weight bearing restrictions. Three of these fractures healed following standard reamed antegrade nailing of the femur, which was relatively uncomplicated, because the condylar component of the fractures had united and the canal alignment had been well preserved by the supracondylar nail. The fourth nonunion healed after conversion to a newer 13-mm diameter supracondylar nail with 5-mm diameter interlocking screws. However, the patient subsequently refractured the healed femur proximal to the nail because of a fall and required insertion of a standard femoral nail.

Initial postoperative alignment was anatomic in 37 of 41 fractures. There were no fractures with varus or valgus deformity greater than 5° and none with apex-anterior or apex-posterior deformity greater than 10°. In one case, reduction was lost in the absence of nail fracture. This patient had a very low fracture of the condyles which precluded placement of a second distal interlocking screw. She developed a 15° valgus deformity which was revised as previously mentioned, with a lateral plate and bone graft.

In spite of the high percentage of severe open fractures and extensive articular comminution (54% open, 54% AO type C), 36 of the 41 knees had at least a 0 to 90° arc of knee motion at final follow-up. This was caused in part by an aggressive approach toward regaining motion when progress with physical therapy was judged to be lagging behind. Three patients underwent surgical lysis of adhesions, while 3 were treated with closed manipulation only. Among the 5 patients with less than 90° of knee motion, one patient had severe preexistent bilateral osteoarthritis with an arc of flexion of the opposite knee of only 30 to 60°; one patient had strong extensor tone in the lower extremities with severe cognitive deficits after a closed head injury; one patient fell and sustained a new coronal split in the condyles that required a second open reduction to correct displacement; and, two patients had severe open fractures complicated by nonunion associated with nail fatigue fracture with need for repeated operations on the knee.

It is difficult to compare the results among these patients to those obtained in previous series using other fixation devices because of the relative severity of the fractures treated, the extent of associated injuries and the evolving design of the supracondylar nail. For example, Leung et al. used antegrade femoral nailing to treat only extraarticular injuries and those intraarticular injuries amenable to percutaneous reduction[8] (overall a less severe spectrum of injury). Although the incidence of nonunion and delayed union in the present series was somewhat higher than found when lateral plate devices were used,[9-12] most of these occurred with the older, failure prone nail design and do not necessarily reflect adversely upon the concept and technique of supracondylar nailing. Measurements of outcome such as ambulatory function, knee range of motion, and pain were compounded by neurologic injuries and other orthopaedic injuries and biased by the high-energy profile of the distal femoral injuries. Nevertheless, it is our impression that the results potentially obtainable by supracondylar nailing are comparable to those obtainable with lateral-plate devices, while the technique offers real

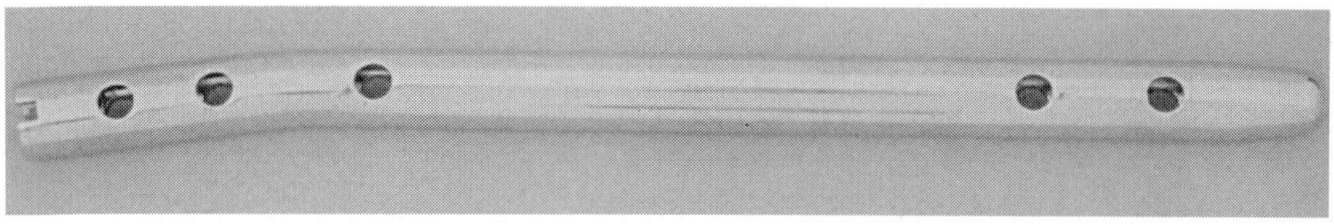

Fig. 11–14. Newly available model of the supracondylar intramedullary nail, which has eliminated the middle holes and subsequently improved in strength for use in more challenging cases where central holes are not essential.

practical advantages in certain clinical situations as previously discussed.

OVERVIEW

At this time, we are cautiously optimistic about the use of the GSH supracondylar nail device in selected patients with supracondylar/intracondylar fractures of the distal femur. The design of the nail and its accompanying instrumentation remain in the evolutionary stages as do the techniques for insertion, which are varied and involve a definite learning curve. We feel that the supracondylar nail provides a valuable resource for the orthopaedic trauma surgeon managing poly-traumatized patients with floating knee injuries and other complicated femoral fractures. Supracondylar nailing holds its greatest advantages for critically injured patients who must be instrumented rapidly with minimal blood loss and operative time. We have found the supracondylar nail to be a valuable tool in managing the population of patients encountered at a Level I trauma center. Extended follow-up will help to determine if there are any long-term adverse effects of the technique upon knee function. A randomized, prospective study comparing the supracondylar nail to the lateral side plate devices is planned in order to objectively assess the relative merits of the two techniques when applied to the same population of patients by the same group of surgeons.

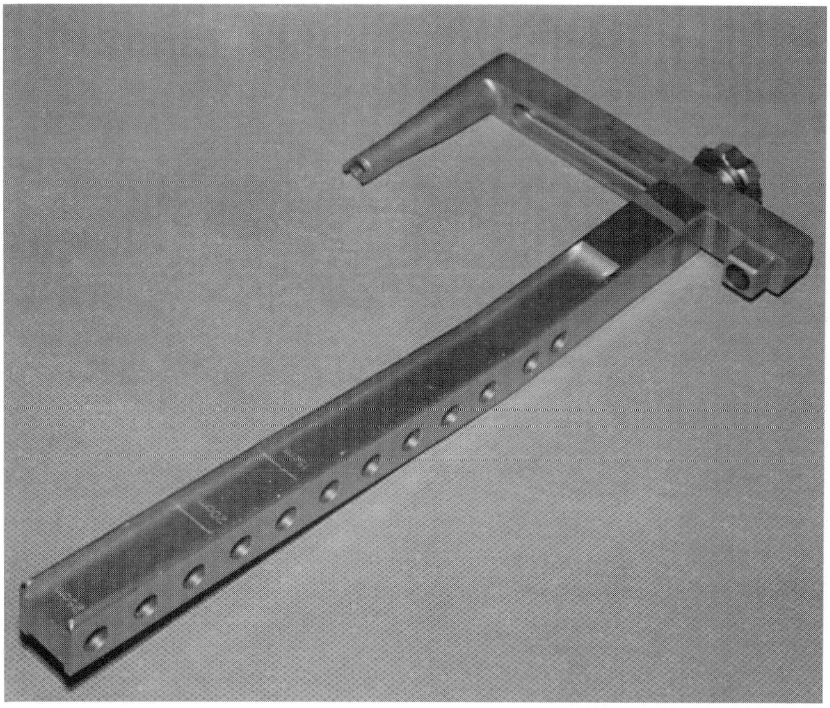

Fig. 11–15. Improved version of insertion and interlocking screw guide for the supracondylar intramedullary nail. The newly designed device will allow positioning of the interlocking screw guide in two different positions to accommodate various size thighs.

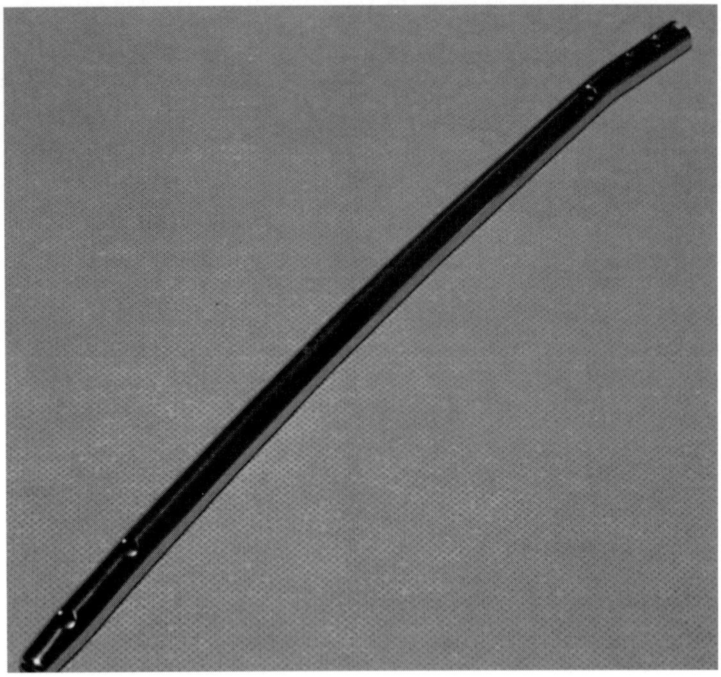

Fig. 11–16. Custom retrograde femoral nail that is 350 mm in length. This nail was designed to address fractures of the diaphyseal region that, for some reason, cannot be addressed through the traditional antegrade method. This is a custom device which is currently in clinical trials.

RECENT DEVELOPMENTS

Failures with the earlier model generally occurred at a hole in the rod adjacent to the fracture. This problem has been adequately addressed by the use of smaller interlocking screws as well as increased rod wall thickness. In another available model, further improvements in strength occurred by including only three distal and two proximal holes which makes a significant portion of the rod solid. The device is now available for clinical use and can provide increased strength for larger patients or, in more demanding situations, when the holes in the center of the rod are not needed (Figs. 11–14 and 11–15).

A custom line of retrograde femoral nails was manufactured to address femoral shaft fractures from 6 cm below the lesser trochanter with insertion through the intercondylar notch (Fig. 11–16). Currently, we are working with these devices to refine techniques and establish indications. The closed section design provides strength with three distal and two proximal holes for interlocking. However, there is no guide for the proximal holes, so a freehand technique is suggested. The distal interlocking screws are inserted with the supracondylar nail guide. This device is not available for general use and is presently going through clinical trials. Preliminary findings show its usefulness for all indications of the supracondylar nail plus diaphyseal fractures occurring in similar circumstances. The standard antegrade femoral nail will remain the gold standard for treating shaft fractures; however, in certain circumstances the retrograde femoral nail will prove to be valuable. A few examples include massively obese patients with diaphyseal fractures and patients with midshaft fractures associated with burns and/or compromised skin in the region of the proximal thigh.

REFERENCES

1. Henry, S.L., Trager, S., Green, S., Seligson, D.: Management of supracondylar fractures of the femur with the GSH intramedullary nail: Preliminary report. Contemp. Orthop. *22*:631–640, 1991.
2. Huckstep, R.L.: The Huckstep intramedullary compression nail. Indications, technique and results. Clin. Orthop. *212*:48–61, 1986.
3. Lewert, A.H., Modny, M.T.: Transfixion rod in condylar and intercondylar fractures of femur. Orthop. Rev. *16*:310–316, 1987.
4. Smith & Nephew Richards, Inc.: Fatigue Testing of the Supracondylar Nail. Tech. Report O.R.:92–22, Memphis, TN.
5. Muller, M.E., Nazarian, S., Koch, P., et al.: The Com-

prehensive Classification of Fractures of Long Bones. Berlin, Heidelberg, Springer-Verlag, 1990.
6. Iannacone, W.M., Bennett, F.S., DeLong, W.G., Born, C.T., Dalsey, R.T.: Initial experience with the treatment of supracondylar femoral fractures using the supracondylar intramedullary nail: A preliminary report. J. Orthop. Trauma *8*:322–327.
7. Gustillo, R.B., Merkow, R.L., Templeman, D.: Current concepts review. The management of open fractures. J. Bone Joint Surg. *72A*:299, 1990.
8. Leung, K.S., Shen, W.Y., So, W.S., et al.: Interlocking intramedullary nailing for supracondylar and intercondylar fractures of the distal part of the femur. J. Bone Joint Surg. *73A*:332, 1991.
9. Chiron, H.S., Casey, P.: Fractures of the distal third of the femur treated by internal fixation. Clin. Orthop. *100*:160–170, 1974.
10. Mize, R.D., Bucholz, R.W., Grogan, D.P.: Surgical treatment of displaced, comminuted fractures of the distal end of the femur. J. Bone Joint Surg. *64A*:871–879, 1982.
11. Olerud, S.: Operative treatment of supracondylar-condylar fractures of the femur. Technique and results in fifteen cases. J. Bone Joint Surg. *54A*:1015–1032, 1972.
12. Slatis, P., Ryoppy, S., Huttinen, V.: AO osteosynthesis of fractures of the distal third of the femur. Acta Orthop. Scand. *42*:162–172, 1971.

12

Lottes Nailing

J. Otto Lottes

Following Küntscher's reports on the first successful intramedullary nailings as a new method for treating fractures, many European surgeons adopted his method.[1,2] At the end of World War II, this technique was introduced to the United States. Although good results were obtained by Küntscher in the nailing of femoral fractures, many surgeons obtained less satisfactory results with the nailing of tibial fractures.[2–4]

After studying the methods used, I soon realized that the U nail, the V nail,[5] and the cloverleaf nail did not adequately stabilize many tibial fractures.[6,9] These nails permitted rotation at the fracture site as the result of weight bearing, thus causing malunion and nonunion. Recognizing the wide proximal metaphysis and somewhat triangular-shaped medullary canal of the tibia, I developed a curved, slightly elastic, tri-flanged nail in 1946. My aim was to construct the nail of a metal that would not be too rigid so that it could be inserted near the tibial tubercle and, after entering the canal, would bend to conform to the canal and then spring back to its original shape after being driven to its full length. The nail was bent on both ends to give extra fixation and to make insertion and removal easier. The shape and flexibility were determined after experimenting with numerous designs. When necessary, casts were applied to supplement the rotational control of the nail. Amputated limbs were used for about 18 months while developing the nail. Repeated changes in shape and hardness of the nails were made before the final nail was selected. When the closed nailing could be accomplished within a reasonably short time in cadaveric tibias, clinical application was begun (Fig. 12–1).[8]

ADVANTAGES OF TIBIAL NAILING

Tibial nailing offers more advantages than does any other procedure for treating fractures of the tibia. Because of the superficial location, a closed nailing can be done quickly and easily, even in the obese patient.[8] Once mastered, the technique can be accomplished within 15 minutes, including time for radiography. One assistant is needed to drive the nail down the canal while the surgeon holds the fracture in reduction. Early postoperative weight bearing in a cast is possible, and full unrestricted weight bearing without a cast begins about 8 weeks after nailing. Because the operative site is located a distance from the fracture site, the complications that occur in open reduction are eliminated.

INDICATIONS

Any fracture within 3 inches below the knee joint and 3 inches above the ankle joint is a candidate for Lottes nailing. Fractures outside this area can be nailed; however, because of the width of the medullary canal, fixation is not as stable as desired, and the patient must accept some displacement (Fig. 12–2). Nailing is not recommended for children with open epiphyses.

TECHNIQUE

Instruments and Implants

1. ⅜-inch end- and side-cutting drill bit or an awl
2. Screwdriver

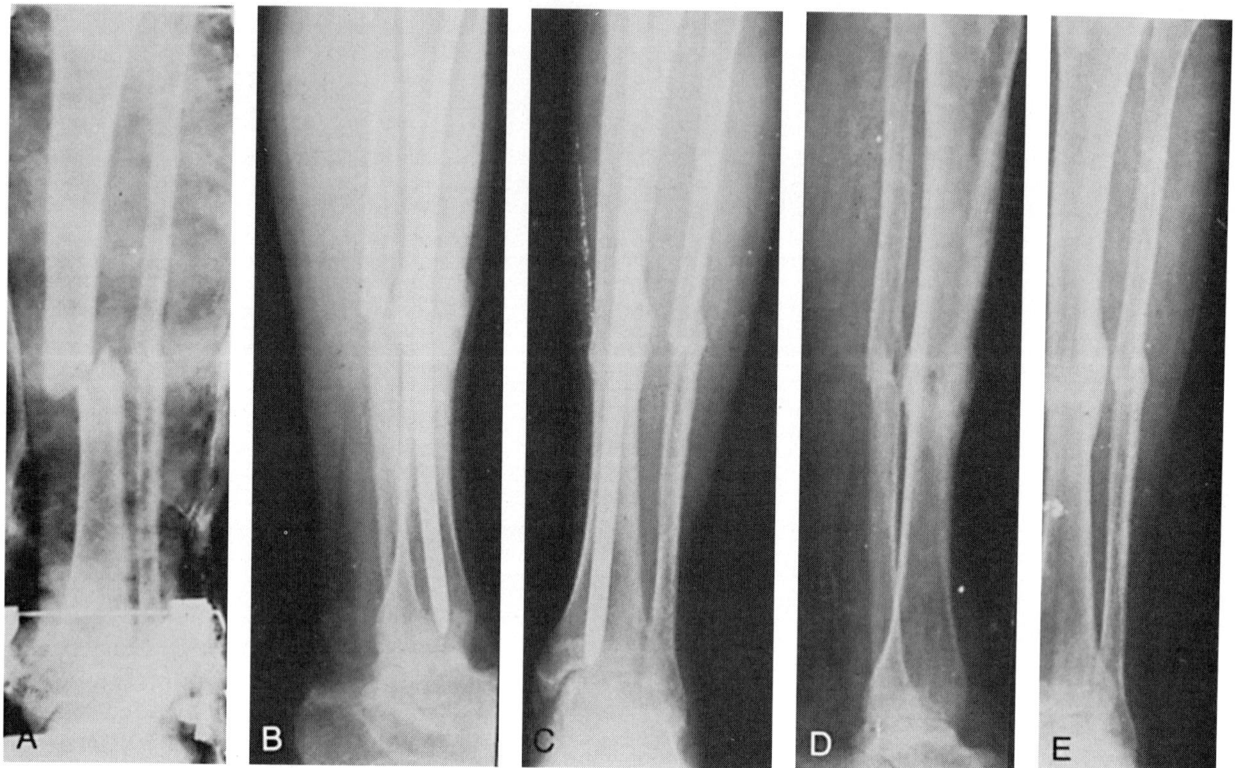

Fig. 12–1. Early nailing. *A*, Slightly oblique midshaft fracture, reduction lost following pins and plaster immobilization. *B,C*, Healing tibia in lateral and AP views 2 months following nailing. *D,E*, Healed fracture following nail removal at 8 months.

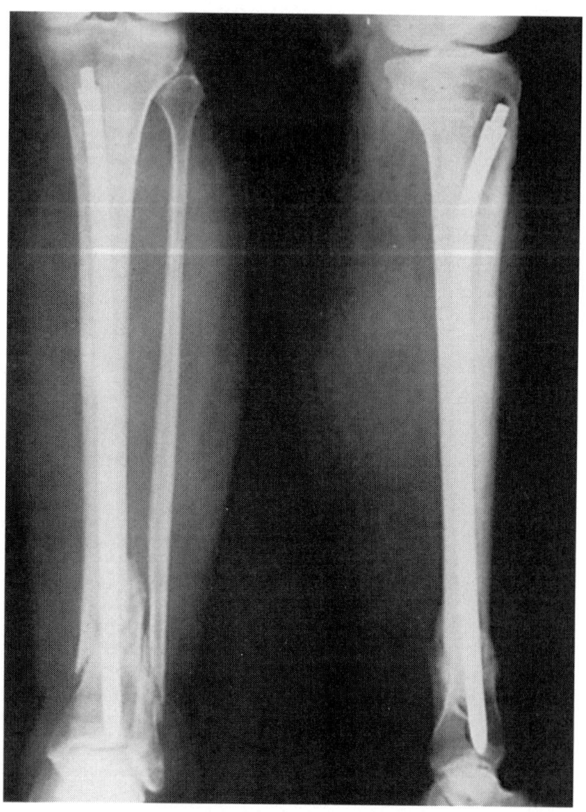

Fig. 12–2. Oblique fracture of distal tibia 3 months following nailing. Varus angulation in this case exemplifies the inability of the nail to control alignment in fractures outside of the isthmic zone.

3. 5/16-inch and 3/8-inch nails
4. 1/2-inch and 1-inch nail extensions
5. Extractor

Measuring for Nail Length

The midpoint of the tibial tubercle is identified. When this area is palpated with the tip of the index finger, a depression in the soft tissues at the base of the tubercle can be felt. The distance is measured from the midportion of the tibial tubercle on the medial side to the palpable tip of the medial malleolus on the uninjured leg. This measurement does not result in the choice of a nail that is too long. Because the nail is curved on both ends and the threaded portion of the nail is outside the canal, the measured length is correct. The tip of the nail ends about 1/2-inch from the ankle joint. The insertion hole is drilled in the previously described area felt by the tip of the index finger.

Position of the Table and Patient

When an open reduction is planned, traction is not necessary. The leg is draped free with the knee bent over the end of the table. When traction is needed, a Collins hitch can be placed around the ankle and extends below the draped leg. The loop of this hitch should extend about 5 inches from the floor. When traction is needed, the foot of the surgeon is placed in the loop of the hitch and downward pressure is applied, thereby distracting the fracture at the fracture site. If the hitch is not used, however, a bone skid can be used to pry the bone ends apart to obtain reduction.

A knee support is more practical in a closed nailing because it holds the fracture in distraction in a fixed stable position. The knee is bent at a right angle, and the leg is positioned at a 45° angle from the floor. The leg is prepped from the ankle strap to above the knee. The leg is abducted about 30° to permit the surgeon to work between the legs. The amount of traction applied must be sufficient to distract the fracture site, and the fracture ends must be allowed to move freely. The rotational deformity can be corrected by palpating the crest of the tibia and realigning the tibia in a straight line. This maneuver can be done even on the obese patient. An incision is made on the medial side of the leg, beginning at about the tip of the distal portion of the patella and carried downward in a straight line to end at about the midportion of the tibial tubercle, about one finger's breadth medial to the tibial tubercle (close to the midportion of the depressed area in which the nail was measured). The upper incision is not cut deeply because the knee joint must not be entered.

Drilling the Hole

Drilling of the hole is the most important step in closed nailings. When the hole is not drilled properly, the insertion of the nail is difficult. The drill is started at right angles to the tibia in the depressed area that was palpated previously. The hole should just touch the base of the midportion of the tubercle. When entering the medullary canal, the drill must continue to turn and should be slanted gradually until it is almost parallel to the axis of the tibial shaft while aiming at the junction of the middle and lower third. When the hole is drilled correctly, the nail can be pushed with a finger down the canal for about 4 inches. If this maneuver cannot be done, drilling should resume. When the hole is not drilled correctly, one of three problems can be encountered: (1) the nail will cut out through the posterior cortex of the tibia, (2) the nail will split the anterior cortex of the tibia (although such an injury will heal and damage does not result, legal problems may occur when the nailing turns out poorly), or (3) the nail will bend, thereby causing recurvation of the tibia.

Insertion of the Nail

The fracture site must be movable before the nail can be driven down the canal; if it is not, more traction should be applied. The nail is driven down the canal with the concave flange in an anterior position until the nail nears the fracture site. The depth of the nail is checked either on the image intensifier or by placing a nail of the same length on the outside of the leg. Then, while the fracture is held in reduction, an assistant drives the nail down about 2 inches beyond the fracture site. After radiographically confirming the portion of the nail in the distal fragment, the nail can be driven home. The nail is driven down until about 1 inch remains outside the canal.

In fractures of the upper third, the distal fragment must be displaced posteriorly about one-half the width of the tibia. When this procedure is not done, the nail exits through the fracture site. The driving of the nail in a young person should be stopped when the pitch of the hammer's blows on the nail gets higher. If driving continues, the nail will get stuck and is difficult to remove. A midthigh cast is applied with the knee straight; a midthigh full-weight-bearing walking cast is substituted in about 10 days. This cast is removed at about the end of 6 weeks, and full weight bearing is started without support. The elderly patient may require support, however. I have no experience with a cast-brace; still, its use may be worthwhile.

Nailing of Open Fractures

In an early series, open fractures were nailed upon admission, if the patient's general condition permitted. Later, because of the lack of operating room personnel, nailings were done when the schedule permitted. To my surprise, the delay did not affect the outcome. The infection rate remained the same, except for patients in whom the original wound had been closed completely at the time of admission. When the skin sutures were removed prior to the nailing procedure and the wound was opened during nailing, the infection rate increased. When the silk skin sutures were left in place until after the nailing procedure, the wound remained closed and the infection rate did not increase.

The time between the onset of injury and the nailing procedure did not affect the infection rate so long as the wound remained closed. An open wound not located at the fracture site was not enlarged to facilitate reduction. Instead, such fractures were nailed by the blind technique. When the open wound was small and damage to tissue was slight, the wound was not debrided but was irrigated profusely. Most of these wounds were about 1 inch in length and were made from "within out" and could be considered clean.

Nailing of Delayed or Nonunited Fractures

If alignment is good and the ends of the bone are not sclerotic, the fracture can be nailed by the closed method. In an established nonunion or open delayed union in a nailed fresh fracture, a 1-inch section of an intact fibula should be excised. In angulated fractures, the fibula should be excised prior to nailing to permit mobilization at the fracture site. When the intact fibula is not resected, the nail often breaks within 2 years. If displacement is evident at the fracture site, or if the bone ends are sclerotic, an open nailing must be done with the use of a *Phemister-type iliac bone graft.* The postoperative care for open fractures is the same as that for closed fractures except that although the cast may not be needed in the closed nailing, it must be used in the open nailing. If the cast is not used, the patient will experience pain when walking. For delayed or nonunited fractures, the cast may be needed for about 1 month longer than is required after primary nailing of fresh fractures.

Infected Fractures

I believe that the nailing of infected nonunited fractures is an alternative approach to be used to avert an amputation when all methods of controlling the infection have failed. The nailing can be done in the routine manner; however, about 1 inch of the fibula must be resected. Surgical trauma is kept to a minimum, and all tissues are raised as one piece. If the alignment is poor or shortening has occurred, an attempt to get length is not made because the trauma to the soft tissues far outweighs any good that might be obtained by restoring length. Sclerotic, portions and all sequestra present are removed. Adequate drainage must be maintained at all times. Skin coverage is not attempted. After applying the usual dressing, a midthigh walking cast is applied and full weight bearing is started. The cast is windowed over the fracture site to permit dressing of the wound. After a few weeks, a new cast is applied and is windowed only when drainage is severe. This method is referred to as the Orr method, and a surprising number of wounds eventually heal with such treatment. Sequestra are removed when present, but the nail is not removed until the fracture has healed. Antibiotics are given as indicated. Healing of these infected fractures generally takes 2 years and chronic osteomyelitis often persists.

Insertion of Two Nails

Two nails can be inserted in wide medullary canals. The second nail, 5/16-inch diameter, is inserted laterally with 1 flange of the small nail inserted between the 2 lateral flanges of the original nail. This small nail does not necessarily have to go much beyond the fracture site, except for fractures of the lower one third for which the nail is driven to within ½-inch of the ankle joint.

Late Malposition

When malalignment has resulted from the bending of a nail, I have straightened the nail in situ by manual three-point bending maneuvers. If bending is associated with refracture, a resection of a portion of the fibula is indicated. Thereafter, the tibia is protected in a walking cast.

Migration of the Nail

If the length of the leg shortens on weight bearing, or if the fracture is located at the junction of the middle and lower one third of the tibia, the nail may back out. The nail may migrate distally and enter the ankle joint if the offset in the nail where it joins the threaded portion catches the tibial cortex. If migration occurs, the nail should be driven back to its original position and anchored with a thin, flat piece of metal about ¾-inch × ½-inch with a ¼-inch hole drilled near 1 of the long ends. After the nail has been repositioned, this metal plate is slipped over the nail. Using a thin os-

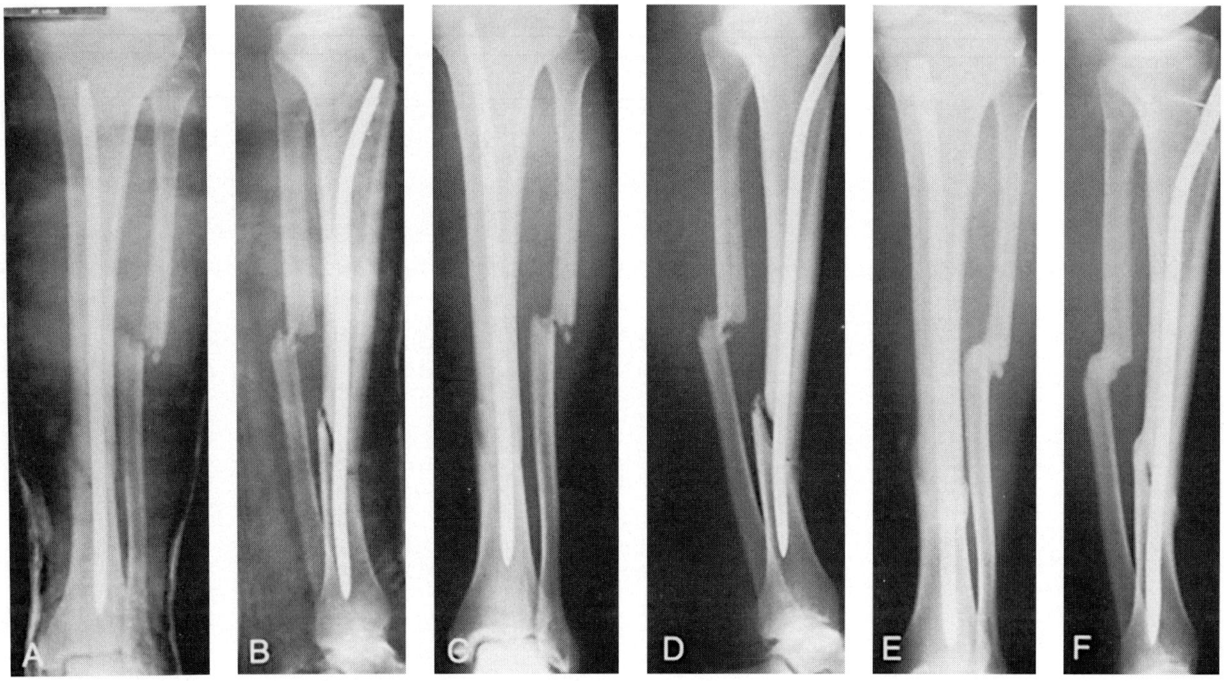

Fig. 12–3. Proximal fixation of a nail that migrated proximally following fixation of a fracture at the junction of the middle and distal thirds. *A,B,* Fracture at the junction of the middle and distal thirds fixed with a Lottes nail, *C,D,* Proximal migration of the nail. *E,F,* Reinsertion of the nail and proximal fixation established with a thin metal plate and a Dobell cap.

teotome, a tract is cut through the outer cortex of the tibia in the path of the thin piece of metal. This thin metal plate is rotated 180°, and a Dobell cap is screwed onto the nail for fixation. This nail can be removed after the fracture has healed by cutting a tract as before. When a blunt instrument is placed against one of the lateral edges in the thin metal sheet, a few blows from the hammer will turn the metal piece around, which then can be removed after removing the cap. The cap may be loosened about one turn prior to turning the flat piece of metal.

Removal of the Nail

During the early nailing procedures, all the nails were removed to check for metal reaction. When none was found, this procedure was discontinued. Now only about 10% of the nails are removed, and only when there is a good reason to do so. The nail should be removed only after the fracture has healed completely, but should be removed within 1 year. After that time, the nail is difficult to remove and may require the removal of a ½-inch section of the anterior cortex of the tibia extending from the insertion site to the midportion of the leg. The difficulty occurs because of the dense layer of bone surrounding the nail. When the nail has a curve at its distal end, this layer of bone blocks the removal of the nail after it has been backed out about 2 inches. When the end of the nail is straight, the nail comes out without much difficulty.

Breaking of the Nail

Breakage occurred in 2 patients approximately 1½ years after nailing. One patient, whose healing was not progressing satisfactorily 5 months after nailing, refused an osteotomy. He continued to refuse osteotomy and continued weight bearing without support until the nail broke 18 months later. Renailing and bone graft were successful.

RESULTS AND COMPLICATIONS

Lottes nailing was used to treat 748 fractures: 349 closed single, 51 closed segmental (double), 9 closed segmental (triple); 214 open single, 50 open segmental (double), 2 open segmental (triple); 57 for delayed or nonunion; and 52 nailed through infection. The distribution of fracture type is presented in Table 12–1. Ages of patients ranged from 13 to 85 years; the average age was 46 years. Most of the 21 bilateral

Table 12–1. Complications in treating fresh fractures*

Nonunions	
409 Closed fractures	2 (0.50%)
266 Open fractures	8 (3.00%)
675 All fractures	10 (1.50%)
Implant failures	
675 All fractures	2 (0.30%)
Deep infections	
409 Closed fractures	3 (0.73%)
206 Open fractures	19 (7.10%)
60 Unspecified fracture type	4
675 All fractures	26 (3.90%)
Amputations	
409 Single closed fractures	3 (0.70%)
675 All fractures	3 (0.40%)
Deaths	
409 Closed fractures	15 (3.60%)
266 Open fractures	13 (4.90%)
675 All fractures	10 (1.50%)

* In the treatment of 57 sterile delayed or nonunited fractures, deep infection occurred in 5.2% and recurrent nonunion occurred in 5.2%. In the treatment of 52 infected nonunited fractures, 5.8% failed to unite and 5.8% required amputation. The remainder united, but often had persistent osteomyelitis. Experience has shown that my tibial nailing technique is highly effective in treating fresh fractures and nonunited fractures. The technique requires, however, attention to the technical details of fracture reduction and nail placement to be routinely successful.

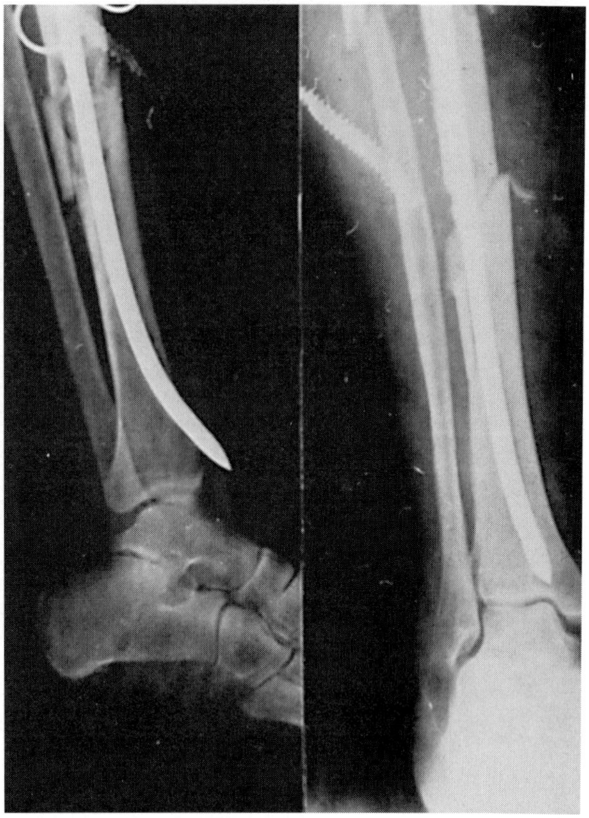

Fig. 12–4. Distal penetration of an excessively long nail driven through the anterior aspect of the distal tibia.

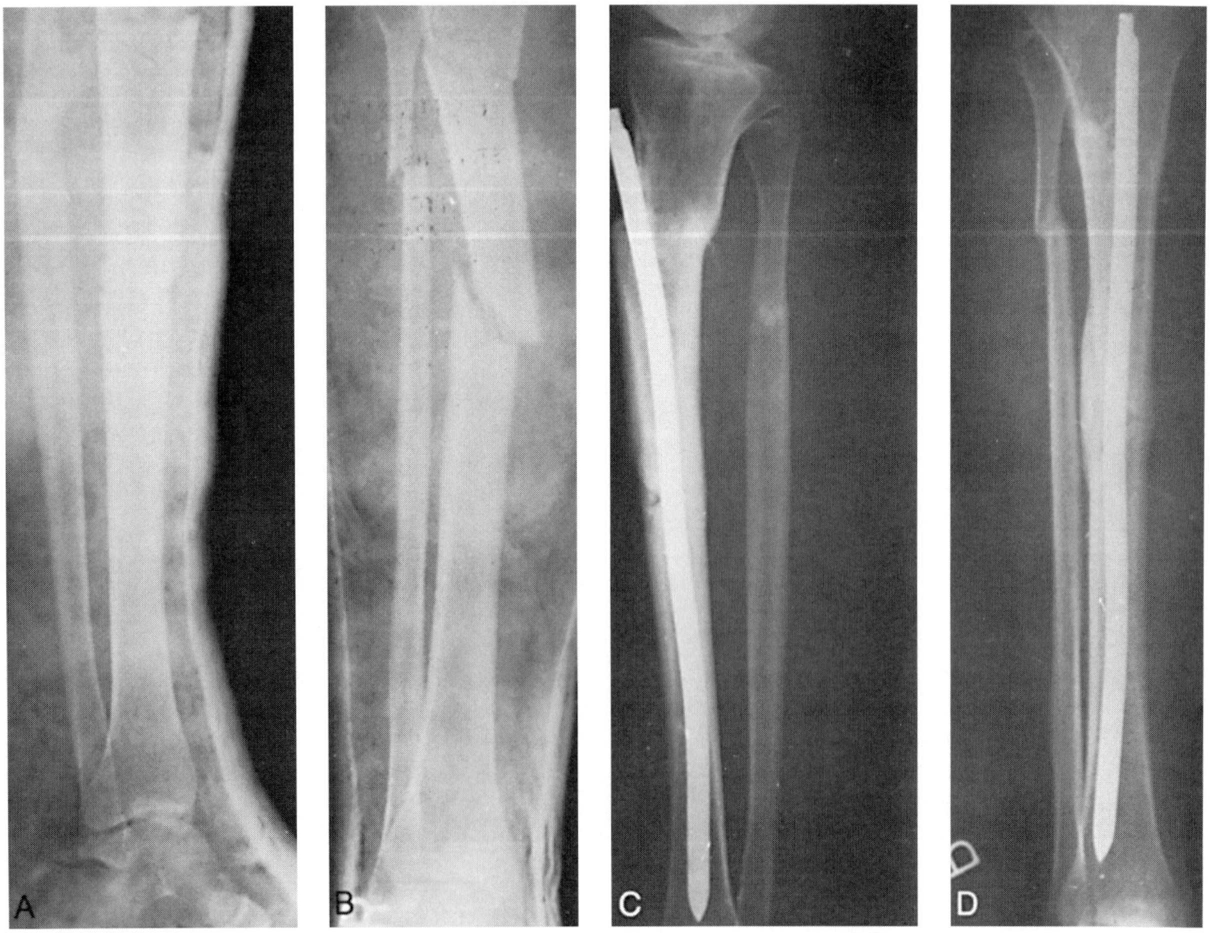

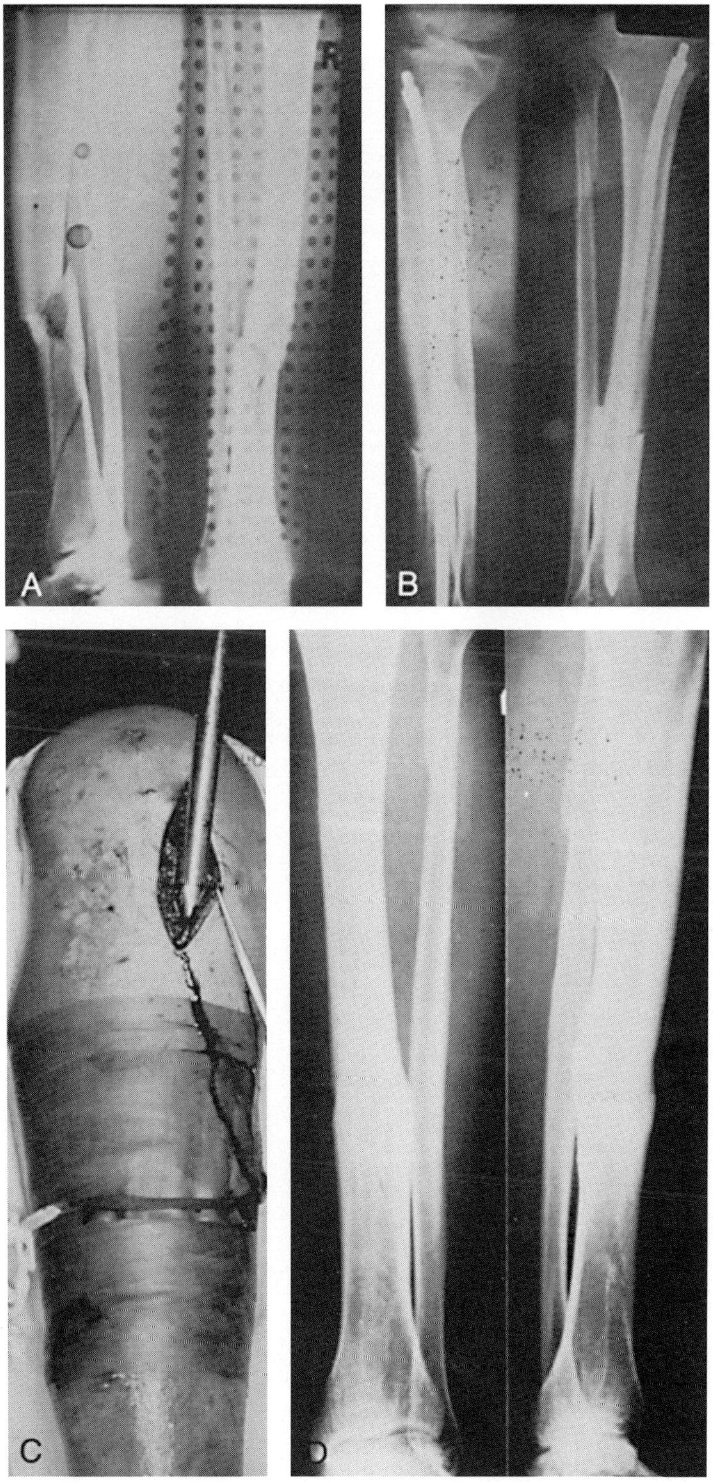

Fig. 12–6. Successful nailing of a comminuted fracture. *A,* AP and lateral views of the fracture. *B,* AP and lateral views of the fracture following nailing. *C,* Use of a sterile esmarch to prevent displacement of the fracture fragments during nailing. *D,* AP and lateral views of the healed fracture following nail removal.

Fig. 12–5. Successful nailing of a segmental fracture with the nail introduced through the proximal fracture site. *A,B,* Lateral and AP views of the segmental fracture. *C,D,* Successful healing of the fracture following nailing with introduction of the nail through the proximal fracture site.

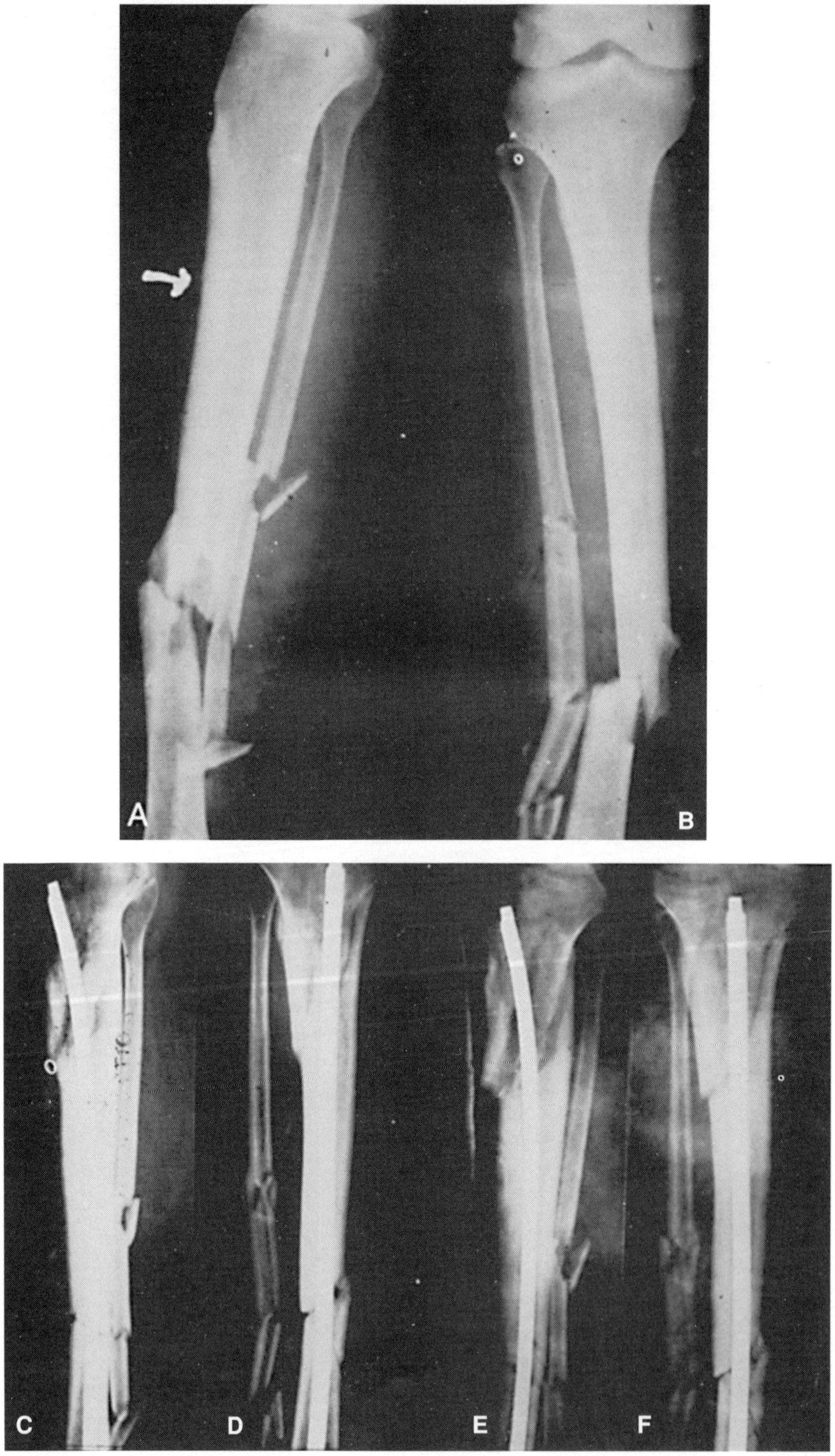

Fig. 12–7. Successful nailing of a comminuted tibial fracture in spite of the intraoperative displacement of the proximal fracture line seen opposite the arrow. *A,B,* Lateral and AP views of the comminuted fracture. *C,D,* Radiograph taken immediately after nailing. *E,F,* Healing fracture 2 months following nailing.

Table 12–2. Distribution of fracture types

Location	*Transverse*	*Oblique*	*Comminuted*	*Butterfly*	*Totals*	*Lost to Follow-up*
		Closed Single Fracture				
Upper third	2	5	16	7	24	1
Mid-third	29	81	158	76	268	39
Lower third	3	41	13	3	57	1
Totals	34	127	187	86	349	41
	(10.0%)	(36.3%)	(53.5%)	(24.6%)		(11.4%)
		Closed Segmental Fracture (Double)				
Upper and mid-third	4	18	7	7	29	4
Mid- and lower third	4	9	9	6	22	3
Totals	8	27	16	13	51	7
	(16%)	(36%)	(48%)	(16%)		(13.7%)
		Open Single Fracture				
Upper third	2	2	6	1	10	—
Mid-third	32	25	115	49	172	30
Lower third	11	12	9	—	32	—
Totals	45	39	130	50	214	30
	(21.0%)	(18.2%)	(60.7%)	(23.3%)		(14.0%)
		Open Segmental Fracture (Double)				
Upper and mid-third	4	11	12	4	27	4
Mid- and lower third	4	7	12	4	23	3
Totals	8	18	24	8	50	7
	(16%)	(36%)	(48%)	(16%)		(14%)
		Delayed or Nonunion				
Upper third	2	4	—	—	6	—
Mid-third	22	20	4	—	46	—
Lower third	2	3	—	—	5	—
Totals	26	27	4	—	57	—
	(45.6%)	(47.3%)	(7.0%)			
		Infected Fractures Nailed Intentionally				
Upper and mid-third	1	1	2	—	4	—
Mid- and lower third	—	3	—	—	3	—
Mid-third	17	3	25	7	45	5
Totals	18	7	27	7	52	5
	(34.6%)	(13.4%)	(51.9%)	(13.6%)		(9.6%)

tibial fractures in this series were nailed in 1 surgical procedure.

Of the closed single fractures, 3 required open nailing because of faulty nailing procedures. Although rare, penetration through the anterior cortex during insertion of the nail occurred when nails were too long or when nails were inserted through incorrectly placed entry portals. Displacement of several linear fractures occurred, and 3 nails were driven into the ankle joint. A thin anchoring piece of metal was added to prevent recurrent ankle penetration.

Results were obtained for 675 fresh fractures. Typical examples of successful cases are seen in Figures 12–6 and 12–7. These included 409 closed and 266 open fractures; 12.9% of patients were lost to follow-up. Of the remaining 588 patients, the frequencies of major complications are listed in Table 12–2. The 3 below-the-knee amputations were performed because of severe vascular and/or nerve damage resulting in numb feet and uncontrollable infections. Symptomatic fat embolism did not occur.

REFERENCES

1. Böhler, L.: Medullary Nailing of Küntscher. Translated by H.Tretter. Baltimore, Williams & Wilkins, 1948.
2. Böhler, L., Böhler, J.: Küntscher medullary nailing. J. Bone Joint Surg. *31A*:295, 1949.
3. Lottes, J.O., Hill, L.J., Key, J.A.: Closed reduction, plate

fixation and medullary nailing of fresh fractures of the leg. A comparative end result study. J. Bone Joint Surg. *34A*:861, 1952.
4. Orr, H.W.: Compound fractures with special reference to the lower extremity. Am. J. Surg. *46*:733, 1939.
5. Küntscher, G.: Recent advances in the field of medullary nailing. Ann. Chir., et Gynaecol. Fenniae *37*: 115, 1948.
6. Rush, L.V., Rush, H.L.: A reconstruction operation for comminuted fracture of the upper one-third ulna. Am. J. Surg. *38*:332, 1937.
7. Rush, L.V., Rush, H.L.: A technique for the longitudinal pin fixation of certain fractures of the ulnar and femur. J. Bone Joint Surg. *21*:616, 1939.
8. Lottes, J.O.: Intramedullary nailing of the tibia. *In* Instructional Course Lectures. Edited by J.W. Edwards. Ann Arbor, American Academy of Orthopaedic Surgeons, *XV*:65, 1958.

13

Reamed and Unreamed Nailing of Tibial Fractures

Samuel G. Agnew and M. Bradford Henley

The indications for intramedullary nailing of open and closed tibial fractures are debated, as both the anatomic criteria and injury criteria are subject to bias. The rationale that more severe fractures may benefit from nonoperative treatment is not valid today. A review of the American Academy of Orthopaedic Surgeons' risk management database for tibial fractures presents thought-provoking data.[1]

Eleven cases resulted in delayed unions or malunion of the tibia. These closed claims resulted in payments totaling $1.2 million. Citing specific reasons of particular importance include inadequate initial reduction, inadequate radiograph follow-up, cast or fixation removed too early, and weight bearing begun too soon. Nine other cases were settled for more than $1 million because of infections, missed associated fractures, or skin loss under a cast. The goal of union is certainly important in treating these injuries, however, it should not be the ultimate goal. What is perhaps more important is the restoration of form and function. These goals should guide the selection of the most appropriate treatment. The scientific database regarding the functional outcome of closed treatment of tibial fractures is sparse. Gamble et al.,[2] citing a 42% complication rate, suggested that closed treatment was not without problems. Their findings were supported by Waddell et al.[3] who found a 66% complication rate. Intramedullary nailing is not without problems either, Koval et al.[24] recently reported a complication rate of 58%, however most of these problems were not treatment altering events.

The decision to stabilize a tibial fracture by intramedullary nailing is becoming less of a dilemma as more data is accrued as to its efficacy and morbidity. The success of nailing is dependent primarily upon the surgeon's judgment, the technique, and the implant employed. It is paramount that these variables match the patient's injury profile, the soft-tissue trauma, the fracture, and the patient's expectations and goals.

The history of tibial implants spans the same half century as its femoral counterpart. Flexible nails (G. Küntscher, K. H. Hackethal, the Rush brothers, and J. Ender) were first used to stabilize diaphyseal injuries. Ender nails for closed fractures were popularized in America through the work of Arsen Pankovich, and later their role in open fracture treatment was reported by Holbrook and colleagues.[4] For many years the Lottes nail was the mainstay for intramedullary tibial fixation. The Lottes nail was the first to incorporate a curved, slightly elastic solid triflanged design.

The evolution of the Küntscher nail for the tibia and its increased rotational control stemmed from modifications made in both design and surgical technique. The Küntscher implant achieved fixation in the diaphysis through elastic expansion of the compressed open section, cloverleaf nail. The application of larger nails was permitted by reaming of the medullary canal. This option improved fracture stability by decreasing the nail's working length and augmenting the nail's endosteal contact.

Second-Generation Nails

Locked tibial nails have expanded the anatomic limitations imposed on previous reamed implants. Initially, few design modifications were made in the devices other then adding proximal and distal holes that permitted insertion of cross-locking screws. Some designs accommodated both anteroposterior screws and medial-lateral screws proximally, while still retaining the general Küntscher design. Other manufacturers added anteroposterior distal screws. These modifications have merit and expand the range of stable fracture fixation to the proximal and distal meta-diaphyseal regions. Other variances in design are open section versus closed section and solid versus cannulated. The open section are perhaps the most forgiving, while the solid design appear to impart greater rotational control.

The availability of a guide rod for which to pass the nail over allows one the ability to asses the eventual placement prior to passage. Perhaps the most radical change in implant design

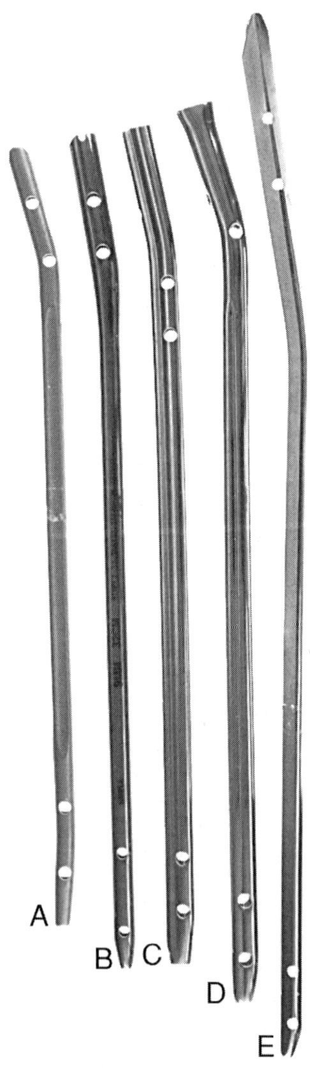

Fig. 13–1. (Left to Right) Tibial nails: *A,* ZMS (Zimmer; Warsaw, IN.); *B,* Uniflex (Biomet; Warsaw, IN.); *C,* Küntscher (Orthopedic Equipment Company); *D,* Grosse-Kempf (Howmedica; Rutherford, NJ.); *E,* AO/ASIF (Synthes; Paoli, PA.).

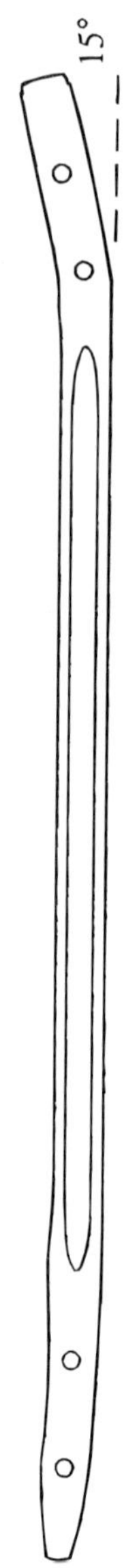

Fig. 13–2. Example of typical proximal bend and degree of bend. (Courtesy of Zimmer; Warsaw, IN.)

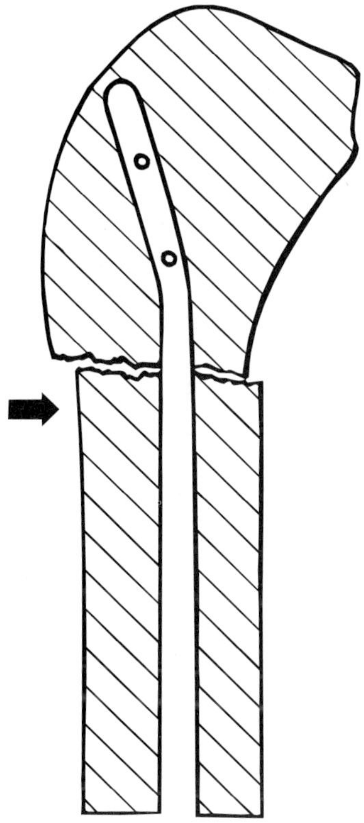

Fig. 13–3. Proposed mechanism of translational deformity with zone II injuries.

came from the work of Stephan Perren and coworkers in Davos, Switzerland.[5] On the basis of anatomic specimens and computed tomography of normal tibiae, the proximal bend in the nail was straightened and moved distally, and the nail's wall thickness was reduced to allow greater flexibility. An additional modification was the creation of slotted holes to permit controlled axial dynamization.

The dilemma of whether every unstable tibial fracture should be surgically addressed is compounded by the choice of implants and the choice of an implant that is appropriate for the situation. Nearly every orthopaedic manufacturer markets a set of tibial nails and each is different. The implants vary in (1) material composition, (2) size, (3) wall thickness, (4) bending stiffness, (5) torsional flexibility, (6) slotting, (7) cannulation, (8) location of the bend, (9) angulation of the bend, (10) tip shape (Figs. 13–1 through 13–3), (11) direction of the locking screw holes, (12) size of cross-locking screw, and (13) insertion/extraction instrumentation. Presently there is no conclusive data to support the superiority of a specific implant. The success or failure of this treatment modality depends primarily on the surgeon.

Small-Diameter ("Unreamed") Locking Tibial Nails

The history of unreamed tibial nails parallels that of present implants. The Lottes tibial nail was inserted unreamed. The advent of unreamed, locking nails introduced another treatment option. The ability to fabricate smaller-diameter (7-, 8-, and 9-mm) implants with smaller locking screws permitted manufacturers to market them as "unreamed nails." It is the small diameters of these nails that permits their insertion without reaming. The term "unreamed" should be applied to the insertion technique and not to the nail.

Recent biomechanical data on tibial nail design suggests that a distally placed bend in the nail may create malalignment at a proximal fracture if the injury is at or above the nail bend (Fig. 13–4).[6] Additionally, the orientation and span of the proximal cross-locking screws affects bending and axial stiffness of the bone-implant composite. Closed section nails, whether cannulated or solid, may be advantageous in the treatment of rotationally unstable tibial fractures because of their higher torsional stiffness.[7]

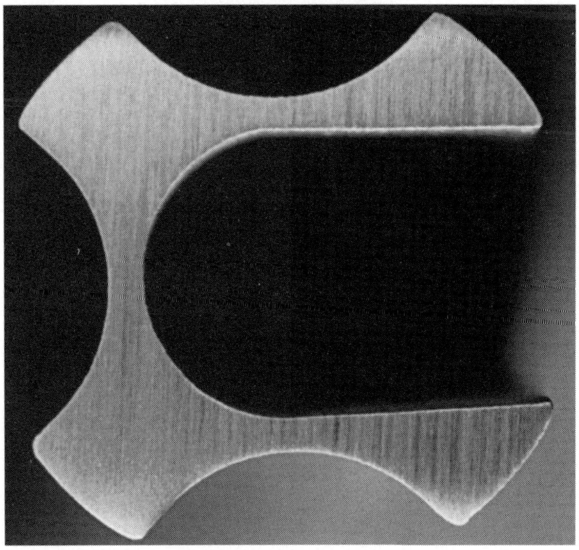

Fig. 13–4. Modification made in classic cloverleaf design to yield greater torsimal rigidity. "M" design of Winquist, Kyle, Zimmer ZMS System. (Courtesy of Zimmer; Warsaw, IN.)

When small-diameter locking nails are inserted without reaming, there may be a relative mismatch between the outer nail diameter and the inner (endosteal) bone diameter at the fracture site. Despite static locking, this mismatch permits motion of the implant within the medullary canal. The working length of a loose-fitting, statically-locked nail is the distance between the proximal and distal locking screws rather than the points of endosteal nail contact. Because these nails may not have a press-fit, forces transmitted across the fracture are borne by the length of the nail and transferred to the bone at the bone-interlocking screw interface. The ability of small-diameter unreamed nails to prevent fracture malalignment is greatly diminished.

The biological effects of reamed and unreamed tibial nail insertion techniques have been investigated recently. Even when small-diameter nails are inserted without reaming, osseous blood flow is reduced. In intact canine tibiae, cortical bone perfusion was reduced by 15 to 55% (avg. 31%) after 3.4-mm cloverleaf nails were inserted without reaming. This was compared to a 45 to 85% (avg. 70%) reduction in cortical perfusion after reaming to 5.3 mm and the insertion of 5-mm nails.[8] Another study used a fractured sheep tibial model to demonstrate a statistically significant reduction in cortical perfusion during and after the insertion of reamed and unreamed statically locked tibial nails, creating a reproducible spiral fracture decreased overall cortical bone perfusion similarly in both groups. Both reaming and nail insertion caused additional decreases in cortical perfusion. However, unreamed nail insertion resulted in a decrease in blood flow which was less than nail insertion with reaming. These findings suggest that violation of the medullary canal without reaming, by using a canal filling nail, disrupts the medullary blood supply but to a lesser degree than with the addition of reaming.[9]

The use of small-diameter locked devices requires a change in philosophy more than merely a change in implant technology. One should achieve anatomic alignment of the tibia prior to insertion of the small diameter nail. This is especially important for fractures outside of the mid-diaphysis. The ability to weight bear needs to be tailored to the implant and fracture personality rather than prescribed empirically. The need for adjunctive stabilization, staged procedures or revision to a larger reamed nail may be part of the original treatment plan.

The data is still inadequate to suggest small-diameter nails as a definitive device for the treatment of every tibial fracture. Biological experiments have shown that these nails are less damaging to the tibial blood supply. This may prove important in the treatment of open fractures and high-energy closed fractures.

Advances have been made in the last decade in all aspects of fracture treatment from the actual implant to the science behind what makes this practice sound. Early on it was thought that delayed nailing, at 3 to 5 days, would be safest in the isolated, unstable injury. However, recent data has been collected by Tischenko[13] and McQueen[14] showing that the rate of compartment syndrome is not increased from early intervention, and the practice is quite cost-effective. The advent of interlocking nails has been singularly the most notable technological advancement for tibial fracture management.

RELEVANT ANATOMY

The tibiae has a wide proximal tibial flare with thin cortices supported by the triangular-shaped medullary canal with slight varus bow. The primary blood supply to the diaphysis is a single nutrient vessel. The nutrient vessel, a branch of the posterior tibial artery enters the posterolateral border of the diaphysis at the junction of proximal and middle one third. The intraosseous path of the artery is traceable into one ascending and two descending vessels.[10,11]

The normal centrifugal endosteal blood supply of the intact bone is well documented and is found to be transiently reversed in situations of acute compromise.[10,11] The preservation or restoration of the muscle envelope and its contributing periosteal blood supply is critical to cortical blood flow and is therefore critical to union.[11]

The muscle envelope surrounding the tibia is eccentric, with the greatest mass of muscle posteriorly and anterolaterally. This eccentricity may create a tethering effect thereby impeding fracture reduction or the maintenance of alignment.

SELECTION OF FRACTURES

Anatomic Indications

The tibia is best thought of as having six anatomic zones (Fig. 13–5). Fractures within zones III and IV can be treated relatively safely

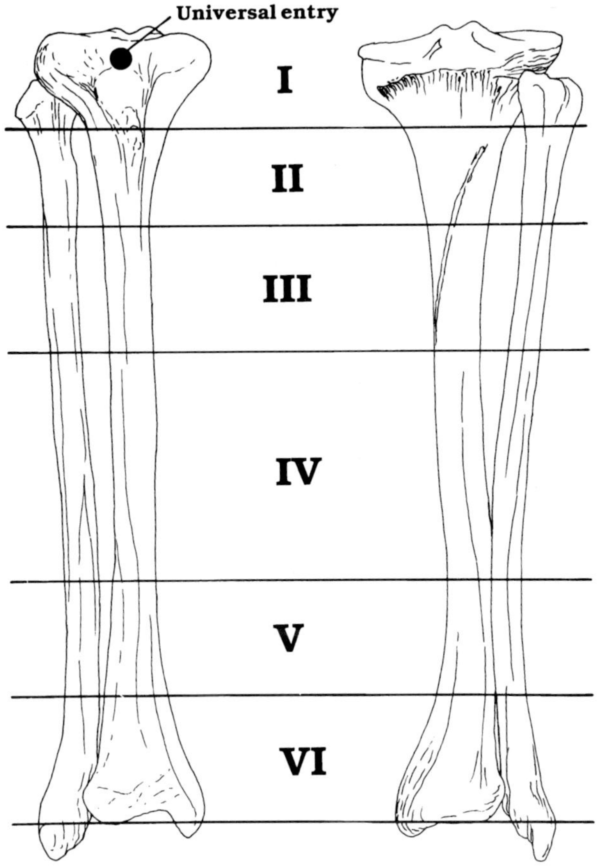

Fig. 13–5. Left-frontal view of tibia with anatomic zones and entry point. Right-hind view of tibial zones. Zone attributes: (I) Tibial head: thin cortices, cancellous bone, periarticular; (II) infratubercular zone: transitional bone, transitional blood flow, strong muscular attachments, thick periosteum; (III) proximal mid-diaphysis: nutrient vessel canal, cortical bone; (IV) mid-diaphysis: average diameter 10.5-mm adult specimens, cortical bond, single vessel blood supply; (V) distal meta-diaphysis: transitional bone, transitional blood flow; (VI) plafond: periarticular bone, thin cortices, cancellous bone (Adapted from Carr J, Sobba D, Bear L: Biomechanics of rigid tibial nail insertion sites. Abstract of VI Annual Meeting OTA, Toronto, 1990. J. Orthop Trauma 5:238, 1991.)

with standard locking nailing technique. Fractures that span zone II or the distal aspect of zone V can be problematic and should not be underestimated simply because the tibia is a subcutaneous bone. The ability to control angulation and translation of fractures in zones II and V are the greatest problem and often require the application of adjunctive reduction techniques.

Injury Profile Indications

Not only will the fracture's anatomic location and configuration determine the rationale for nailing, but the patient's injury profile will aid in the decision process (Fig. 13–6). Specific injuries best treated by the stabilization of tibial fractures are as follows:

- High-energy, closed fractures
- Floating knee injuries
- Polytrauma: associated pelvic, acetabular, or spine fractures
- Elevated compartment pressures requiring fasciotomy or compartment syndrome
- Fracture of tibia and fibula at same level
- Open tibial fractures: Gustilo types I, II, IIIa, and IIIb
- Low-energy fractures which cannot be controlled by nonoperative methods

Patients presenting with any of these injury profiles are treated with early if not immediate stabilization, which can be safely achieved with intramedullary nailing. Patients with open fractures presenting even 12 to 16 hours

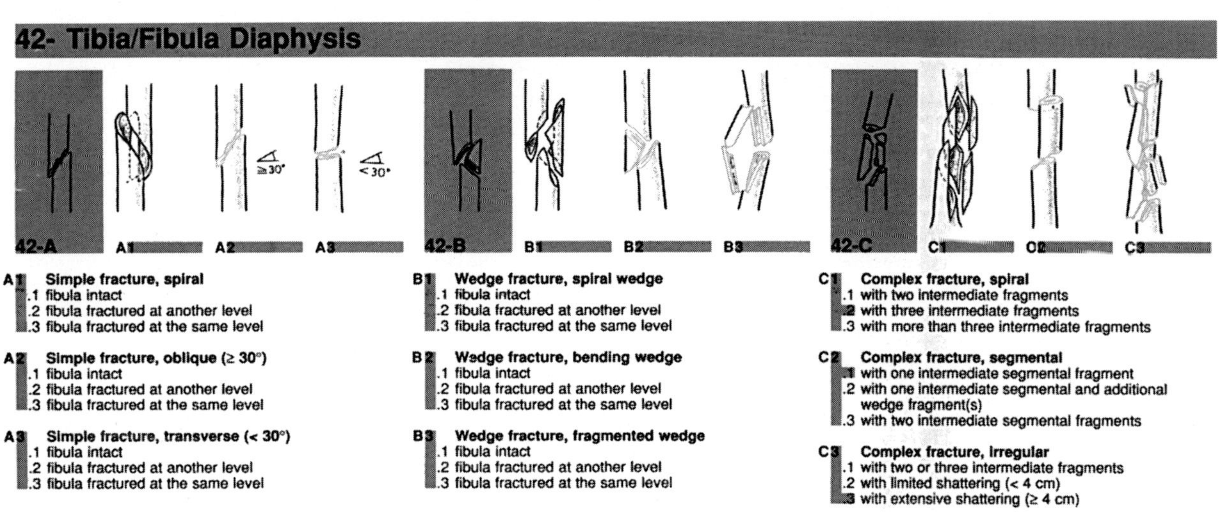

Fig. 13–6. OTA classification of diaphyseal tibial fractures (Courtesy of Springer-Verlag; New York, NY.)

from injury may still be candidates for stabilization provided appropriate antibiotics have been administered early on and a thorough debridement is planned in accordance with the stabilization.[12]

PREOPERATIVE PLANNING

Assuming the decision to treat a fracture with an intramedullary device, one must proceed with a suitable plan. Templating of the fracture with a Küntscher ossimeter or other radiological ruler is important. This will guide the selection of implant length and diameter. It is important to estimate nail length to assure an adequate nail selection before committing to the procedure. An estimate of maximum nail diameter can be made from the lateral radiograph. This is especially important if the nail is to be inserted unreamed. The inner (endosteal) diameter of medullary canal should be gauged at it's narrowest dimension (usually mid-distal, third junction).

Fracture Reduction and Reduction Aids

In distinction to the femur, the tibia has a relatively short and distally placed isthmus. Insertion of an intramedullary nail across a femoral fracture will generally result in satisfactory fracture alignment with the exception of limb rotation. This is also true for fractures in tibial zones III and IV. Unfortunately, many tibial fractures fall outside of this isthmic region and may require adjunctive reduction measures. Helpful tibial fracture reduction aids include fracture tables, fracture (femoral) distractors, pointed bone forceps (Weber clamps), Schanz pins, Kirschner wires, lag screws, unicortical plates, and fibular osteosynthesis. When treating isolated tibial fractures, the use of a fracture table or a fracture distractor are the best aids to successful nailing.

OPERATIVE TECHNIQUES

Fracture Table or Fracture (Femoral) Distractor

The salient points of successful nailing are discussed to prevent iatrogenic problems (Table 13–1). With the patient in a supine position, one must remember to place the limb in slight internal rotation to allow the tibia to be in a neutral rotational posture. This can be accomplished by placing the ipsilateral buttock on a rolled towel. If the fracture table is used, taping the thigh to the post is helpful in maintaining internal rotation and adduction. This will permit the acquisition of 90° orthogonal (true AP and medial-lateral) fluoroscopic images. Ideally, the limb should be positioned with the hip flexed 70 to 90°, adducted 10 to 20°, the knee flexed 80 to 90°, and the ankle in neutral rotation (Fig. 13–7). If the foot is perpendicular to the floor in this position on the fracture table, the rotation of the tibia is generally neutral. The typical iatrogenic deformity when a nailing is performed with the limb free is fracture recurvatum and internal rotation of distal fragment. Rotational and angular deformities are not tolerated by most active patients. Five degree variations from the opposite extremity appear to be the limit of acceptance for most patients.

The angulation of a fracture cannot be assessed accurately with present day fluoroscopic devices. In part this is because of the small size of the radiograph receiver and the tendency for optical aberrations. To minimize imaging problems, the C-arm should always be at a 90° angle to the limb. The limb should be imaged along

Table 13–1. Common tibial nailing technique

Aids for Reduction	*Advantages*	*Disadvantages*
Fracture table	Ultimate control	Time-consuming setup
	Distal locking facilitated	Traction side effects
	One surgeon	Difficult with associated injuries
Limb free	Associated injury care facilitated	Poor alignment assessment
	Potentially faster	Requires second assistant for distal locking
Fracture distractor	Ease of insertion	Can create deformity
	Traction without encroaching popliteal space	Cross-locking requires assistant
	Depth gauge for nail length	Learning curve

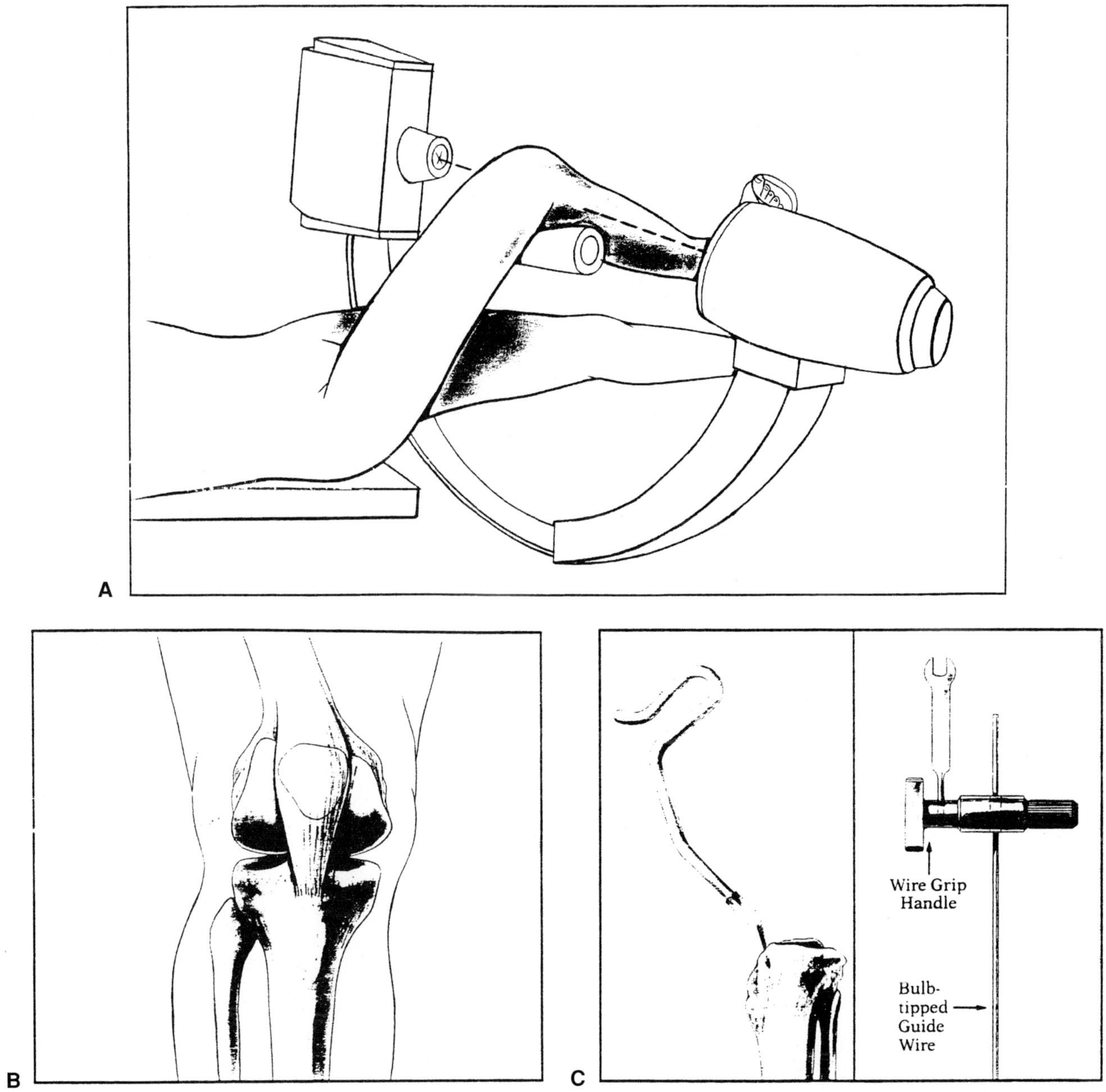

Fig. 13–7. *A,B,C,* Surgical technique for intramedullary nailing of the tibia using a fracture table. (Courtesy of Zimmer; Warsaw, IN.)

its longitudinal axis by translating the base of the unit and not by pivoting the unit's C-arm.

The application of some traction is frequently necessary to reduce the fracture. The foot of the injured extremity is taped to the foot plate of the fracture table. Two- or 3-inch cloth tape is attached to the skin after the application of Benzoin. The tape is placed caudal to the tips of the malleoli, around the heel, and over the dorsum of the foot. Calcaneal traction pins are generally not necessary if performed acutely.

Stabilization of fractures within 24 hours of injury lessens the traction force required for reduction compared to fractures treated in a delayed fashion. This is another reason to expedite tibial fracture treatment. Delaying treatment permits contraction of the soft-tissue envelope with concomitant limb swelling and shortening. This can be a source of iatrogenic problems as increased compartment pressures have been documented with higher traction forces.[13] Other investigators[14] found that pro-

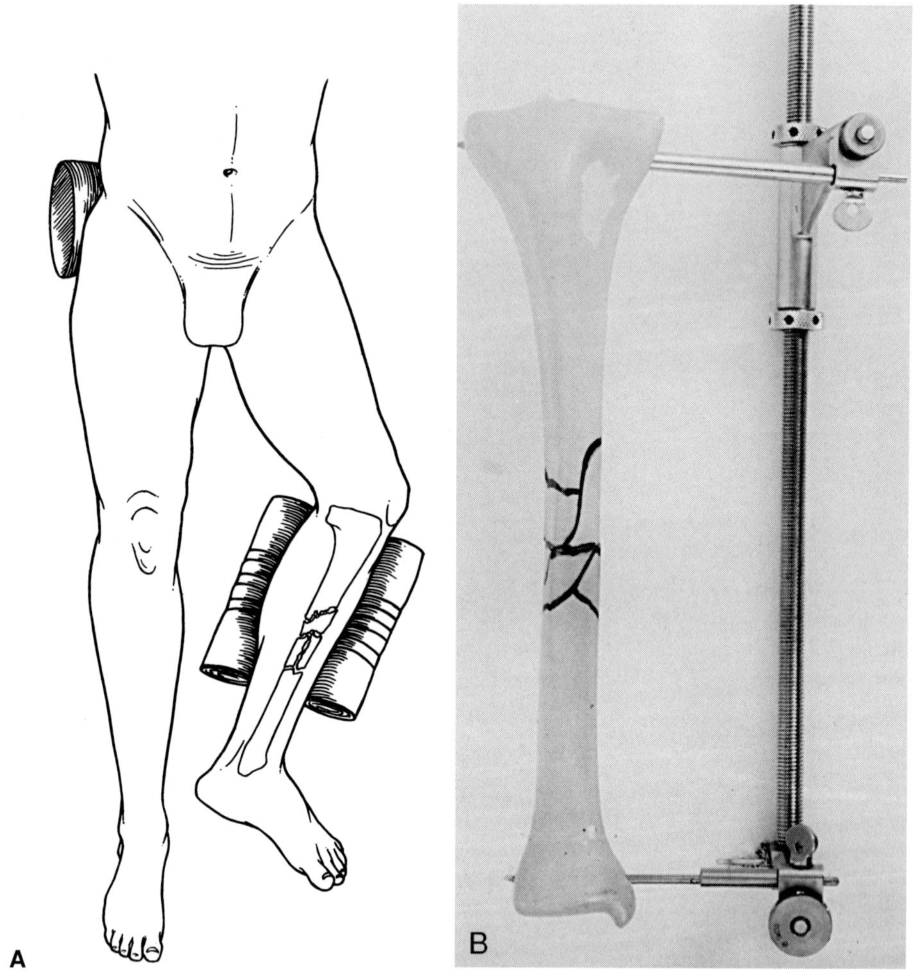

Fig. 13–8. *A,* Operative position of limb prior to placement of fracture distractor. (From Duwelius, P.: Intramedullary locked tibial nailing: A new technique. J. Orthop. Trauma *6*:90–95, 1992.) *B,* Frontal view of correct application of distractor (Synthes, Paoli, PA). (From Duwelius P.: Intramedullary locked tibial nailing. J. Orthop. Trauma *6*:90–95, 1992.) *(Figure continues)*

longed traction and manipulations are maneuvers that may create pressure complications with greater frequency than reaming or actual nail insertion.

Large traction forces can be generated by a fracture table. Traction should be used only as necessary and for short periods to prevent a sustained strain on an injured limb's compartments. The inadvertent placement of the proximal counter traction device in the popliteal space will occlude arterial and/or venous blood flow as well as permit nerve compression. The use of such devices as the fracture distractor[15] (Fig. 13–8) creates a more controlled traction environment without compromising the popliteal space. Traction can be limited to a single limb segment. This device has the added advantage of being both a traction device and fracture reduction tool. The use of this tool requires care to avoid angulatory deformity. The proximal Schanz pin should be inserted parallel to the knee joint in the posteromedial tibial plateau. It is best placed under C-arm guidance from the medial side in the posterior plateau region. The distal Schanz pin is inserted in the posteromedial metaphysis, just above the tibial plafond. On an AP image,[15] it should be inserted parallel to the ankle joint. The disadvantage of nailing a tibia with the limb free or with a distractor is that distal locking may be more difficult. Insertion of the distal cross-locking screws in a limb that is not rigidly secured may require the use of an extra assistant or limb stabilizing jig.

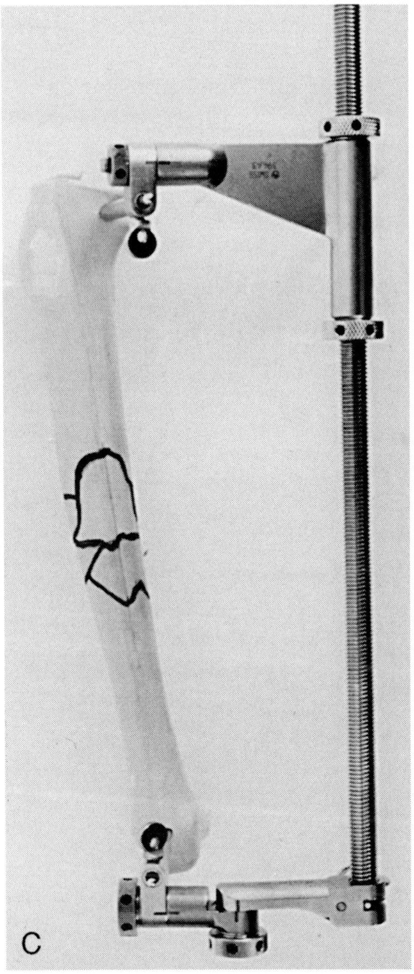

Fig. 13–8. *(continued) C,* Lateral view of same distractor showing AP orientation of proximal Schanz screw.

Fibular Osteosynthesis

The reduction and stabilization of a concomitant fibula fracture poses some theoretical concerns. The work of Teitz et al.[16] hypothesizes that an intact fibula may prevent timely tibial union and tends to create varus malunion in the younger population. The injuries for which fibular osteosynthesis is proposed are quite different. Fractures of the tibia and fibula at the same level and other high energy fractures with disparate tibia and fibular fracture levels were not the scope of that study. The primary restoration of the fibula length and rotation offers many distinct advantages. Tibial fractures involving zones IV, V, and VI, especially if associated with bone loss and a fibula fracture in the same region, may be indirectly reduced by fibular stabilization. Fractures of the fibular diaphysis and metaphysis may be stabilized with plates, or if they are axially stable, with intramedullary implants. In acute leg fractures, the restoration of fibular length, alignment, and rotation will reduce indirectly the tibial fracture and restore ankle architecture. If the tibia has bone loss or proceeds to a delayed union or nonunion, the restoration of fibular anatomy facilitates reconstruction by a posterolateral bone grafting procedure.

Double-Pointed Bone Reduction Forceps (Weber Clamps) and Schanz Pins

The use of small, large, and quadrangular-shaped double-pointed bone reduction forceps is often necessary to reduce and securely stabilize fractures in all zones outside of the isthmus. T-handled [Jacob's] chucks attached to unicortical Schanz pins also permit fracture manipulation and reduction. Although infrequently used for closed fractures, these instruments are a vital part of the fracture surgeon's armamentarium. Double-pointed reduction forceps and Schanz pins can be placed either percutaneously or under direct exposure. Often several forceps are necessary to reduce and then neutralize comminuted fractures with multiplanar deformities.

Kirschner Wires

The use of provisional Kirschner wire stabilization can be a helpful method of stabilizing a fracture prior to nail insertion. Careful planning of wire placement is necessary to prevent an obstruction to nail passage.

Composite Stabilization—Provisional

Provisional fracture reduction may require a more rigid construct than that provided by pointed forceps or Kirschner wires to maintain proper alignment during nail insertion. A unicortical 3.5 dynamic compression plate can be used for provisional stabilization in diaphyseal and meta-diaphyseal fracture patterns. This is particularly useful in open fractures with concomitant periosteal stripping. The traumatic wound or surgical exposure used for irrigation and excisional debridement generally permits safe application of a plate in an extraperiosteal or subperiosteal location. The average cortical screw length to permit nail insertion is 8 to 12 mm. In open fractures this technique is particularly helpful in quickly restoring anatomic alignment and providing sufficient provisional stabilization to permit unreamed small-diameter nail fixation. These plates are removed after completion of the nailing procedure.

Composite Stabilization—Definitive

The use of lag screws, antiglide plates and push (spring) or pull plates may help to maintain unstable reductions in zones II, III, and V.[17]

Tourniquets

A pneumatic tourniquet should never be used for reamed intramedullary nailing. Even if a nail is to be inserted without reaming, the inflation of a tourniquet should be discouraged. A tourniquet may be applied to the thigh and inflated only to control excessive bleeding during the excisional debridement of an open fracture, but this is a rare occurrence. The creation of additional tissue hypoxia, by a no-flow state in an injured extremity has no scientific merit. (One would not run their car engine without oil in the crankcase.)

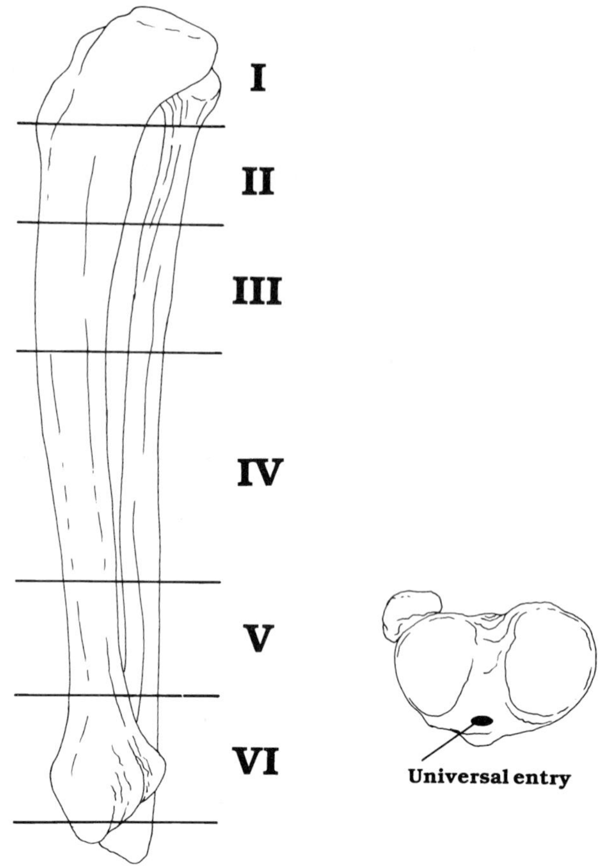

Fig. 13–9. *A*, Lateral view of tibia with anatomic zones depicted. *B*, Coronal view of tibial head with recommended starting point.

Entry Site

The tibia's starting point has not been considered an issue, but, in fact, an incorrectly placed entry portal can be a source of fracture site deformity or may lead to additional fracture comminution. The cadaveric studies of Carr et al.[19] found the ideal point to be more proximal than previously described by Lottes, and described the "universal" entry originally depicted by Alms (Fig. 13–9).[20] The recommended skin incision is centered on the inferior pole of the patella and extends from just proximal to the tibial tuberosity to the middle of the patella. The preferred osseous entry site is accessed through an incision along the medial border of the patella ligament which is then retracted laterally. A patellar ligament splitting approach can be used in patients with very proximal fractures (zone II). In certain fracture patterns, translating the starting point laterally (by 5 to 10 mm) may be of benefit in lessening the valgus deformity that frequently accompanies fractures in this zone especially if the proximal segment has a short lateral wall.

The medial-lateral starting position is determined on an AP fluoroscopic image by extending the longitudinal mid-axial line of the medullary canal cranially. In the coronal plane, the entry point coincides with the "soft spot" at the intersection of the tibial plateau and the anterior metaphyseal cortex. Frequently, the distal extent of the retropatellar ligament's fat pad must be partially released and retracted posteriorly. Entry into the metaphysis is made using a 2.5-mm-diameter guide pin inserted at an angle coincident with that of the proximal bend (Herzog curve) of the nail. The C-arm fluoroscope is used to confirm placement of the guide pin in both AP and medial-lateral planes. The entry portal is enlarged with an 8- or 9-mm cannulated drill or reamer. Alternatively, the metaphysis may be opened with a curved awl. However, the latter technique does not permit correction of selected entry site after the metaphysis has been opened.

Fractures in zone V require accurate guide rod placement in the center of the tibial plafond on both AP and lateral images to prevent angulatory deformity. It is helpful to use a cannulated nail which can be inserted over a guide rod. Some small-diameter nails and solid unreamed nails are not fully cannulated and therefore they do not permit their insertion over a guide wire. This may make their insertion into a zone V fracture more difficult as confirmation of fracture reduction and limb alignment requires continuous fluoroscopic monitoring.

CROSS-LOCKING

As with the femur, all acute unstable tibial fractures should be statically locked. Most surgeons have abandoned distal interlocking targeting devices and use the freehand technique. As with the distal femoral screws the use of radiolucent drill drives facilitates this part of the procedure. Securing the limb to prevent rolling will facilitate cross-locking. An additional aid to cross locking screw insertion is the creation of laser-guided C-arms (Fig. 13–10), as the beam is co-linear with the laser one has directional cues without radiation exposure. With most nail screw combinations, a 12° margin of error from true perpendicular is available to permit safe screw passage without binding on the hole.

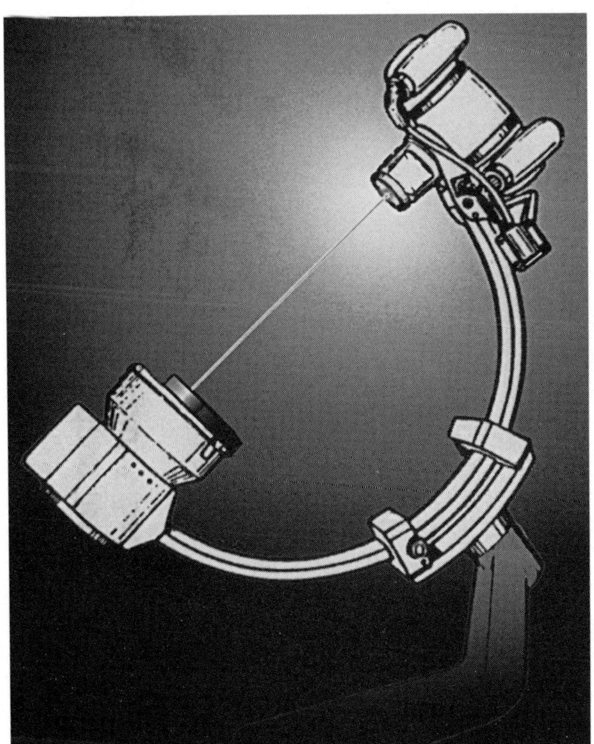

Fig. 13–10. Laser targeting device. Class II laser is co-axial with center of C-arm beam allowing one to "site" distal locking without use of radiation. (Courtesy of Randal R. Trecha, M.D.)

The screw chosen should be 2 to 4 mm longer than measured by a depth gauge. This will assure that the screw's tip will protrude through the opposite cortex; it is helpful also in case an interlocking screw breaks in its midportion during the period of fracture healing, removal is simplified by the precaution. After the extraction of the head portion of a broken screw, a blunt impactor is introduced through the vacant screw hole in the media tibial cortex and abutted to the remaining portion of the screw tip. The screw can usually be impacted through the lateral cortex. A small incision should be made over the protruding portion and then the broken screw tip can be extracted with pliers.

CONTROVERSIES

Reamed vs Unreamed

The decision to use a reamed or unreamed technique is debated because of the lack of clinical data on unreamed nail technique. No prospective randomized study exists comparing the use of the two devices. The unreamed device is marketed as a solution to problems seen with external fixation of open tibial fractures not medullary fixation of fractures. It was not intended to be a permanent device. Most surgeons did not accept the idea of temporary fixation, and the unreamed nail gained rapid use as the definitive treatment for most open tibial fractures. Biological and early clinical data support the use of small-diameter nails in open fractures types I, II, and IIIa.

Solid vs. Cannulated; Closed Section vs. Open Section

All types of nail designs currently exist, with no one design showing clear superiority in clinical trials. For the small-diameter nails the solid design was found to have higher torque stiffness and in selected reports found a lower mechanical failure rate. However, Haas et al.[20] found an alarmingly high incidence of elevated compartment pressures when using this nail, 42%, as compared to 1.6% by McQueen. The hypothesis is perhaps solid implants or even sounds may create too much medullary pressure, and this is dissipated in the surrounding compartments. The Edinburgh group used cannulated reamed nails with lower incidence of pressure related problems.

Nail breakage continues to be a great concern, and therefore the removal of a broken nail should be reconciled. A surgeon should not implant what he or she cannot remove safely. Solid and closed section nail removal can be quite frustrating and special equipment may be necessary.

PITFALLS AND COMPLICATIONS

Poor Starting Point

Biplanar imaging of the proposed starting point should always be performed to assure proper placement. The typical error is distal translation of the starting point to a location at or below the universal entry site described by Alms[19] and Carr.[20]

Iatrogenic comminution can result from too low an entry angle into the tibia, thereby fragmenting the thin anterior cortex and undermining the tuberosity. Similarly, too acute an entry angle may lead to posterior cortical penetration.

Lateral tracking tendencies created by the knee extensor mechanism may result in lateral metaphyseal penetration or additional fracture comminution. The patella itself can be a source of deformity during the procedure. As the guide pin or nail is inserted into the proximal tibial metaphysis the implant tends to be pushed medially by the patellar ligament and patella (the patella may sublux laterally) causing the advancing nail tip to aim laterally. The path of the guide pin, hand-held reamers, and the nail must be monitored radiographically to prevent iatrogenic metaphyseal penetration or additional fracture site comminution.

Implanting the wrong size nail occurs very infrequently, but may result from erroneous labeling of the package from either the hospital or manufacturer. Check the size of your reamers and the nail by passing them through sizing templates.

Nail Incarceration

This is becoming less and less of a problem with the increasing popularity of the smaller-diameter nails. The average nail diameter of the adult tibia when reviewing 110 patients was 10.5 mm, therefore the need or want to implant a nail of greater size may not be necessary or justified.[22] Should this occur, a longitudinal osteotomy, centered about the point of incarceration will free the implant.

Fracture Malalignment

Fracture malalignment is still possible in all planes with a medullary device and should not be accepted. High quality radiographs showing both knee and ankle joints should be obtained while one is in the position to effect a change should it be needed.

Valgus-procurvatum appears to be a phenomenon particular to fractures of the proximal zone of the tibia. Particularly problematic are injuries spanning zones II to III. Fractures in this proximal meta-diaphyseal region tend to develop translational, and angulatory deformities (Fig. 13–11), especially if they are stabilized with small-diameter nails. Combined valgus and procurvatum malalignments are frequent. The etiology of this biplane deformity

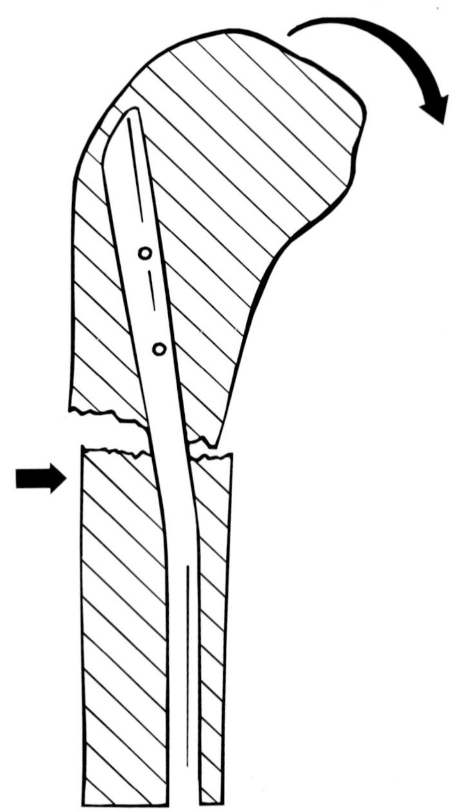

A

Fig. 13–11. *A,* Proposed mechanism of combined procurvation/translational deformity with zone II injury. *(Figure continues)*

is still incompletely understood. This may be caused by a number of factors working in concert. Traction on the extensor mechanism, tethering by the strong posterior leg muscle envelope, nail design, and a posteriorly directed nail insertion path in the proximal metaphysis may contribute to procurvatum at the fracture site. The effects tethering of the eccentric anterolateral muscle envelope, nail shape, starting point, and insertion path may all contribute to the valgus deformity seen with proximal zone fractures. Fracture malalignment may also occur when the fracture is proximal to the sagittal plane bend of the tibial nail.

These deformities are not benign. Fracture reduction should be obtained prior to nail insertion for all tibial fractures. This is especially important for fractures in zones II, III, and V. Fracture reduction must be maintained during nail insertion and during the insertion of proximal and distal locking screws. Expecting a tibial nail to effect reduction for every fracture is an exaggeration of the role of the device.

In rare cases, the procurvatum deformity cannot be corrected without full knee extension. Relaxing the quadriceps muscle and extensor mechanism reduces the bending moment that may contribute to the apex anterior deformity. This may require removal of the insertion instrumentation and proximal targeting guide. Freehand insertion of both proximal cross-locking screws is recommended in this situation.

Angulatory malalignment of the distal metadiaphyseal zone may occur because of the lack of a lateral hinge when the fibula is fractured. The use of small-diameter nails implanted without prereduction will not correct the deformity (Fig. 13–12). The use of large-diameter nails not centered in the plafond on biplane images may even exaggerate the deformity.

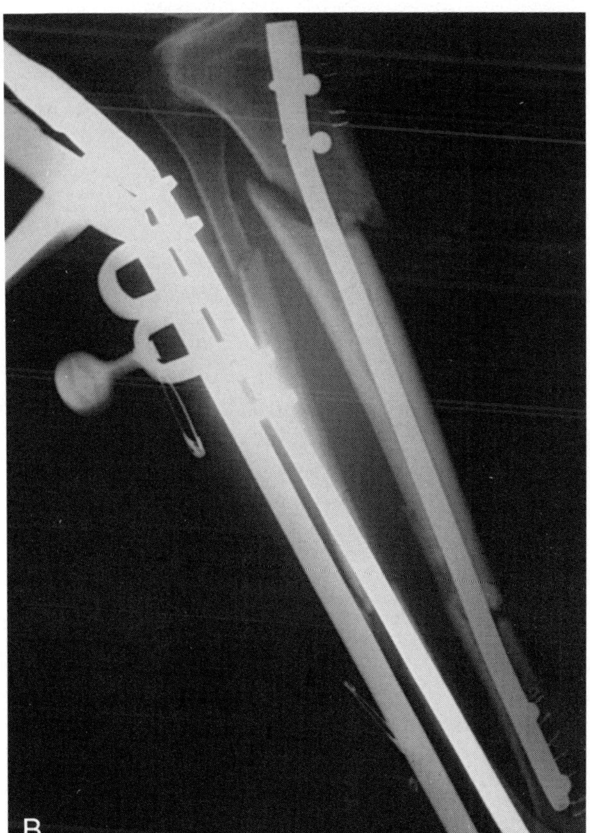

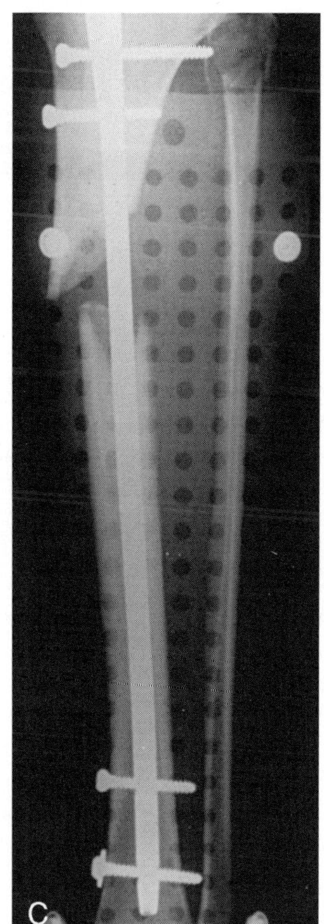

Fig. 13–11. *(continued) B,* Clinical example of deformity. *C,* Clinical example of valgus deformity. (Courtesy of M.L. "Chip" Routt, Jr., M.D.)

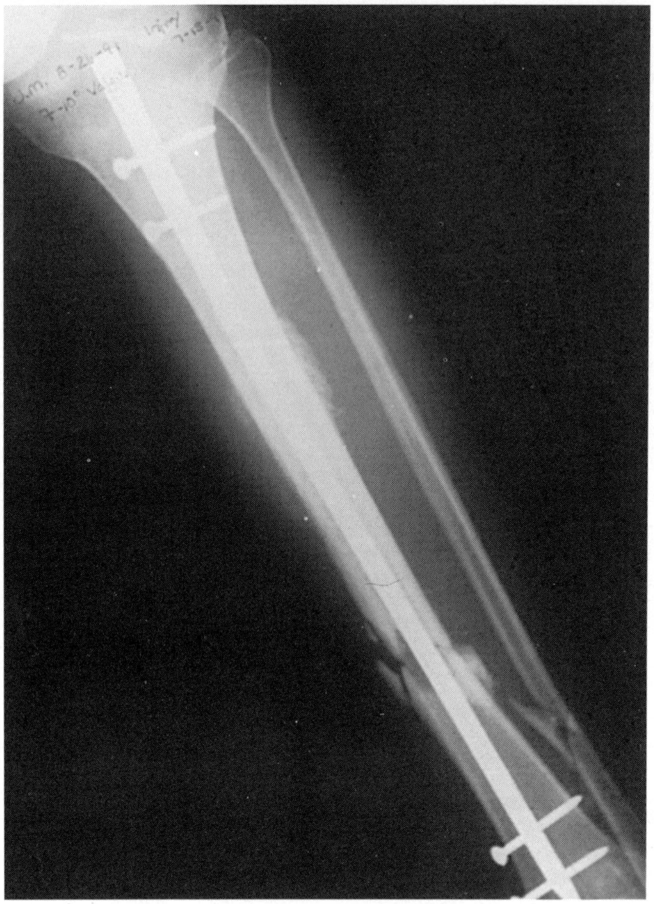

Fig. 13–12. Clinical example of infraisthmal valgus position despite medullary rod placement.

Fracture Distraction

Distraction at the fracture site can occur with mechanical traction or the use of tight-fitting nails in fractures above the narrowest portion of the isthmus. The nail will bind in the distal segment and transport it distally as it is advanced. This can be corrected by the "backslap" technique in which the nail is first locked distally and retracted with the extraction device until the limb is at anatomic length. For comminuted tibial fractures or fractures with bone loss, use the fibular fracture as a guide to appropriate limb length. All mechanical traction must be removed (e.g., traction table or femoral distractor) prior to nail retraction. Appropriate nail length must be confirmed again so that it is not prominent proximally. A nail that is not fully inserted into the metaphysis may cause patellar tendon irritation.

Compartment Syndrome

The creation of increased compartment pressure cannot be avoided completely, but the factors most commonly associated with increased pressure have been identified. Severity of injury, manipulation of the limb, traction, limb positioning, use of intramedullary sounds, or large reamers may all contribute to increased intracompartmental pressure. Continuous traction is responsible for increased pressure in both the deep posterior and anterior compartments. The study by McQueen demonstrated the physical implantation of a cannulated nail did not appear to cause pressure problems. The act of reaming, however, may be a contributor to increased compartment pressure, as intraosseous pressures exceeding 500 mm Hg have been measured in canine models.[22] Fractures above the isthmus may be at great risk for pressure-generated complications.[22,23]

It is recommended that all patients sustaining high energy injuries that are to undergo medullary nailing should be monitored objectively before and after nailing for elevated compartment pressures.

Patellar Tendonitis

No hard data is present regarding the actual incidence of significant tendonitis, Koval reported 22% from the Shock Trauma study (Maryland Shock Trauma Center). The incidence may be skewed because of the tendon-splitting approach employed in 42 of the 60 patients reviewed.[24]

Peroneal Palsy

Iatrogenic neurapraxia is a result of traction and manipulation, and the longer the delay to surgery, the greater the traction one must apply. It is also possible, though not confirmed, that some neurapraxia findings may have been the result of missed compartment syndromes.[26,27]

Malunion

Rotatory and angulatory malunion are still possible with intramedullary nailing, however the correction of such deformities when not accompanied by a transitional component is made simpler.

Nonunion

A review of the recent literature on tibial fractures treated with intramedullary nailing revealed the nonunion rates presented in Table 13–2. The variables that remain in the surgeon's control as surgeon are alignment and iatrogenic insults (i.e., traction, manipulation, timing of surgery). If these insults are kept to a minimum and ankle motion is quickly restored whereby ambulation can be safely done without increased stress to the device-bone construct nonunion rates of 1 to 4% can be expected.

Table 13–2. Union rates following tibial nailing

Author	*Nonunion (%)*	*Comments*
Holbrook[4]	10	Ender's
Santoro[35]	3	(65 grade II, III fractures)
DiPasquale[33]	3	
Puno[30]	2	
Klemm[37]	1	
Bone[32]	1	
Melis[35]	7	(16 patients)
Zucman[31]	12	(Flexible nails)
Solheim[36]	4	
Koval[24]	5	
Court-Brown[28]	1	
Court-Brown[29]	10	(IIIa, IIIb)

Infection

Increasingly lower infection rates continue to be reported for all fracture soft-tissue injuries with types IIIb and IIIc injuries being 10 to 25% and closed fracture infection rates being less then 2%. Adequate debridement remains the mainstay to infection prophylaxis, with avoidance of over-reaming an adjunct to the debridement. It is thought that solid nails will have a lower infection rate then cannulated because of the avascular zone created by the hollow core of the cannulated nail. The preliminary reports from Riemer et al. support this theory.[25]

POSTOPERATIVE COURSE

Loss of ankle motion loss is considered to be the source of great morbidity for these patients and may contribute to prolonged healing times. The restoration of both ankle and knee motion is one of the primary goals of post operative rehabilitation.

Because of the injury and soft-tissue treatments and bone treatments, all patients are placed in a short leg splint to relax the compartments for 48 to 72 hours. Prior to hospital discharge, the splint is removed. For stable fractures, the patient may be placed in a removable orthosis to permit range of motion exercise and to perform daily hygiene and wound care. Unstable fractures are placed in a short leg cast for 2 to 4 weeks. Patients with small-diameter nails are permitted only touch-down weight bearing. Partial weight bearing is permitted for patients whose fractures are treated with nails of at least 10-mm diameter if their knee and ankle range of motion approximates 90% of the uninjured limb. Patients are taught extrinsic stretching and active range of motion exercises to all foot and leg muscle groups. Progressive weight bearing is deferred until provisional healing is confirmed radiographically and joint range of motion remains acceptable.

ADJUNCTIVE PROCEDURES/DEFERRED INTERVENTIONS

Adjunctive procedures are required to facilitate bone healing, particularly with complex tibial fractures or fractures with bone loss. Dynamization with or without bone grafting is occasionally necessary despite the use of intramedullary nails. At the time of soft-tissue coverage or delayed primary closure of open fractures, antibiotic-impregnated PMMA beads may be inserted as space holders in bone defects. These defects are later filled with autogenous iliac crest cancellous bone graft after healing of the soft-tissue envelope, generally 4 to 8 weeks after wound closure.

Revision or "exchange" nailing as it has come to be known, must be considered part of the original treatment plan when using small-diameter nails. Exchange nailing should be considered if adequate consolidation is not occurring by 12 to 14 weeks in the unstable fracture pattern. Exchange to a reamed nail can facilitate healing while potentially allowing patients to advance their weight bearing status because of the larger-diameter nail.

Dynamization of tibial nails is done with far more regularity in our clinical practice than for femoral nails. Dynamizaton is still an inexact science, as the timing is still unclear. The experience with small-diameter nails is that they tend to "auto-dynamize" as early as 12 to 14 weeks postoperatively by fatiguing through the screws. The screw breakage rate of larger-diameter nails is considerably lower, as the forces are not borne entirely by the screw and the diameter of the screw will be larger with a larger nail. Kassman et al. recommended dynamization and bone grafting at 6 weeks for unstable fractures treated with unreamed technique.[26] Whereas, Georgiadis and coworkers did not demonstrate an increased rate of union in the canine model and concluded the routine dynamization of tibial nails may not be necessary.[27]

One should not delay intervention if clinical and radiographic signs of delayed union exist 12 to 16 weeks after insertion of a small diameter intramedullary nail. Because the average time to union of an *open* tibial fracture is 26 weeks, delaying intervention until one meets the 9 month criteria of nonunion is no longer justified.

REFERENCES

1. An Advanced Risk Management Program for Use in the Treatment of Tibia Fractures ed. by the AAOS Committee on Professional Liability. Park Ridge: AAOS, 1989.
2. Gamble, W.E., Clayton, M.L., Leidholt, J.D., Cletcher, J.O.: Complications following treatment of tibial fractures with weight bearing. J. Bone Joint Surg. *54A*:1342, 1972.
3. Waddell J.P., Reardon, G.P.: Complications of tibial shaft fractures. Clin. Orthop. *178*:173–178, 1983.
4. Holbrook, J.L., Swiontkowski, M.F., Sanders, R.: Treatment of open fractures of the tibial shaft, Ender nailing vs external fixation: Prospective randomized comparison. J. Bone Joint Surg. *71A*:1231–1238, 1989.
5. Muller, M.E., Allqöwer M., Schneider R., Willenegger H.: Manual of Internal Fixation: Techniques recommended by AO/ASIF group. 3rd Edition. Springer-Verlag, Berlin, 1990, pp. 290–296.
6. Henley, M.B., Meier, M., Tencer, A.F.: Influences of some design parameters on the biomechanics of the unreamed tibial nail. J. Orthop. Trauma *7*:311, 1993.
7. Schandelmeir, P., Krettek, C. Haas, N. Tscherne, H.: Biomechanical & calculated stiffness in the implant complex of eight locked tibial nails. Proceedings of the LIX AAOS/ORS Annual Meeting, San Francisco, 1993, p. 572.
8. Klein, M.P.M., Rahn, B.A., Frigg, R. Kessler, S., Perren, S.M.: Reaming versus nonreaming in medullary nailing: Interference with cortical circulation of the canine tibia Arch. Orthop. Trauma Surg. *109*:314–316, 1990.
9. Schemitsch, E.H., Kowalski, M., Swiontkowski, M.F., Senft, D.: Effects of reamed versus unreamed locked intramedullary nailing on cortical bone blood flow in a fractured sheep tibia model. Proceedings of IX Annual OTA Meeting, New Orleans, LA 1993.
10. McNab, I., DeHaas, W.G.: Role of periosteal blood supply in healing fractures of tibia. Clin. Orthop. *105*: 27–33, 1974.
11. Strachan, R.K., McCarthy, I., Fleming, R., Hughes, S.P.F.: Role of tibial nutrient artery. J. Bone Joint Surg. *72B*:391–394, 1990.
12. Patzakis, M.K., Wilkins, J.: Factors influencing infection rate in open fracture wounds. Clin. Orthop. *243*: 36–40, 1989.
13. Tischenko, G.J., Goodman, S.B.: Compartment syndrome after intramedullary nailng of the tibia. J. Bone Joint Surg. *72A*: 41–44, 1990 and Shakespeare, et al.: J. Bone Joint Surg. *64B*:498, 1982.
14. McQueen, M.M., Christie, J., Court-Brown, C.M.: Compartment pressures after intramedullary nailing of the tibia. J. Bone Joint Surg *72B*: 395–397, 1990.
15. Rubinstein, R.A., Jr., Green J.M., Duwelius, P.J.: Intramedullary interlocked tibial nailing: A new technique (Preliminary Report). J. Orthop. Trauma *6*:90–95, 1992.
16. Teitz, C.C., Carter, D.R., Frankel, V.H.: Problems associated with tibia fractures with intact fibulae. J. Bone Joint Surg. *62A*:770–776, 1980.
17. Benirschke, S.K., Henley, M.B., et al.: Proximal 1/3rd tibial fractures: Solutions. Presented at the LX Annual AAOS, New Orleans, 1994.
18. Mast, J., Jakob, R., Ganz, R.: Planning and reduction technique in fracture surgery. Springer-Verlag, Berlin, 1989, pp. 243–244.
19. Carr, J., Sobba, D., Bear, L.: Biomechanics of rigid tibial nail insertion sites. J. Orthop. Trauma *5*:238, 1991 (Abstract of VI Annual Meeting OTA, Toronto, 1990.
20. Alms, M.: Medullary nailing of the shaft of the tibia. J. Bone Joint Surg. *44B*:329–339, 1962.

21. Haas, N., Kretteck, C., Schandelmaier, P., Frigg, R., Tscherne, H.: A new solid unreamed tibial nail for shaft fractures with severe soft tissue injury. Injury *24*: 49–54, 1993.
22. Agnew, S.: Personal Communication, 1994.
23. Winquist, R.: Personal Communication, 1994.
24. Koval, K.J., Clapper, M.F., Brumback, R.J., Ellison, P.S., Jr., Poka, A., Bathon, G.H., Burgess, A.R.: Complications of reamed intramedullary nailing of the tibia. J. Orthop. Trauma *5*:184–189, 1991.
25. Reimer, B.L., Butterfield, S.L.: Comparison of reamed and nonreamed solid core nailing of tibial diaphysis after external fixation. J. Orthop. Trauma *7*:279–285, 1993.
26. Kassman, S., Bone, L., Stegemann, P., France, J.: Delayed union with unreamed tibial rods. J. Orthop. Trauma *6*:507, 1992 Abstract from VII OTA Annual Meeting, Seattle, WA 1991.
27. Georgiadis, G., Minster, G., Moed, B.R.: Effects of dynamization after intramedullary tibial nailing: Experimental study in dogs. J. Orthop. Trauma *4*:323–330, 1990.
28. Court-Brown, C.M., Christie, J., McQueen, M.M.: Closed intramedullary tibial nailing: Its use in closed and type I open fractures. J. Bone Joint Surg. *72B*:605–611, 1990.
29. Court-Brown, C.M., McQueen, M.M., Quaba, A.A., Christie, J.: Locked medullary nailing of open tibial fractures. J. Bone Joint Surg. *73B*:959–964, 1991.
30. Puno, R.M., Teynor, J.T., Nagano, J., Gustilo, R.B.: Critical analysis of results of treatment of 201 tibial shaft fractures. Clin. Orthop. *212*:113–121, 1986.
31. Zucman, J., Maurer, P.: Two level fractures of the tibia: Results in 36 cases treated by blind nailing. J. Bone Joint Surg. *51B*:686–692, 1969.
32. Bone, L.B., Johnson, K.D.: Treatment of tibial fractures by reaming and intramedullary nailing. J. Bone Joint Surg. *68A*:877–886, 1986.
33. DiPasquale, T., Helfet, D.H., Sanders, R., Howey, T., Zinar, D., Pompan, D., Brooker, A.: The treatment of open and/or unstable tibia fractures with an unreamed double-locked nail. Orthop. Trans. *13*:273, 1989.
34. Santoro, V.M., Henley, M.B., Benirschke, S.K., Mayo, K.A.: Prospective comparison of unreamed interlocking IM nails versus half pin external fixation in open tibia fractures. Proceedings of VI Annual OTA Meeting, Toronto, CA 1990.
35. Melis, G.C., Sotgiu, F., Lepori, M., Guido, P.: Intramedullary nailing in segmental tibial fractures. J. Bone Joint Surg. *63A*:1312–1318, 1981.
36. Solheim, K., Bø, S.: Intramedullary nailing of tibial shaft fractures. Acta Orthop. Scand. *44*:323–334, 1973.
37. Klemm, K. W., Borner, M.: Interlocking nailing of complex fractures of the femur and tibia. Clin. Orthop. *212*: 89–100, 1986

14

Flexible Intramedullary Nailing of Humeral Shaft Fractures

William R. Dobozi and Robert F. Hall, Jr.

Fractures of the shaft of the humerus account for approximately 1% of all fractures treated. The majority of these fractures are treated successfully without operation by a hanging cast,[1,2] coaptation splints,[3–5] functional bracing,[6] traction, or sling and swathe.[7] Nonunion is rare, and infection is uncommon when conservative measures are used.[6,8–10]

Open reduction and internal fixation by compression osteosynthesis is not the treatment of choice for humeral shaft fractures, even by the most ardent advocates of the AO method. The incidence of nonunion and complications with this procedure is twice that seen with nonoperative treatment.[11]

Medullary fixation rarely has been indicated for humeral shaft fractures, because in most reported series, the results of medullary fixation have been inferior to those of either closed treatment or open reduction and plating. Most intramedullary nails are round and straight and fail to control rotation at the fracture site, thus often resulting in nonunion (Fig. 14–1).

Rush described the use of curved flexible intramedullary nails for humeral shaft fractures. Hackethal was the first to advocate the use of multiple flexible rods to better control rotation at the fracture site and to increase union rates in long bone fractures.[12] Recently, the Ender nail was made smaller so that closed multiple flexible pin fixation could be accomplished with curved nails. Both the curve of the nails and the use of multiple nails appear to enhance fixation and union rates. This chapter reviews our experiences with this technique for the fixation of humeral shaft fractures.

MECHANISM OF INJURY

Falls on the outstretched arm or flexed elbow, direct violence, gunshot wounds, crushing injuries, and even throwing episodes all can lead to fractures of the humeral shaft. Many of these fractures are comminuted and open. Muscle forces often result in displacement and angulation, which can make treatment by closed means difficult.

The muscle forces that act on the humeral shaft influence the type of fracture displacement seen at different levels of the humerus. Fractures below the surgical neck but above the pectoralis major insertion cause the proximal fragment to abduct and rotate externally, whereas the deltoid muscle causes shortening to occur. The pectoralis major also may pull the shaft medially. Fracture reduction by closed methods is difficult to achieve in these injuries (Fig. 14–2). Fractures above the deltoid insertion but below the pectoralis major insertion result in adduction of the proximal fragment and abduction and shortening of the distal fragment. Fracture reduction is difficult to achieve by closed methods in this fracture type also. Finally, fractures below the deltoid insertion result in shortening and displacement caused by pull of the deltoid and coracobrachialis on the proximal fragment and by pull of the biceps and triceps on the distal fragment.

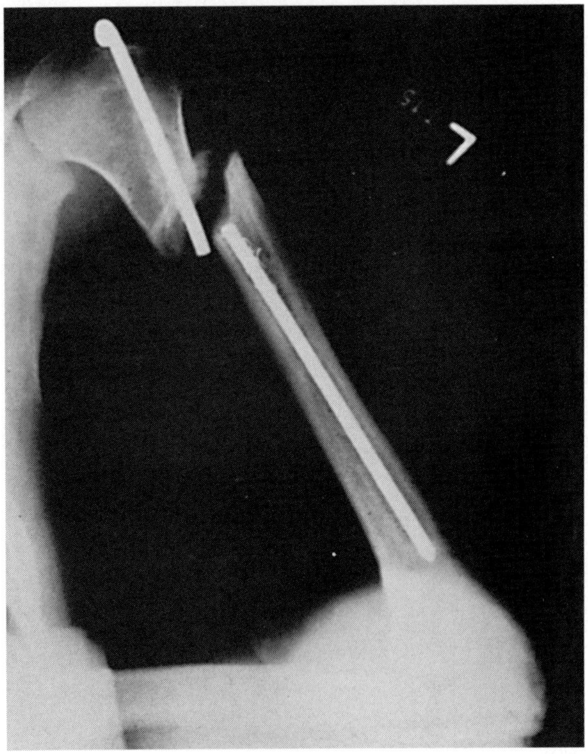

Fig. 14–1. Nonunion and implant failure following Rush pin fixation of an open proximal humerus fracture. Poor rotational control at the fracture site provided by the single straight nail resulted in a nonunion.

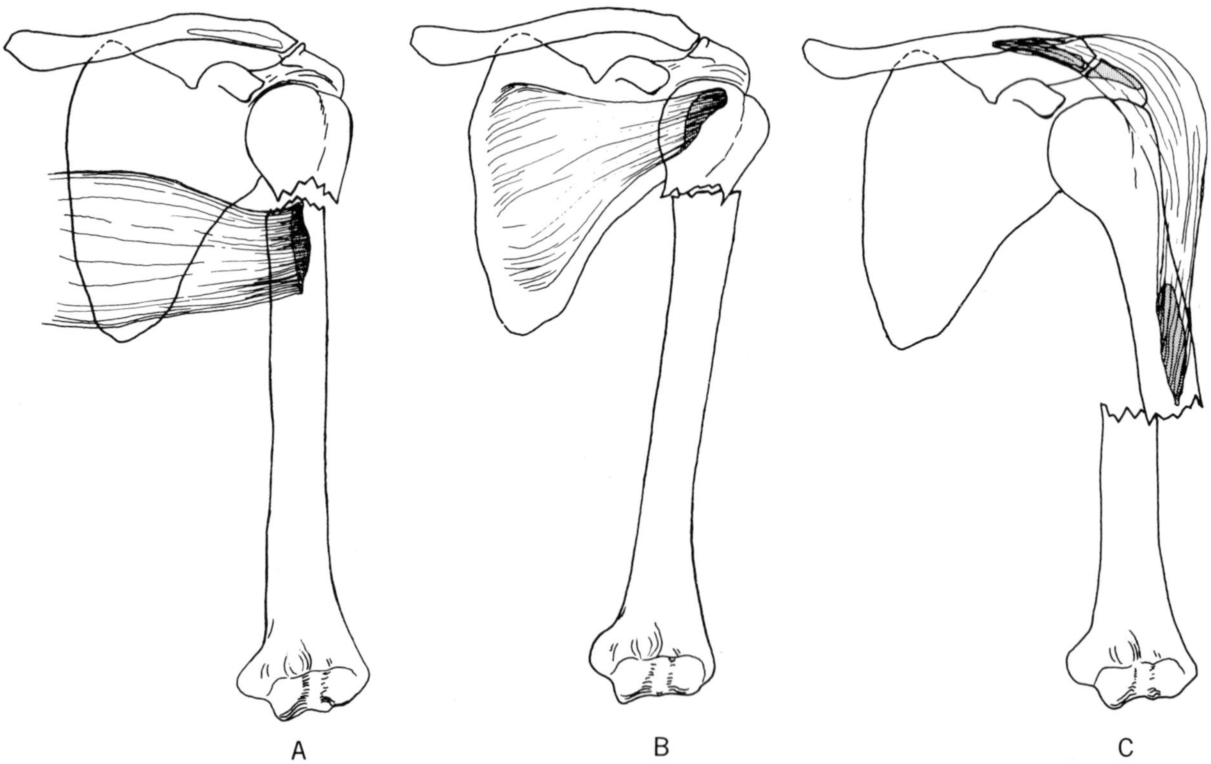

Fig. 14–2. *A,* A fracture located below the surgical neck region but above the pectoralis major insertion becomes displaced because of muscular forces. Maintaining a satisfactory closed reduction is difficult (see Fig. 14–13). *B,* A fracture located below the pectoralis major insertion but above the deltoid insertion also becomes displaced due to muscular forces. Closed methods of treatment can produce an unsatisfactory result. *C,* The most common location for a fracture of the humeral shaft is located below the deltoid insertion. Muscular forces result in shortening and angulation. Treatment using gravity is often successful.

INITIAL EVALUATION AND MANAGEMENT

Displaced fractures of the humeral shaft are easily diagnosed. A gentle examination of the extremity usually reveals motion at the fracture site, crepitus, and shortening. A complete evaluation of the vascular and neurologic status of the involved extremity, especially of radial nerve function, is mandatory with humeral shaft fractures. Impairment of radial nerve function is the most common neural injury. All data should be recorded to establish a baseline should neural or vascular injury occur following fracture reduction or surgical intervention. Radiographic evaluation of the humerus must include the shoulder joint and the elbow joint. Careful evaluation for comminuted longitudinal splits in the bone must be made before considering treatment by intramedullary nailing. If the comminution is increased while driving in the nails, poor fixation may result. After evaluation, all fractures should be splinted. Simple coaptation splints can be applied readily. These splints dramatically relieve pain and are our treatment of choice. The patient then can be mobilized without risk of further fracture displacement, which could result in vascular or neural damage.

INDICATIONS

In 1933, Caldwell provided a conservative method for the treatment of humeral shaft fractures that has stood the test of time. The hanging arm cast and all other variations of "gravity control" of the humerus are effective in treating the majority of humeral shaft fractures. Several indications for flexible nailing, however, follow:

1. Poor reduction of the fracture following conservative treatment with 20° or more angulation in any plane.
2. The recumbent polytraumatized patient.
3. The noncompliant patient.
4. The morbidly obese patient.
5. Bilateral humeral shaft fractures.
6. Gunshot fracture with or without associated radial nerve injury.
7. Segmental fractures.
8. Facilitation of walking with a crutch.
9. Pathologic fractures.
10. Associated vascular injury of the arm.

OPERATIVE TECHNIQUE

The smaller size of the intramedullary cavity of the humerus relative to that of long bones in the lower extremity requires adjustment in the length and diameter of the intramedullary nails to be used. A radiographic survey of 50 normal adult humeri revealed that the average length of the intramedullary canal is 30.4 cm and that the average diameter is 9.9 mm. Nail lengths therefore should vary from 20 to 32 cm, whereas nail diameters smaller than the standard 4.5 mm are desirable.

At present, nail diameters of 3.2, 3.5, and 4 mm are available commercially for use in the humerus. The insertion and extraction instruments similarly must be downsized to accommodate these smaller nails. Control of nail rotation during insertion is mandatory for a successful closed procedure. Rotational maneuvers with the larger standard insertion instruments allow too much slack for efficient control and may damage the eye of the nail during insertion. Finally, the extractor hook must be smaller to allow its insertion into the eye of the nail for proper removal.

Because the humerus is a non-weight bearing bone with a surrounding muscle mass that is considerably smaller than that of the femur or tibia, a strong tendency of humeral conformity to the shape of the nails placed within the intramedullary canal has been noted. Nails designed in both C and S shapes are available and desirable. When placed together within the canal, such nails alleviate this problem, and a straighter bone is evident in the postoperative radiograph.

Comminuted fractures of the humerus, when treated with flexible intramedullary nails, tend to collapse and shorten, thereby leading to protrusion of the nail. In the lower extremity, this problem is solved with adjunctive fixation, which helps to hold the bone to length while the fracture heals. This fixational aid is unnecessary and undesirable in the humerus because of the proximity of the nerves and arteries in this location. Rather, multiple nails of smaller diameter can be placed in the canal and packed snugly to allow multiple points of fixation and to resist collapse of the fracture. When 3.2-mm nails are used, 3 nails can be placed in the 10-mm canal, which is the average size of the intramedullary canal in the humerus.

Nails may be placed through either one of

two portals in the humerus, depending on the location of the fracture. Retrograde nailing is performed through a portal at the posterior aspect of the distal humerus directly above the olecranon fossa; this portal is indicated for fractures within the middle and proximal thirds of the humerus. Antegrade nailing is performed through a portal at the greater tuberosity and is indicated for fractures within the distal third of the humerus.

Retrograde Technique

Patient Positioning

The patient can be placed in either a supine or a lateral decubitus position on the operating table. For patients placed in the supine position, a pad is attached to the railing of the table and is placed against the chest wall below the axilla (Fig. 14–3). The pad allows lateral traction of the arm without pulling the patient off the table. A tourniquet may be applied to the proximal third of the arm, if desired. Before finalizing the position of the patient on the table, the humerus is scanned with the image intensifier to ensure that the humeral head can be seen in its entirety. The maneuvers necessary to obtain reduction of the humerus then are rehearsed.

When the lateral decubitus position is used, the patient is secured in the lateral position in the same manner as that used for a total hip replacement. The image intensifier then is brought over the top of the patient and is lowered to the level of the fractured humerus (Fig. 14–4); it then can be swung proximally or distally to scan the entire humerus. The image heads are draped sterilely following prepping and draping of the patient.

Surgical Approach

After proper sterile preparation with the arm draped freely, a 4-cm midline longitudinal incision is made over the posterior distal third of the humerus and is directed toward the olecranon fossa. After incising the triceps fascia, the muscle is dissected bluntly. The posterior humerus is bared with a periosteal elevator, and the initial drill hole is placed 3 to 4 cm

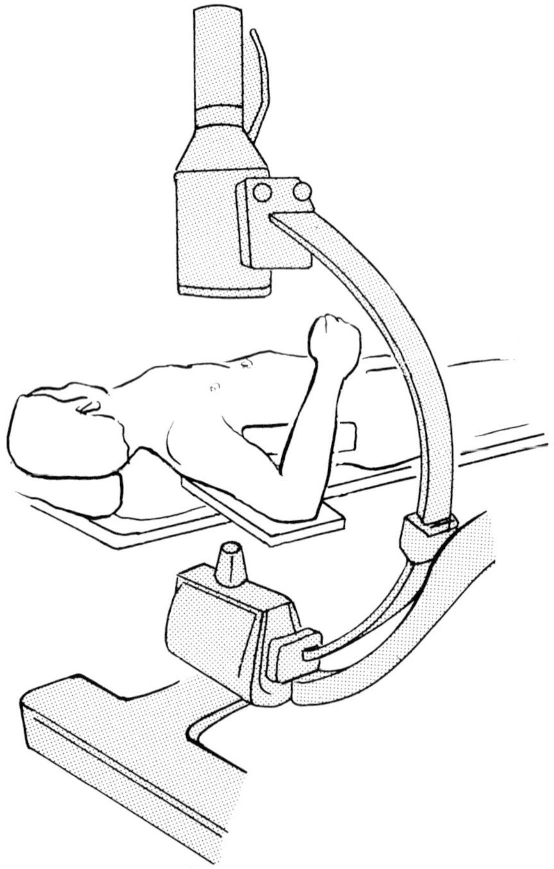

Fig. 14–3. Position of the patient and placement of the image intensifier for a flexible intramedullary nailing performed with the patient in the supine position. Note the pad placement against the lateral chest wall which provides counterpressure during fracture reduction.

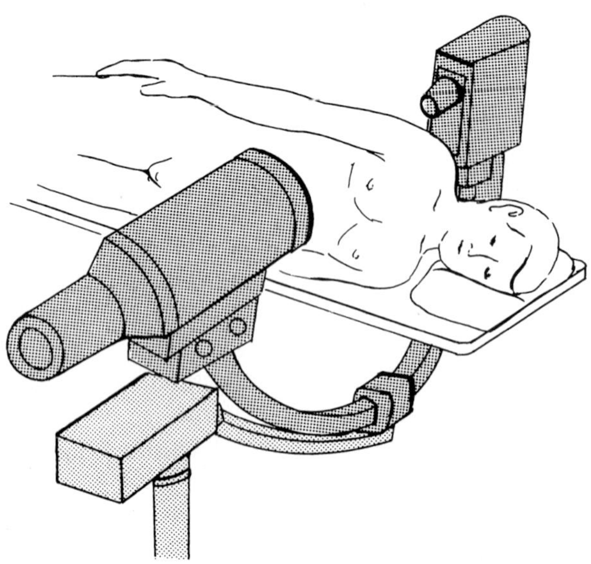

Fig. 14–4. Position of the patient for a nailing performed using a lateral decubitus position. Note how the image intensifier is placed horizontally under the patient. The image heads are then covered with sterile drapes prior to surgery.

above the olecranon fossa (Fig. 14–5). A hemostat is placed within the drill hole, and a lateral image is taken to check the placement of the drill hole. The hole should be 1 to 2 cm above the termination of the intramedullary canal. Three additional drill holes are placed in tandem and longitudinally along the posterior humerus; a 2- to 3-mm bone bridge is left between each drill hole. Power equipment and sharp drill bits facilitate penetration of the bone because the humeral cortex is thick in this area, even in the elderly patient. The drill holes are connected with a gooseneck double-action rongeur or burr, and an elliptically shaped portal measuring ½ × 3 cm is fashioned. The edges of the portal are enlarged with a Kerrison rongeur. The entry point should accommodate four 3.2-mm nails. If additional nails are desired, the entry point can be enlarged by making an additional drill hole proximally and repeating the procedure. Care should be taken to avoid stretching of the radial nerve with retractors because the nerve is not visualized during the procedure.

Nail Insertion

A C nail of approximate length is selected and placed next to the humerus while an assistant pulls the arm out to length. The humeral head is visualized with the image intensifier, and if the length is satisfactory, the nail is placed within the intramedullary canal and is driven across the fracture site while the assistant uses the maneuvers previously rehearsed for closed reduction. Long butterfly, long oblique, and comminuted fractures often are difficult to traverse. Engagement of the proximal fragment can be facilitated by driving the nail to the proximal long spike of bone of the distal fragment and then by using a 360° sweeping motion of the insertion device while visualizing with the image intensifier operating in the fluoroscopic mode. When the proximal spike is engaged with the nail during this motion, the nail purchases and rotates the proximal fragment. The nail then can be driven to its proper final position 1 cm distal to the subchondral bone of the humeral head (Fig. 14–6). In this way, the length of the nail may be checked again, and if satisfactory, the nail is withdrawn to within several centimeters of the fracture site. An additional C nail and one or two S nails are added by hand through the entry portal and are driven proximally across the fracture site in 2-cm increments. All the nails are driven farther in a similar fashion until they reach their final destination (Fig. 14–7). The nails should fill the canal snugly but not rigidly. Some motion at the fracture site is expected and is de-

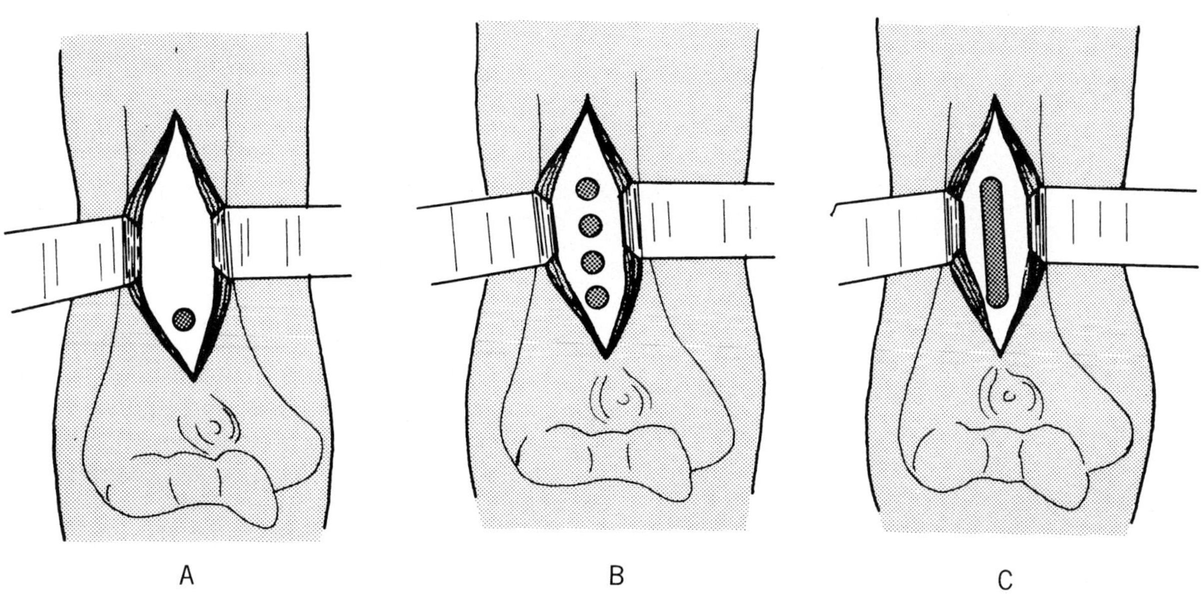

Fig. 14–5. *A*, For retrograde intramedullary nailing, a standard triceps splitting approach is used. *B*, One-quarter inch (5-mm) drill holes are placed in tandem starting 3 to 4 cm above the olecranon fossa. Three or more drill holes are necessary. *C*, The drill holes are connected with a rongeur, creating an ellipse-shaped entry portal 0.5 cm by 3 cm.

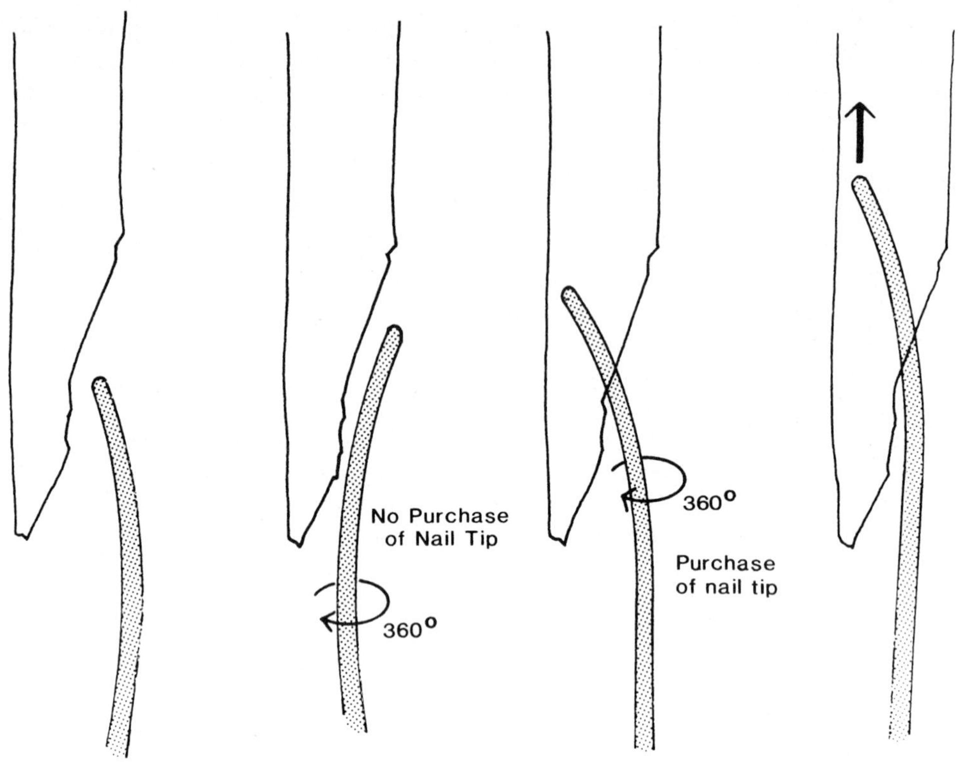

Fig. 14–6. Technique for engaging the proximal fragment in long oblique fractures. The nail is driven to the level of the proximal fragment and then rotated 180° while the image intensifier is kept on. When the proximal fragment is engaged it will rotate with the nail. Then the nail can be driven to its final position.

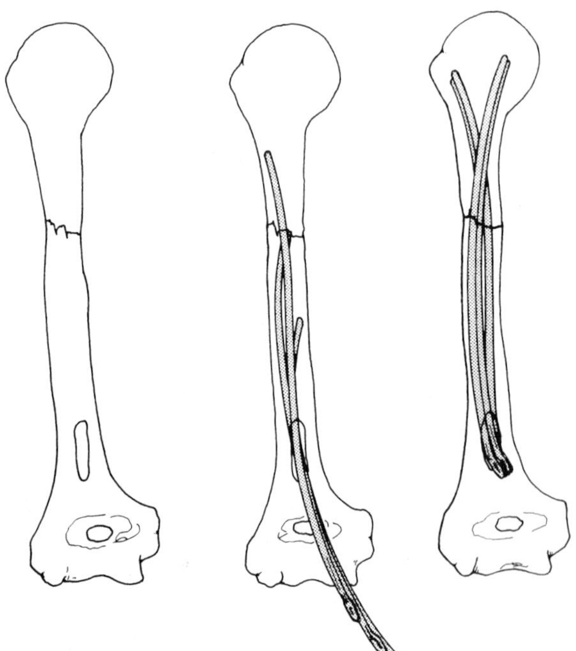

Fig. 14–7. In a simple transverse fracture, the fracture is reduced and the appropriate size nail is driven across the fracture site under image control. Remaining nails (C and S types) are driven across the fracture and then all nails are driven to their final position in the humeral head.

sired because it promotes periosteal callus formation about the fracture. A balance of C- and S-shaped nails allows maintenance of a more satisfactory reduction. Finally, a compression dressing is placed about the fracture site.

Antegrade Technique

The same principles advocated in retrograde nailing apply also to antegrade nailing. The only difference is the entry portal. After positioning the patient and rehearsing the reduction, the patient is prepared properly and is draped. An incision is made over the anterior deltoid; it starts at the tip of the acromion and is carried distally no farther than 1½ inches to avoid injury to the terminal portion of the axillary nerve (Fig. 14–8). After blunt dissection through the deltoid, the periosteum is stripped over the anterolateral humeral metaphysis. A 5-mm drill hole is placed at the lower portion of this area, which coincides with the distal portion of the incision. The portal is enlarged with an awl and Kerrison rongeur to accommodate 3 or 4 nails (Fig. 14–9). The portal may be enlarged if necessary. The nails are

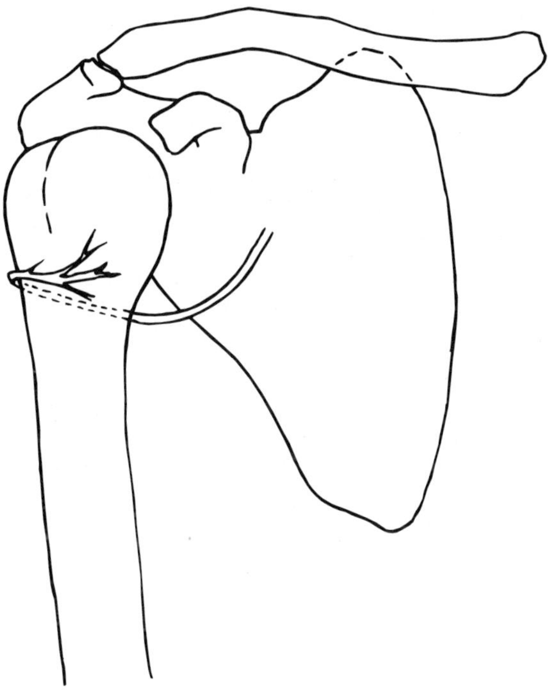

Fig. 14–8. For an antegrade nailing, an anterior deltoid splitting incision is used. The approach must not violate the terminal portion of the axillary nerve located in the distal aspect of the operative incision.

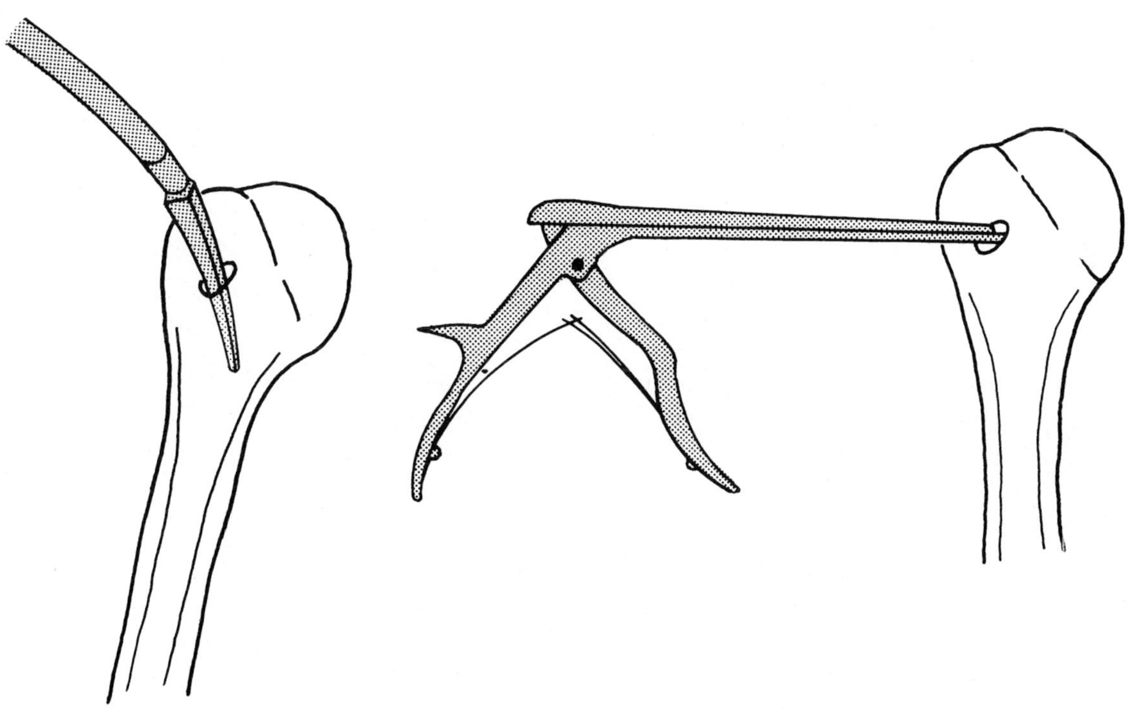

Fig. 14–9. The entry portal is located anterolateral and distal to the greater tuberosity. The portal is enlarged with either an awl or a Kerrison rongeur.

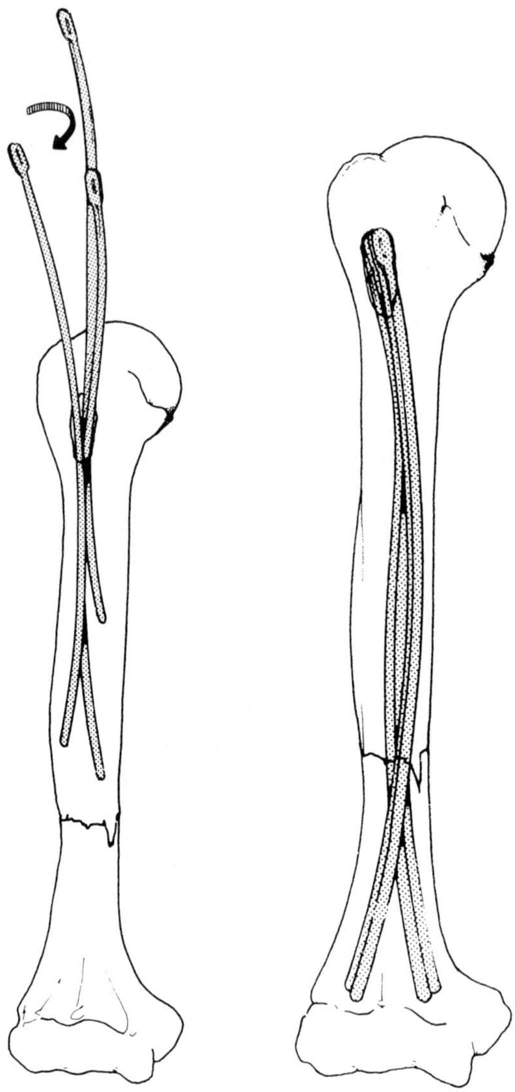

Fig. 14–10. *A,B,* Antegrade nail insertion for distal third fractures. A balance of C and S nails are driven distally to the fracture site. The fracture is then reduced and the nails driven into the distal fragment as far as possible without violating the olecranon fossa.

placed within the intramedullary canal and are driven in the fashion previously described. Great care must be taken to obtain the appropriate length. All nails should be 1 to 2 cm below the tip of the greater tuberosity and along the side of the metaphysis. This location prevents acromial impingement of the nails when the shoulder is abducted. The nail tips should be directed as far distally as possible without violating the olecranon fossa (Fig. 14–10).

POSTOPERATIVE REHABILITATION

Plaster splints, casts, and slings are unnecessary in the postoperative period. Rather, early range-of-motion exercises are advocated and are initiated the day following operation. If the patient is unconscious, passive range-of-motion exercises can be performed at the bedside. Otherwise, the patient performs these exercises with a therapist. Particular attention is directed to flexion and extension of the elbow. Active and passive shoulder abduction exercises also are encouraged. The therapy continues until a full range of motion is achieved in both joints, usually about 6 weeks after operation.

PATHOLOGIC LESIONS

The humerus is the second most common bone involved with metastases.[13–15] Because the humerus is a non-weight bearing structure, it often becomes substantially involved by the metastatic process before symptoms appear. Therefore, most patients do not consult the physician until fracture already has occurred. The goals of the orthopedic surgeon in treating patients with humeral pathologic fractures are palliative relief of pain and return of function to the involved extremity. Methods of fixation previously employed for the humerus include Rush pin fixation,[16] plates and screws (with and without augmentation with methyl methacrylate cement),[15] and tumor resection with replacement by custom-made prostheses.[15] Flexible intramedullary nails for fixation of humeral pathologic lesions offer a closed method of stable fixation with minimal operative morbidity to the patient. The nails can be used for both prophylactic stabilization and fixation after fracture. Painful pathologic lesions from the surgical neck region to the distal third of the humerus that have not fractured can be nailed prophylactically by retrograde or antegrade techniques, depending on the location of the lesions (Fig. 14–11). Criteria for closed nailing of these lesions include painful lesions unresponsive to radiation therapy or those with greater than 50% cortical destruction in which fracture may be imminent. Two 4-mm nails or four 3.2-mm nails are sufficient for stabilization. Stabilization following a pathologic frac-

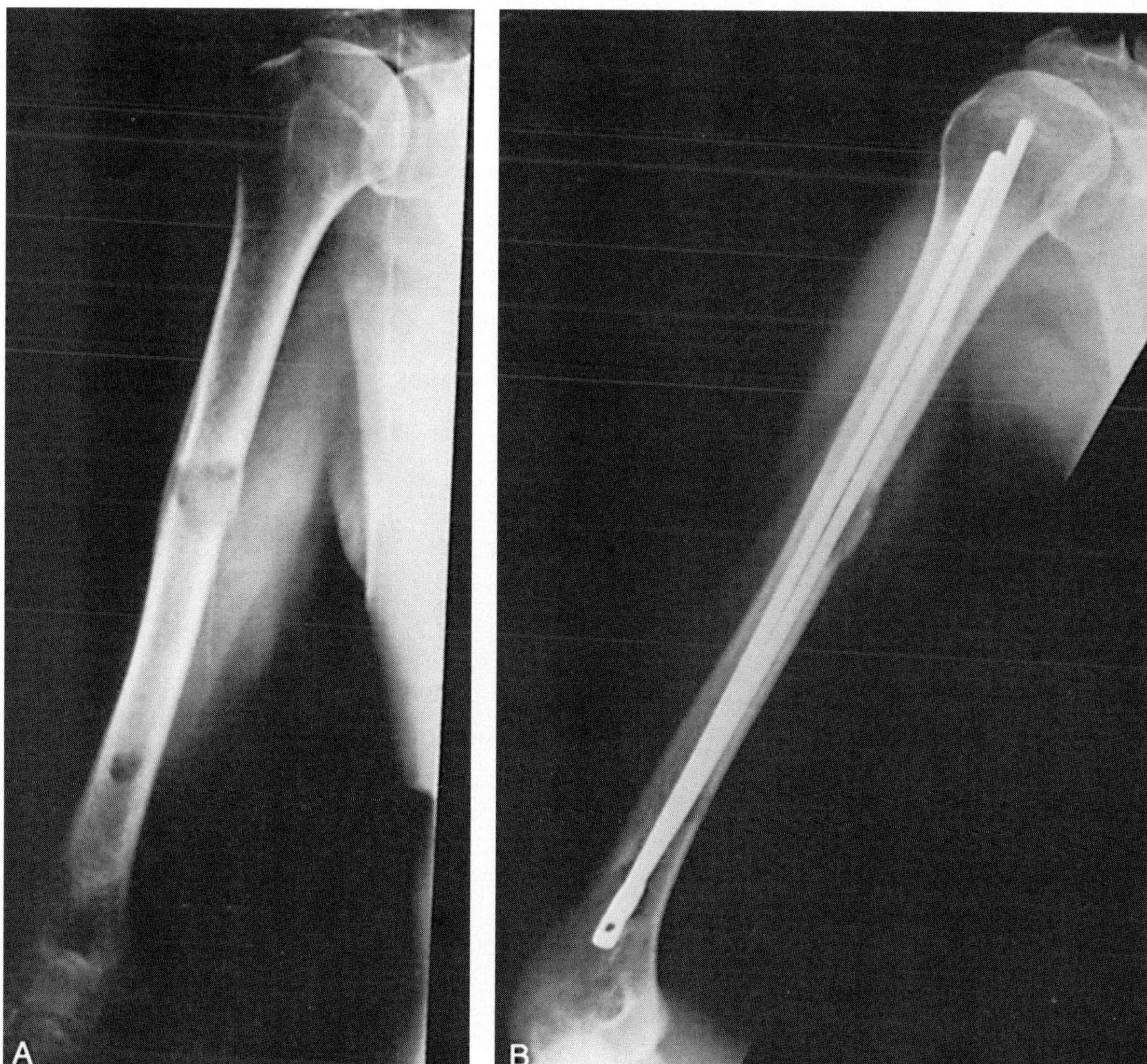

Fig. 14–11. *A,B,* Impending pathologic fracture of the humerus caused by breast metastases. It was treated by closed retrograde intramedullary nailing using two 4-mm diameter nails. Radiation therapy to the lesions was begun immediately after the operation.

ture is indicated for a patient who is medically able to undergo an operative procedure and general anesthetic. Fractures in the humerus from below the surgical neck region to the distal third can be treated by antegrade or retrograde nailing, depending on the location of the lesions, as discussed previously (Fig. 14–12). Large lytic lesions may require curettage and addition of bone cement around the nails to secure fixation. The fracture is opened first, and the tumor is curetted. The nails then are passed across the fracture, and finally, bone cement is placed around the nails up and down the canal, if possible.

Radiation therapy can be started immediately in prophylactically nailed lesions and in fractures that have been nailed closed, if the tumor is well away from the site of the entry portal. In pathologic fractures, the radiation dosage must be decreased so that healing can take place. In lesions that have been opened, curetted, and cemented, radiation therapy should be delayed for at least 2 weeks (until the wound has healed) to prevent dehiscence. Postoperative physical therapy includes range-of-motion exercises of the shoulder and elbow joints.

In conclusion, pathologic lesions can be treated successfully by closed intramedullary nailing in the majority of patients. Relief of pain, restoration of function to the extremity, and decrease in length of the hospital stay are provided to patients treated by this method. Radiation therapy to the pathologic lesion can be continued or started immediately after operation in the majority of patients.

SPECIAL PROBLEMS

Neural and vascular complications are the two immediate problems that can occur with fractures of the humerus. Injury to the radial nerve is the most common complication.[17–22]

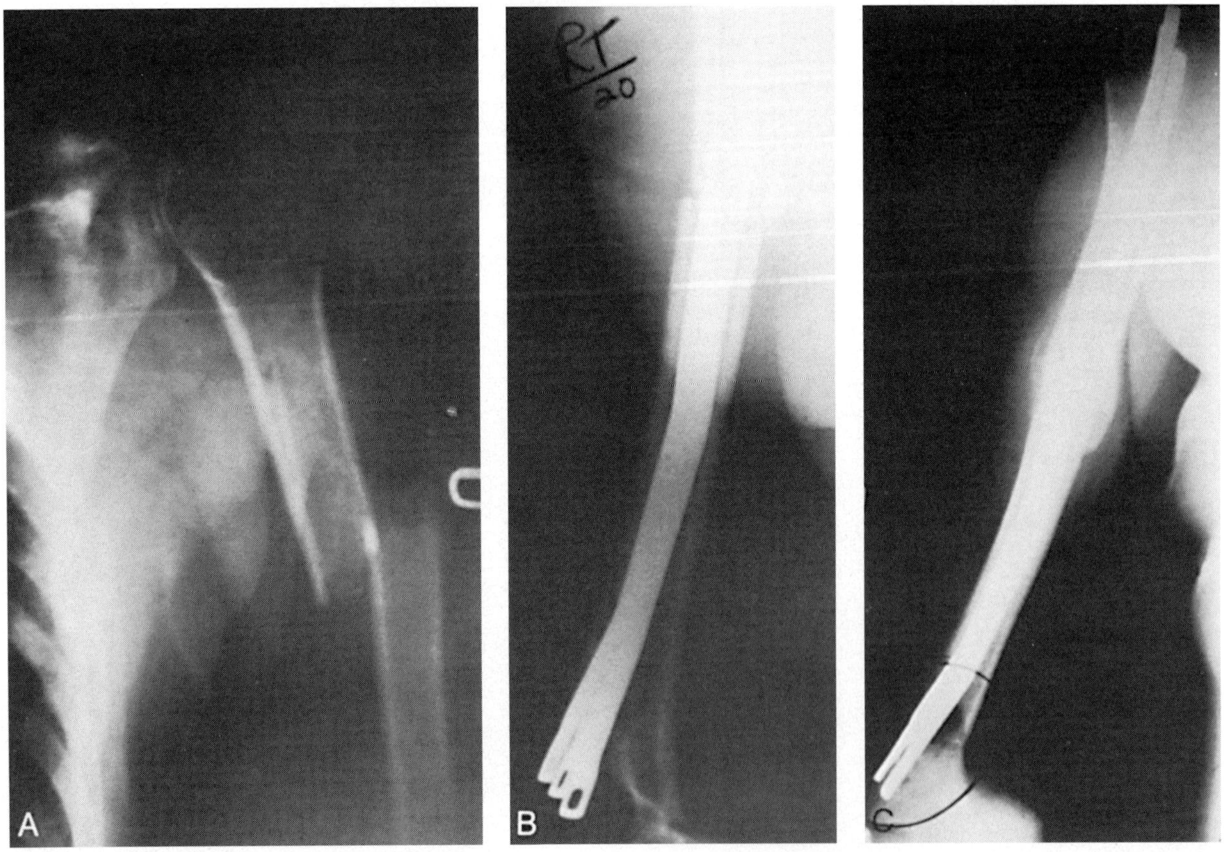

Fig. 14–12. *A,B,* Pathologic fracture of the middle third of the humerus treated by closed retrograde nailing. Three 4-mm diameter nails were used. *C,* Fracture is healed at 9 months. No fractures occurred at the distal entry portal despite the larger than necessary entry portal that was made. (Courtesy of Arnold Cohen, M.D.)

The nerve can be injured either prior to the operative treatment or during the surgical procedure by traction on the nerve during closed reduction and intramedullary nailing or by direct injury to the nerve during open reduction. Conservative treatment of the injury is the rule. If nerve entrapment in the fracture site is suspected, open exploration is warranted. Care must be taken when inserting flexible intramedullary nails. Because they are curved, the nails can migrate out of the fracture site into the soft tissue, thereby causing direct trauma to the radial nerve where it is close to the bone as it courses around the humerus. Gentle passage of the nail under image control is necessary.

Fractures of the humerus that involve vascular injury are an orthopedic emergency. Rapid stabilization of the bone, even in comminuted fractures, can be obtained with flexible intramedullary nails. When the fracture is closed and time permits, closed nailing is performed prior to arterial repair. Open fractures with arterial injury require debridement, nailing, and vascular repair, in that order. These procedures usually can be accomplished in rapid succession. Vascular repair should be performed by a peripheral vascular surgeon working in concert with the orthopedic surgeon.

Delayed union and nonunion of fractures of the shaft of the humerus can occur.[23] Nonunion usually is seen in transverse fractures or in those with marked displacement and associated soft- tissue interposition. Distraction at the fracture site caused by the use of a hanging cast

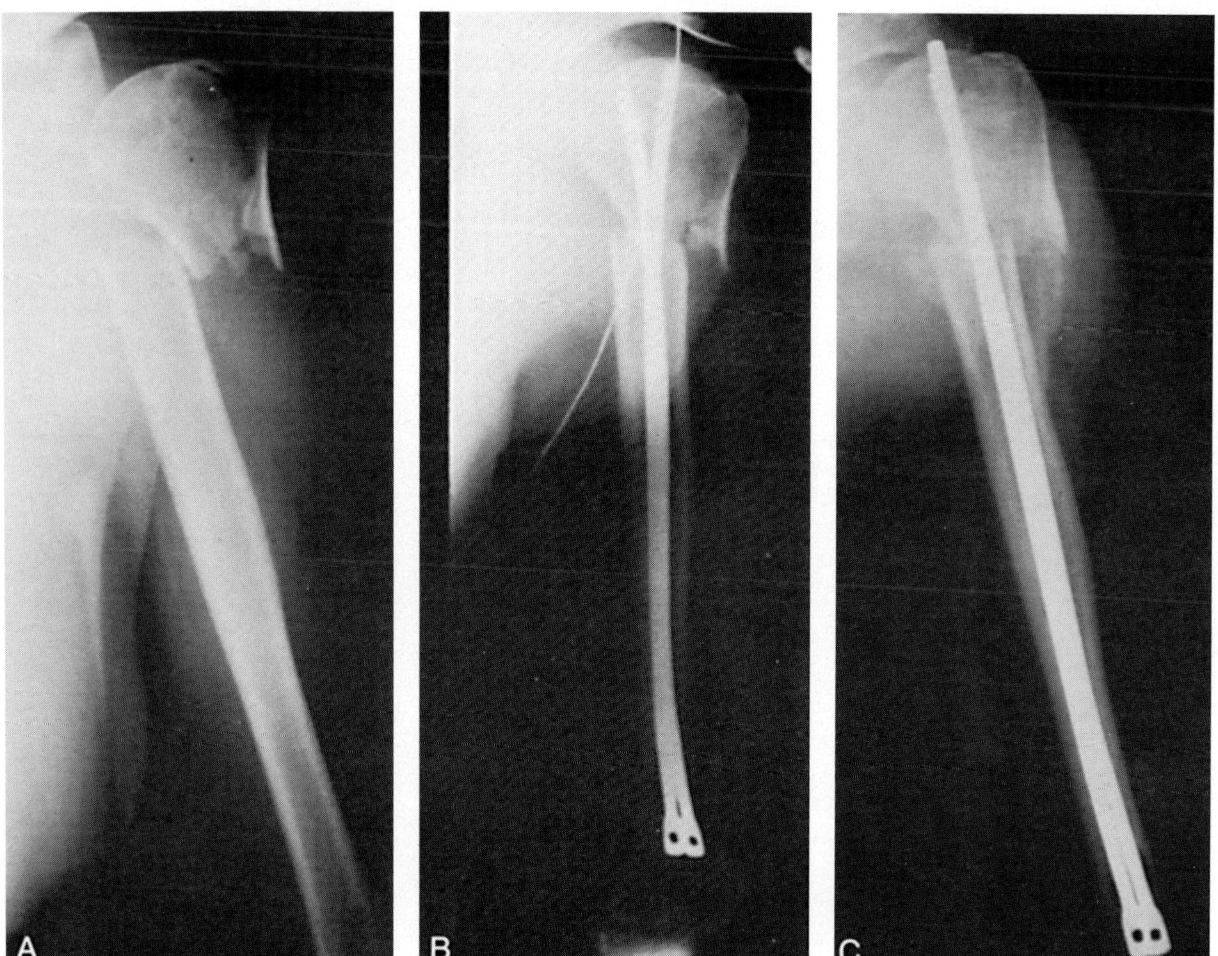

Fig. 14–13. *A*, Proximal third fracture of the humerus with marked displacement. The pectoralis major is the primary deforming force in this fracture (see Fig. 21–2). *B*, The fracture was reduced and treated by closed retrograde nailing using two 4-mm diameter nails. *C*, Fracture is healed at 6 months. Shortening caused the 1-mm penetration of the nail tip through the humeral head. The nails were removed and full shoulder motion was regained.

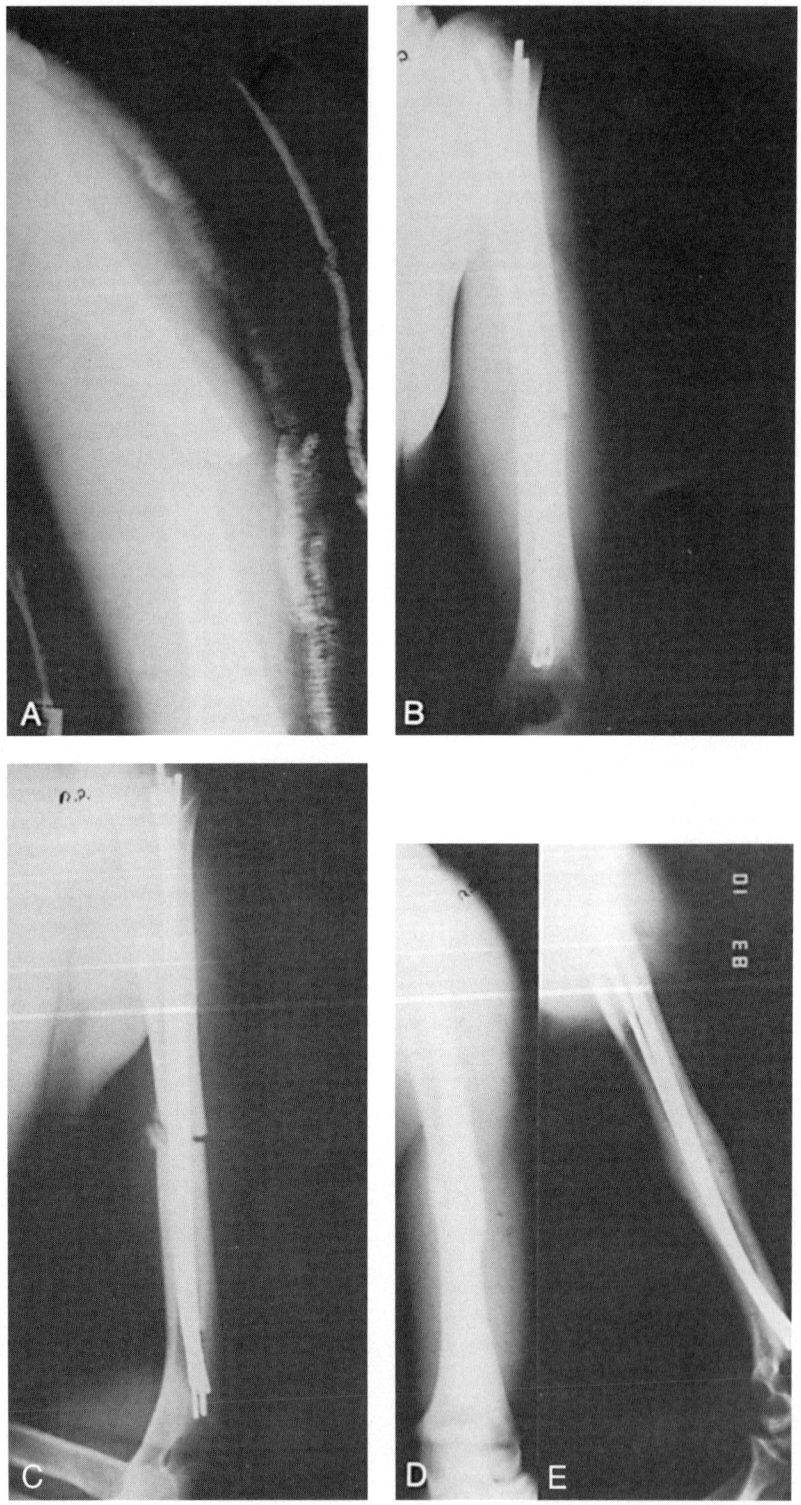

Fig. 14–14. *A*, Middle third fracture in which the alignment could not be maintained satisfactorily. *B,C*, Closed retrograde nailing restored alignment. Four 3.2-mm nails were used (two C and two S nails). *D,E*, Fracture is well healed at 8 months.

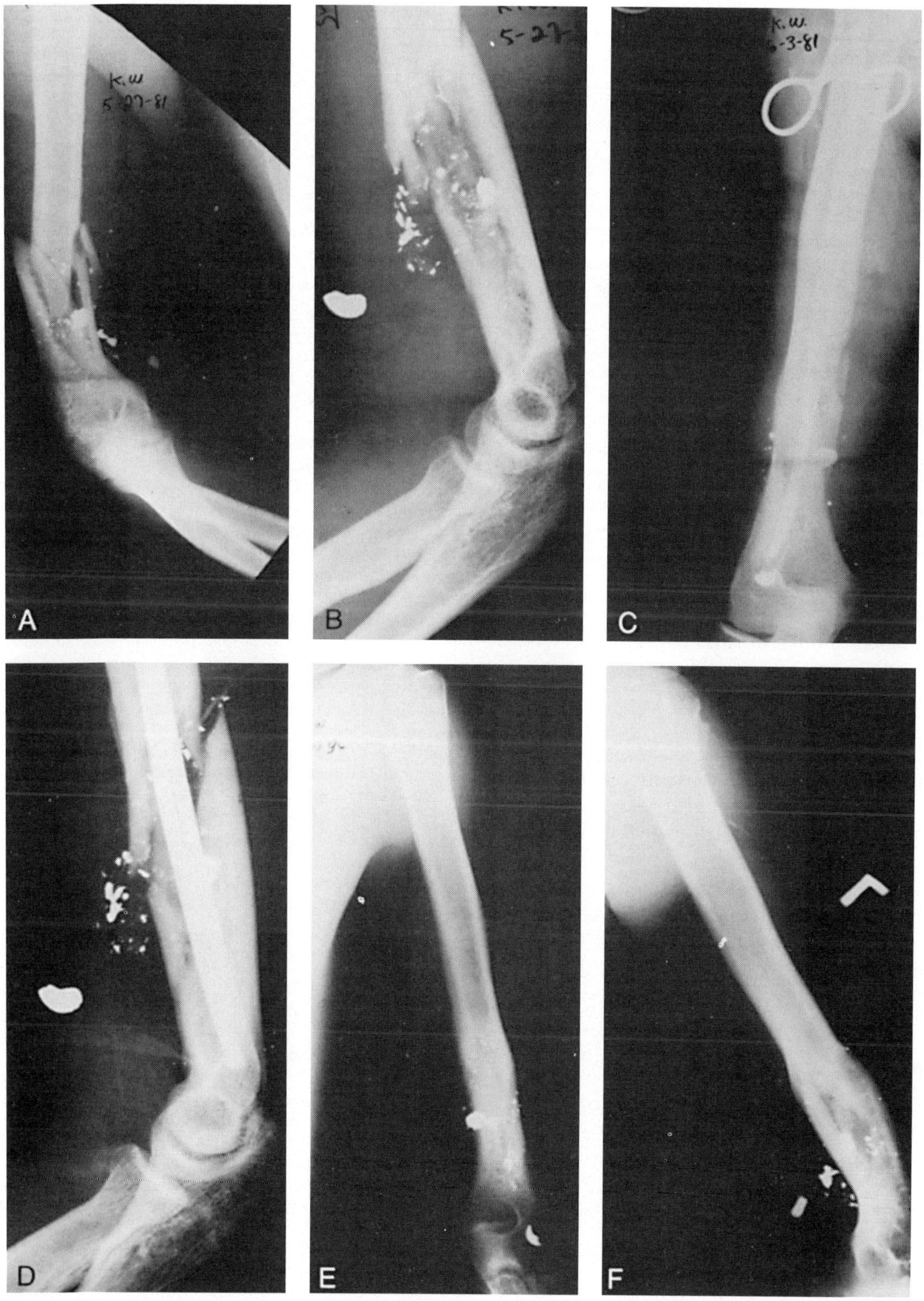

Fig. 14–15. *A,B,* AP and lateral radiographs of a comminuted distal third gunshot fracture. The neurovascular status was normal. *C,D,* Closed antegrade nailing was performed. *E,F,* The nails were removed after the fracture had healed because of nail retreat and shoulder pain.

that is too heavy also can lead to nonunion. Open reduction of the fracture with stripping of the bone and rigid fixation often contributes to nonunion. Flexible intramedullary nailing eliminates these problems by allowing anatomically correct fracture reduction by closed methods.

CLINICAL EXPERIENCES

A prospective study of 85 patients treated at Cook County Hospital, Chicago, Illinois follows.[24] This series included 63 men and 22 women who ranged in age from 17 to 72 years; the average age was 36 years. Of the fractures, 81 were closed, including 2 pathological fractures, and 6 were open (5 grade I and 1 grade III). Twenty-two gunshot fractures were included in the series. Of the fractures, 27 were located in the proximal third of the humerus (Fig. 14–13). Twenty-five were in the middle third (Fig. 14–14), and 34 were in the distal third (Fig. 14–15). All patients underwent operation within 5 days of injury.

Results

The average healing time was 7.2 weeks. Nonunion of one fracture occurred and there were no infections or malunions. Six of the nine preoperative radial nerve palsies healed spontaneously. Three of the nerves were severed by missiles and needed further treatment. Nail back-out caused pain in 8 patients and 5 were revised. The average loss of complete extension of the elbow was 4° and flexion of the elbow was 132°.

SUMMARY

Flexible intramedullary nailing of humeral shaft fractures provides an excellent alternative method of fixation for problem fractures in this region. The indications for intramedullary nailing should be followed strictly; the majority of fractures of the humerus require nonoperative treatment. The technique of nailing is simple to learn, requires downsized nails (4, 3.5, and 3.2 mm diameters), and has a low complication rate. This technique should be added to the physician's operative techniques for stabilization of problem fractures of the humeral shaft.

REFERENCES

1. Caldwell, J.A.: Treatment of fractures of the shaft of the humerus by hanging cast. Surg. Gynecol. Obstet. *79*: 421, 1940.
2. Thompson, R.G., et al.: The treatment of humeral shaft fractures by the hanging cast method. J. Int. Coll. Surg. *43*:52, 1975.
3. Hunter, S.: The closed treatment of fractures of the humeral shaft. Clin. Orthop. *164*:192, 1982.
4. Klenerman, L.: Fractures of the shaft of the humerus. J. Bone Joint Surg. *48B*:105, 1966.
5. Comfort, T.H.: The sugartong splint in humeral shaft fractures. Minn. Med. *56*:363, 1973.
6. Sarmiento, A., et al.: Functional bracing of fractures of the shaft of the humerus. J. Bone Joint Surg. *59A*:596, 1977.
7. Gelchrist, D.K.: A Stockinette-Valpeau for immobilization of the shoulder girdle. J. Bone Joint Surg. *49A*:750, 1967.
8. Spak, I.: Humeral shaft fractures. Acta Orthop. Scand. *49*:234, 1978.
9. Balfour, G., Mooney, V., Ashby, M.: Diaphyseal fractures of the humerus treated with a ready-made fracture brace. J. Bone Joint Surg. *64A*:11, 1982.
10. Holm, C.: Management of humeral shaft fractures: Fundamental nonoperative technique. Clin. Orthop. *71*: 132, 1970.
11. Rüedi, T., Moshfegh, A., Pfeiffer, K.M., Allgöwer, M.: Fresh fractures of the humerus—Conservative or operative treatment. Reconstr. Surg. Traumatol. *14*:65, 1974.
12. Hackethal, K.H.: Dee Bundel-Nageling. Wien, Springer-Verlag, Berlin, 1961.
13. Albright, J., Gillespie, T., Butaud, T.: Treatment of metastasis. Semin. Oncol. *7*:4, 1980.
14. Douglass, H., Shukla, S., Mindell, E.: Treatment of pathological fractures of long bones excluding those due to breast cancer. J. Bone Joint Surg. *58A*:1055, 1976.
15. Harrington, K., et al.: Methyl methacrylate as an adjunct in internal fixation of pathological fractures. J. Bone Joint Surg. *58A*:1047, 1976.
16. Stewart, M.J., Hundley, J.M.: Fractures of the humerus: A comparative study in methods and treatment. J. Bone Joint Surg. *37A*:861, 1955.
17. Holstein, A.L., Lewis, G.: Fractures of the humerus with radial nerve paralysis. J. Bone Joint Surg. *45A*: 1382, 1963.
18. Pollack, F., et al.: Treatment of radial neuropathy associated with fractures of the humerus. J. Bone Joint Surg. *63A*:239, 1981.
19. Mast, J., Spiegel, P., Harvey, J.P., Harrison, C.: Fractures of the humeral shaft. Clin. Orthop. *112*:254, 1975.
20. Garcia, A., Jr., Maeck, B.H.: Radial nerve injuries in fractures of the shaft of the humerus. Am. J. Surg. *99*: 625, 1960.
21. Mann, R.J., Neal, E.G.: Fractures of the shaft of the humerus in adults. South. Med. J. *58*:264, 1965.
22. Kettlekamp, D.B., Alexander, H.: Clinical review of radial nerve injury. J. Trauma *7*:424, 1967.
23. Fisher, D.E.: Nonunions of the humeral shaft. Minn. Med. *55*:395, 1972.
24. Hall, R.F., Pankovich, A.M.: Ender nailing of acute fractures of the humerus. J. Bone Joint Surg. *69A*:558, 1987.

15

Intramedullary Nailing of the Humerus

Barry L. Riemer

Most fractures of the humeral diaphysis are well managed by nonoperative techniques, by functional bracing in particular. Fractures reliably unite. Minor rotational or angular deformities are well tolerated. Indications for internal fixation include arterial injuries, pathologic fractures, floating elbows, selected open fractures (including gunshot wounds), and blunt polytrauma patients.

The results of plate fixation have been satisfactory. Union rates approaching 100% have been reported. When studied, shoulder motion has rarely been significantly affected.[1–5] Intramedullary fixation of the humerus has gained acceptance slower than the femur or tibia because of the successful record of plates and the lack of linear extraarticular access.

The Division of Orthopaedic Fractures at Allegheny General Hospital became interested in intramedullary fixation of the humerus. Our service treats blunt polytrauma patients and those referred with complex single-system fracture problems. Though plates are a reliable means of achieving union for isolated fractures, they have several disadvantages. Particular humerus fracture management goals in blunt polytrauma patients are access to the chest and ambulation on crutches. The exposure for plate application requires an extended dissection of the arm, causing pain in the critical immediate posttrauma period. Plates are an eccentric extraosseous device precluding weight bearing prior to union. Over half the patients with humeral shaft fractures seen on our service sustain either pelvic or lower extremity fractures requiring ambulation on their fractured humeri. Furthermore, plates carry a significant risk of iatrogenic nerve injury, particularly with metal removal when there is a risk of refracture as well.[3]

Though virtually all of our patients have an indication for internal fixation based on their associated injuries, approximately 25% of our humeral fractures are treated conservatively. Low-energy fractures in thin patients can often be sufficiently braced that even crutch ambulation or bed-to-chair transfers are possible without fixation. The results of functional bracing in our patients are inferior to those of other reports with a nonunion rate of approximately 20%, probably caused by increased functional demands. However, the nonunions have been easily reconstructed once patients have completed rehabilitation.[6]

A significant clinical experience has been reported with flexible nails. Union rates are high, approximately 94%, though these rates are not quite as reliable as plate fixation. Flexible nails are useful for low-energy and simple geometry fractures. They are an excellent technique for fractures of the surgical neck of the humerus where proximal fixation can be precarious.[7,8]

Locked humeral nailing is in its early stages. Techniques, indications, and results have varied widely. An array of biomechanically different implants are available and reported series are small. The investigators have had a particular interest in locked humeral nailing, the Seidel nail in particular, to expand closed intramedullary nail techniques to complex fracture problems and to allow immediate humeral weight bearing.

IATROGENIC AND TRAUMATIC NEUROVASCULAR INJURIES

Traumatic radial nerve palsies with fractures of the humeral shaft are not generally an indication for nerve exploration and internal fixation. The investigators recommend radial nerve exploration and internal fixation in open fractures and high-energy closed fractures of the humeral shaft with radial nerve injuries.[3,9–11] Median and ulnar neuropathies are rare and, when associated with fractures of the humeral shaft, are an indication for exploration and fixation.

When a humeral fracture that requires intramedullary fixation has an associated partial or complete radial nerve palsy, the authors recommend a nerve exploration at least 2 cm above and below the fracture to be certain that the nerve is not trapped between the bone ends. Further exploration of the nerve is not necessary, provided the nerve can be documented to be intact. The soft-tissue envelope of the humerus should be disturbed as little as possible. The periosteum should not be elevated from the bone and gentle retraction of the thin soft-tissue layer between the nerve and bone is critical. Every attempt to retain a closed technique of the humerus should be made.

The Holstein-Lewis fracture of the humerus can trap the radial nerve. With newer antegrade locked nail techniques, it is amenable to intramedullary fixation and when internal fixation is needed, it is another indication for nerve exploration and closed nailing irrespective of the clinical presence or absence of radial nerve symptoms. The following three criteria define the Holstein-Lewis fracture (Fig. 15–1): the fracture is in the distal third of the humerus, (2) a lateral spike is present, and (3) the fracture is displaced into varus. In these cases, a closed manipulation under general anesthesia should not be attempted and an open nailing should be performed.[10]

If while close reducing a fracture for intramedullary nailing bone crepitation cannot be felt or fracture ends cannot be brought into adequate apposition, the fracture should be opened to be certain that there is not soft tissue and, in particular, a nerve entrapped. The authors have performed 126 humeral nailings, 61 flexible and 65 locked using these criteria for nerve exploration. No cases of iatrogenic, radial, median, or ulnar neuropathies have been seen.

Iatrogenic neurologic complications have resulted from the use of intraoperative skeletal or skin traction devices.[12] The humerus is easy to grip distally by the condyles. The soft-tissue envelope is sufficiently thin so that manual reduction is simple.

A slight risk exists with late entrapment of nerves in fracture callus. The investigators have seen this complication twice, once with functional bracing and once with flexible nail techniques, this complication may present with locked nails also. This is a complication that would be obviated with plates which significantly inhibit callus formation. Both proximal and distal locking screws can injure neurovascular structures and will be discussed with their surgical techniques.[12]

Osseous Anatomy

The humeral head is not analogous to the femoral head, where excellent screw purchase can be obtained. The humerus bears very little weight and stress is not born in a repetitive pattern, obviating any reliable areas of dense trabecular bone for screw purchase. All fixation (nails, plates and screws, and flexible nails) have a precarious hold in the proximal humerus. Whenever possible locking should be accomplished through purchase in the dense bone of the humeral neck, avoiding the humeral head.

The shape of the humerus is generally straight. Minor variations can easily be accommodated by flexible nails. However, locked nails are far more stiff. Minor variations in the shape of the humerus can incarcerate nails or reamers.

In the AP view, the humerus is straight. The medullary canal is in line with the lateral edge of the articular surface of the humerus and the acromion. In the lateral view, there is an anterior bend at the distal end of the medullary canal. The distal taper of the medullary canal places mechanical stress on power reamers. If a bent guide rod is inserted to act as a reduction tool, it can incarcerate a reamer or prevent it from advancing distally. The bone of the distal

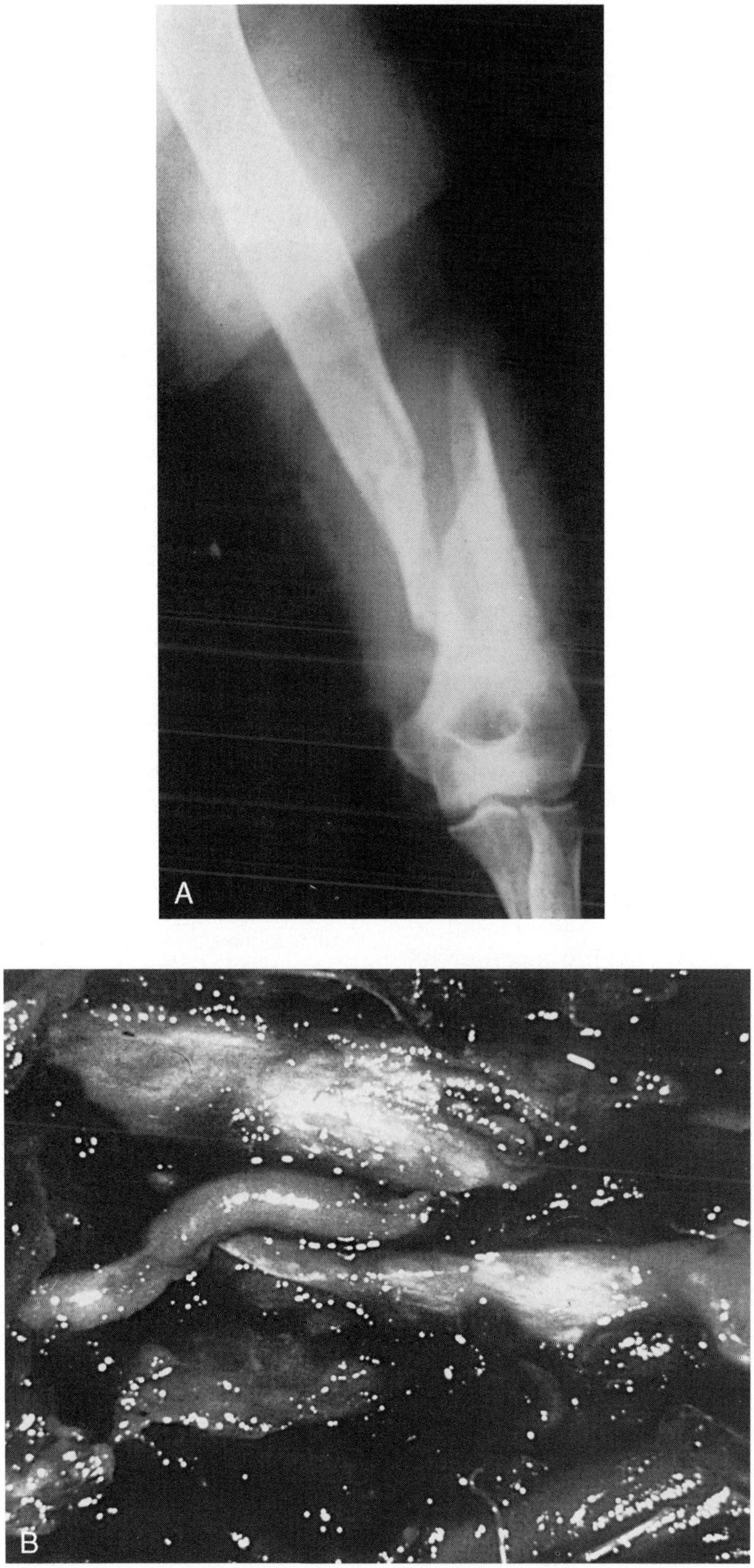

Fig. 15–1. *A,* A Holstein-Lewis fracture characterized by distal third, a lateral spike, displaced into varus. The patient presented with no radial nerve symptoms. This fracture geometry is amenable to current locked nail techniques. *B,* A radial nerve exploration was performed prior to internal fixation. The radial nerve was noted to be tented across the lateral spike. A closed nailing would have damaged the radial nerve.

humerus is hard, and there is not a flare to decompress the pressure head of power tools. The authors have experienced significant clinical difficulties reaming tight humeri. The investigators have used six different systems including four flexible systems, two with narrow cores and wide-cutting fins to decompress the canal, and two rigid systems from total hip arthroplasty sets. None could reliably cut the bone of a narrow humerus. The bone is also short. If a guide backs out in the humerus, it can easily be delivered into the soft tissues through the fracture site allowing power tools to be guided out of the bone.

Biomechanics

The biomechanical differences between flexible and locked nails are obvious. Flexible nails provide axial stability in stable fracture patterns, and at best, fair rotational stability. Of particular interest in the humerus are the differences between screw-locked nails and the Seidel nail. Screw-locked nails have excellent rotational and axial stability once both screws engage in the holes of the nails. Several current nails have slots rather than screw holes, allowing for several millimeters of axial movement and several degrees of free rotation prior to achieving excellent stability. The Seidel nail, in contrast, has an internal locking mechanism that applies an interference fit between the implant and the endosteal bone. There is immediate mild rotational stability and excellent axial stability. The rotational stability, however, is inconsistent and often not maintained. Though biomechanically very different, the variant of fixation that will best allow fracture union is unclear.[13–15]

SURGICAL TECHNIQUE: LOCKED NAILS

Preoperative Planning

Reaming the humerus has been shown to increase complication rates. Whenever possible, a nail diameter that can be accommodated without reaming should be chosen.[6] Preoperative canal diameter measurements should be made on both AP and lateral views, because the shape of the medullary canal is not always round. The smaller of the two measurements should be used to determine the competency of the medullary canal. Measurements should be made at the most distal end of the canal that would be used for reaming or nail insertion (Fig. 15–2).

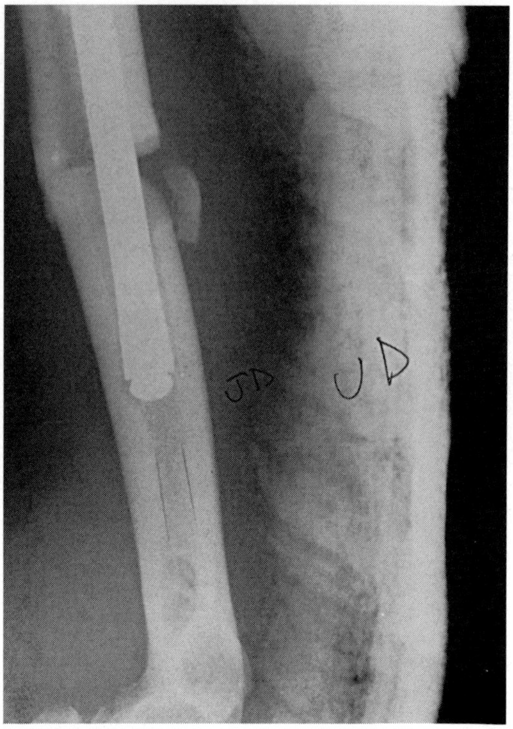

Fig. 15–2. Lateral radiograph showing the appropriate level for canal diameter measurements, at or just beyond the distal end of the nail. The lesser canal diameter measurement on AP and lateral radiographs is accepted. Measurements are made between the pencil lines shown drawn in the distal canal. A 9-mm Seidel nail has been inserted. Note the endosteal beveling created by reaming. In this case, the reamer could not be advanced beyond the beveling. This patient has developed a recalcitrant nonunion (see Fig. 15–19).

Positioning[15]

The patient is positioned on a radiolucent table. Traction is not applied to the arm to avoid iatrogenic nerve palsies.[16] The fluoroscope is set on the side opposite the surgeon. The patient is positioned to the side of the table opposite the surgeon allowing the fluoroscope to reach across the chest to the fractured arm. The contralateral arm is abducted or tucked tightly at the patient's side. A roll is placed behind the operative scapula. This is necessary to elevate the fracture from the table. Shoulder extension of approximately 30° also brings the humeral head out from under the acromion, allowing access to the humeral head (Fig. 15–3).

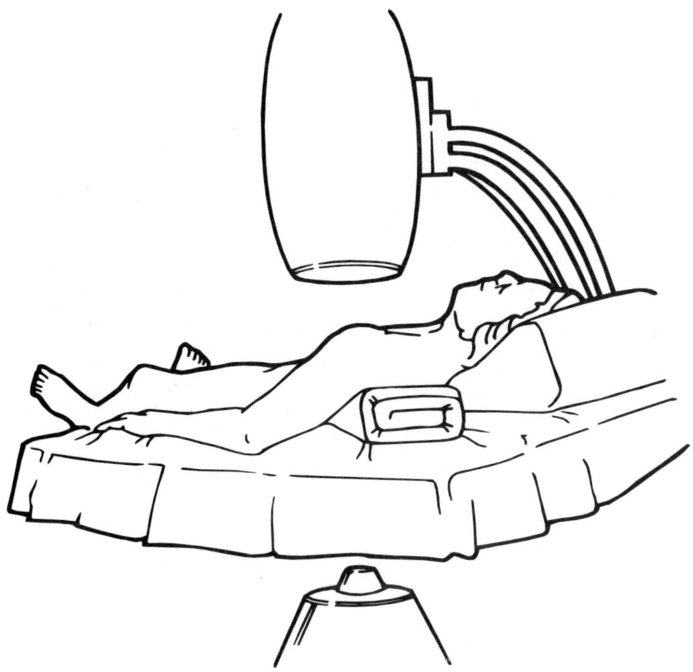

Fig. 15–3. The patient is positioned to the contralateral side of the table with a roll beneath the operative scapula. A fluoroscope can reach the operative humerus from the contralateral side, allowing the surgeon to operate on the humerus while not changing positions to accommodate the fluoroscope. (Courtesy of Homedica; Rutherford, NJ.)

Great care is taken to be certain that any nail is buried below the substance of the humeral head. With the shoulder extended, it is possible to not obtain an adequate profile of the nail within the substance of the humeral head. If there is any question, the fluoroscope should be obliqued to obtain an adequate AP view of the humeral head, accommodating the 30° extension of the shoulder (Fig. 15–4).[12]

Entry Portal

The variety of locked intramedullary nails can be divided into two general designs, each of which has different indications and techniques for insertion and application into the proximal humerus. First are nails that are straight (in the AP plane), including the Seidel nail (with an apex anterior bend), the Biomet nail, the Tru-Flex nail, and the straight Küntscher nails.

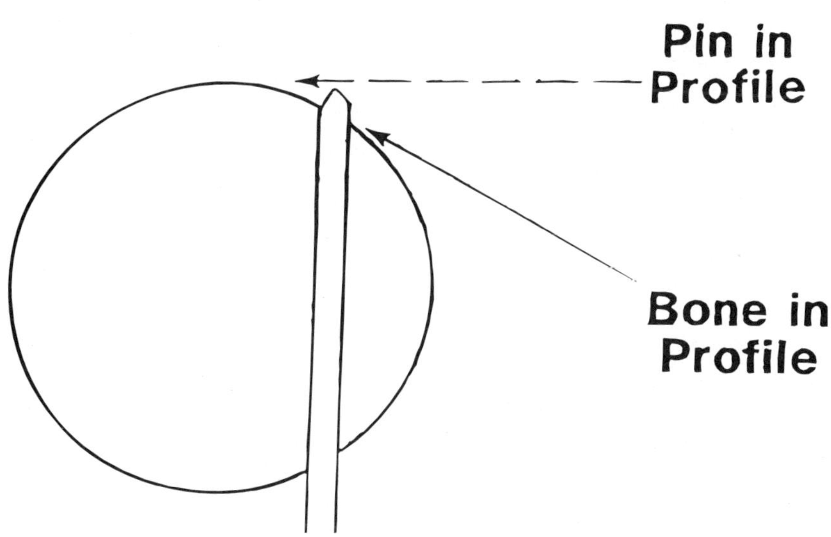

Fig. 15–4. A nail inserted eccentrically into a round bone can appear to be within the bone while actually protruding, unless an appropriate view showing the bone in profile is obtained.

Other nails have an apex medial bend including the Russell-Taylor nail, Alta nail, AO nail, and tibial nails inserted into the humerus. If a nail with an apex medial bend is inserted with the bend anterior, the principles of a straight nail insertion must be applied.

Straight (In The AP Plane) Locked Nails

The advantage of straight nails lies in their applicability to fractures of the proximal humerus. An entry portal in line with the medullary canal is used. Nails can be inserted through proximal fractures, only requiring an area for screw purchase. However, straight nails require an articular starting point and violation of the rotator cuff as potential disadvantages.

The Anterior Acromial Approach[17]

An incision is made over the anterior half of the acromion (Fig. 15–5). The deltoid muscle is split in line with its fibers. With the shoulder extended 30°, most of the humeral head is delivered from underneath the acromion. The coracoacromial ligament is cut in its entirety through this incision and is critical to prevent stiffness. An incision is made in line with the fibers of the rotator cuff, 1 cm medial to the greater tuberosity, avoiding the avascular lateral tendon. The incision is planned in line with the medullary canal of the humerus. This places the starting portal at the lateral edge of the articular surface. A large cut scores the bone. If reaming is required, a ball-tip guide rod is inserted. If the nail is to be inserted unreamed, a nail or guide rod is inserted.

Apex Medial Bent Nails

The advantage of apex medial bent nails is their insertion through the greater tuberosity. Neither the rotator cuff nor the joint are violated. A several centimeter cuff of proximal humeral circumference however is needed to guide nails down the medullary canal, obviating their use for very proximal fractures.

Apex medial nails are inserted through the greater tuberosity (Fig. 15–6). An incision is made over the lateral deltoid. An awl is used to enter the bone of the greater tuberosity. Because this is an eccentric starting point, a cuff of intact proximal humeral shaft must be present to guide the nail down the canal of the bone.

Proximal Locking Screws

All antegrade locked nailing requires proximal locking to avoid proximal migration and impingement. Cross-locking screws in the upper humerus are most safely accomplished with lateral to medial screws.[12]

Proximal locking of humeral nails is easily accomplished with jigs. The bone is soft and starting points are easily obtained. A significant risk of neurovascular injury, however, exists with improper technique. The axillary artery and vein lie within 3 cm and slightly posterior to the medial cortex of the surgical neck of the humerus. Whether transverse or oblique downward screws are employed, the vessels are at risk with over penetration of drill bits (Fig. 15–7). In osteopenic bone, the medial cortex cannot be felt well and drilling should be done under fluoroscopic control.

The axillary nerve is at particular risk with proximal humeral locking. The axillary nerve courses around the humeral neck, on the posterior surface of the humerus it is in one main trunk. The nerve lies close to the bone and, particularly when the humerus is internally rotated, is tethered to the bone. The main trunk of the nerve is vulnerable to anterior to posterior drill bits and screws. If the nerve is damaged along the posterior surface of the humerus, most of the deltoid will be paralyzed with significant functional impairment.

Along the lateral humerus, the nerve has arborized into multiple branches. If a branch of the nerve is damaged, at most, weakness of a small part of the deltoid, of questionable significance, will result. Branches of the deltoid can be protected by making a longitudinal incision over the lateral humerus, inserting a curved hemostat to the bone, and spreading longitudinally retracting small branches of the axillary nerve. Drill guides can then be inserted between the teeth of the hemostat, protecting the small branches of the nerve.

Danger to the lateral axillary nerve can also be avoided by obliquely downward-oriented screws starting above the nerve. However, screw heads around the upper edge of the greater tuberosity can impinge, and a more distal nail insertion point must be employed or the screw head must be buried. However, any screw protruding beyond the medial cortex can impinge upon the axillary nerve with internal rotation of the humerus. Metal protruding be-

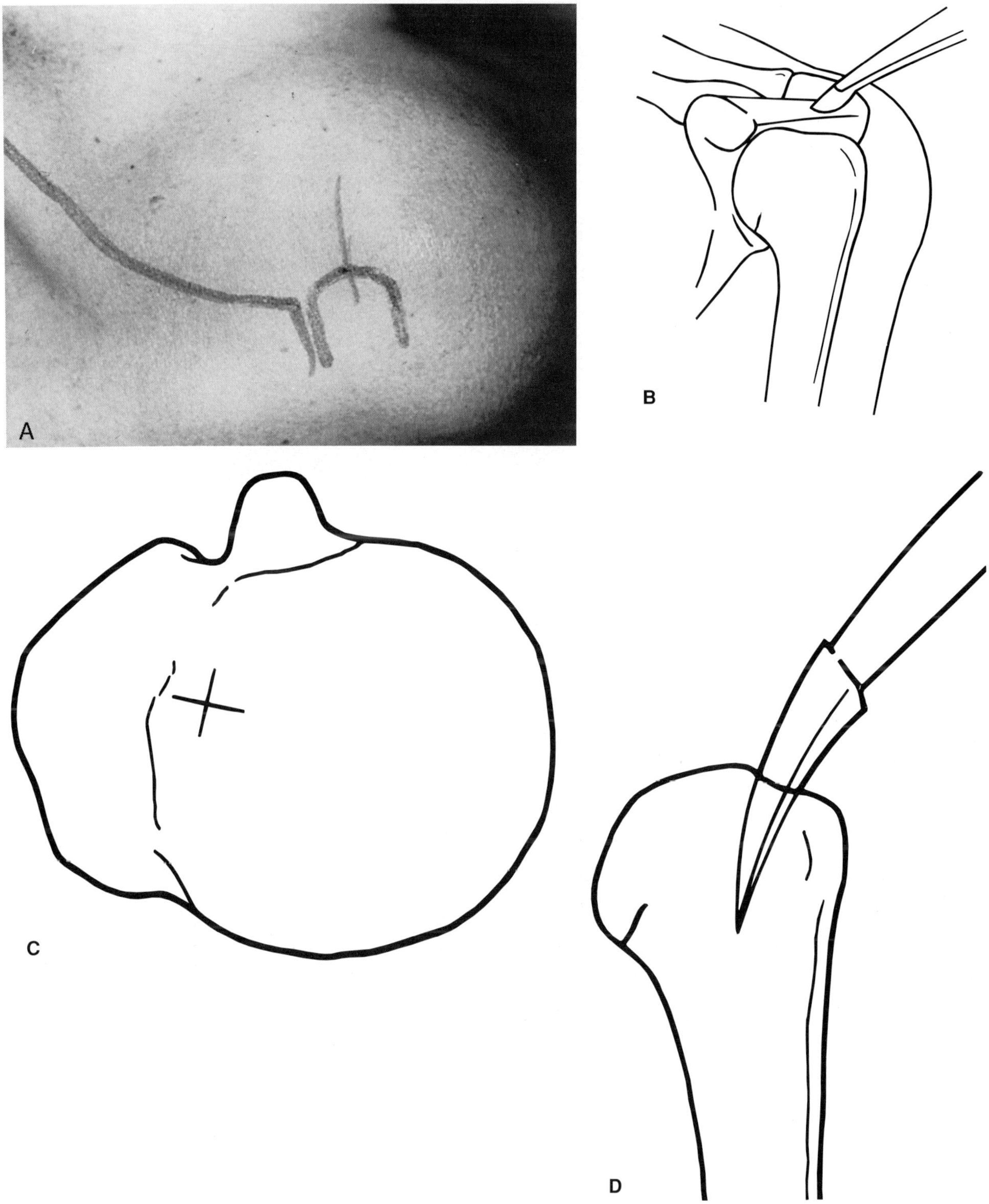

Fig. 15–5. *A,* Incision for insertion of straight nails. An incision is made over the anterior half of the acromion. This places the dissection over the coracoacromial ligament which is transected with the exposure. *B,* The coracoacromial ligament is transected. The rotator cuff is incised in line with its fibers directly above the medullary canal of the humerus. *C,* Entry point for a straight nail into the canal of the humerus. *D,* An awl creates a large hole in the humeral head that will not eccentrically guide a stiff nail. (Courtesy of Howmedica; Rutherford, NJ.)

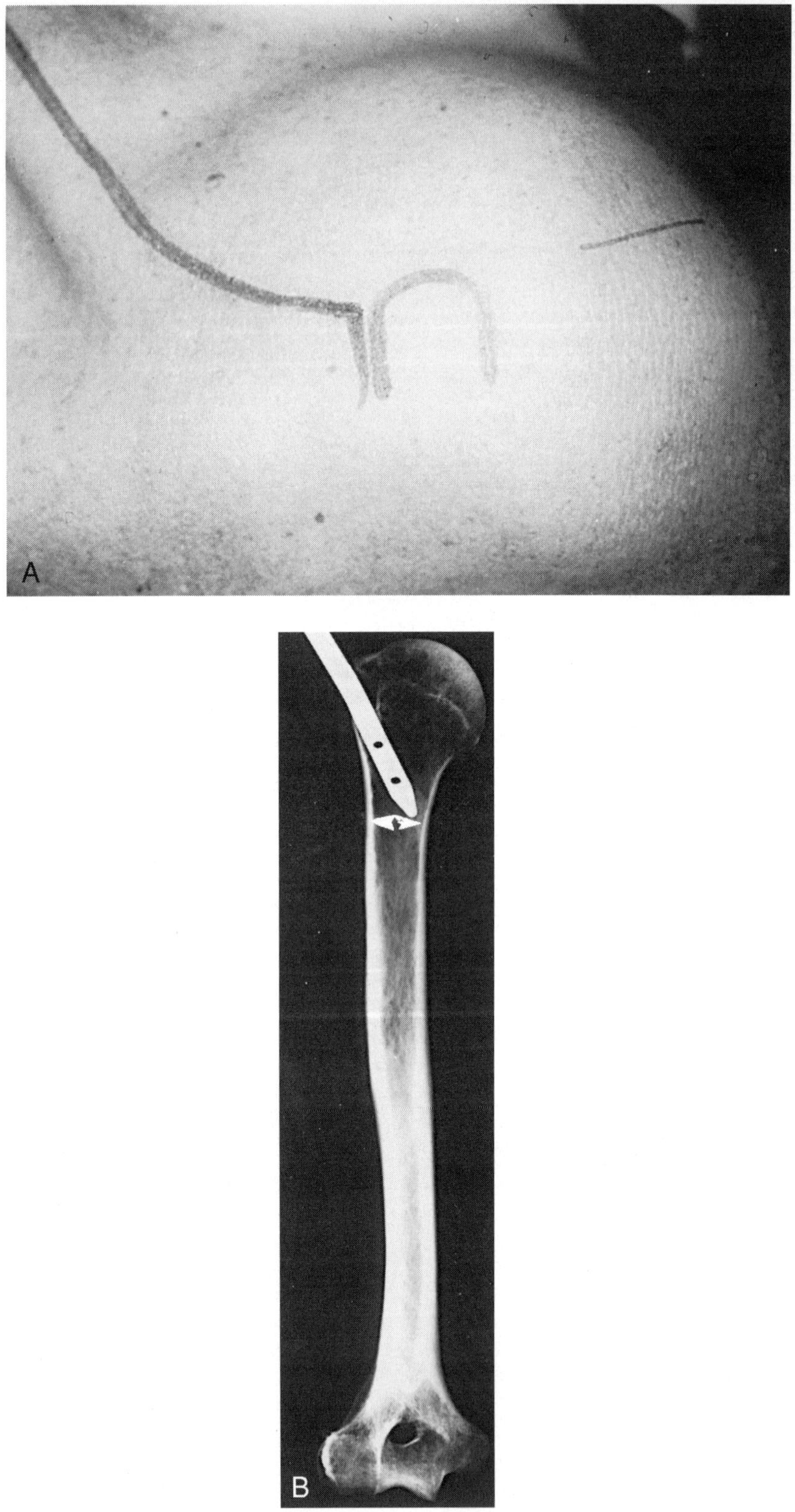

Fig. 15–6. *A,* Incision for insertion of apex medial bent nails through the greater tuberosity. *B,* A locked nail is inserted through the greater tuberosity. It strikes the medial cortex. A sufficient cylinder of upper humerus must be intact to deflect the nail into the distal canal (arrows). Such nails cannot reliably be inserted into bone when a fracture is present above the level marked by arrows.

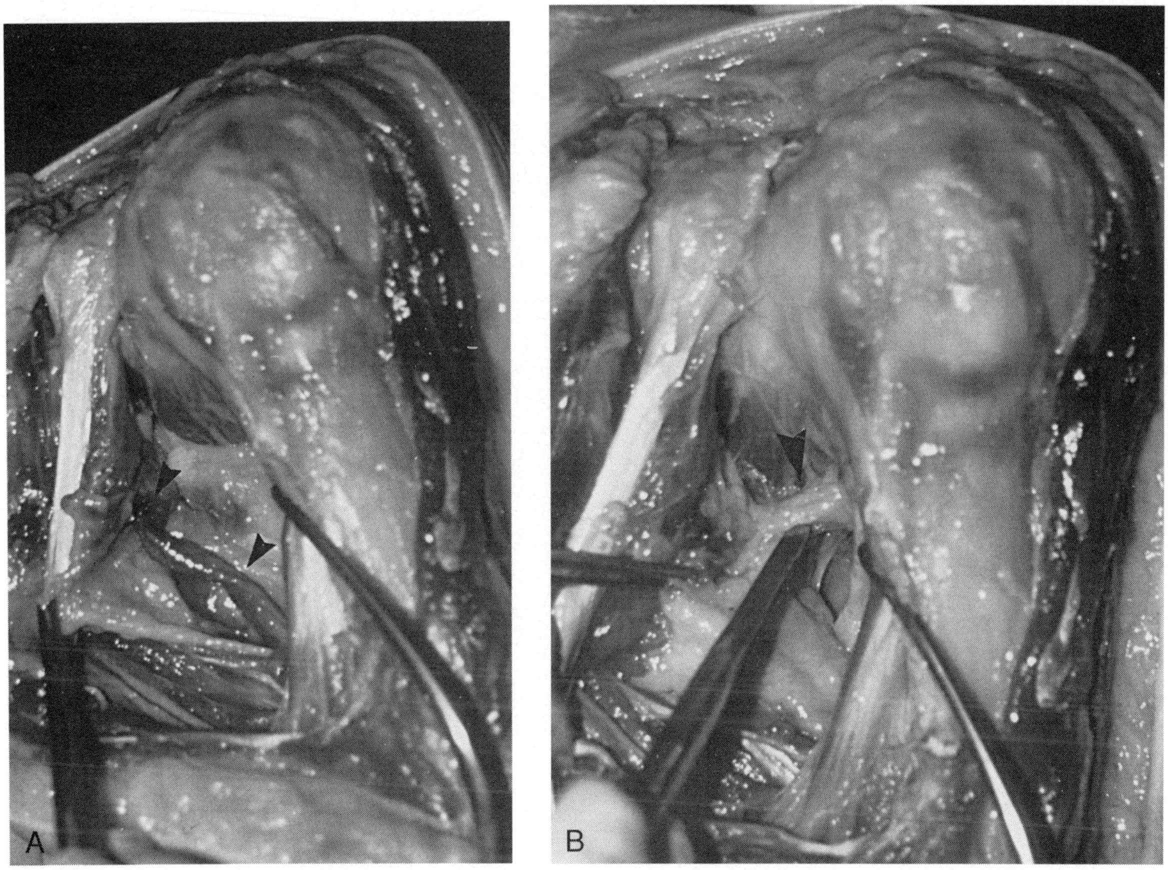

Fig. 15–7. *A,* A shoulder is viewed from the front. The deltoid muscle has been reflected and the conjointed tendon retracted. Note that the axillary artery and vein course parallel to the medial humeral neck and are equally at risk with transverse or oblique downward-oriented locking screws. *B,* The axillary nerve is seen coursing around the neck of the humerus. As it exits the quadrilateral space and lies posterior to the humerus, it is in one main trunk. An injury to the nerve at this level will paralyze the deltoid. *(Figure continues)*

yond the medial cortex should therefore be avoided.

Distal Locking

The Seidel nail locks distally by retraction of a ball retrograde into the substance of the nail (Fig. 15–8). The distal nail is cut into phalanges that spread against the endosteum. Distal locking is accomplished by inserting the screwdriver into the end of the nail and rotating counter clockwise. Fluoroscopy is not employed to assess distal locking. The phalanges are spread until the spreading screw becomes tight. There is often a "popping" sound as the screw becomes tight. This provides at best fair rotational control but excellent axial control.

Unlike the femur, tibia, or proximal humerus, distal screw locking in the humerus is performed through dense cortical bone. The drill must be centered exactly over the hole of the nail. Minor angular corrections to penetrate the nail by routing the bone with the side of the drill are not possible. A slightly wider exposure to the bone is often helpful, possibly placing surrounding nerves at risk from retraction (Blasier, personal communication).

The technique of AP locking from an anterior approach, involves a 2-cm incision lateral to the biceps tendon allowing adequate retraction and control of the drill (Fig. 15–9). The muscle is retracted after blunt dissection. The only neurovascular structures in the plane of fixation are small cutaneous branches of the musculocutaneous nerve that will innervate the lateral forearm skin. The nail must be inserted so that the holes lie lateral to the biceps tendon. Minor rotational errors can align locking holes medial to the biceps tendon, placing at risk the brachial artery and median nerves.

Lateral to medial screws should be used with caution. An incision is made over the lateral

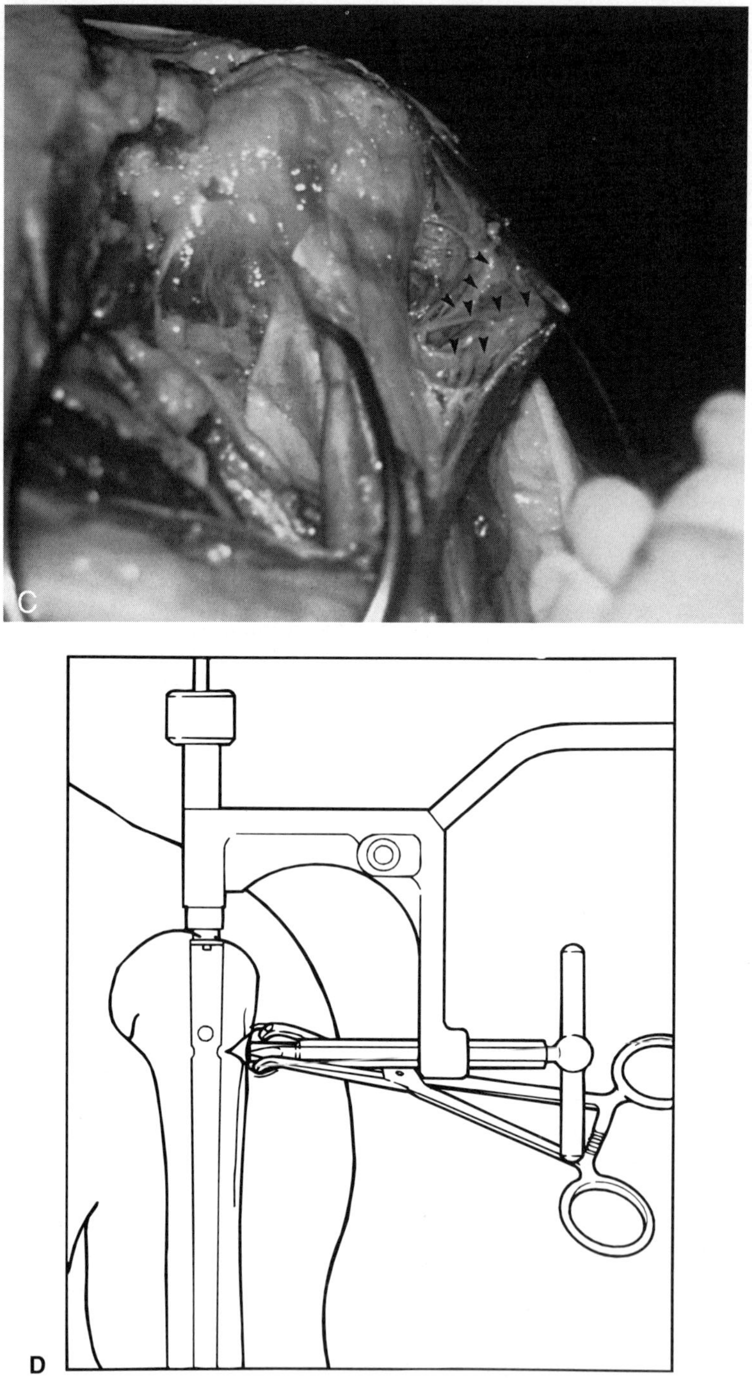

Fig. 15–7. *(continued) C,* The axillary nerve has reached the lateral humerus and has arborized into, in this case, three branches. Damage to one of these branches will at most weaken a portion of the deltoid. *D,* A hemostat is inserted to the bone and spread longitudinally to protect the arborized fibers of the axillary nerve. A drill guide can be inserted between the teeth of the hemostat and held to the bone preventing nerve branches from being harmed by power tools. (Courtesy of Howmedica; Rutherford, NJ.)

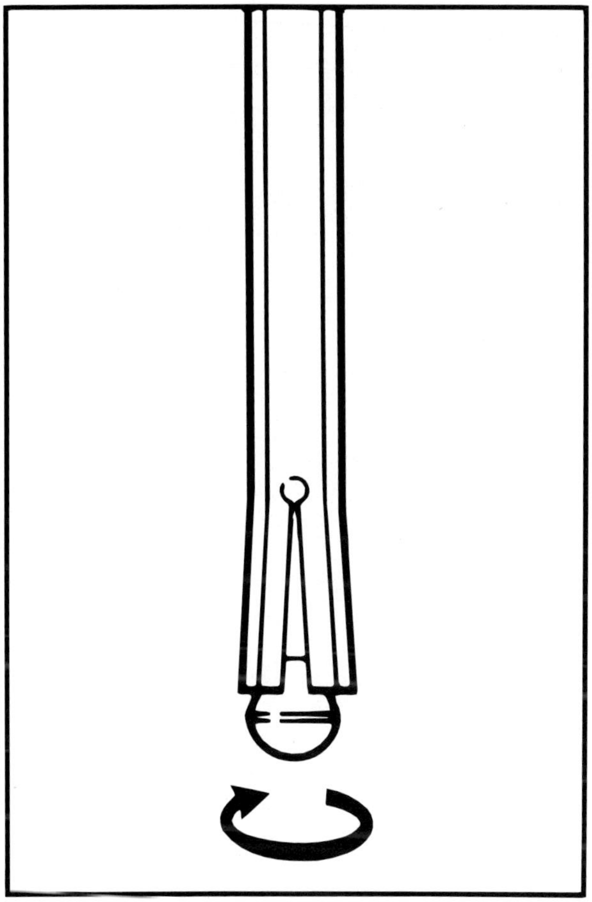

Fig. 15–8. The Seidel nail locks by retraction of a ball into the substance of the nail, spreading phalanges against endosteal bone. (Courtesy of Howmedica; Rutherford, NJ.)

humerus and the biceps and brachio-radialis are retracted anteriorly. A significant incidence of iatrogenic radial nerve palsies have been reported with this technique (Blasier, personal communication). Further, the bone is dense and curved making accurate drilling difficult.

Retrograde Locked Nail Techniques

Retrograde techniques cannot be used for fractures in the distal third of the humerus. The entry portal must begin above the olecranon fossa and be beveled proximally. Because this is a nonlinear entry portal, a cuff of intact bone above the entry portal must guide the nail proximally. The stiffer the nail inserted, the longer the length of the intact collar of bone must be. This is a major deficit into the routine use of retrograde nailing, as many fractures that are easily amenable to antegrade nailing are within this zone (Fig. 15–10).

Any of the above groups of nails can be inserted retrograde. It is critical, however, to choose only nails that are flexible enough to accommodate a nonlinear entry portal.[18] Design as well as material properties of the nail must be considered. The Seidel nail, made of stainless steel and available only in a 9-mm diameter, has no retrograde application. The nail is so stiff, that it cannot be directed reliably into the ec-

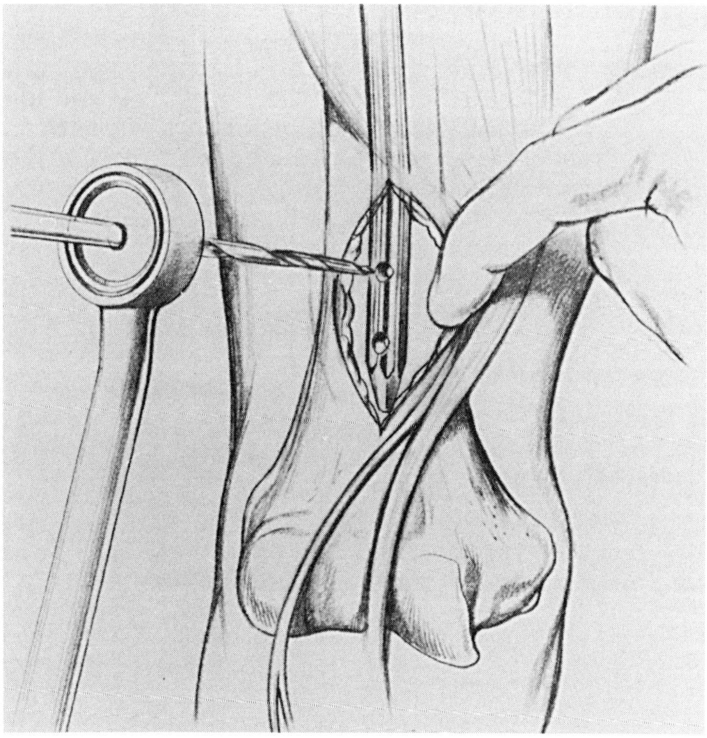

Fig. 15–9. An incision is made lateral to the biceps tendon. The only neurovascular structures in this area are cutaneous branches of the musculocutaneous nerve coursing to the lateral forearm. Care must be taken with nail insertion to orient the locking screws to this position. If the nail is internally rotated, locking screws may present on the medial side of the biceps tendon, placing the brachial artery and median nerve at risk. (Courtesy of Howmedica; Rutherford, NJ.)

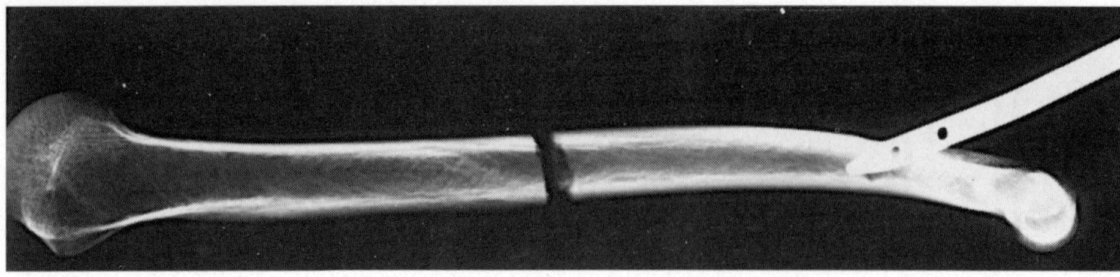

Fig. 15–10. A locked nail is inserted retrograde entering the bone eccentrically above the olecranon fossa. A sufficient intact cylinder of distal humerus must be present to guide the nail into the medullary canal of the bone. The length of the necessary cylinder depends upon the stiffness of the nail being inserted.

centric medullary canal of the bone. However, the stainless steel Russell-Taylor nail, in a 7-mm diameter is sufficiently flexible to accommodate a retrograde posterior entry portal. Nails such as the Alta and AO humeral nails are fabricated from titanium alloys. The increased flexibility of titanium makes them more amenable to a retrograde technique than a stainless steel nail of a comparable diameter.

The patient is positioned either supine with a traction device through the olecranon or in a prone position. An incision is made just proximal to the olecranon fossa. A drill is used to enter the bone of the distal humerus. The drill must be oriented proximally to allow a bevel into the dense bone of the distal humerus, entering the medullary canal obliquely to allow nail insertion. Retrograde techniques are discussed in greater detail under flexible nails.

Proximal locking of retrograde nailings can be dangerous. Posterior/anterior proximal locking at the level of the humeral neck is contraindicated to avoid damage to the main trunk of the axillary nerve. The bone of the humeral head does not allow consistent screw purchase.[18] Metal protruding through the anterior

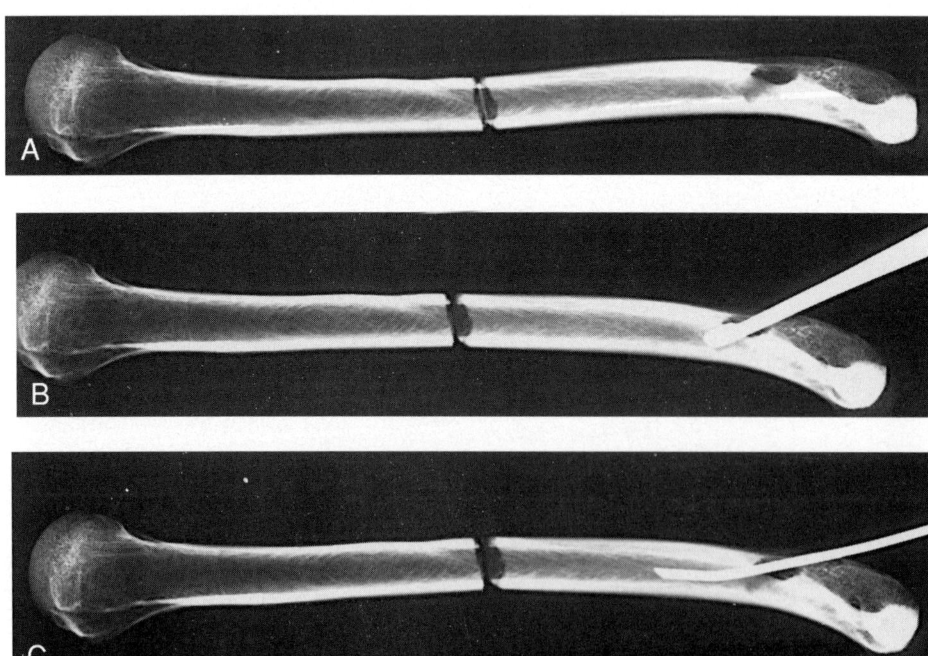

Fig. 15–11. *A,* A large drill hole is made in the posterior humerus above the olecranon fossa, beveled proximally. *B,* A curette further bevels the posterior endosteal cortex, decreasing the angle for nail insertion. *C,* A Rush nail is inserted. The nail deflects against the anterior cortex. An intact cylinder of bone above the entry drill hole is necessary to guide the nail proximally. *(Figure continues)*

or posterior humeral head can block shoulder motion or enter the joint with rotation, possibly causing articular damage.

Flexible Nails: Surgical Technique

Flexible nails depend on three-point fixation. Two or more curved flexible nails are necessary to achieve adequate stability of the bone and a functional brace is frequently needed for additional support. Because the nails are malleable, and three-point fixation is needed, a nonlinear entry portal is advisable. Nails can be inserted antegrade through drill holes in the greater tuberosity or retrograde through a hole above the olecranon fossa.

We prefer that the patient be positioned prone for retrograde nailing. A large drill hole, beveled proximally is made above the olecranon fossa (Fig. 15–11). A curette is used to bevel

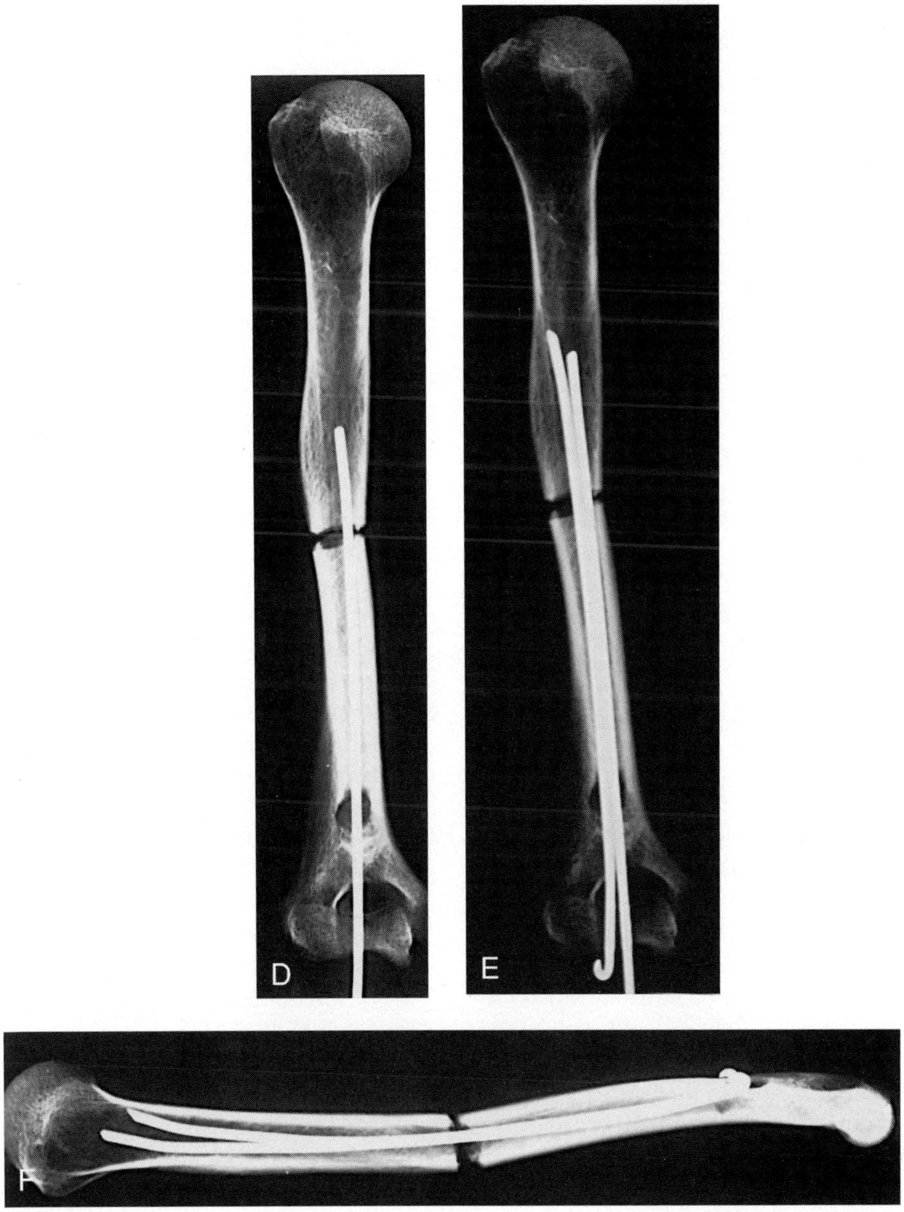

Fig. 15–11. *(continued) D,* The first nail is inserted until it just crosses the fracture site.The nail is not advanced beyond this point as it could cross the canal and block the introduction of a second nail. *E,* The second nail is introduced to a similar depth, and each is sequentially tapped into the proximal humerus. *F,* The fixation is complete. Two divergent nails have entered the canal of the bone and the hooks of the rush nails are lying against the proximal edge of the entry drill hole.

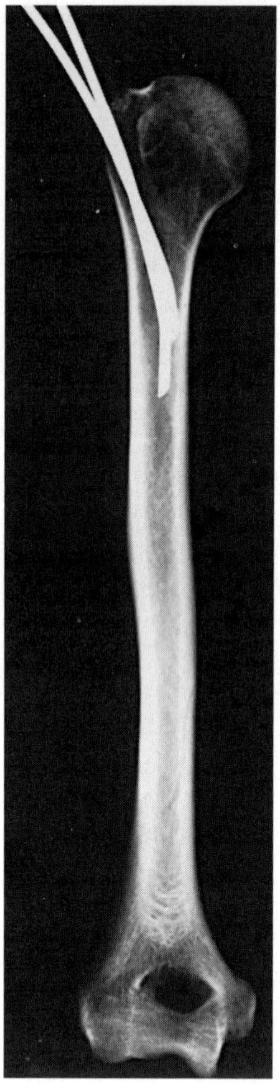

Fig. 15–12. Two flexible nails have been inserted through the greater tuberosity deflecting against an intact cylinder of upper humerus. Nails are driven sequentially into the canal to avoid one nail blocking the canal, preventing advancement of the second.

the posterior endosteal cortex and a Rush nail is inserted. Note the apex anterior bend that is applied. An intact cuff of distal humerus as indicated, is needed to guide the nail proximally. The first nail is inserted until it crosses the fracture site. The nail should not be inserted completely, as the curve of the nail can cross the medullary canal and block insertion of the second nail. The second nail is inserted to a similar depth. The nails are sequentially tapped until the hooks of the Rush rods engage the posterior cortex. If Hackenhal or Ender nails are inserted, they can either be left protruding outside the hole in the posterior distal humerus or can be bent into the canal distal to the insertion hole. Nails left prominent can irritate the triceps. Nails bent into the distal canal can be very difficult to remove.

For antegrade insertion, the patient is positioned supine, as described for antegrade locked nailing. An incision lateral to the acromion is made spreading the deltoid exposing the greater tuberosity. Either single drill holes or an awl is used to open the bone of the greater tuberosity. First one curved flexible nail (Fig. 15–12) is inserted until it crosses the fracture site and enters the distal fragment. Because the canal tapers, nails can become incarcerated distally. For this reason a second nail is inserted prior to complete impaction of the first nail, similar to the retrograde technique.

Proximal Shaft and Humeral Neck Fractures

There are many intramedullary techniques for proximal humeral fractures, but there are few reported series. Nails straight in the AP plane do not require a cuff of intact proximal humerus, and, therefore, are more applicable to the upper humerus. The Seidel nail, for example, requires only a cuff of medial calcar of bone remaining on the proximal fragment (Fig. 15–13).

Flexible or apex medial bent nails, inserted through the greater tuberosity, require an intact cuff of bone, or fractures can be tipped into varus (Fig. 15–14). Locked bent humeral nails, therefore, have little utility for humeral neck fractures. Flexible nails inserted through the greater tuberosity often require ancillary tension bands wiring of the greater tuberosity to the shaft to prevent varus, obviating the advantages of closed intramedullary nailing techniques.

The bone of humeral head does not accommodate screw purchase well. The Mouradian nail, for example, requires that screws purchase in the soft bone of the proximal humerus, precluding its utility in other than young patients with hard bone. The Mouradian nail is, further, inserted through the greater tuberosity, potentially fragmenting the lateral cortex.

The investigators use the Hackethal technique for humeral neck fractures. The difference between Hackethal's and Ender's or Rush's techniques lies in the number and diameter of nails inserted. The investigators use multiple 2-mm, 12-inch long Kirschner wires. The principle of the Hackethal technique is to fill the medullary canal with multiple wires. This is a

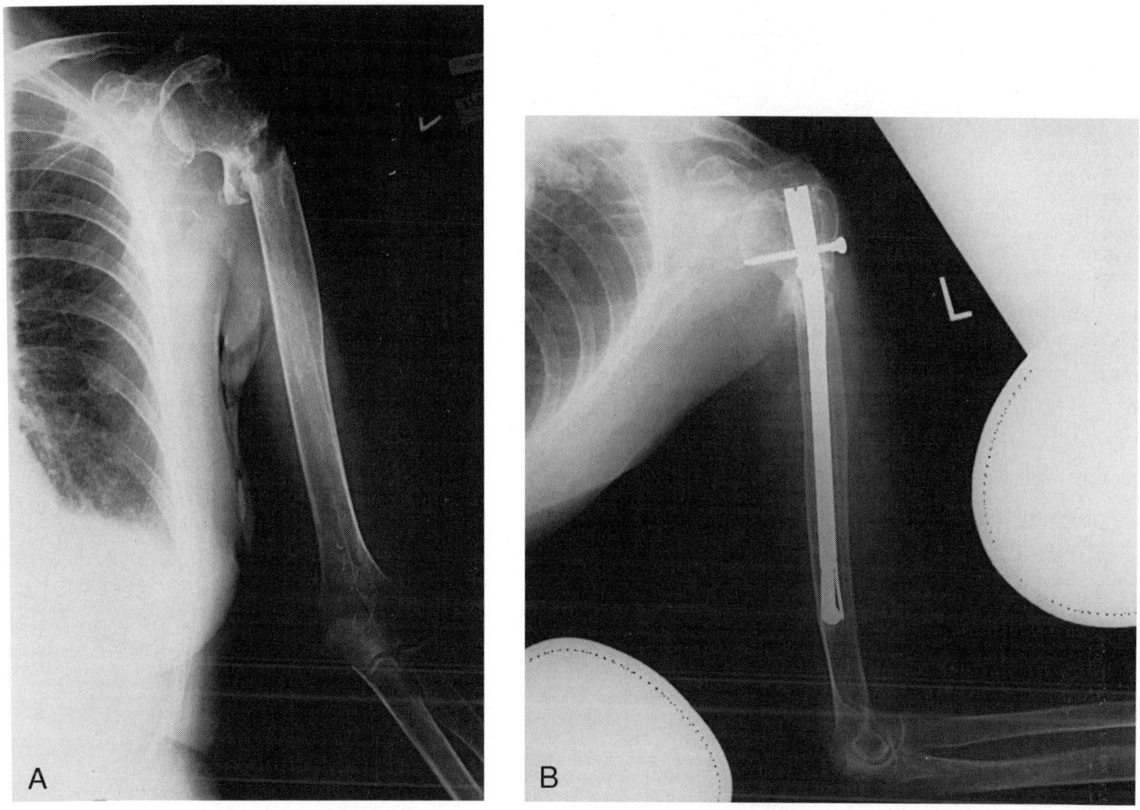

Fig. 15–13. *A,* AP radiograph of a proximal humeral nonunion. Note the varus positioning of the proximal fragment. An intact "calcar" of medial humeral neck is present. A straight nail can correct this deformity. *B,* Postoperative radiograph showing that a straight nail, through a standard entry portal, has straightened the nonunion. The intact medial calcar is used to gain purchase with proximal locking screws.

more demanding technique for diaphyseal fractures than either Rush or Ender nails but is without clinical benefits. However, it is a far superior technique for humeral neck fractures, because it allows the delivery of multiple nails diverging into the humeral head.

The identical entry portal for retrograde flexible nailing is used. Multiple nails are bent in divergent directions and driven into the humeral head. A critical point is to avoid penetration of the nails through the bone of the upper humerus (Fig. 15–15). If, under fluoroscopy over-penetration is seen, the involved nails should be removed and repositioned and not simply retracted. Hackethal nails are very thin and tend to move within the canal. Once a track through the humeral head is made, nails can migrate proximally while the fracture line settles allowing for late shoulder penetration. It is imperative, especially with a prone patient, using the retrograde technique that the surgeon be cognizant of the anatomy of the main trunk of the axillary nerve. Every attempt should be made to perform closed reduction on the fracture prior to inserting the first nail. An exposure to openly reduce a humeral neck fracture from posterior brings the surgical exposure perpendicular to the axillary nerve.

Retrograde locked nails can also be used for humeral neck fractures. Care must be taken, again, to avoid the main trunk of the axillary nerve as it courses along the back of the humeral neck with locking screw or open reduction techniques. Protrusion of screws behind the head of the humerus, further, might be difficult to visualize under fluoroscopy. These can enter the shoulder joint with rotation, damaging articular cartilage. The Seidel nail is too stiff to be inserted retrograde, and there is no alternative self-locking nail available.

A second generation, 8-mm Seidel nail is currently under early clinical evaluation. It is a straight nail that allows two screws to enter obliquely upward into the substance of the

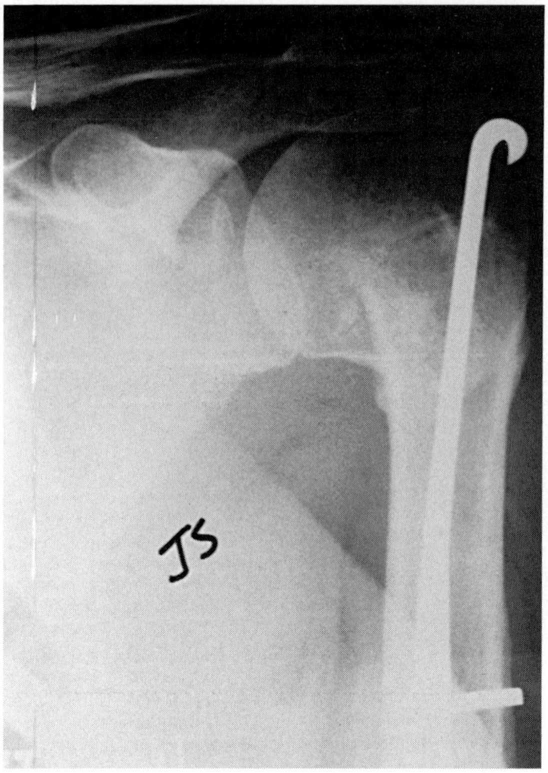

Fig. 15–14. A humeral neck fracture has been repaired by a flexible nail inserted through the greater tuberosity. The nail has tipped the fracture into varus. An alternative would be the use of flexible nails with tension band wiring holding the greater tuberosity to the humeral shaft. This exposure would obviate many of the advantages of closed nailing.

humeral head. To avoid some of the difficulties of the soft bone of the humeral head, screws purchase in the nail itself. The same nail, because it is straight, can be turned 180° in order to have one screw oriented obliquely downwards, obviating the necessity for a second inventory. Distal locking is accomplished with a modified Seidel technique. Experience with this implant is currently limited (Fig. 15–16).

Distal Humeral Fractures

Fractures within the last 4 cm of the humeral canal have not been generally considered amenable to intramedullary nailing techniques. Antegrade flexible nails can migrate proximally losing fixation. Fractures can toggle, making screw locking difficult. There is a risk of displacing cortical cracks. The Seidel nail has been particularly useful for these fractures, provided the canal diameter is adequate. Intramedullary nailing of very distal humeral fractures should be reserved for experienced surgeons. The internal distal locking mechanism applies gentle pressure to the endosteum. The investigators have stabilized fractures where only half the length of the distal spreading mechanism has crossed the fracture site (Fig. 15–17). Preoperative planning is critical to

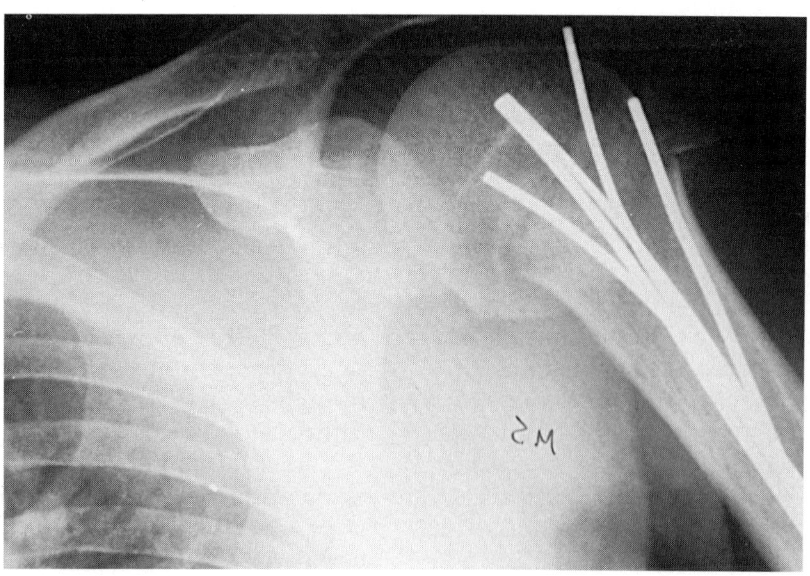

Fig. 15–15. A humeral neck fracture is repaired by multiple diverging fine Kirschner wires (Hackethal technique). Note the nail protruding above the humeral head. This was noted intraoperatively and the nail was retracted. As the fracture settled, however, the nail migrated proximally again. When nails are seen protruding above the humeral head, they should be removed and replaced to avoid proximal migration through a tract.

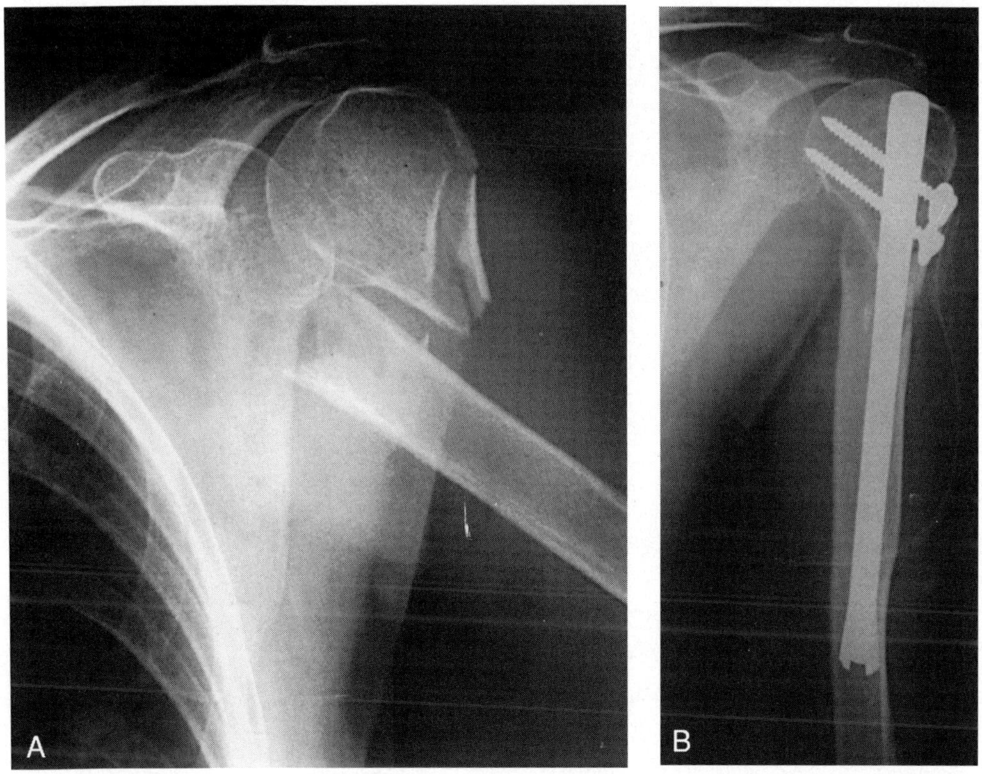

Fig. 15–16. *A,* AP radiograph of a displaced surgical neck fracture. *B,* A "second generation" straight Seidel humeral nail has been inserted with upward screws. The same nail can be rotated 180° allowing the screws to be oriented downward. Experience with this nail is preliminary at the time of this writing. (Courtesy of Dr. Gilbert Tagelund; Strasbourg, France)

select nail length and determine that an adequate distal diameter is present for nail insertion.

CLINICAL RESULTS OF INTRAMEDULLARY NAILING OF THE HUMERUS

For intramedullary nailing of the humerus to have a role, there must be clinical advantages over plate fixation. Plates have union rates approaching 100%,[1,3–5,19] which are not seen with intramedullary nail techniques. The advantages of intramedullary nail fixation are minimal dissection, load bearing, including the ability to use crutches or bed-to-chair transfers, and the fixation of comminuted and very proximal and distal fractures.

Flexible Nails

When indicated, flexible nails have an acceptable rate of union, approaching 95%. Infection rates are low. Ultimate shoulder function is rarely a concern, though shoulder motion recovery requires up to 5 months. They are useful for mildly comminuted fractures which often require a brace for support.

Flexible nails tend to back out of the bone. With an antegrade technique, this can cause shoulder irritation requiring premature removal or necessitating an inconvenient metal removal post union. Retrograde migrating nails can irritate the triceps and the supracondylar entry portal can fracture. Migrating nails, further, can back out across the fracture site losing reduction.[2,7,20]

RESULTS OF LOCKED INTRAMEDULLARY NAILING

There are few reports of clinical results following locked intramedullary nailing of humeral diaphyseal fractures. The investigators initially reported, along with several others,

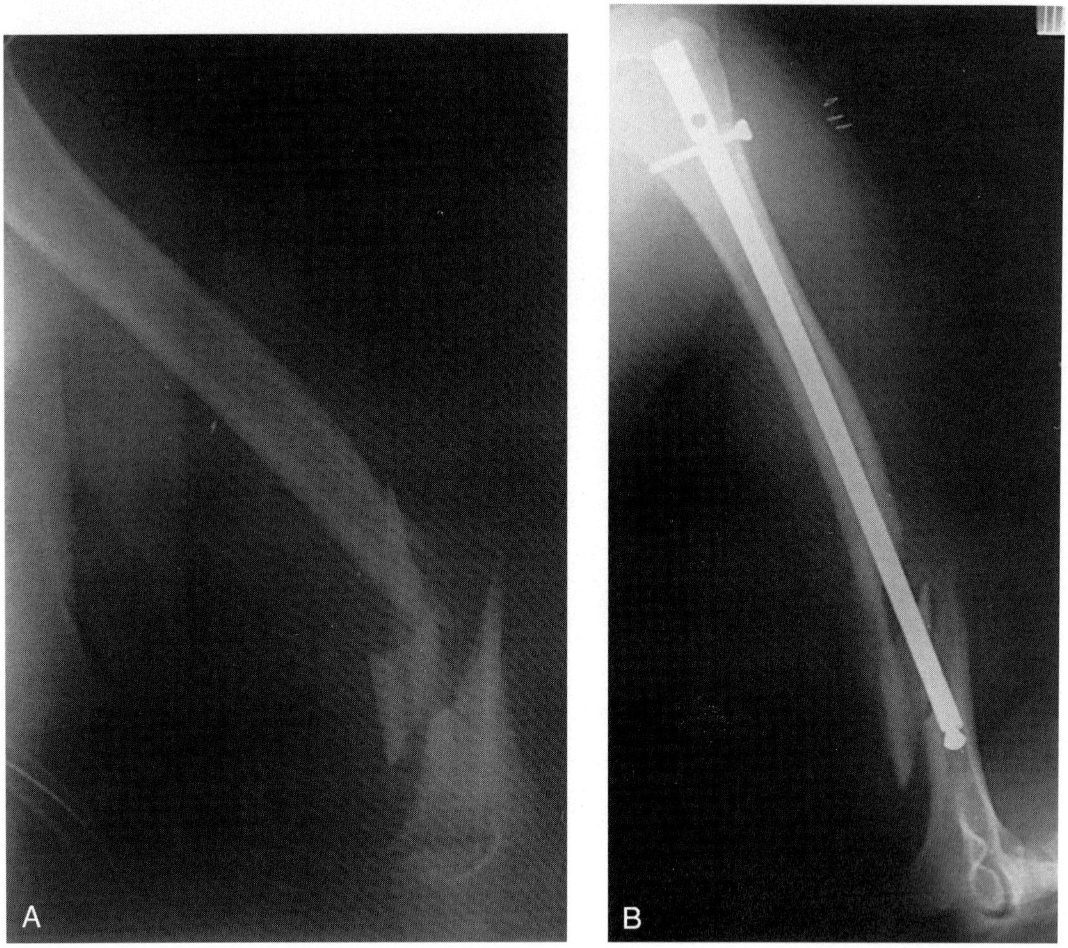

Fig. 15–17. *A*, Preoperative radiograph of a comminuted distal humerus fracture in a 6 foot 10 inch polytrauma patient. *B*, Two weeks post fixation. The longest Seidel nail available has been inserted. Note that only half the distal spreading mechanism has entered the distal fragment. The spreading screw has begun to loosen. *(Figure continues)*

success using the Seidel nail to treat acute fractures of the humerus. There were no infections. Union rates were high.[15,21,22] However, further experience demonstrated complications not originally seen, particularly when Seidel nail insertion required reaming.[6,23] The Seidel nail is available, at this time in only a 9-mm diameter. Insertion of the nail into a narrower canal obviously requires reaming. When reaming was required, significant complications were encountered.

We retrospectively grouped our patients into those with radiographic canal diameters of less than or equal to 9 mm and greater than or equal to 10 mm without regard to radiographic magnification. Body habitus did not correlate with canal diameter. When the Seidel nails were inserted into bones of narrow canal diameter (less than or equal to 9 mm), a 58% complication rate of infection, nonunion, and iatrogenic comminution jeopardizing distal fixation was encountered. When the same nail was inserted into humeri with canal diameters of greater than or equal to 10 mm, only one minor complication was encountered.

We believe that this was caused by reaming. In each case in the narrow canal diameter group reaming was difficult, generating significant heat and requiring cleaning every few millimeters to advance down the canal of the bone. All nails destroy the endosteal blood supply of bone; reaming, in particular excessive reaming, damages the endosteal architecture and prevents revascularization. This can lead to infection and nonunions (Fig. 15–18). Furthermore, reaming thins the cortex, potentially leading to

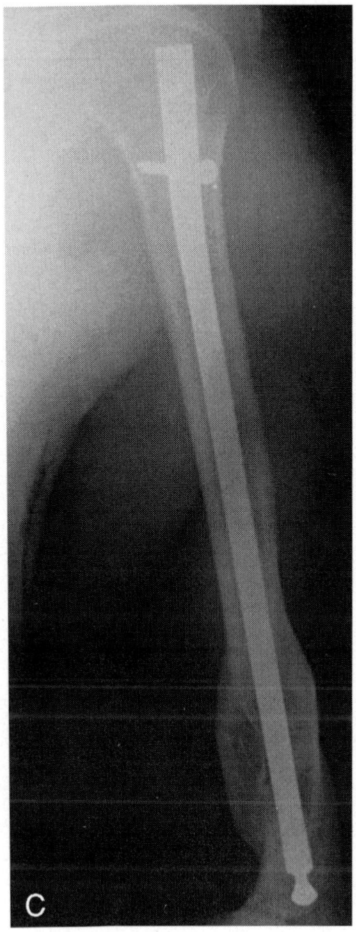

Fig. 15–17. *(continued) C,* The fracture has united in spite of loosening the distal screw lock.

iatrogenic comminution with the insertion of a stiff nail (Fig. 15–19). Whenever possible, nails should be inserted without first reaming the humerus with power tools. Sounding the canal with a hand tool or reamer will not significantly alter union or infection rates or propagate iatrogenic comminution.

Russell has reported consistently excellent results.[16] The Russell-Taylor nail is available in a variety of diameters, so most of these nails can be inserted without reaming. Because this is an apex-medial bent nail, it cannot reliably stabilize very proximal fractures and screw locking limits its distal utility. The straight Seidel nail, in contrast, can stabilize shaft fractures as well as very proximal and distal ones.

The Seidel distal spreading mechanism is seen to fail radiographically approximately 20% of the time.[6] If this mechanism radiographically fails 20% of the time, it must be loose even more frequently without being radiographically measurable. Failure of the distal spreading mechanism does not seem to relate to other complications such as nonunion or infection. This calls into question whether distal locking or an interference fit in the narrowing distal canal is necessary.

Shoulder Motion

Whether an articular or greater tuberosity entry portal is used for antegrade medullary humeral nailing, an adequate return of shoulder function can be anticipated, provided aggressive rehabilitation is employed. Shoulder motion and the rate of return have not been well studied with functional bracing or plate techniques. The anterior acromial approach, the preferred technique for antegrade insertion of straight (in the AP plane) nails, violates the shoulder joint, rotator cuff, and the lateral articular cartilage. Apex-medial bent locked nails[16] and flexible nails inserted through the greater tuberosity, do not violate the shoulder. Similar shoulder function, has been observed with each technique.[12] Minor deficiencies in ultimate shoulder motion without clinical significance have been seen. The rate of return of shoulder function with locked or flexible intramedullary nailing has varied between immediate return and return after 6 months. In our series with the Seidel nail, the average interval to plateau of shoulder function was 17 weeks. Similar findings have been noted with locked or flexible nails inserted through the greater tuberosity, without violating the shoulder.[20] This clearly, therefore, is not caused by violation of the rotator cuff but is caused either by the original trauma or the slight motion seen with all current nails. The same may be true with functional bracing or plate fixation but has not, as yet, been examined.

The key to any antegrade nail insertion involves either using an extraarticular entry portal or decompressing the shoulder by transecting the coracoacromial ligament (Blasier, personal communication).[12,17] In the originally described Seidel technique, nails were inserted lateral to the coracoacromial ligament. This did not allow linear access to the medullary canal. For a nail to gain access to the medullary canal, it required levering against the lateral fibers of the coracoacromial ligament, tearing the lateral aspect of the ligament, and potentially causing inflam-

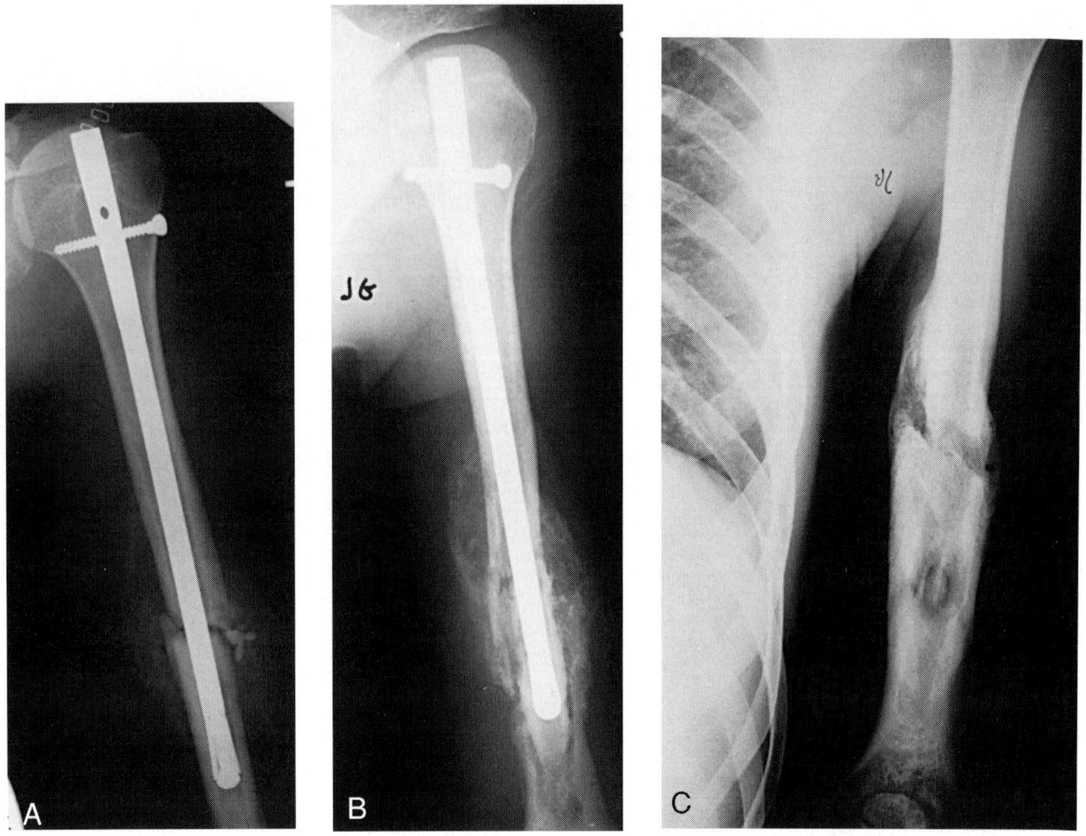

Fig. 15–18. Two weeks post Seidel fixation of a grade II open transverse fracture, periosteal callus has begun to form. Insertion of this nail required reaming. Note the canal measurement is less than the diameter of the nail. Reaming was difficult. *B,C,* The fracture became infected but has united with significant periosteal reaction and near separation of the bone of the distal humeral shaft from the metaphysis. Following metal removal, a sequestrum was identified in the distal canal. Control of this infection required multiple debridements and sequestrectomies.

mation and impingement. A 50% rate of permanent shoulder stiffness was observed with this technique.[23] With transection of the coracoacromial ligament, a 95% rate of excellent shoulder function has been reported. The factors that most likely jeopardize ultimate shoulder function are traumatic or iatrogenic neurologic injuries, not surgical technique.[12,17]

Our early experience with the Seidel nail involved fragile insertion equipment that has now been redesigned. Faulty equipment sometimes forced us to allow nails to remain above the level of the humeral head, protruding through the substance of the rotator cuff. Other authors have noted the same complication caused by technical or equipment errors. If patients can tolerate the impingement while the nails are in place, shoulder motion will reliably return following metal removal. Only if patients are significantly uncomfortable should the nail be exchanged or driven deeper into the substance of the humeral head.

Infections

There is little experience and few publications on treating infected humeri following intramedullary nailing. This is a particular concern, as the upper end of the nail enters the shoulder joint and there is a potential for proximal migration of infected material. Removal of an infected implant through to the shoulder joint can track debris into the shoulder. We have treated only 5 infected humeral nailings, and none had secondarily infected the shoulder. This is not an adequate experience to be

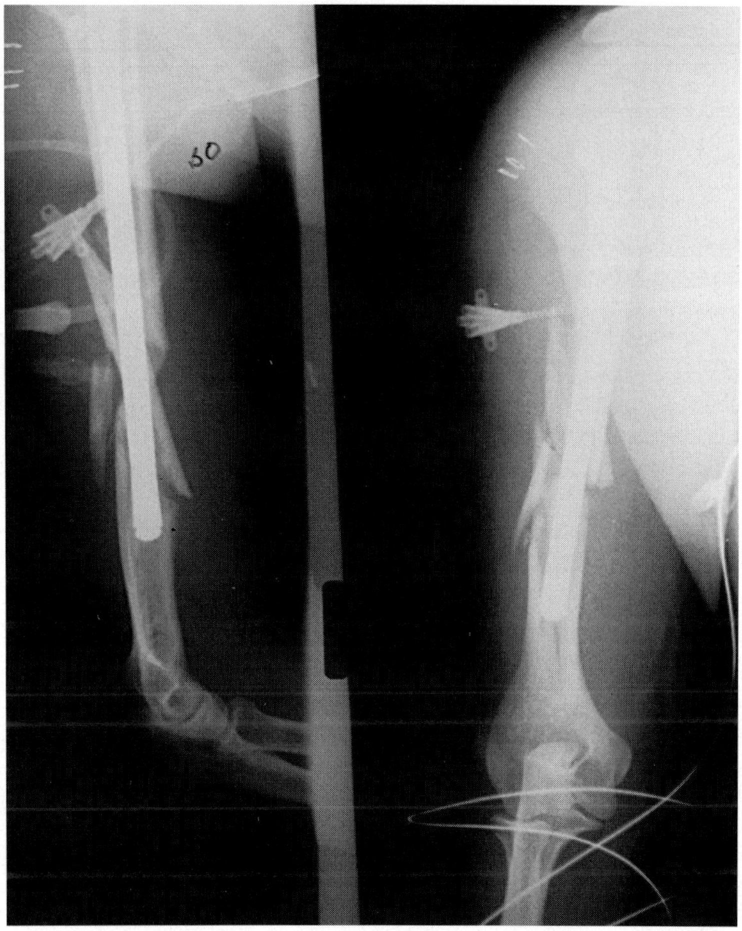

Fig. 15–19. A Seidel nail has been inserted into a comminuted fracture in a thin female blunt polytrauma patient. Reaming the distal fragment was difficult. Upon nail insertion, the bone split beyond the tip on the nail. The fracture was maintained in a brace until union.

certain that the shoulder will not be at risk. Intramedullary nails should be used with caution in fractures that are at high risk for septic complications.

Geriatric Patients

Humeral fractures in the geriatric population, especially in elderly women, pose particular difficulties. Pendulous breasts deform the humerus into varus. Obesity and loose skin turgor make brace fitting difficult and soft bone can make fixation precarious. The Seidel nail has been particularly helpful in this population. The medullary canal is generally wide and nail insertion does not require reaming. Driving the nail through soft cancellous bone impacts sufficient bone into the end of the nail so that with spreading, the distal locking mechanism holds well. Proximal cross-locking screws must be drilled under fluoroscopic control to prevent over penetration with drill points.

Pathologic Fractures

Like geriatric patients, most cancer patients are elderly with soft, wide bone. The immediate goal is stabilization and ambulation on crutches. A slow return of shoulder function is not a great clinical concern. Humeral nails, the Seidel nail in particular, is ideal for this population. Patients are very comfortable immediately following surgery. They are able to use their arms for daily function in the immediate

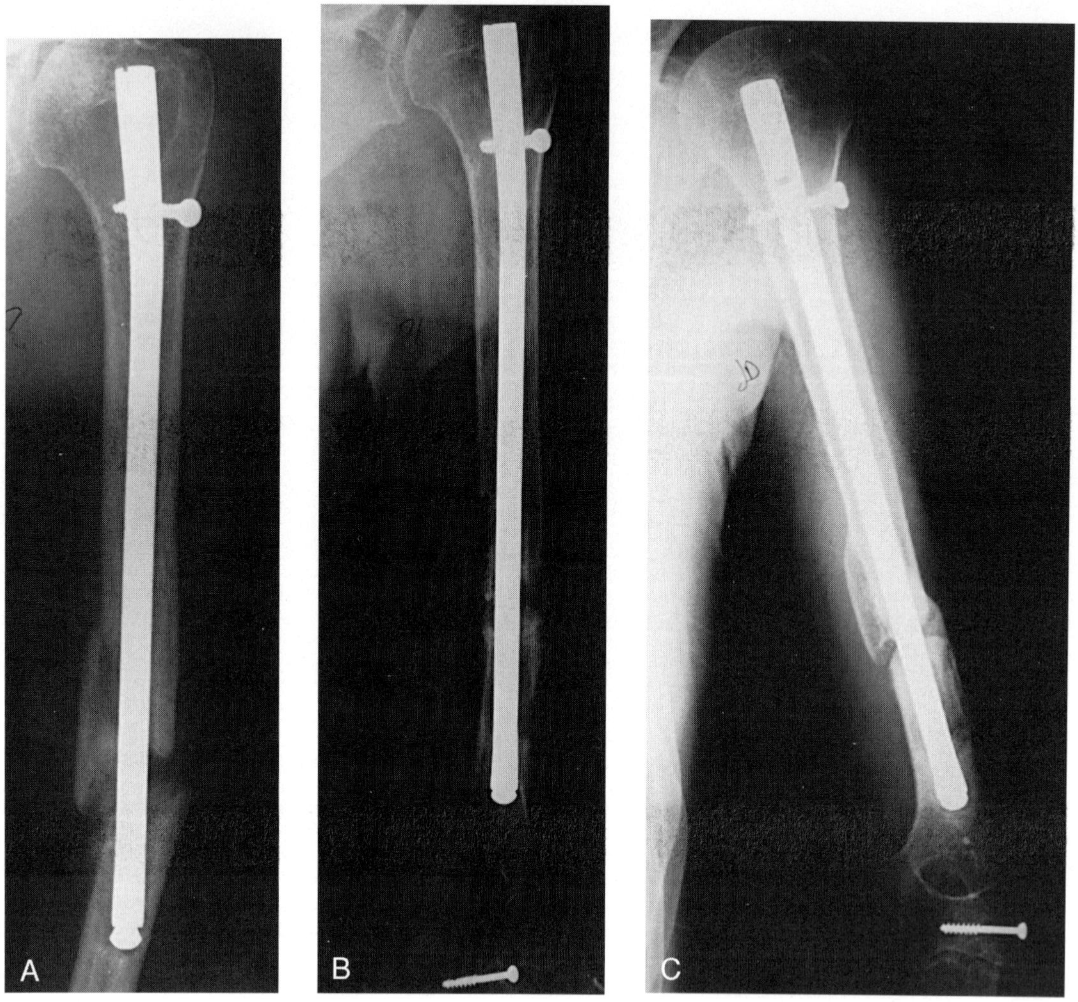

Fig. 15–20. *A,* (Follow-up radiograph of the patient in Fig. 15–2.) A nonunion of the humerus has developed. Note the degree of bony erosion in the distal canal, making further surgery precarious. *B,* An exchange nailing has been performed. The fracture still has not united. Even in the osteopenic bone of a nonunion, reaming of the distal fragment was difficult. *C,* An open bone graft has been performed following unsuccessful exchange nailing and the fracture has united.

postoperative period with no external support.

Nonunions Following Intramedullary Nails

As interest in intramedullary nailing has increased, difficulties have been encountered treating the failures of intramedullary nailing. Unlike the tibia and femur, exchange nailings alone do not seem to be sufficient. Bone grafting or plate fixation is required. When an exchange nailing of the humerus is performed, subjectively, there is not the same grinding of endosteal bone that might act as a bone graft. The bone instead is hard. Loose intramedullary fixation the Seidel nail in particular erodes significant bone, making reconstructions precarious (Fig. 15–20).

CONCLUSION

For intramedullary nailing of the humerus to have a role, it must compete with the results of plates. Shoulder motion, with proper technique, is a minor concern. Distal, proximal, and comminuted humeral fractures with adequate bone stock for locking are well managed by intramedullary techniques. Simple-geometry, midshaft fractures requiring surgery in patients who do not require humeral weight bearing, may be optimally treated by plates. Reaming should be avoided.

Closed nailing techniques should be employed whenever possible. Any patient with any neurologic injury who requires intramedullary nailing, should have a nerve exploration. The Holstein-Lewis fracture is an indication for nerve exploration prior to nailing, even without radial nerve symptoms.

REFERENCES

1. Bell, M.J., Beauchamp, C.G., Kellam, J.K., McMurtry, R.Y.: The results of plating humeral shaft fractures in patients with multiple injuries: The Sunnybrook experience. J. Bone Joint Surg. *67B*:293–296, 1985.
2. Brumback, R.J., Bosse, M.J., Poka, A., Burgess, A.R.: Intramedullary stabilization of humeral shaft fractures in patients with multiple trauma. J. Bone Joint Surg. *68A*: 960–970, 1986.
3. Dabezies, E.J., Banta, C.J. II, Murphy, C.P., D'Ambrosia, R.D.: Plate fixation of humeral shaft for acute fractures, with and without radial nerve injuries. J. Orthop. Trauma *6*:10–13, 1992.
4. Dameron, T.B. Jr, Grubb, S. A.: Humeral shaft fractures in adults. South. Med. J. *74*:1461–1467, 1981.
5. Vander Griend, R., Tomasin, J., Ward, E. F.: Open reduction and internal fixation of humeral shaft fractures: Results using AO plating techniques. J. Bone Joint Surg. *68A*:430–433, 1986.
6. Riemer, B.L., Foglesong, M.E., Burke, C.J. III., Butterfield, S.L.: Complications of Seidel intramedullary nailing of narrow diameter humeral diaphyseal fractures. Orthopedics *17*:19–29, 1994.
7. Henley, M.B., Chapman, J.R., Claudi, B.F.: Closed retrograde Hackethal nail stabilization of humeral shaft fractures. J. Orthop. Trauma *6*:18–24, 1992.
8. Lehmann, M., Kirschner, P.: Elastic intramedullary nailing in the treatment of fractures of the humerus Presented at the American Academy of Orthopaedic Surgeons, Annual Meeting, February 20–25, 1992, Washington, DC.
9. Bostman, O., Bakalim, G., Vainionpaa, S., et al.: Immediate radial nerve palsy complicating fracture of the shaft of the humerus: When is early exploration justified? Injury *16*:499–502, 1985.
10. Holstein, A., Lewis, G.B.: Fractures of the humerus with radial nerve paralysis. J. Bone Joint Surg. *45A*: 1382–1388, 1963.
11. Pollock, F.H., Drake, D., Bovill, E.G., et al.: Treatment of radial neuropathy associated with fractures of the humerus. J. Bone Joint Surg. *63A*:239–243, 1981.
12. Riemer, B.L., D'Ambrosia, R.: The risk of injury to the axillary nerve, artery, and vein from proximal locking screws of humeral intramedullary nails. Orthopedics *15*:697–699, 1992.
13. Henley, M.B., Monroe, M., Tencer, A.F.: Biomechanical comparison of methods of fixation of a midshaft osteotomy of the humerus. J. Orthop. Trauma *5*:14–20, 1991.
14. Kellam, J., Beverland, D., Broskhuyse, H., et al: The anatomy and biomechanics of locked humeral nails Presented at the Orthopaedic Trauma Association Sixth Annual Meeting combined with the Canadian Orthopaedic Association Trauma Symposium Toronto, Ontario, Canada, 1990.
15. Riemer, B.L., Butterfield, S.L., D'Ambrosia, R., Kellam, J.: Seidel intramedullary nailing of humeral diaphyseal fractures: A preliminary report. Orthopedics *14*: 239–246, 1991.
16. Russell, T.A., Simard, J., Taylor, J.C., et al.: Interlocking intramedullary nailing of humeral shaft fractures. Orthop. Trans. *16*:334, 1992.
17. Riemer, B.L., D'Ambrosia, R., Kellam, F.J., Butterfield, S.L., Burke, C.J. III.: The anterior acromial approach for antegrade intramedullary nailing of the humeral diaphysis. Orthopedics *16*:1219–1223, 1993.
18. Ingman, A.M., Waters, D.A.: Locked intramedullary nailing of humeral shaft fractures. Implant design, surgical technique, and clinical results. J. Bone Joint Surg. *76B*:23–29, 1994.
19. Foster, R.J., Dixon, G.L. Jr., Bach, A.W., Appleyard, R.W., Green, T.M.: Internal fixation of fractures and nonunions of humeral shaft: Indications and results in a multi-center study. J. Bone Joint Surg. *67A*:857–864, 1985.
20. Hall, R.F., Pankovich, A.M.: Ender nailing of acute fractures of the humerus. A study of closed fixation by intramedullary nails without reaming. J. Bone Joint Surg. *69A*:558–567, 1987.
21. Haberneck, H., Orthner, E.: A locking nail for fractures of the humerus. J. Bone Joint Surg. *73B*:651–653, 1991.
22. Seidel, H.: Humeral locking nail: A preliminary report. Orthopedics *12*:219–226, 1989.
23. Robinson, C.M., Bell, K.M., Court-Brown, C.M., McQueen, M.M.: Locked nailing of humeral shaft fractures. J. Bone Joint Surg. *74B*:558–562, 1992.

16

Intramedullary Nailing of the Forearm

Daniel M. Zinar, Dana Street, and Mark Wolgin

The concept of an implant traversing the full length of the medullary canal was used in the forearm before it was used in the femur. Schöne employed silver rods in both the radius and ulna in 1913.[1] Other early investigators of intramedullary nailing of the forearm were the Belgian group of Lambotte, Danis, and Joly.[2] Steinmann pins were initially used and their use was reported again by Lambrinudi and Dickson in the 1940s.[3,4] Larger pins were used by Rush in the late 1930s, [5,6] followed by the use of even larger nails by Küntscher and Böhler in the early 1940s.[7–9]

Treatment with Kirschner wires had advantages over plating in terms of less surgical trauma, shorter operative times, and a smaller residual scar. However, the resulting nonunion rates of 17% were unacceptably high; nonunion resulted from too flexible an implant and an inability to fill the canal, which allowed shortening and rotation in certain fractures. A trend toward larger and stronger nails began first with threaded 3-mm Steinmann pins followed by 4- and 5-mm U-shaped Küntscher nails.[10] The larger nails could not be inserted at the radial styloid as the more flexible smaller nails had been; so an insertion point at Lister's tubercle was used, as recommended by Küntscher and Böhler.[11] The change in insertion point created problems with rupture of the extensor pollicis longus tendon. In addition, the Küntscher nails often distracted and bound tightly in both fracture fragments and were prone to breakage.

Rush rods of both ⅛-inch (3-mm) and ³⁄₁₆-inch (4.5-mm) were used, but frequent problems still arose concerning backing out of the nails and lack of rotational control that resulted in high nonunion rates.[12] In 1954, the Street nail was developed in an attempt to improve rotational control (Fig. 16–1). A square pattern was used similar to Schneider's principle of a square nail in a reamed canal (Fig. 16–2).[13–15,26] Experimental testing of the holding power revealed that a bite of 0.005 inch of the corners into the cortex of bone would control 14 foot-pounds of torque per linear inch of canal length. Essential to the success of this technique is the use of a correlated nail and reamer size to give this amount of bite to avoid incarceration or splitting of the distal fracture fragment. This nail design was used predominantly in all our clinical studies that were performed until 1984. Sage introduced his triangular nail that helped control rotation, and in 1959 he reported a nonunion rate of 6.2% in 81 fractures.[16] Marek, using the von Saal square nail[55,56] reported no nonunions or infections in 32 of 35 patients in 1961.[18] The Schneider forearm nail with four flutes produced healing in all but 6.4% of 125 fractures treated without bone grafting, as reported by Cotler in 1971.[19]

In 1984, Tibone modified the Street nail by using a titanium alloy instead of stainless steel, providing greater flexibility and increased fatigue strength to the new implant. In addition, the male stud on the driving end was modified to a female end, permitting flush seating of the

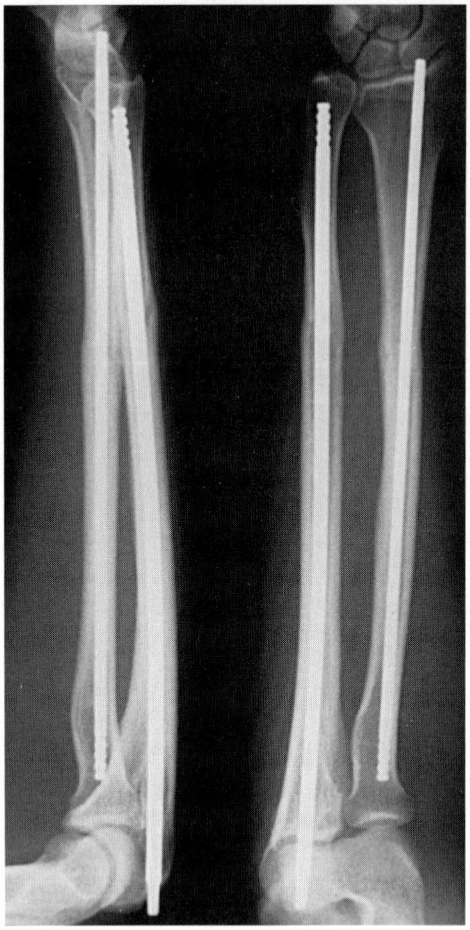

Fig. 16–1. The 3-mm Street square nail used in the radius and the 4-mm Street nail used in the ulna. Note self-broaching distal end and threaded proximal end with male stud.

Table 16–1. History of forearm nailing

Author	*Union Rate (%)*
Smith/Sage (1957)	79
Sage (1959)	93
Marek (1961)	100
Cotler (1971)	93
Street (1986)	93
Zinar (1992)	97

nail to minimize local mechanical irritation from the tip of the nail at the wrist or elbow. Intramedullary reamers were also modified to minimize problems with breakage or cortical penetration. Minimal clinical experience was reported with this nail.[20]

In 1988, the square nail was further modified by enlarging the proximal end of the nail to allow for improvements in the nail driver (Fig. 16–3). A titanium material was continued for the implant, but the reamers were again modified to a side-cutting design with a blunt tip to minimize cortical perforation. Some problems with driver stud breakage were noted with this nail system. As improvement in rotational control was gained with square nailing, clinical results improved. Table 16–1 summarizes the results of forearm nailing over the past four decades.

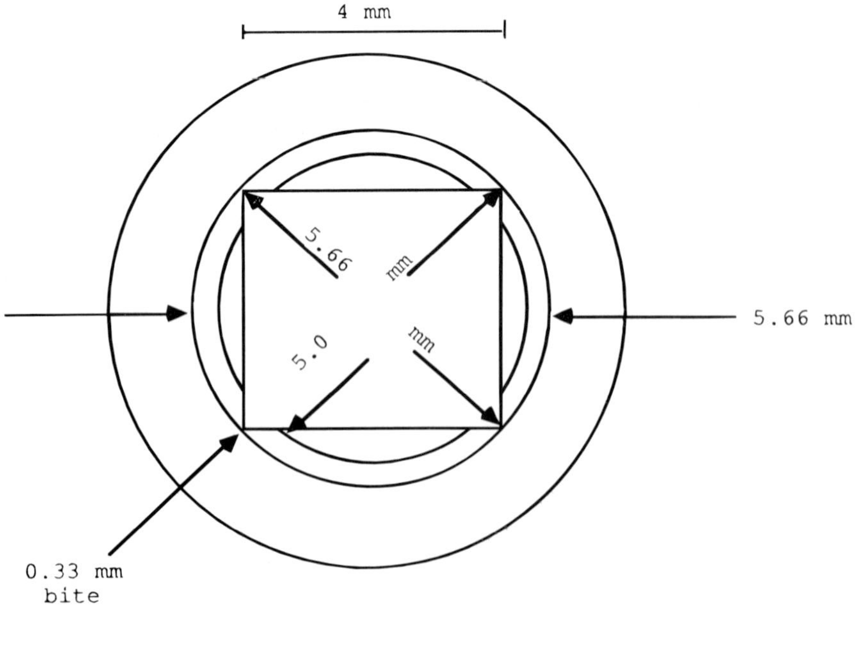

Fig. 16–2. Diameter of reamed hole vs. diameter of 4-mm nail: outer circle equals full nail diameter, inner circle equals reamer diameter. The 0.33-mm bite of nail corners into the cortex.

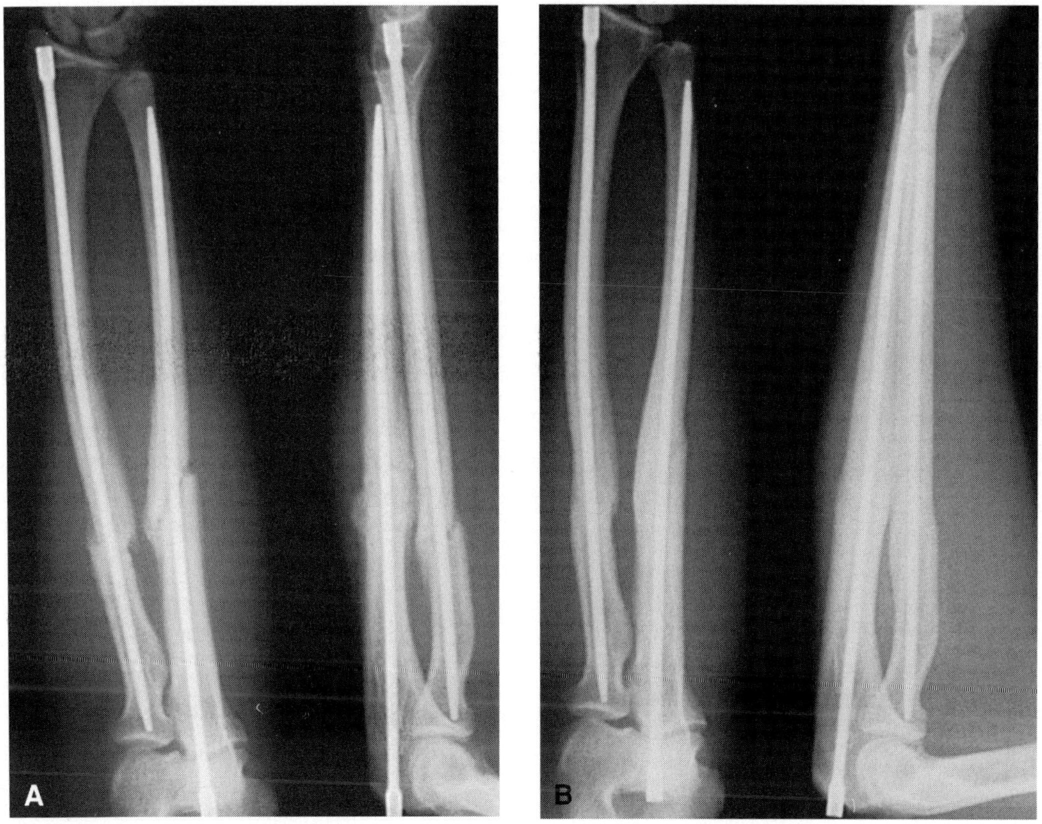

Fig. 16–3. *A,B,* Modified titanium square nail used to treat both bone forearm fracture. Recessed threads within proximal end of nail to allow for flush seating of implant.

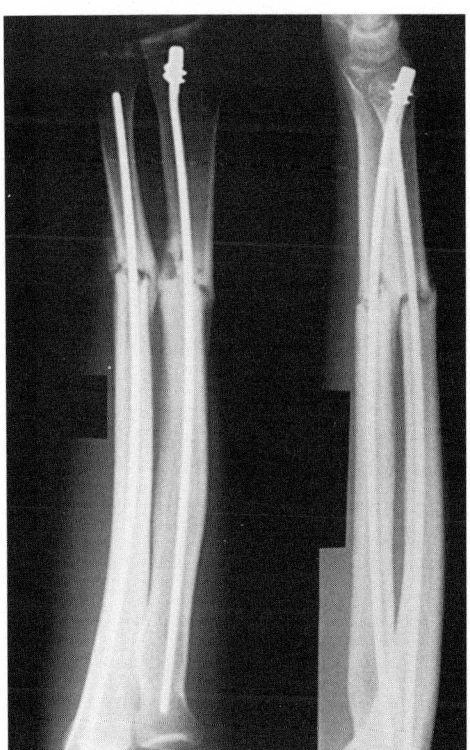

Recent developments include preliminary testing of "interlocking" forearm nails, which are similar to compression-type nails developed by Hoek in the 1960s.[21,22] Both a screw-type and interference-type interlocking mechanism are being evaluated in clinical trials (Fig. 16–4). In Europe, DePedro has reported on 20 cases of an interlocking-type nail used successfully in the ulna.[23] These nails may expand the role of forearm nailing as did the advent of interlocking nails in the femur, tibia, and humerus.

INDICATIONS FOR FOREARM NAILING

Closed Fractures

Closed fractures include any adult diaphyseal fracture of the radius and/or ulna with at least 5 cm of intact proximal or distal bone, with angulation of more than 10° or subluxation of the proximal or distal radial-ulnar joint.

Fig. 16–4. Interlocking-type of nail with interference fit of threaded-locking cap into bone at proximal end of nail.

Open Fractures

Primary intramedullary fixation can be performed in all patients with grade I, II, and IIIa [24] open fractures after initial debridement. Type IIIb and IIIc open fractures may require external fixation or plate and screw fixation because of the need for significant wound care and soft-tissue reconstruction without postoperative immobilization.

SURGICAL TECHNIQUE

In most patients, even those who have multiple injuries, the operation is recommended to be performed as soon as possible. The sooner the procedure is performed, the better the chance of success of closed nailing.

One potential advantage of forearm nailing is the ability to obtain stable internal fixation without opening the fracture site. Before the advent of image intensification in 1967, most fractures were nailed with an open technique. Some single-bone ulnae were performed blind, because they were easily palpated for alignment. The choice of open or closed technique depends on the time from injury to surgery, the degree of fracture comminution and displacement, and the experience of the surgeon. Early in our series, all nailings were done on a radiolucent arm board with the image intensifier. During the last several years we have used a modified finger-trap setup as a forearm fracture table (Fig. 16–5).

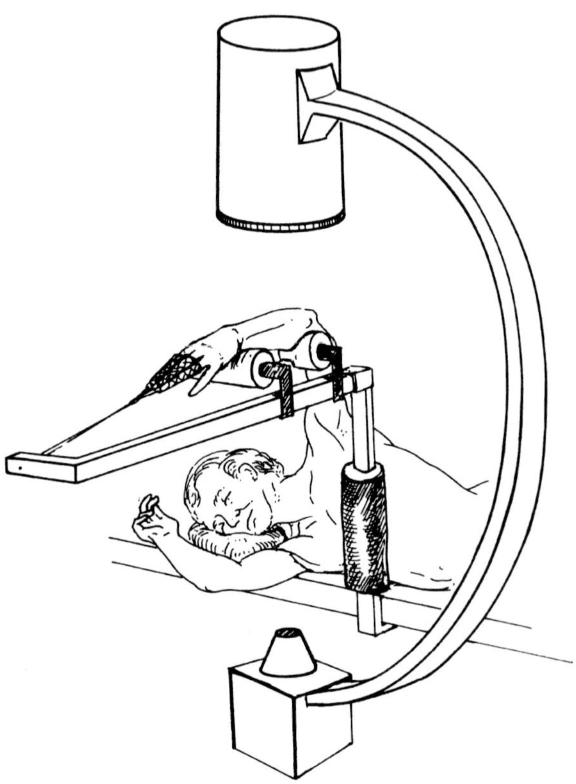

Fig. 16–5. Forearm traction fracture table designed to attach to regular operating room table with patient in lateral decubitus position.

Several companies including Zimmer, Dow Corning Wright, Biomet, Howmedica, and Applied Osteo have manufactured either a square forearm nail or a locking nail designed to provide rotational control. Each manufacturer has their own set of instruments with details of insertion specific to each. The general principles will be outlined here. Nails come in sizes ranging from 18 to 30 cm in 1- to 2-cm increments.

PREOPERATIVE PLANNING

Radiographs are reviewed to determine proper nail length and diameter. Three methods are available to determine the correct nail length: (1) measurement of the patient's intact arm with a tape from the olecranon to the ulnar styloid and then subtracting 1 cm, (2) intraoperatively taking a nail of known length and using the image intensifier against the affected bone and applying traction to keep the bone out to appropriate length, or (3) preoperatively using available radiographic templates with known magnification parameters. Because the radial head is often difficult to palpate, the radial length can also be determined by subtracting 2 cm from the ulnar length.

Proper size reamers are essential to successful nailing and must be available. The narrowest portion of the intramedullary canal may range from 2 to 7 mm. Obtaining a measurement of this diameter will determine if reaming of the medullary canal is necessary prior to rod insertion. If reaming is necessary, then over-reaming by 0.5 to 1 mm to prevent nail incarceration may be necessary in select cases. If the nail is not locked, then it must have a snug fit to provide stable fixation.

CLOSED NAILING

The surgical technique has not changed significantly since its original description by Street.[15] Either a 3- or 4-mm nail can be used, depending on the size of the intramedullary canal. If both bones are fractured, the radius is approached first. A 1.5-cm incision is made just lateral to Lister's tubercle at the distal radius. After incising the skin, the soft tissues are spread to avoid damage to neurovascular structures. The interval between the short and long radial wrist extensors is identified. Care is taken to identify the distal edge of the radius to avoid inadvertent insertion through the scaphoid. The canal is entered at the dorsal margin of the radius with a 2-mm pilot drill, with the drill bit shifting from a vertical position to a horizontal position to avoid penetration of the volar cortex. Flexion of the wrist over a stack of towels is helpful to prevent this complication.

If necessary, the canal should be overreamed by 0.5 to 1 mm to prevent rod incarceration or fracture distraction. Certain nails are prebent to conform to the natural dorso-radial bow. This may require a separate right and left nail for the radius, but not for the ulna, depending on the manufacturer. The ulnar rod may be turned 180° for either right or left arm to conform to the normal proximal lateral bow. Often, the 3-mm nails are flexible enough to conform to the radial bow without prebending the nails, but if a 4-mm nail is being used, then prebending is recommended to preserve the normal radial bow. Three millimeter nails can be prebent if desired.

Because the ulna bows toward the radius in the proximal third, the point of insertion for the ulna is toward the radial side of the olecranon, about 5 mm from the lateral cortex. It is essential to properly prepare the ulnar canal distally with the reamer to prevent distraction at the fracture site, which could lead to nonunion.

Whether open or closed nailing is performed, both fractures should be prepared before either bone can be nailed; otherwise, the stability of the nailed bone could make reduction of the other fracture difficult. When closed nailing is performed, the rotational control obtained by the hold of the nail is less mandatory than for open nailing, because of the preservation of soft-tissue attachments and the subsequent maintenance of circulation to any intermediate fracture fragments.

POSTOPERATIVE CARE

Postoperatively, the forearm is immediately placed in a bulky soft dressing that includes plaster splints that support the wrist, hand, and elbow. As soon as the swelling has decreased, a long-arm cast is applied. Stable fractures in reliable patients are immobilized for 2 weeks in a long-arm cast. Unreliable patients and/or unstable fracture patterns are continued for an additional 2 weeks. Formal physical therapy is usually not necessary to regain motion. Activities of daily living usually can be performed within 2 weeks of cast removal.

Table 16–2. Evaluation of forearm nailings

	Prospective Study (%)	*Retrospective Study (%)*
Union rate	97	93
Excellent/good results	92	83
Intra-op complications	5	9
Post-op complications	6	15

CLINICAL RESULTS

At Los Angeles County Harbor/UCLA Medical Center both retrospective and prospective reviews have been done to evaluate forearm nailings. Table 16–2 summarizes these results.

RETROSPECTIVE STUDY

To evaluate the effectiveness of the Street square forearm nail, the records of 195 unselected consecutive patients with 264 fractured forearm bones, between 1962 and 1988, were reviewed retrospectively. Only those cases followed until union or nonunion was established were included in the study. Minimum follow-up was 6 months, with an average follow-up of 23 months. Twenty four percent of the cases were open fractures and 25% were high-energy injuries with bony comminution and marked soft-tissue trauma. Primary bone graft was used in 15% of the cases after 1976 but in none of the cases before this time.

Results were tabulated using the criteria of Anderson.[25] Fifty-eight percent of the results were excellent, 27% were satisfactory, 7% were unsatisfactory, and 8% were failures. The nonunion rate was 6.8%. Operative complications occurred in 9.4% of forearm nailings. Postoperative complications occurred in 15.2% of forearm nailings. These complications are detailed in Table 16–3.

Table 16–3. Complications

	Retrospective Study (%)	*Prospective Study (%)*
Intraoperative		
Increased comminution	2	1
Cortical perforation	2	1
Transient nerve palsy	2	1
Broken reamer bit	2	1
Joint penetration by nail	2	0
Postoperative		
Impingement	4	3
Nail migration	6	2
Infection	2	0
Re-fracture	1	0
Rupture E.P.L.	1	0
Myositis ossificans	1	0
Synostosis	1	0

Bony union was defined as the presence of bridging callus and the absence of focal tenderness at the fracture site by 12 months (Fig. 16–6). Time to union for patients in this study was estimated to be 6.2 months for fractures of the ulna and 6.4 months for fractures of the radius. While the time to union may seem long, it is deceiving, because following their initial period of casting, patients were allowed to resume full unprotected activities with the exception of heavy lifting and twisting. Function of the extremity is restored long before radiographic consolidation of the fracture fragments is achieved.

A case was declared a nonunion if there was failure to progress after 12 months or if an additional operative procedure was required to effect union. Eleven of the 13 ulnar nonunions occurred in midshaft comminuted fractures that underwent open nailing without bone grafting.

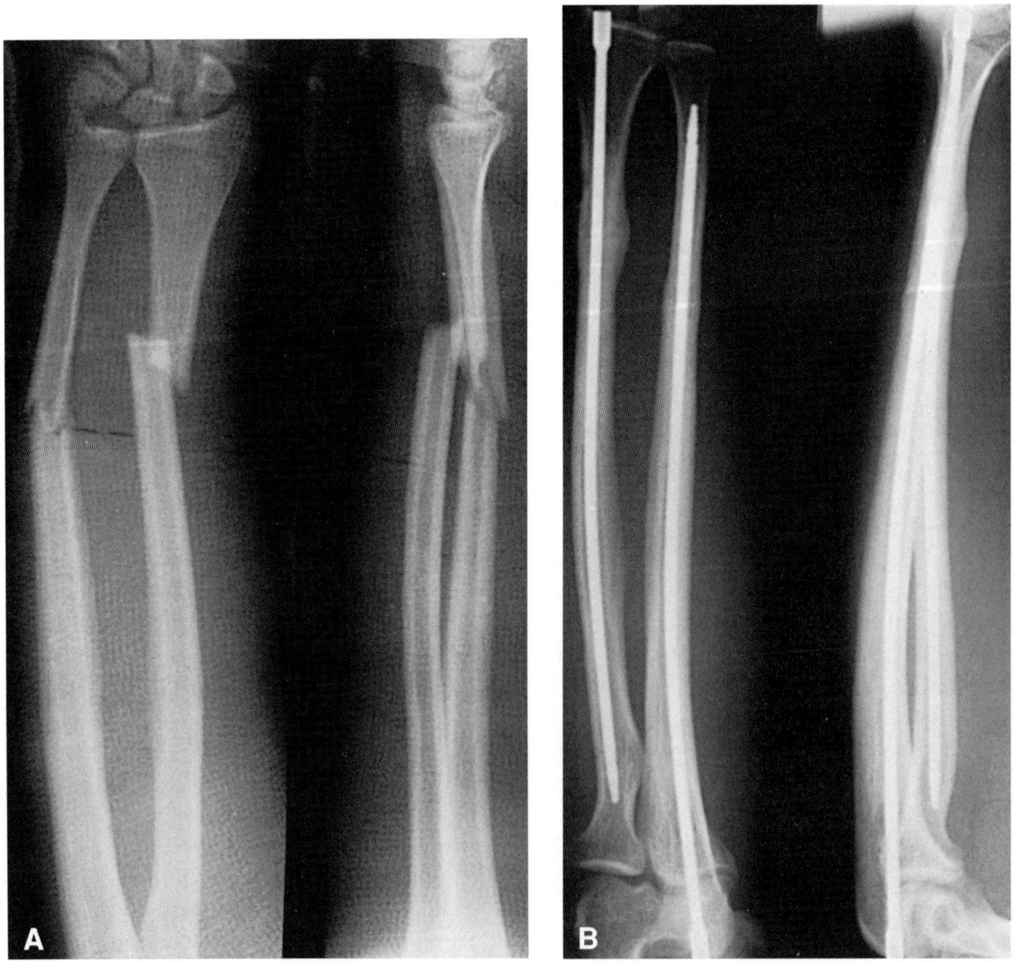

Fig. 16–6. *A,B,* Radial and ulnar fracture treated with closed nailing at 3 months with bridging callus at both fractures.

Four of 5 radial nonunions were distal to the junction of the mid-distal third, where rotational control is less than optimal secondary to the flaring of the metaphyseal bone.

PROSPECTIVE STUDY

This study was designed to evaluate, standardize, and improve the technique and indications for forearm nailing in a prospective fashion. In 1988, the following entry criteria were established: (1) all patients must be skeletally mature, (2) all patients must have diaphyseal forearm fractures with at least 5 cm of intact proximal or distal radius or ulna, and (3) the senior surgeon (D.M.Z.) must be present for all surgeries.

Based on our retrospective study, our goal was to minimize preventable complications by standardizing and refining existing surgical techniques and adapt a more aggressive approach toward bone grafting of comminuted fractures that require open nailing.

In 65 patients (90 diaphyseal fractures) at least one bone was rodded. Five patients were lost to follow-up. Six patients with 6 radial fractures and 2 patients with 2 ulnar fractures were excluded because there was not at least 5 cm of intact distal or proximal bone. Two patients were excluded because the supervising surgeon was not available. These 10 patients were treated with plate and screw form of osteosynthesis. Fifty patients with 75 fractures were followed for at least 6 months; they form the basis of this report.

The average age of patients was 31 years (range 14 to 72 years). There were 38 male and 12 female patients. Of the 75 radii and ulnae fractures, 2 radii and 1 ulna had a segmental fracture; so, the total number of fractures was 78. Of these 78 fractures, 75 were treated with intramedullary fixation, while the other 3 patients with both bone fractures had hybrid fixation with ulnar nailing and plating of the radius, because less than 5 cm of intact distal radius was present. Each fracture was evaluated separately, making 75 fractures available for review.

Twenty five patients had fractures of both the radius and ulna. Of the thirteen isolated radial fractures, 10 were Galeazzi fractures; of the 12 isolated ulnar fractures, 10 were Monteggia fractures. The incidence of each fracture was recorded using the fracture classification system of the Orthopaedic Trauma Association (Figs. 16–7 and 16–8). Twenty seven (36%) of

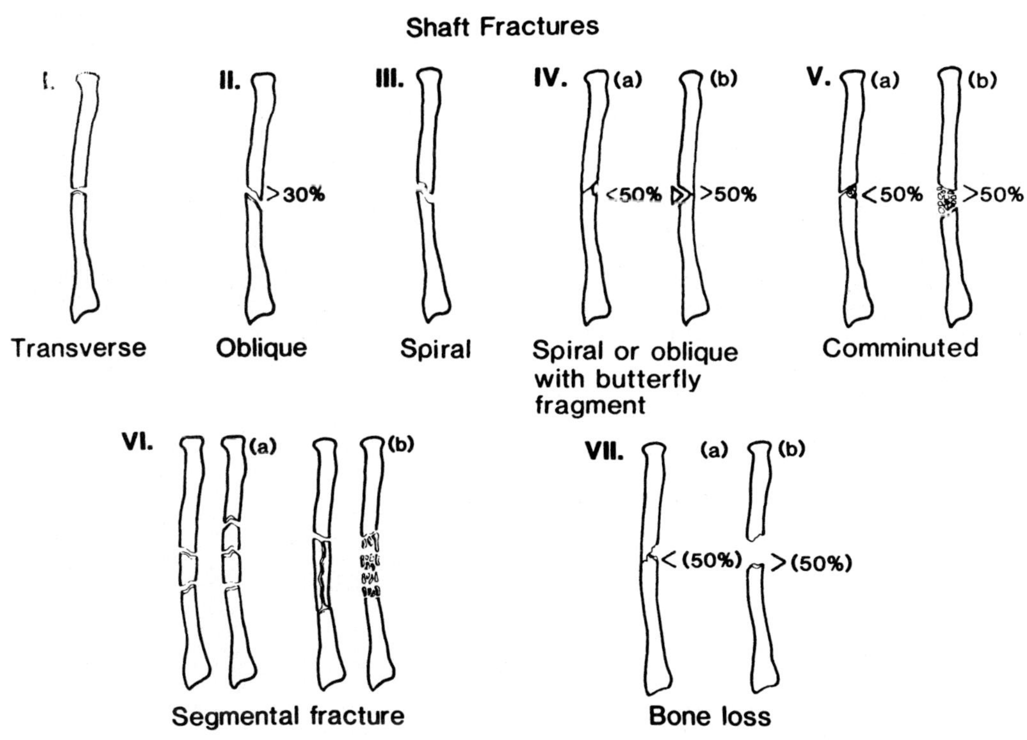

Fig. 16–7. Orthopaedic Trauma Association classification system of diaphyseal fractures of the forearm. (From Chapman, M.W., Gordon, J.E., Zissimos, A.G.: Compression-plate fixation of acute fractures of the diaphyses of the radius and ulna. J. Bone Joint Surg. *71A*:159-169, 1989.)

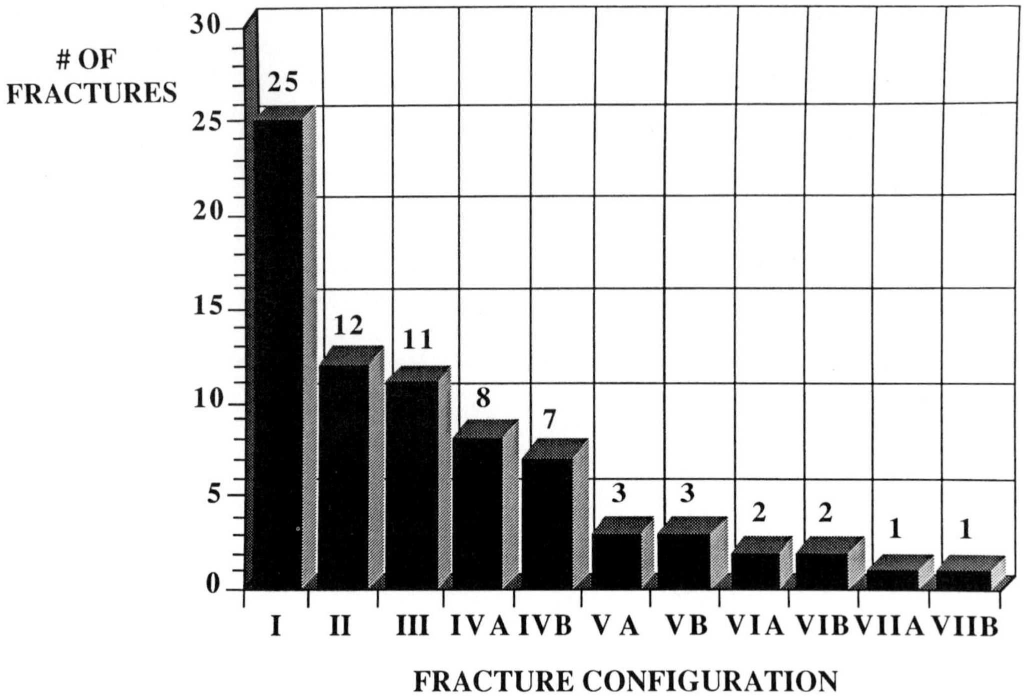

Fig. 16–8. Incidence of fracture pattern in prospective forearm study.

the fractures were comminuted, categories IV through VII, 60 were closed (88%), and 15 were open (12%). The open fractures were further classified according to the system of Gustilo et al.[24] Most of these were low-grade open fractures, Type I or II.

Twenty eight (37%) of the fractures were found in patients who had multiple injuries; twenty five (33%) were found in patients who had one or more concomitant fractures of the ipsilateral upper extremity. The mechanism of injury included motor vehicle accidents (53%), falls (27%), assault (14%), and low-velocity gunshot wounds (6%). No high-velocity missile wounds were included.

Two patients had a concomitant vascular injury (Fig. 16–9). One patient had successful repair of a radial artery laceration and the other had ligation of an ulnar artery laceration. Ten patients had an associated neurological injury. Six radial, 2 ulnar, and 2 median nerves were damaged. One of the ulnar nerves and 1 of the radial nerves were lacerated. Both were repaired, but only the radial nerve had any appreciable return of function at 14 months. Neuropraxia was identified preoperatively in 2 median nerves, 5 radial nerves, and 1 ulnar nerve preoperatively. There was complete re-

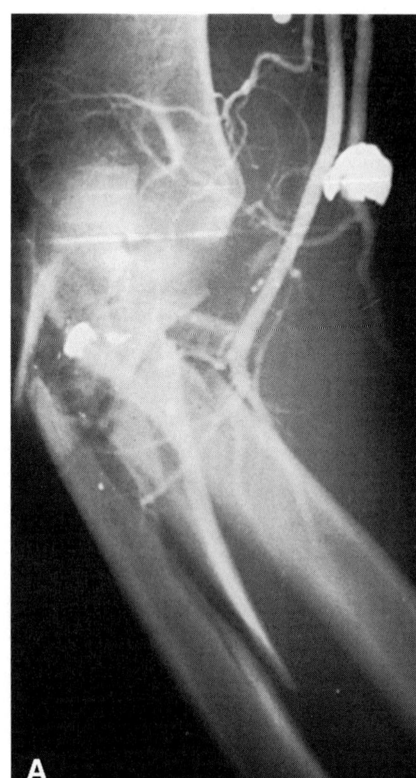

Fig. 16–9. *A,* Highly comminuted proximal fractures of ulna and radius with vascular injury/compartment syndrome. *(Figure continues)*

covery in 1 median nerve, 4 radial nerves, and 1 ulnar nerve.

OPEN FRACTURES

For patients with open fractures, cefazolin sodium is given intravenously in the emergency room, along with tetanus prophylaxis where necessary. After irrigation and debridement of the wound, internal fixation is performed, as described for the closed technique. If the canal diameter allows, inserting the nails without reaming is preferred. The traumatic wound is left open with closure of the elective surgical incision. Antibiotics are administered for 48 hours.

In this study, wounds were closed between 5 to 10 days. The wound was closed primarily in all 9 grade I open fractures and by delayed primary closure in the 3 grade II injuries. The one patient with a grade IIIa injury required a split-thickness skin graft. Closed fractures, with severe comminution that required open nailing, or low-grade open fractures that had bone defects or comminution, were bone grafted at the time of delayed primary wound closure using iliac crest cancellous bone. Fifteen of the 75 fractures (20%) underwent bone grafting, all with fracture comminution of grade IV or higher.

A 3-mm rod was used in 80% of fractures and a 4-mm rod was used in the remainder of patients. Thirty fractures were nailed on the day of injury, 10 were nailed within 48 hours of injury, 15 were nailed between 3 to 7 days, 14 were nailed between 7 to 14 days after injury, and 6 were nailed more than 2 weeks after injury.

Union occurred in 97.5% of fractures. The average time to radiographic union was 18

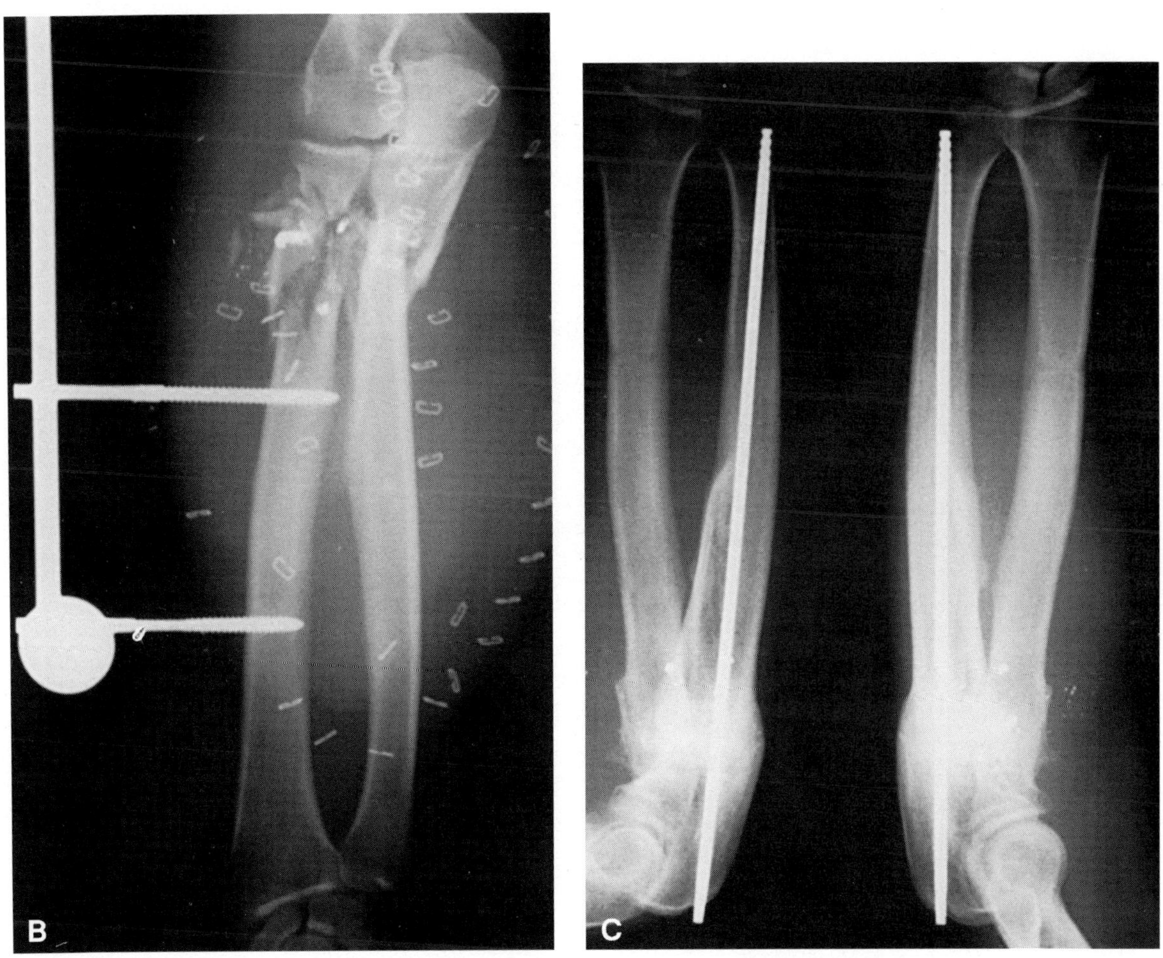

Fig. 16–9. *(continued) B,* Temporary external stabilization across elbow for revascularization and soft-tissue coverage. *C,* Closed ulna nailing done 10 days postinjury; the fracture healed with synostosis and no evidence of infection.

weeks (with a range of 12 to 30 weeks). Of the 38 fractures treated with a closed technique and the 15 fractures bone grafted, 100% united. Using the criteria of Anderson,[25] the functional results were 70% excellent, 22% satisfactory, 5% unsatisfactory, and 3% failures.

ADOLESCENT FOREARM NAILING

Children aged 10 to 14 with displaced diaphyseal forearm fractures represent a difficult subset of patients to treat. The surgeon is often unclear about whether to treat the fracture as a pediatric fracture, with the forgiving nature and remodeling potential that characterizes most younger patients with forearm fractures, or to treat them as an adult with internal fixation. The indications for operative management of forearm fractures in the skeletally immature patient are rare: (1) inability to obtain or maintain a closed reduction, (2) management of a floating elbow injury, (3) or skeletal stabilization to allow for management of significant soft-tissue injuries.

Displaced or unstable fractures can be treated with intramedullary nailing similar to the technique described previously for adults in which the distal-radial physes or proximal-ulnar physes are closed. If the distal-radial or proximal-ulnar physes are open, then closed Rush pin nailing as described by Blasier [26] and Amit [27] is preferred. Many investigators report excellent results with minimal complications using similar techniques.[28,29] Because of fairly rapid fracture healing, the nails can be removed after only 6 to 8 weeks (Fig. 16–10). If the tip of the pins are left under the skin, then they may be left in place longer if they are not causing significant irritation. Cast immobilization during the initial 4 to 6 weeks is recommended be-

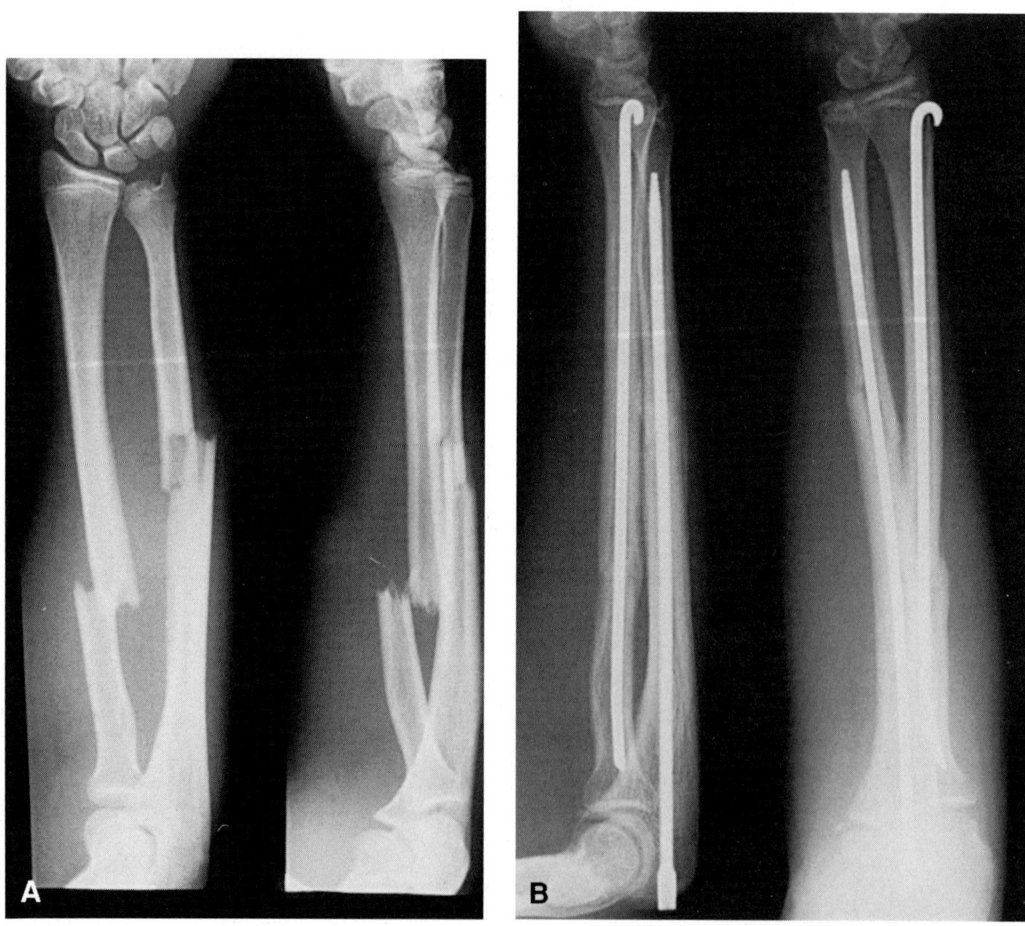

Fig. 16–10. *A,* A 13-year old with displaced radial/ulnar fracture. *B,* Closed nailing with Rush rod in radius, square nail in ulna. *(Figure continues)*

cause of the lack of good rotational control. Although this technique does require a second minor surgery for pin removal, its advantages over open reduction, as with adult forearm nailing, include maintenance of a stable anatomic reduction, minimal exposure with lowered risk of nerve injury or infection, minimal periods of convalescence and disability, less risk of refracture, and far less residual scarring and disfigurement.

COMPLICATIONS

As outlined in Table 16–3, the complications can be divided into two main groups. The first and largest group occurs at the time of nailing and is related to technique. The second group occurs during the time in which the fracture unites or fails to heal and involves the character of the fracture, the holding power of the nail, and the behavior of the patient.

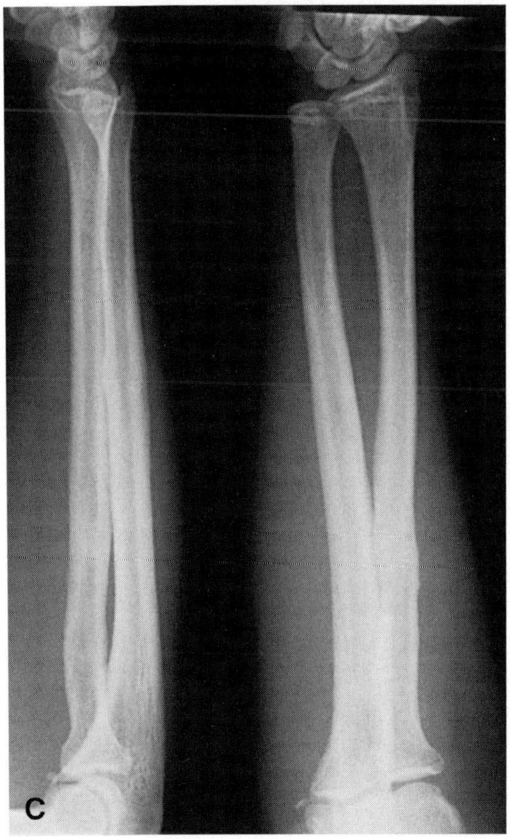

Fig. 16–10. *(continued) C,* Excellent clinical result at 3 months.

Intraoperative Complications

Nail Incarceration

As with any intramedullary nailing, care must be taking in selecting the correct size implant to fit the patient's anatomy. Careful preoperative review of good quality radiographs is essential to avoid both nail incarceration and/or splitting of a fracture fragment. Sometimes the 3-mm nail can be inserted without reaming but frequently preparation of the canal by overreaming 0.5 to 1 mm is necessary in patients with small canals (Fig. 16–11). This will also prevent increased comminution at the fracture site either by eliminating extension of incomplete fracture lines or creation of new fractures.

Impingement

Pain may result when the nail is not seated sufficiently, causing mechanical irritation at either the wrist or elbow. This may be caused by a nail that is too long, so that the nail cannot be driven in further without penetration of the joint (Fig. 16–12). More often, the nail is the correct length but care is not taken to fully seat the nail (Fig. 16–13). The design modification from a male-threaded stud on the original Street nail to a recessed female driving end on the current titanium nail allows for flush seating of the implant. Attention to these details is important, because if the implant does not cause any discomfort after the fracture is healed, then nail removal is often not necessary.

Cortical Perforation

Cortical perforation can occur either during placement of the entry hole into the intramedullary canal or during preparation of a tight canal with the reamers. A conventional drill is used to make the entry portal hole. Care must be taken in the radius to have sufficient palmar flexion of the wrist over a bump of towels to prevent inadvertent cortical penetration of the volar cortex. By modification of the reamers to a blunt tip and side-cutting thread only, the problem of perforation during canal reaming has been eliminated. Reaming in 0.5-mm increments can minimize the likelihood of perforation of the cortex by the reamers.

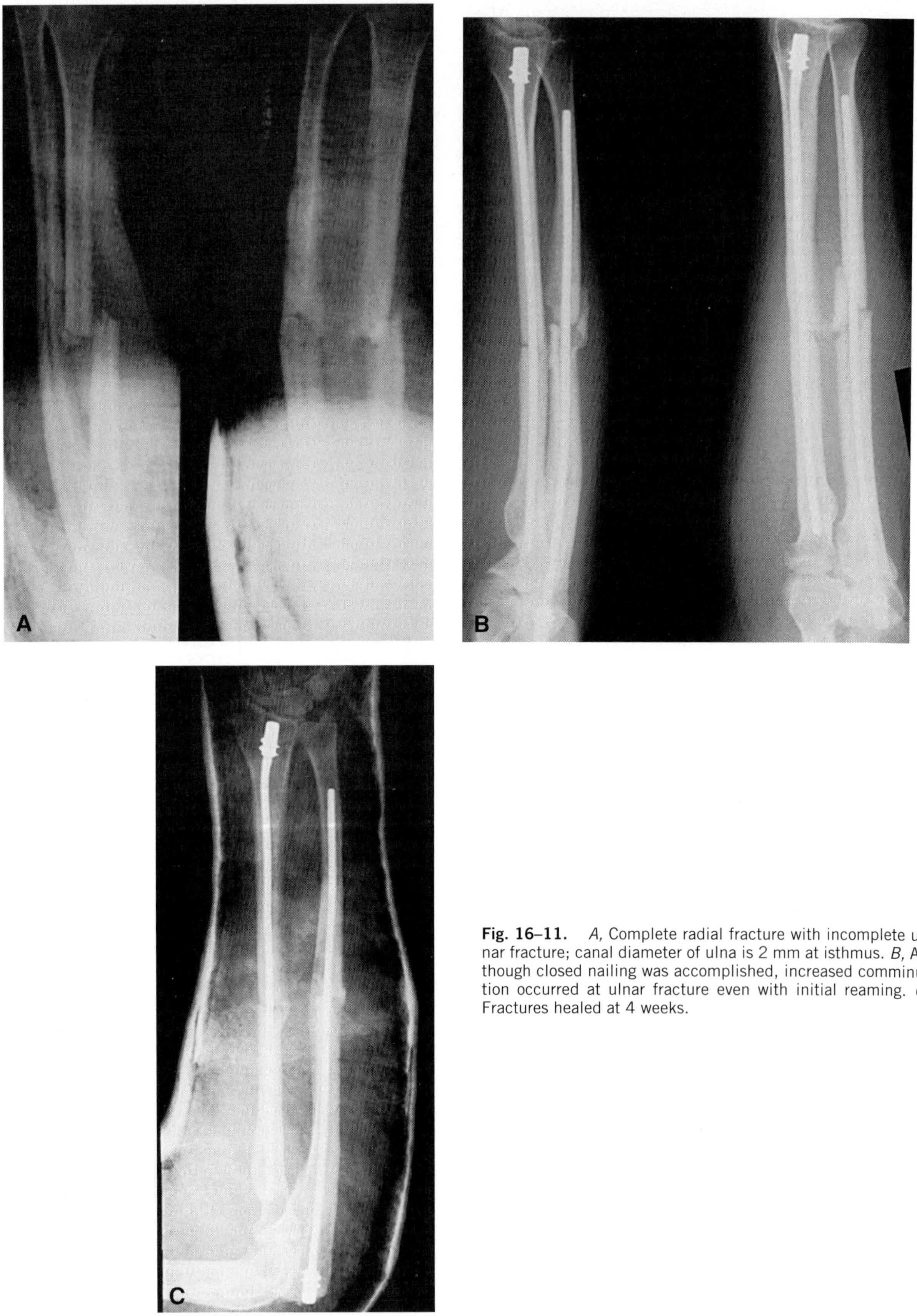

Fig. 16–11. *A,* Complete radial fracture with incomplete ulnar fracture; canal diameter of ulna is 2 mm at isthmus. *B,* Although closed nailing was accomplished, increased comminution occurred at ulnar fracture even with initial reaming. *C,* Fractures healed at 4 weeks.

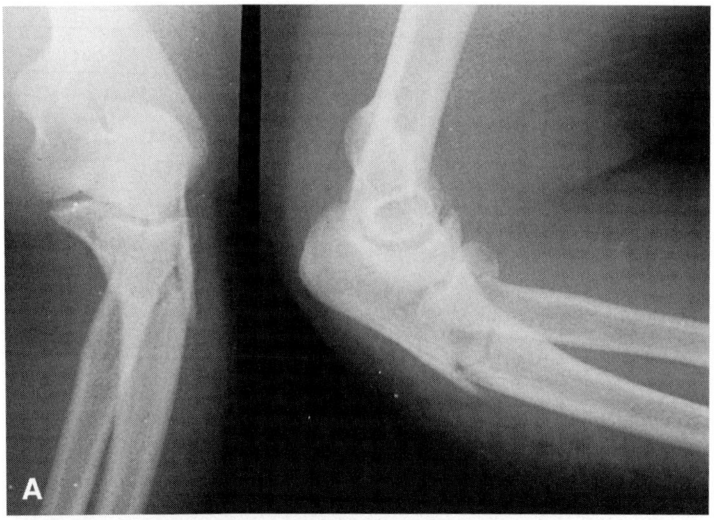

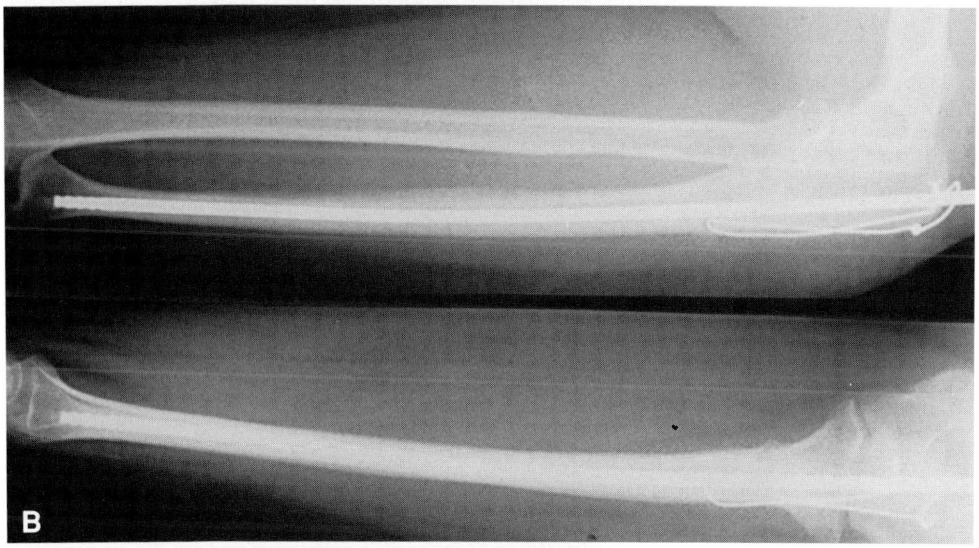

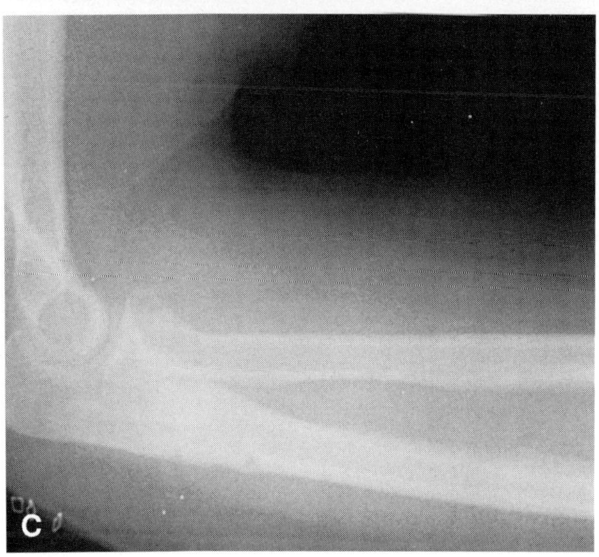

Fig. 16–12. *A*, Monteggia variant with proximal ulnar fracture associated with radial neck fracture. *B*, Treatment with closed Street nail supplemented with tension band. *C*, Despite nail being too long fracture healed with excellent function. A nail of correct length may have prevented need for nail removal.

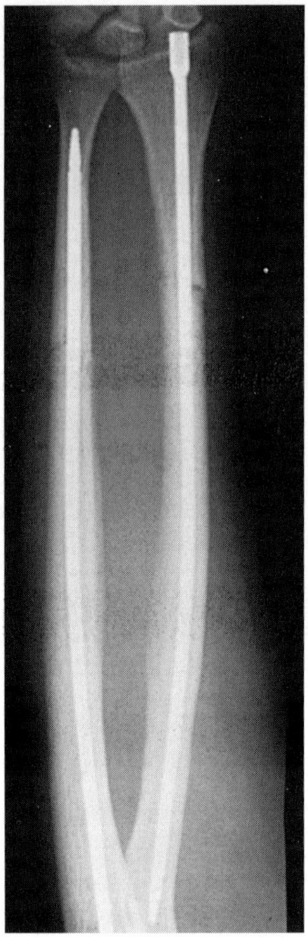

Fig. 16–13. Radial nail with incomplete seating may cause irritation at wrist. Nail is correct length but not driven fully during final seating.

Postoperative Complications

Nail Migration

When nail migration occurs, this complication will usually be seen within the first several months after nailing. Failure to fully impact a fracture at the time of nailing, placement of a short nail, or insertion of a 3-mm nail in a large canal will predispose a nail migration. The snugness of the nail in the canal is not as mandatory in closed nailing as in open nailing, because the soft-tissue support encourages early healing and enhances fracture stability. The least favorable combination is a short, loose-fitting nail in a highly comminuted fracture that has a propensity for shortening. The advent of interlocking-type nails may reduce the incidence of this complication.

Patient Behavior

The routine use of a cast for 2 to 4 weeks protects the patient from a false sense of security after the pain has subsided. The early callus can be disrupted by the vigorous patient who engages in strenuous activity or by the elderly patient who falls. Once the callus begins to consolidate at about 4 weeks, stimulus during ordinary use seems to enhance the healing. The overprotective patient delays not only rehabilitation of the hand and wrist, but also to some extent, fracture healing.

Reliable patients with stable fracture patterns are often only protected for only 2 weeks in a long-arm cast. This is especially true if closed nailing has been accomplished, because of the additional stability gained by the intact soft-tissue envelope.

Infection

Although infection is rarely seen in closed nailings, it still remains a problem in the occasional iatrogenic infection in open nailings, as well as in open fractures. As with any infection after intramedullary nailing, the nail should not be removed until the fracture has united. The fracture will usually continue to drain until the nail is removed. Surgical drainage should be performed if necessary, and appropriate antibiotics should be administered until the acute inflammatory process is quiescent.

For open fractures, delayed closure of the traumatic wound is essential for prevention of infection. The forearm, particularly the ulna, is less likely to bridge with callus formation while active drainage exists. This situation is analogous to the tibia and possibly may be caused by the presence of less surrounding soft tissue than seen in other bones like the femur. All infections seen in our series cleared promptly after the infection was controlled by drainage, antibiotics, and nail removal after the fractures healed. No bone grafting was necessary to promote union in these cases. Rarely, if a loose nail is associated with infection, renailing can be done with a more snug-fitting, larger nail to promote stability.

Nail Removal

Occasionally a nail is removed before 1 year, and then it is only recommended if the patient

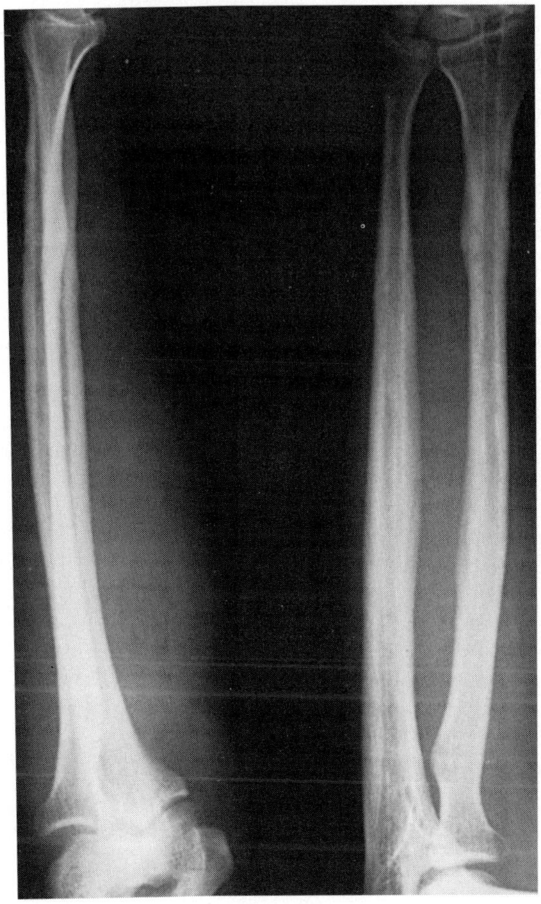

Fig. 16–14. After nail removal from both bone fracture, no protection of forearm is needed, as risk of refracture is minimal with good periosteal callus at fracture sites.

is symptomatic. If the nail is placed properly, it will rarely cause irritation at the wrist or elbow. If necessary, removal is usually a minor and simple procedure that can be performed as an outpatient through only a 1 to 2 cm incision. Unlike the precautions necessary after plate removal, after rod removal the risk of refracture is minimal and there is no need for protection of the forearm (Fig. 16–14). Even with the correct instrumentation, occasionally nail removal is difficult or impossible. The threads may be stripped or significant excavation of bone may be required to expose a sufficient portion of nail in order to place the extractor. In these rare situations, if the nail is short enough, it may be driven out of sight to avoid mechanical irritation or may be broken off. The patient must be informed that the potential exists for failure to successfully achieve nail removal prior to recommending the procedure.

DISCUSSION

Nonoperative treatment of displaced, adult diaphyseal fractures does not produce acceptable clinical results.[30,31] Intramedullary fixation of forearm fractures with either a square nail or an interlocking-type nail has many advantages over plate fixation. The control of rotational forces is essential for adequate fracture stability. With the square nail, bite into the cortex of a circumferentially reamed canal protects against the strong torque loads in the forearm. Although at this time no clinical results have been reported, the advent of interlocking-type nails may enhance this stability even more and obviate the need for any postoperative immobilization. The nails also provide some space for restoration of the endosteal blood flow.

Because the rod is stress-sharing, as opposed to stress-shielding (which occurs with plate fixation), the peripheral callus that forms may lead to a biomechanically stronger union.[32] Despite the occasional abundant callus formation, no mechanical block to forearm rotation has been seen (Fig. 16–15). Even in those cases rodded open, the disruption to the periosteal blood supply is less than that with plating and, consequently, more favorable to fracture healing.

Despite the advantages of intramedullary fixation reported by many investigators,[33–38] satisfactory results are still achieved with plate fixation.[25,39–48] Good results in our series were obtained when a hybrid technique was used with plate fixation of the radius and nailing of the ulna or vice versa (Fig. 16–16). This technique was used when the radius or ulnar fracture was too distal (i.e., less than 5 cm from the joint) for adequate fixation with a nail. From experience we learned that certain radial fractures at the junction of the metaphysis and diaphysis were not suitable for nailing because of the inadequate purchase on the distal fragment. The new generation of interlocking nails may prove successful in expanding the role of forearm nailing to include these very distal fractures.

Bone grafting was not used in any fractures in our clinical study prior to 1976. Since 1976, iliac crest bone graft was used in only 15% of cases (Fig. 16–17). All cases that were bone grafted were nailed using an open technique; bone grafting is not necessary in closed nailing. Both Chapman[41] and Anderson[39] advocated liberal bone grafting in comminuted fractures. Their studies included bone grafting rates of

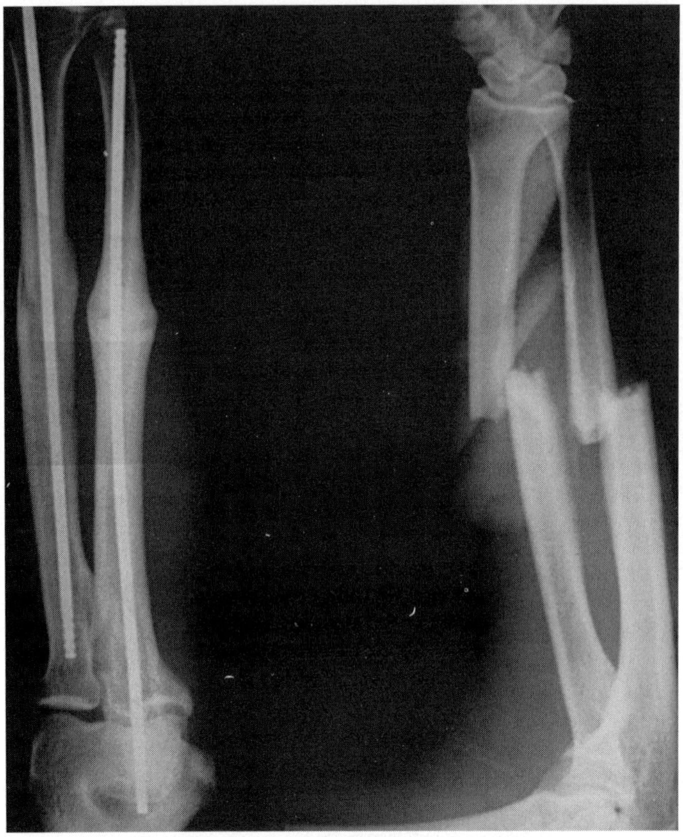

Fig. 16–15. Despite abundant callus formation, forearm rotation is normal in this both bone fracture.

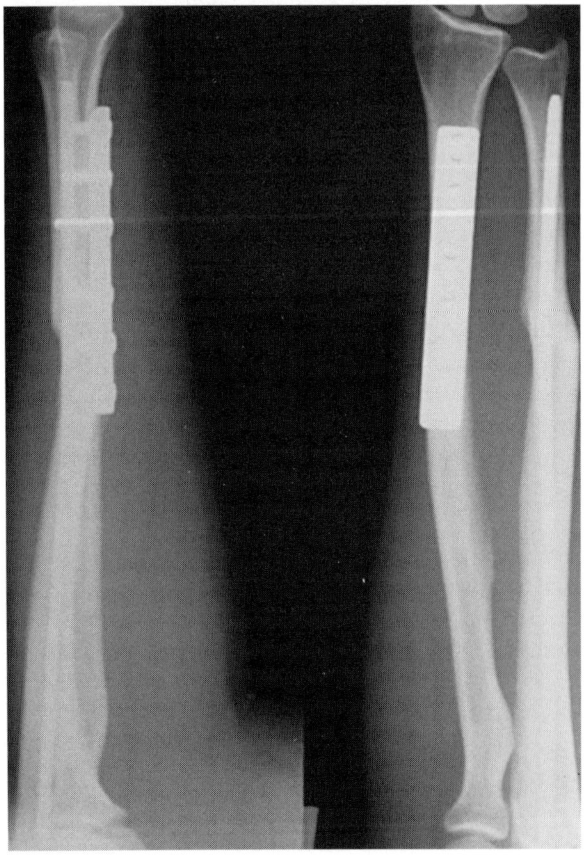

Fig. 16–16. Hybrid fixation used successfully with plating of distal radial fracture and blind nailing of ulna.

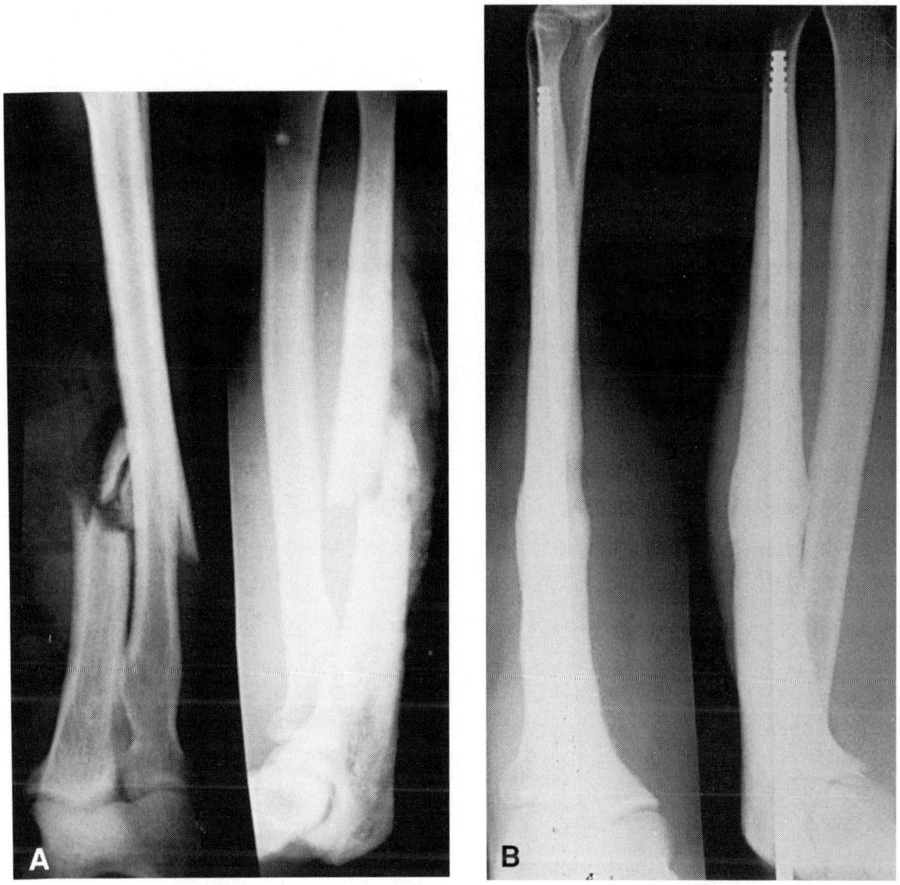

Fig. 16–17. *A*, Comminuted open ulnar fracture treated with 4-mm Street nail and cancellous grafting. *B*, Healed fracture with good functional result at 1 year postinjury.

53% and 27% respectively. The aggressive use of bone grafting may be a factor in such excellent rates of union. This is in contrast to the Swiss group who used bone grafts in only 7% of their cases.[43]

Refracture after forearm nailing is a rare complication that occurred only 4 times in our series of over 339 fractures, producing a rate of 1.2%. In all cases, the rods were removed prematurely, less than 8 months after insertion. Removal of forearm rods is not necessary unless the patient is symptomatic. When indicated, the procedure can be done through a small incision as an outpatient without the need for postoperative protection or immobilization. The high rate of complications, including refracture with or without plate removal, has caused some investigators to discourage the routine removal of plates or to delay this procedure for at least 2 years (Fig. 16–18).[39,42,49–55] Intramedullary nailing also eliminates the additional problem of forearm refractures in the competitive athlete who is involved in contact sports.

The restoration of the normal radial bow is important in restoring forearm function. The effect of malunion of the radial diaphysis has been demonstrated.[56] The preservation of this anatomy is built into some rods that are prebent during manufacturing. However, the 3-mm nails are generally flexible enough to conform to this radial bowing even without significant prebending. (Fig. 16–19) If a larger nail is to be used, then a prebent nail or prebending a straight nail is important in improving final function.

The rate of 92% of patients experiencing good and excellent functional results in this series of forearm nailings is comparable to recent reports of forearm plating.[41] The improvements are largely attributable to increased success of closed nailing. With increasing experience,

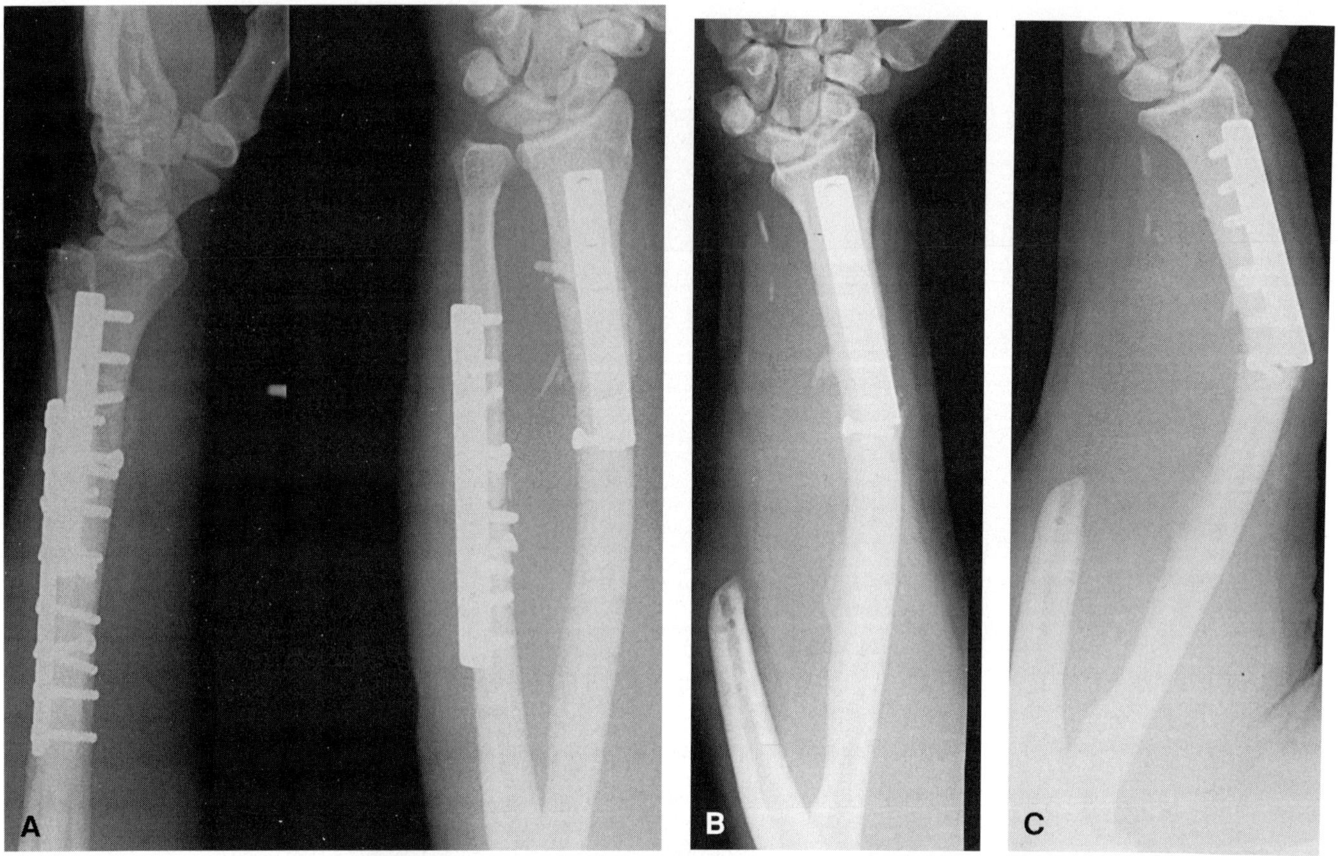

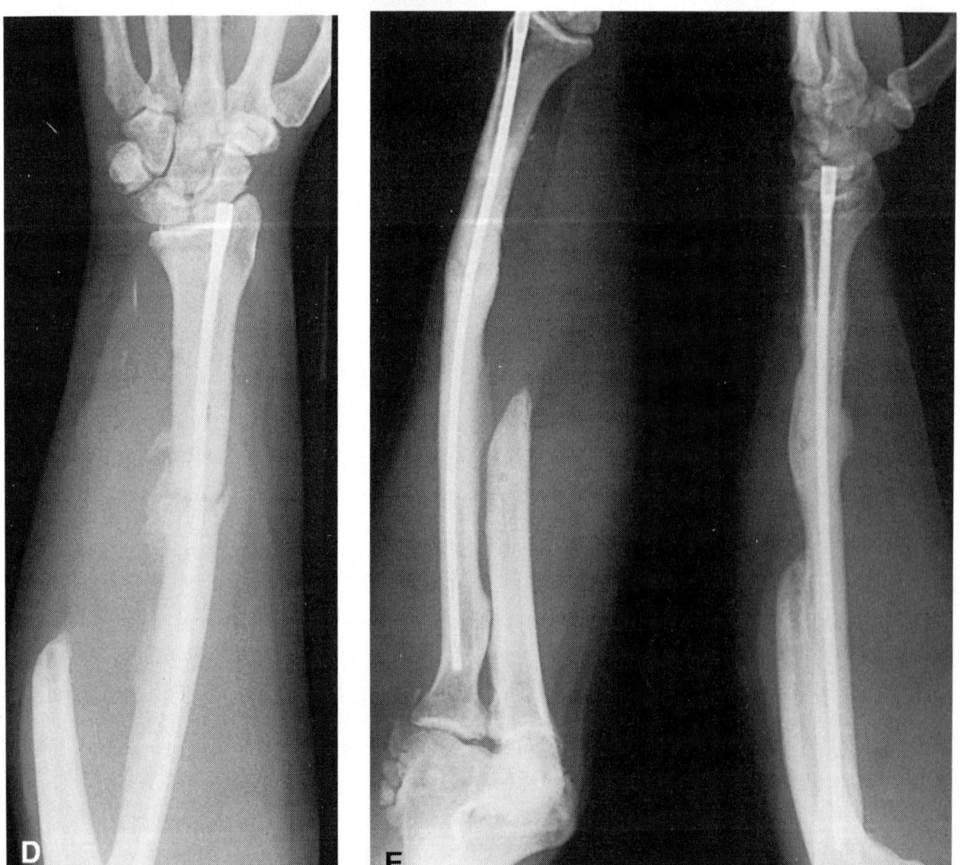

Fig. 16–18. *A,* Open radial/ulnar fracture treated with plate/screw osteosynthesis *B,* Persistent infection caused resection of ulna. *C,* Eighteen months later while playing golf, patient refractured at proximal end of plate. *D,* Plate removal, open nailing, and cancellous bone grafting done. *E,* Final result with good function and healing at 1 year post-nailing.

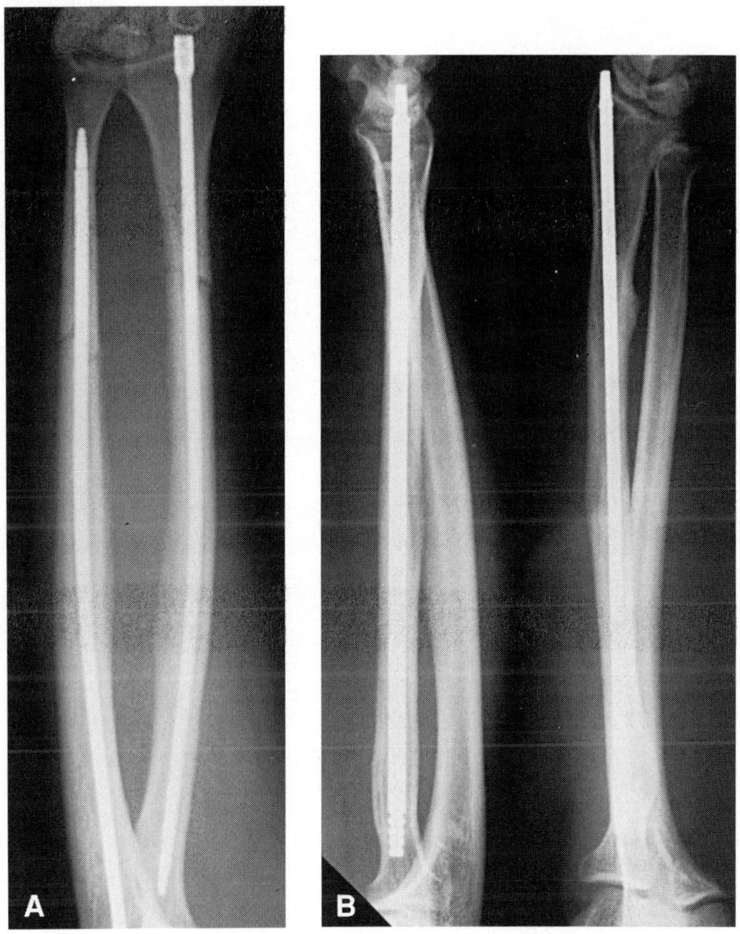

Fig. 16–19. *A,* Preservation of normal radial bow with a 3-mm titanium nail. *B,* Larger nails, if not prebent, may cause some loss of normal radial bow.

closed nailing can be performed more frequently. For the surgeon who is unfamiliar with the technique, experience is best first gained with simple single bone fracture patterns such as the isolated displaced ulnar fracture or Monteggia fracture. (Fig. 16–20). More complex patterns including segmental fractures are particularly well suited for nailing as further experience is gained (Fig. 16–21). The recent additional use of a forearm fracture table, similar to that designed by Street in 1979,[57] and the decrease in time from injury to surgery have helped in the goal of accomplishing closed nailings. Bone grafting is recommended for comminuted fractures in which open nailing is necessary. Although the long

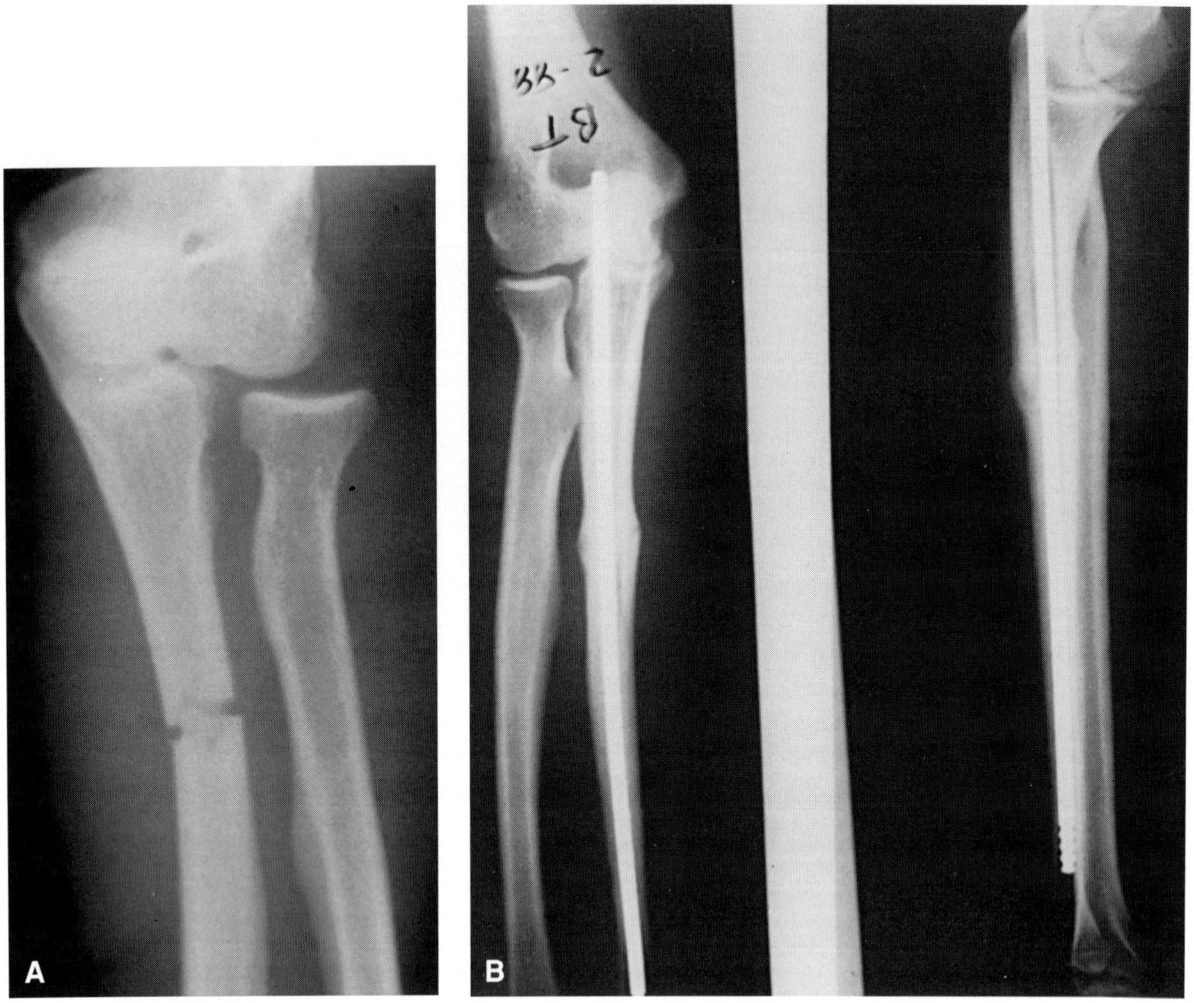

Fig. 16–20. *A,B,* Monteggia fracture; subluxation amenable to closed nailing with Street nail and subsequent healing.

time to radiographic union with forearm nailing has been criticized, restoration of extremity function occurs long before radiographic consolidation.

SUMMARY

Intramedullary nailing of the forearm requires the same attention to detail as do other nailing techniques of long bones. As technology has progressed in the last several years with improved instrumentation and better implants, the complications previously associated with this technique have been minimized. These advances have also increased the success of closed nailing to well over 75%. The advantages of forearm nailing are maintenance of stable anatomic reduction, minimal exposure with lowered risk of nerve injury or infection, minimal periods of convalescence and disability, less risk of refracture, and significantly less scarring and disfigurement. For these reasons, the popularity of intramedullary of the forearm is on the rise. Forearm nailing represents an excellent alternative to plate fixation of the forearm and is the method of choice for the majority of diaphyseal forearm fractures. Careful preoperative planning, precise technique, and instrumentation improvements will allow the surgeon to obtain gratifying functional results with intramedullary nailing of the forearm as it has for the femur, tibia, and humerus.

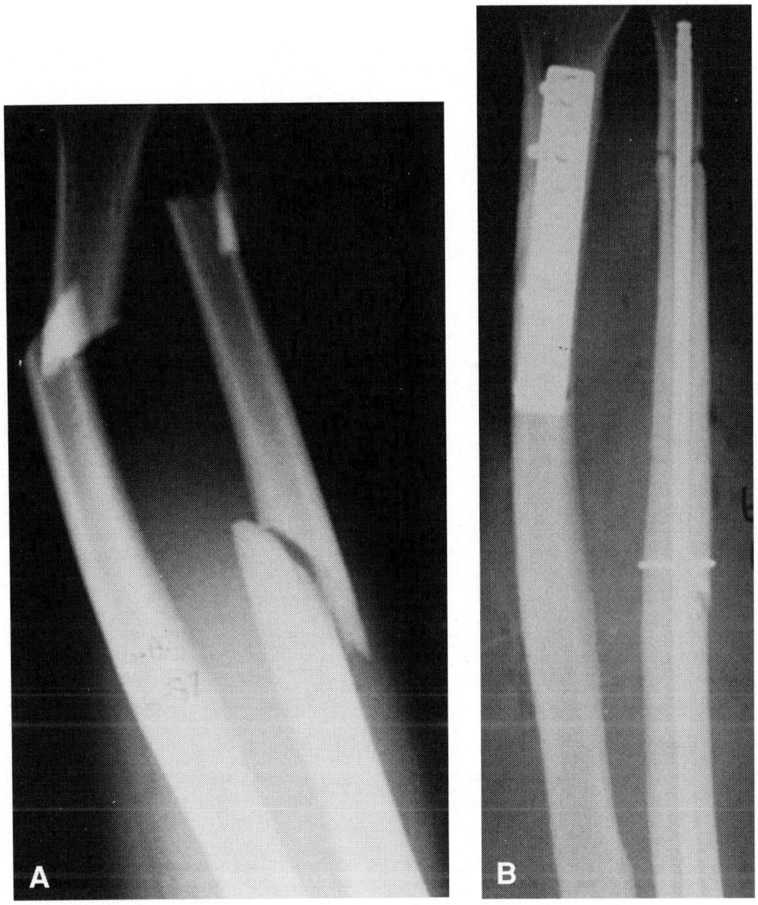

Fig. 16–21. Segmental ulnar fracture treated early in series with open nailing. Radial fracture plated at initial surgery by different surgeon.

REFERENCES

1. Street, D.: Intramedullary forearm nailing. Clin. Orthop. *212*:219, 1986.
2. Soeur, R.: Intramedullary pinning of diaphyseal fractures. J. Bone Joint Surg. *28*:309, 1946.
3. Dickson, J.A.: Intramedullary fixation of certain fractures of both bones of forearm: report of two cases. Cleve. Clin. Q. *11*:62, 1944.
4. Lambrinudi, C.: Intramedullary Kirschner wires in the treatment of fractures. Proc. R. Soc. Med. *33*:153, 1940.
5. Rush, L.V., Rush, H.L.: Reconstruction operation for comminuted fracture of the upper third of the ulna. Am. J. Surg. *38*:332, 1937.
6. Rush, L.V., Rush, H.L.: Technique for longitudinal pin fixation of certain fractures of the ulna and of the femur. J. Bone Joint Surg. *21*:619, 1939.
7. Böhler, L.: Die Technik der knochenbruchbehandlung im Frieden und im Kriege. Wien, Wilhelm Maudrich, 1945.
8. Böhler, L.: Medullary nailing of Küntscher. Translation by H. Tretter. Baltimore, Williams & Wilkins, 1948.
9. Küntscher, G., Maatz, R.: Die Technik der Marknagelung. Leipzig, Thieme, 1945.
10. Haebler, C.: Experiences with the marrow nail operation according to the principles of Küntscher. Part I. U.S. Naval Med. Bull. *49*:459, 1949.
11. Hall, R.H., Bugg, E.I., Vitolo, R.E.: Intramedullary fixation of fractures of the forearm. South. Med. J. *45*:814, 1952.
12. Von Saal, F.: Review of complications in intramedullary nailing. J. Bone Joint Surg. *32B*:717, 1950.
13. Street, D.M.: Medullary fixation of fractures. *In* Monographs on Surgery—1950. Edited by B.N. Carter. New York, T. Nelson & Sons, 1949.
14. Street, D.M.: Medullary nailing in the treatment of industrial injuries. Indust. Med. Surg. *21*:485, 1952.
15. Street, D.M.: Medullary nailing of forearm fractures. J. Bone Joint Surg. *39A*:715, 1957.
16. Sage, F.P.: Medullary fixation of fractures of the forearm. J. Bone Joint Surg. *41A*:1489, 1959.
17. Von Saal, F.: Personal Communication, 1953.
18. Marek, F.M.: Axial fixation of forearm fractures. J. Bone Joint Surg. *41A*:1099, 1961.
19. Cotler, J.M., Ingemi, B.J., Prabhakar, M.P.: Experience with Schneider nailing in forearm fractures. J. Bone Joint Surg. *53A*:1228, 1971.
20. Tibone, J.: Personal Communication.
21. Hoek, K.: Personal Communication, 1993.
22. McFarlane, A.G., MacDonald, L.T.: Parameters of the ulnar medullary canal for locked intramedullary nailing. J. Biomed. Eng. *13*:74, 1991.
23. DePedro, J.A., Garcia-Navarrete, F., DeLucas, F.G., Otero, R., Oteo, A., Stern, L.L.: Internal fixation of ulnar fractures by locking nail. Clin. Orthop. *283*:81, 1992.

24. Gustilo, R.B., Anderson, J.T.: Prevention of infection in the treatment of one thousand and twenty five open fractures of long bones. J. Bone Joint Surgery, *58A*:453, 1976.
25. Anderson, L.D.: Compression plate fixation and the effect of different types of internal fixation on fracture healing. J. Bone Joint Surg. *47A*:191, 1965.
26. Blasier, R.D., Salamon, P.B.: Closed Intramedullary Rodding of Pediatric Adolescent Forearm Fractures. Op. Tech. Orthop. *3*:128-133, 1993.
27. Amit, Y., Salai, M., Checkik, A., et al.: Closing intramedullary nailing for the treatment of diaphyseal forearm fractures in adolescence: A preliminary report. J. Pediatr. Orthop. *5*:143–146, 1985.
28. Lascombes, P., Prevot, J., Ligier, J.N., Metaizeau, P., Poncelet, T.: Elastic stable intramedullary nailing in forearm shaft fractures in children: 85 cases. J. Pediatr. Orthop. *10*:167, 1990.
29. Roy, D., Crawford, A.: Operative management of fractures of the shaft of the radius and ulna. Orthop. Clin. North Am. *21*:245, 1990.
30. Key, J.A., Conwell, H.E.: The Management of Fractures, Dislocations and Sprains. St. Louis, C.V. Mosby Co., 1934.
31. Knight, R.A., Purvis, G.D.: Fractures of both bones of the forearm in adults. J. Bone Joint Surg. *31A*:755, 1949.
32. Rand, J.A., An, K.N., Chao, E.Y., Kelly, P.J.: A comparison of the effect of open intramedullary nailing and compression-plate fixation on fracture-site blood flow and fracture union. J. Bone Joint Surg. *63A*:427, 1981.
33. Maatz, R., Lentz, W., Arens, W., Beck, H. (Eds.): Intramedullary Nailing and Other Intramedullary Osteosynthesis. Translated by K. H. Mueller. Philadelphia, W.B. Saunders, 1986, p. 260.
34. Ritchey, S.J.: Rigid medullary fixation of forearm fractures. South. Med. J. *51*:852, 1958.
35. Smith, H., Sage, F.P.: Medullary fixation of forearm fractures. J. Bone Joint Surg. *39A*:91, 1957.
36. Wolgin, M., Zinar, D.M.: Intramedullary Fixation of Forearm Fractures using the Street Square Forearm Nail. American Academy of Orthopaedic Surgeons. New Orleans. 1990.
37. Zanasi, R., Franceschini, F., Rotolo, F., Romano, P., Galmarini, V., Zanasi, L.: Intramedullary Osteosynthesis—4. Küntscher Nailing in the Ulna. Ital. J. Orthop. Traumatol. *16*:369–378, 1990.
38. Zinar, D., Wolgin, M., et al.: Prospective Evaluation of Forearm I.M. Nailing. American Acadamy of Orthopaedic Surgeons. Washington D.C. 1992.
39. Anderson, L.D., Sisk, T.D., Tooms, R.E., Park, W.I. III: Compression-plate fixation in acute diaphyseal fractures of the radius and ulna. J. Bone Joint Surg. *57A*: 287, 1975.
40. Boyd, H.B., Boals, J.C.: The Monteggia lesion. A review of 159 cases. Clin. Orthop. *66*:94, 1969.
41. Chapman, M.W., Gordon, J.E., Zissimos, A.G.: Compression-plate fixation of acute fractures of the diaphyses of the radius and ulna. J. Bone Joint Surg. *71A*:159, 1989.
42. Dodge, H.S., Cady, G.W.: Treatment of fractures of the radius and ulna with compression plates. A retrospective study of one hundred and nineteen fractures in seventy-eight patients. J. Bone Joint Surg. *54A*:1167, 1972.
43. Drake, J., Jupiter, J.B., Claudi, B., Allgower, M.: Compression plate fixation of diaphyseal forearm fractures. Read at American Academy of Orthopedic Surgeons Meeting, Atlanta, February 1988.
44. Grace, T.G., Eversmann, W.W.: Forearm fractures: Treatment by rigid fixation with early motion. J. Bone Joint Surg. *62A*:433, 1980.
45. Kraus, B., Horne, G.: Galeazzi fractures. J. Trauma, *25*: 1093, 1985.
46. Moore, T. M., Klein, J.P., Patzakis, M.J., Harvey, J.P., Jr.: Results of compression-plating of closed Galeazzi fractures. J. Bone Joint Surg. *67A*:1015, 1985.
47. Naiman, P.T., Schein, A.J., Siffert, R.S.: Use of ASIF compression plates in selected shaft fractures of the upper extremity. A preliminary report. Clin. Orthop. *71*:208, 1970.
48. Teipner, W.A., Mast, J.W.: Internal fixation of forearm diaphyseal fractures: Double plating versus single compression (tension band) plating—A comparative study. Orthop. Clin. North Am. *11*:381, 1980.
49. Deluca, P.A., Lindsey, R.W., Ruwe, P.A.: Refracture of bones of the forearm after the removal of compression plates. J. Bone Joint Surg. *70A*:1372, 1988.
50. Hidaka, S., Gustilo, R.B.: Refracture of bones of the forearm after plate removal. J. Bone Joint Surg. *66A*: 1241, 1984.
51. Labosky, D., Cermak, M.B., Waggy, C.: Forearm fracture plates: To remove or not to remove. J. Hand Surg. *15A*: 294, 1990.
52. Langkamer, V.G., Ackroyd, C.E.: Internal fixation of forearm fractures in the 1980's: lessons to be learnt. (abstr., proceedings) J. Bone Joint Surg. *72B*:530, 1990.
53. Langkamer, V.G., Ackroyd, C.E.: Safe forearm plate removal: Fact or fallacy? J. Bone Joint Surg. *71B*:875, 1989.
54. Rosson, J.W., Petley, G.W., Shearer, J.R.: Bone structure following plate removal from the forearm. J. Bone Joint Surg, *72B*:1092, 1990.
55. Rumball, K., Finnegan, M.: Refractures after forearm plate removal. J. Orthop. Trauma *4*:124, 1990.
56. Schemitsch, E., Richards, R.: The effect of malunion on functional outcome of fractures of both bones of the forearm in adults. J. Bone Joint Surg. *74A*: 1068, 1992
57. Street, D., Plut, J., Wood, W.: Intramedullary Forearm Nailing. American Academy Orthopaedic Surgeons Exhibit. 1979.

17

Applications for Reamed Intramedullary Nails in the Treatment of Femoral Nonunions

Keith Mayo

The use of intramedullary nailing techniques for femoral nonunions is generally restricted to diaphyseal applications. For the purposes of this discussion, we will consider the zone beginning 2 cm below the lesser trochanter and extending distally to 10 cm proximal to the knee joint. Fortunately, because of a circumferential muscle envelope and redundant blood supply, nonunions in this area are rare. Closed reamed nailing, the treatment of choice in most clinical settings, results in delayed or nonunion rates of less than 1%.[1–6] Open nailing techniques have shown nonunion rates that average 2.1%.[7] Plate fixation is complicated by nonunion in as many as 5 to 7% of patients.[8,9–14] Open fractures, particularly those with grade III soft-tissue injuries and/or segmental bone loss, are more prone to proceed to nonunion regardless of treatment modality.[13,15,16] Higher infection rates in these open injuries reflects greater devascularization and wound contamination and further increases the risk of nonunion.

Factors beyond the initial injury severity may contribute to the occurrence of nonunion. Surgical devascularization of the fracture site can occur with open nailing or plating techniques. Supplementary circlage wiring with intramedullary nailing and plating techniques that value anatomic reduction above fracture site blood supply have both been associated with higher nonunion and infection rates.[17,18] This does not indict the technique as much as it does the technician. Clearly both open nailing and plating can be carried out in a biologically conservative manner to achieve the goals of relative stability and restoration of length and alignment at minimal cost to fracture site vascularity. Although the interlocking nail has made open nailing now primarily of historical interest, plating indications persist in a variety of clinical settings and must take these factors into account. An additional technical mistake that may predispose a nonunion is fracture stabilization in a distracted position. Although this is most frequently seen with statically locked nails, it can also occur with plating.

General patient condition may also play a role in progress to union. This is primarily true in patients with multiple trauma or burns, where a catabolic state can easily occur unless parenteral or enteral nutrition is initiated early. Rarely, metabolic bone disease may play a role in the occurrence or persistence of nonunion.

A possible future concern is nonunion rates with unreamed interlocking femoral nails. The pulmonary effects of reaming, particularly in the multiply injured patient, have provided one stimulus for the use of these nails.[19,20] Another area of interest in this regard is open fractures. Theoretically, less damage to the endosteal blood supply may enhance healing. Perhaps offsetting this advantage is the loss of the autogenous grafting effect of reaming. Early clinical results with the unreamed interlocking nail are conflicting.[8,21,22] Given the relatively low frequency of nonunion with both techniques, it will take a large clinical series to document significant differences.

CLINICAL, RADIOGRAPHIC, AND LABORATORY EVALUATION

Most patients with femoral diaphyseal fractures will radiographically demonstrate some fracture callus within 6 to 8 weeks of injury and cortical bridging by 6 months.[1,4,5,23] This is the basis for the somewhat arbitrary definition of nonunion. Common sense dictates that patients who show slow, but continued progress toward union beyond this limit can be appropriately further observed if symptoms permit.

The history in most cases of femoral nonunion is straightforward. The mechanism may be revealing with regard to the amount of energy dissipated in the injury. Details of open fracture management such as timing of debridements, stabilization, and wound closure can be relevant. History of prolonged or recurrent drainage or systemic symptoms can be suggestive of occult infection. Pain complaints are variable. Individuals with hypertrophic nonunions, especially those with intramedullary nails in place, may have minimal discomfort. However, most patients will relate significant, localized discomfort, which is increased by weight bearing. Those patients who have not begun weight bearing may have discomfort with muscle force alone such as straight leg raising. Some patients are able to appreciate motion at the nonunion site. Deformity, when obvious, may be a major presenting complaint.

The directed physical exam begins with an assessment of leg length. This is done indirectly by assessing iliac crest height in the standing patient. Pelvic obliquity is corrected by measured blocks on the side of the perceived short limb. This method may be unreliable in the obese patient or in cases where there is posterior pelvic ring malunion. Hip or knee flexion contractures also present potential sources of error, thus making assessing clinical evaluation difficult. In these cases radiographic techniques may become the primary assessment modality. Alignment is also initially measured clinically. This is a triplane evaluation of varus-valgus, flexion-extension, and torsion. The latter is best appreciated using prone rotation profiles if the hip joints are unaffected. Wound status, muscle atrophy, and joint contractures are noted. A detailed lower extremity neurologic exam is routine. Gait abnormalities may be complex and reflect pain, deformity, and muscle weakness.

Radiographic evaluation must at least include full-length AP and lateral plane radiographs. If there is significant deformity present in the frontal or sagittal planes, comparison views of the opposite femur should be obtained for planning purposes. Alteration in weight bearing axis is best appreciated on a full length hip to ankle weight bearing comparison AP view. Some computed tomographic software packages will also provide this image with an extended scout view, but supine position may introduce artifact. Computed tomography is more routinely used for measurement of leg length and rotation if there is doubt about accuracy of clinical assessment. If significant hip or knee flexion contractures exist, metered lateral projections of the femur are the best guide to length. Occasionally, fluoroscopy may be useful to guide positioning for plain films for preoperative planning in complex deformities or rarely to direct aspirate or biopsy in cases of suspected infection.

Nuclear medicine scans using gallium- and indium-labelled white cells have been advocated for evaluation of potential nonunions. However, they are expensive and rarely provide pivotal information that cannot be derived from history, exam, simple laboratory values, and the radiographic assessment outlined above.

The laboratory assessment should always include a sedimentation rate as a general screen for subclinical infection. Additional evaluation will depend on the clinical setting. Patients who have had multiple system trauma and a prolonged convalescence may warrant a nutritional analysis as a baseline and to direct management of negative nitrogen or caloric balance. Occasionally, a workup for metabolic bone disease is warranted. This usually occurs in the case of aseptic nonunion refractory to appropriate prior surgical management. The patient at risk is generally female, middle-aged, or older and may have a history of other fractures with minimal trauma. Screening laboratory as well as tetracycline labelled biopsy may be needed in these situations. Treatment of the underlying bone disease must then precede further surgical intervention.

SURGICAL MANAGEMENT OF SYMPTOMATIC NONUNION

Overview

Numerous techniques have been reported for the management of femoral diaphyseal nonunions. Debridement and grafting with plaster (spica) immobilization has been relatively unsuccessful in achieving union and are complicated by muscle atrophy and joint contracture.[24–26] Electrical stimulation also appears to be poorly adapted to the problem of femoral nonunion.[27,28] External fixation, though complicated by pin tract morbidity, has a limited treatment role in the setting of active infection as discussed below.[29–33] The majority of modern reports of treatment of femoral shaft nonunions deal with plate or intramedullary nail osteosynthesis techniques, variably augmented with grafting techniques. Comparison between these often dissimilar series is difficult, but in general, intramedullary nailing has been more successful and attended by fewer complications.[11,12,34–36,38,47]

Limitations of Intramedullary Nail Technique

There is a natural temptation to extend the use of intramedullary nails to nonunions of the metaphyseal-diaphyseal junction or beyond. When there is minimal distortion of anatomy and good bone quality present, this may be successful, particularly with third-generation locking or reconstruction nails.[39] However, peritrochanteric and supracondylar nonunions are generally better managed by condylar blade plates which provide better metaphyseal fixation and precise restoration of anatomic and weight bearing axes.[11] This is particularly important in the young patient or in the patient with pre-existing lower extremity arthrosis.[40] Occasionally, it may actually be prudent to shift the weight-bearing axis through intentional varus or valgus at the fracture site, in light of known symptomatic arthritis. Deferred full weight bearing is usually required for nonunions in this area, regardless of implant, and the additional morbidity of plating is small.

Obliteration of the medullary canal in long-established nonunions of the femur is another relative contraindication to the use of intramedullary nailing. This most frequently occurs in the setting of prior traction treatment, in which there is bayonet apposition. Surgical treatment in this setting requires an extensive exposure for mobilization and restoration of length and alignment. Although it may be technically possible to recreate the medullary canal, the additional sacrifice of the blood supply at the nonunion site may outway the advantages of intramedullary stabilization. In this now relatively unusual context, plate fixation may be the best choice.

Starting-point errors inherited from a primary nailing attempt are another source of difficulty. In cases where the nonunion is in the middle or distal third of the diaphysis, it may be safe to use a poorly-placed entry point for renailing if one takes into account the increased insertional forces required and overreaming is increased 0.5 to 1.0 mm. Alternately, a new (correct) starting point may be initiated if a large-diameter nail has not been used initially and an adequate bridge of intact bone remains between the two. When this bridge fails, a trough is created and may compromise proximal fixation, even with reconstruction nails. There is also the theoretical increased risk to femoral neck and head blood supply with two starting points adjacent to the superior retinacular anastomosis. However, the major concern arises in fractures of the proximal third. In these instances, reestablishment of alignment is frequently impossible unless the nail entry point is corrected. When this is not possible, significant malreduction may persist and the chance of achieving union is reduced. Use of the condylar blade plate, while technically demanding, becomes the best salvage in this setting (Fig. 17–1).

Surgical Technique

Thorough preoperative planning based on the above outlined evaluation is critical. Tactics for correction of deformity, if present, must be detailed. Surgical positioning is a matter of surgeon preference based on experience. I prefer the lateral position for nonunions of the proximal two thirds and the supine position with a soft support under the lumbar spine for cases involving the distal third. A fracture table with articulated leg holders may be used, but I

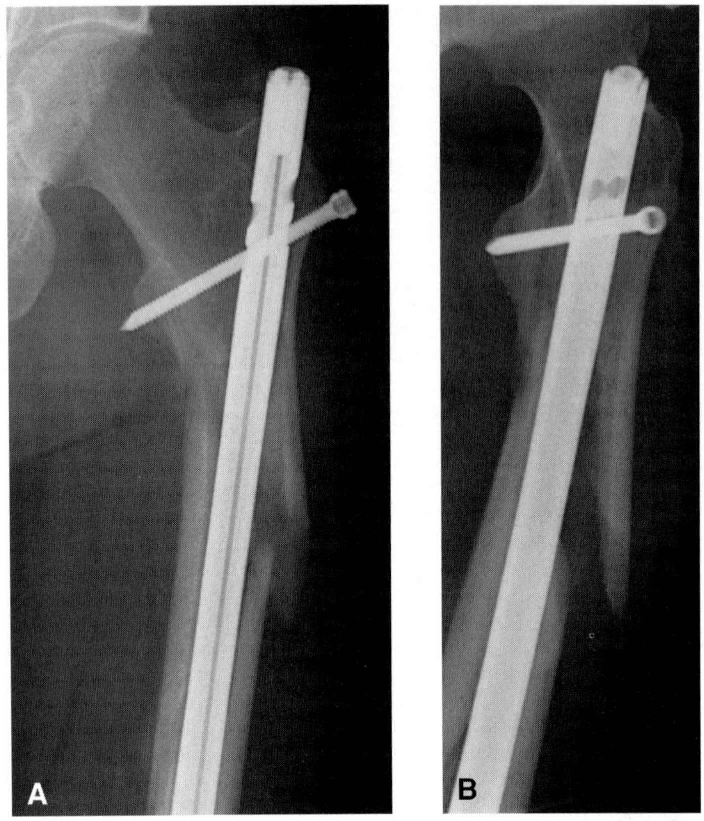

Fig. 17–1. *A,B,* AP and lateral views of a 32-year-old man who sustained this closed segmental subtrochanteric fracture 6.5 months prior. He was treated by open nailing technique with extensive dissection and use of a statically locked nail, which was inserted through a lateral and anteriorly malpositioned starting point. A large posteromedial shaft butterfly fragment has united and the patient is left with a painful nonunion in varus and slight flexion. *(Figure continues)*

have opted for a standard radiolucent table which will allow biplanar fluoroscopic access to the pelvis and lower extremity. The involved extremity and buttock are prepped and draped with the limb free. A starting-point incision is made in the routine manner and enlarged as necessary to accommodate the proximal locking jig of an interlocking nail chosen by preoperative planning.

The most straightforward case involves exchange nailing of a nonunion which is in acceptable position (Fig. 17–2). Preservation of rotational alignment should be assured by parallel proximal and distal fragment Kirschner wires. These are most easily placed posteriorly at the level of lesser trochanter and distally in the lateral femoral condyle. The old femoral nail and locking screws are then removed. Strategies and instrumentation for removal of broken implants must be anticipated. Broken screws can usually be removed by limited open techniques and nails with intramedullary extraction tools. These techniques preserve the closed nature of the procedure. Once the old implants have been removed, the leg may be gently manipulated to disrupt fibrous tissue at the nonunion site and promote local neovascularization. Sufficient reaming is then carried out to allow passage of a nail 2 mm larger. When bone loss is not present, use of a dynamic proximal and distal locked nail is preferred to allow impaction with weight bearing at the nonunion and still guarantee rotational control.

The sequence is similar in the case of failed but not malaligned plate fixation. Surgical exposure of the nonunion is limited to the extent required for implant removal. Reestablishment of a patent canal is accomplished with

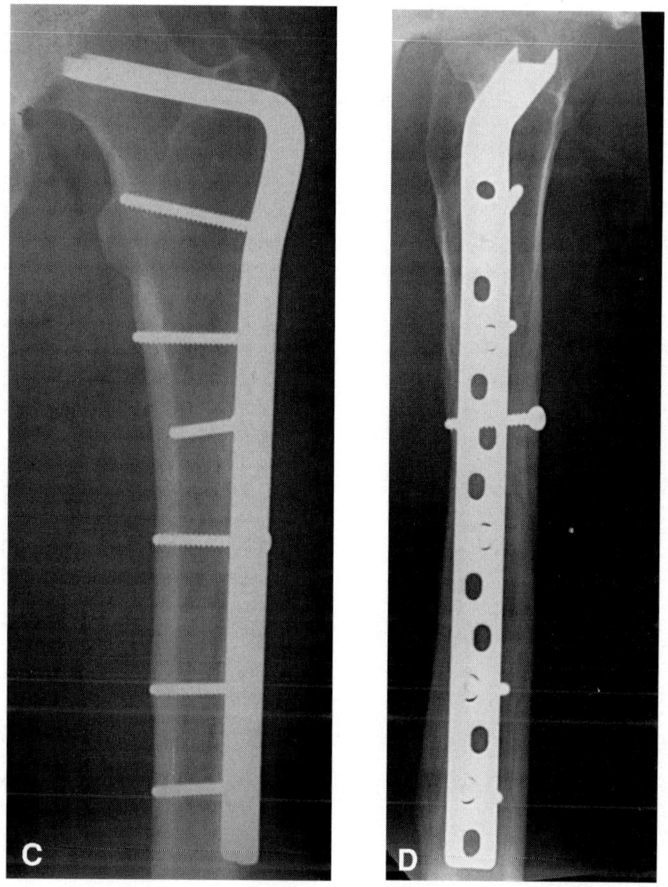

Fig. 17–1. *(continued) C,D,* Because of the proximal location, varus malposition, and significant starting point error, this problem is best managed by 95° condylar blade plate as shown. This is the appearance 6 months postoperatively with pain-free solid union and anatomic reconstruction of the proximal femur. The patients weight bearing was limited to 20 kg for the first 8 weeks. Otherwise there were no postoperative restrictions.

medullary awls and osteotomes, thus minimizing dissection.

When malposition and nonunion are combined, operative intervention becomes progressively more challenging. Shortening of more than 1 cm and malrotation or angulation of more than 10 to 15° may have functional sequelae.[41] Rotational malalignment is the easiest deformity to manage and can often be accomplished closed or with percutaneous mobilization of the nonunion (Fig. 17–3). The desired correction can be established between proximal and distal Schanz screws using a sterile goniometer prior to implant removal. Derotation is then carried out around a guide rod and locked with the AO-ASIF Universal Distractor (Synthes; Paoli, PA) until the new interlocked nail is in place.[42]

As deformities become more complex, surgical exposure of the nonunion becomes unavoidable. The approach is usually mid-lateral, with elevation of the vastus lateralis anteriorly off the intermuscular septum. The deep dissection is performed in a manner that preserves as much periosteal blood supply as possible. Rarely, a repeat medial approach with mobilization of the superficial femoral artery and anterior retraction of the vastus medialis and rectus femoris is required. This occurs in the setting of prior open fracture with arterial repair and medial plate stabilization. Next, old implants are removed as noted above and the nonunion is mobilized to facilitate restoration of length, as well as frontal and sagittal plane alignment. The universal distractor becomes even more valuable in these cases of complex

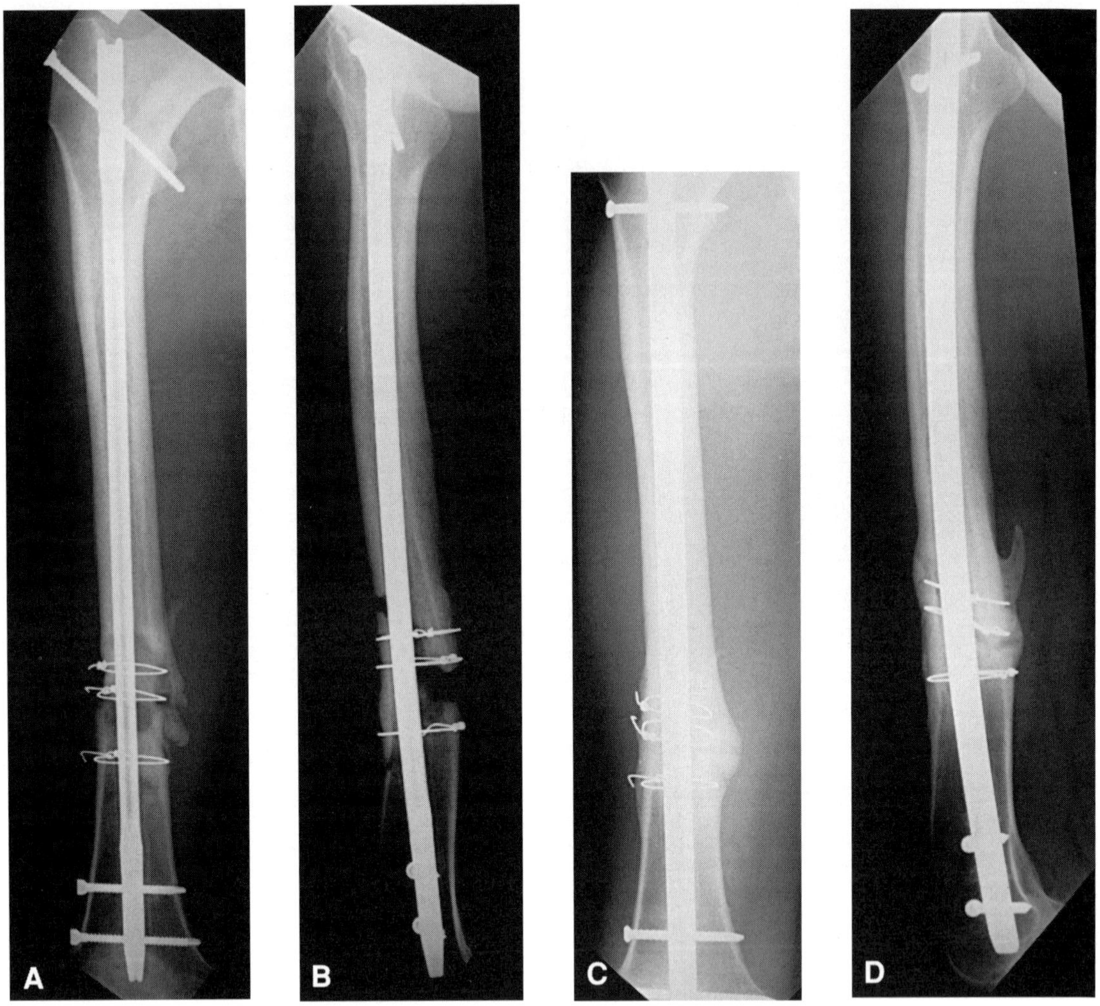

Fig. 17–2. *A,B,* Radiographs of a closed distal diaphyseal femur fracture in a 29-year-old man 8 months after open, statically locked nailing which was "augmented" by circlage wires. Alignment is satisfactory but the patient continues to have weight bearing pain. *C,D,* Appearance 4 months after exchange static locked nailing with 2-mm larger-diameter nail. Union has occurred rapidly and the patient is asymptomatic.

deformity. Single stage length restorations of 3 to 5 cm can be safely carried out.[41] It is not necessary or desirable to extensively debride the nonunion site.[35,38] After restoration of triplanar alignment and length, the medullary canal is then recanulated, reamed, and a statically locked nail inserted.

The success of closed technique for treatment of most femoral diaphyseal nonunions [35,36,38] has narrowed the discussion of bone grafting techniques and indications to those cases with segmental defects and/or complex deformities requiring open realignment. Closed medullary autogenous cancellous grafting of segmental defects has been described in the acute fracture setting,[43] but its applicability in the nonunion environment is uncertain. This leaves open grafting techniques as the primary treatment modality.

When the defect is small, Judet[30,31] achieved excellent results with local osteoperiosteal grafting alone. As the size of the defect increases, spanning cancellous autograft becomes necessary. Allograft impregnated with bone morphogenic protein has also been used successfully,[41] but is not widely available at this time. As a general rule, when an open procedure is required, cancellous autografting is appropriate and adds little to operative morbidity when performed carefully.

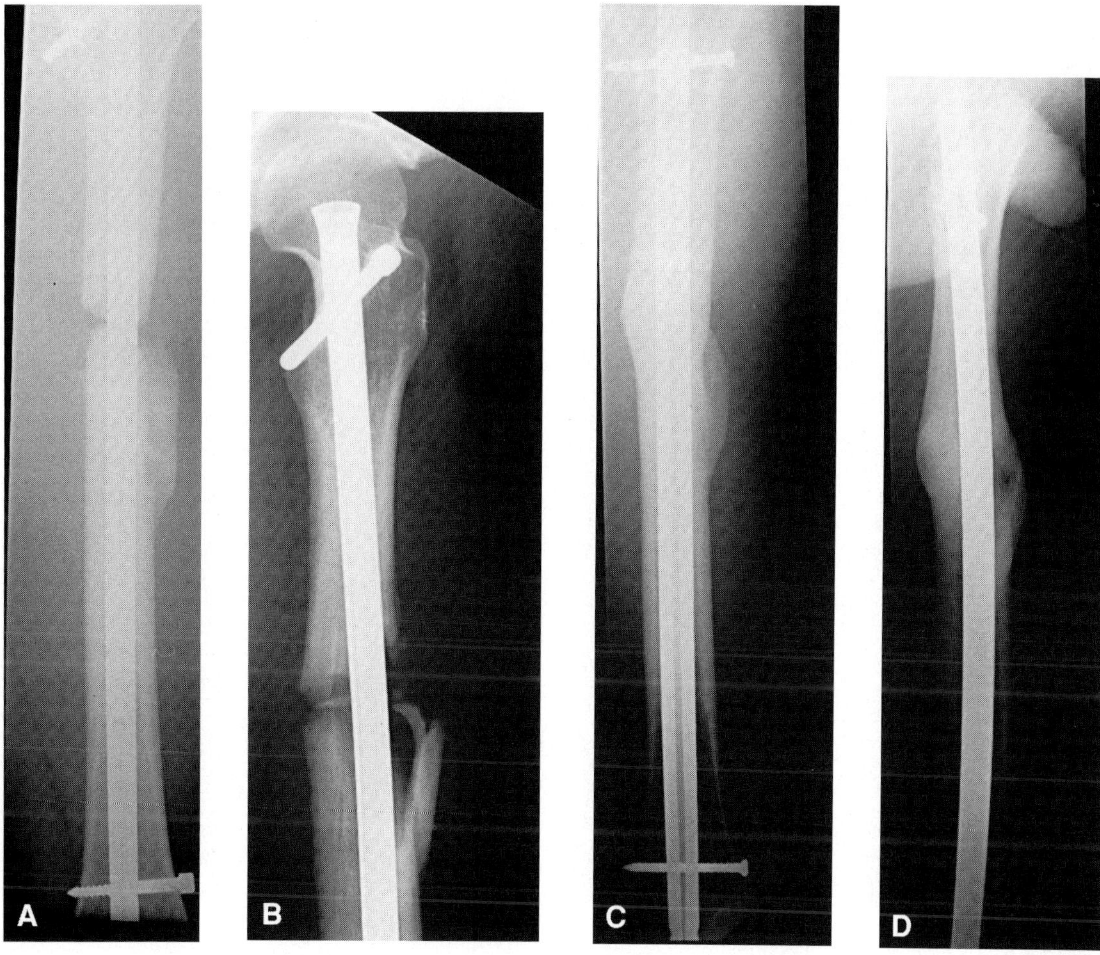

Fig. 17–3. *A,B,* A 24-year-old male pedestrian struck by a car sustained this grade IIIa open fracture 7 months prior. He was treated by primary irrigation, debridement, and stabilization with a reamed 12-mm statically locked nail. His wound was closed on a delayed basis and he had no subsequent drainage or other evidence of infection. He was nailed in slight distraction and both clinical exam and computed tomography show 20° of external rotation at the fracture site. *C,D,* Radiographic appearance 6 months following percutaneous fibrolysis, rotational correction, and repeat medullary nailing with dynamic proximal and distal locked implant.

Treatment of Infected Nonunions

The presence of infection may seriously complicate management of even the most anatomically routine nonunion. Intramedullary nailing technique can still be used successfully, but may require multiple surgical interventions with intermittent-use suppressive antibiotics. The initial procedure calls for removal of previous implants with adequate decompression of any deep abscess pockets followed by reamed nailing. Extensive primary debridement is not needed unless there are radiographically obvious sequestra. Early use of suction-irrigation systems[44,45] has been replaced by suction drains alone. Bone grafting, if necessary, is delayed until active wound drainage has abated. The use of adjunctive antibiotic beads may be helpful in some cases and most patients will need several weeks of parenteral perioperative antibiotics. Despite these interventions, drainage may persist until union has been achieved and the implants are removed. This drainage, while bothersome, may be protective in preventing further abscess formation and systemic illness. When the latter do occur, repeated surgical decompression may be necessary. The success rate of achieving union in this unfortunate milieu is a surprisingly high (80 to 90%).[37,38,44–46] After union is achieved, it may be prudent to remove the nail and ream the medullary canal to remove any contaminated

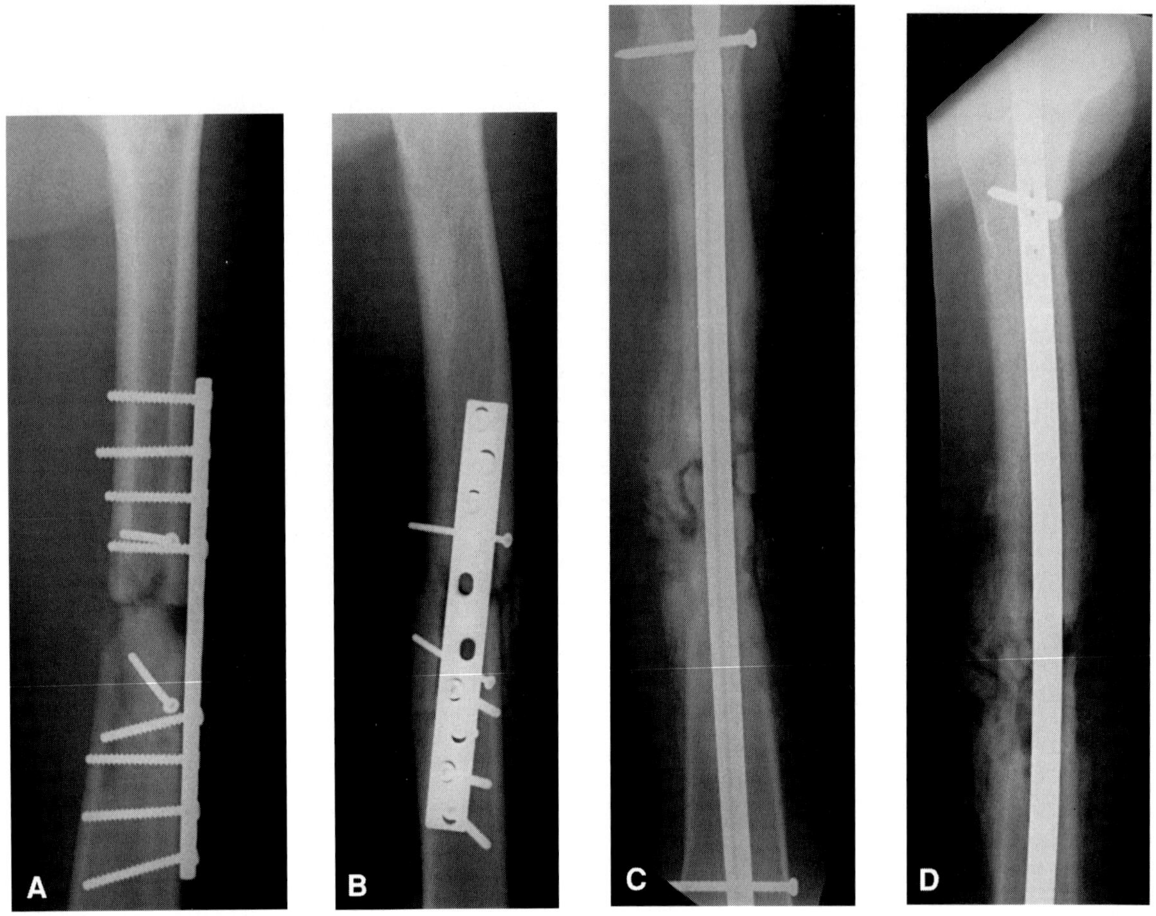

Fig. 17–4. *A,B,* A 22-year-old man sustained this grade IIIa open fracture in a motorcycle accident 4.5 months prior. Plate stabilization was elected in the presence of ipsilateral open tibia fracture and multiple system trauma. The wound healed after delayed closure, but there is clear failure of radiographic progress toward union. *C,D,* This is the appearance of the femur 3 months after plate removal and stabilization with a 12-mm reamed nail. Deep infection with *S. aureus* was discovered at the time of plate removal. Local debridement and lavage preceded nail placement. The wound was closed primarily over suction drains. Two weeks of intravenous antibiotics were followed by 6 weeks of oral therapy. *(Figure continues)*

implant membrane. In addition, the patient may benefit from debridement of obvious sequestra and bone grafting at sites of tenuous union (Fig. 17–4). This combination of measures usually is successful in producing a dry wound and union of adequate strength. However, an accurate term for the underlying osteomyelitis is more likely quiescent than cured.

Alternative treatment modalities for infected nonunions have been used. Extensive debridement accompanied by depot or systemic antibiotics, external fixation, and delayed bone grafting has produced reasonably good union rates.[29,30–32] However, local morbidity from pin tract sepsis and extensor mechanism scarring is a major detractor. Knee joint contracture may be significant enough to warrant quadricepsplasty in some patients and poor cosmetic outcome is almost universal.

Modified plating techniques have also been successfully adapted by some surgeons for the treatment of infected nonunions.[33,37] These protocols call for a similar sequence of debridement, stabilization, local and/or systemic antibiotics, and bone grafting.

The ultimate decision regarding management techniques for the infected femoral nonunion is based on multiple factors including bacteriology, methods of previous surgical treatment, presenting signs and symptoms, and general patient condition. A multidisciplinary approach may be helpful with input from plastic

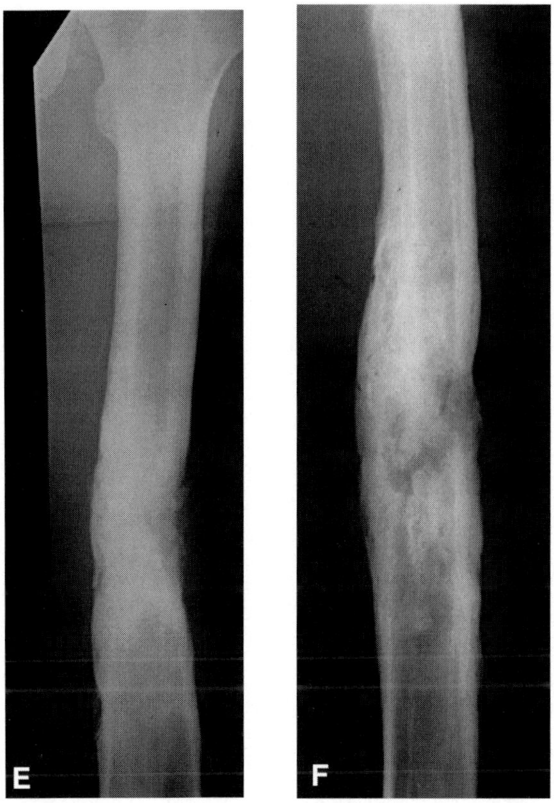

Fig. 17–4. *(continued) E,F,* Final appearance 26 months following nail placement. The nonunion healed with persistence of a small sinus tract and the nail was removed after an 18-month interval. At the time of implant removal, the sinus tract was excised and lateral cortical sequestrum was removed, followed by placement of antibiotic beads. Four weeks later the beads were removed and autogenous grafting was carried out. The wounds healed and no further drainage has occurred.

surgery regarding complex wound problems and a surgical infectious disease consultant, when the bacterial isolates are unusual or extended antibiotic treatment is required. In selected cases, it may be necessary to employ different modalities sequentially to achieve union, such as a brief period of external fixation following debridement followed by definitive stabilization with intramedullary nail or plate.

SUMMARY

Nonunions of the femoral diaphysis are a relatively uncommon problem. Treatment presents a wide spectrum of clinical challenges from the nearly routine exchange nailing of a well aligned hypertrophic nonunion to the staged management of an infected nonunion with segmental bone loss. The same implant may be used in both cases, but the level of surgical experience and technical expertise required to produce a successful outcome is far different. In general, intramedullary nailing techniques are well suited to this clinical setting, but the individual surgeon must make a prudent choice about his own involvement on a case by case basis.

REFERENCES

1. Brumback, R.J., Uwagie-Ero, S., Lakatos, R.P., et al.: Intramedullary nailing of femoral shaft fractures. Part II: Fracture-healing with static interlocking fixation. J. Bone Joint Surg. *70A*:1453–1462, 1988.
2. Carr, C.R., Wingo, C.H.: Fractures of the femoral diaphysis. A retrospective study of the results and costs of treatment by intramedullary nailing and by traction and a spica cast. J. Bone Joint Surg. *55A*:690–700, 1973.
3. Christie, J., Court-Brown, C., Kinninmouth, A.W.G., Howie, C.R.: Intramedullary locking nails in the management of femoral shaft fractures. J. Bone Joint Surg. *70B*:206–210, 1988.
4. Kempf, I., Grosse, A., Beck, F.: Closed interlocking intramedullary nailing. Its application to comminuted fractures of the femur. J. Bone Joint Surg. *67A*:709–720, 1985.
5. Winquist, R.A., Hansen, S.T., Jr., Clawson, D.K.: Closed intramedullary nailing of femoral fractures: A report of five hundred and twenty cases. J. Bone Joint Surg. *66A*: 529–539, 1984.
6. Zuckerman, J., Veith, R., Johnson, K., et al.: Treatment of unstable femoral shaft fractures with closed interlocking intramedullary nailing. J. Orthop. Trauma *1*: 209–218, 1987.
7. Chapman, M.W.: The role of intramedullary fixation in open fractures. Clin. Orthop. *212*:26–34, 1986.
8. Allgöwer, M., Ehrsam, R., Ganz, R., et al.: Clinical experience with a new compression plate "DCP". Acta Orthop Scand *36*(suppl.):277–279, 1969.
9. Gant, G.C., Shaftan, G.W., Herbsman, H.: Experience with the ASIF compression plate in the management of femoral shaft fractures. J. Trauma *10*:458–471, 1970.
10. Magerl, F., Wyss, A., Brunner, C., et al.: Plate osteosynthesis of femoal shaft fractures in adults: A follow-up study. Clin. Orthop. *138*:62–73, 1979
11. Müller, M.E., Thomas, R.J.: Treatment of nonunion in fractures of long bones. Clin. Orthop. *138*:141, 1979.
12. Murray, W.R., Lucas, D.B., Inman, V.T.: Treatment of nonunion of fractures of long bones by the two-plate method. J. Bone Joint Surg. *46A*:1027, 1964.
13. Riemer, B.L., Butterfield, S.L., Burke, C.J., Mathews, D.: Immediate plate fixation of highly comminuted femoral diaphyseal fractures in blunt polytrauma patients. Orthopedics *15*:907–916, 1992.
14. Rüedi, T., Luscher, N.: Results after internal fixation of comminuted fractures of the femoral shaft with DC plates. Clin. Orthop. *138*:74, 1979.
15. Brumback, R.J., Ellison, P.S., Poka, A., et al.: Intramedullary nailing of open fractures of femoral shaft. J Bone Joint Surg. *71A*:1324–1330, 1989.
16. Lhowe, D.W., Hansen, S.T.: Immediate nailing of open fractures of the femoral shaft. J. Bone Joint Surg. *70A*: 812–820, 1988.
17. Baumgaertel. F., Gotzen, L.: The biological plate osteosynthesis in multi-fragment fractures of the para-ar-

ticular femur. A prospective study. Unfallchirurg *97*: 78–84, 1994.

18. Tscherne, H., Haas, N., Krettek, C.: Intramedullary nailing combined with cerclage wiring in the treatment of fractures of the femoral shaft. Clin. Orthop. *212*:62–67, 1986.
19. Pape, H.C., Regel, G., Dwenger A., et al.: Influence of thoracic trauma and primary femoral intramedullary nailing on the incidence of ARDS in multiple trauma patients. Injury *24*:82–103, 1993.
20. Wenda, K., Runkel, J., Degreif, G., et al.: Pathogenesis and clinical relevance of bone marrow embolism in medullary nailing—demonstrated by intraoperative echocardiography. Injury *24*:73–81, 1993.
21. Hutson, J.J., Zynch, G.A., Latta, L.: Unreamed nine millimeter femoral nailing. A prospective randomized comparison with reamed twelve millimeter femoral nails. Presented at the Orthopaedic Trauma Association Annual Meeting, Los Angeles, California, September 22–24, 1994.
22. Moed, B.R., Watson, J.T.: Retrograde unreamed intramedullary nailing of fractures of the femoral shaft in the multiply injured patient. Presented at the Orthopaedic Trauma Association Annual Meeting, Los Angeles, California, September 22–24, 1994.
23. Klemm, K., Börner, M.: Interlocking nailing of complex fractures of the femur and tibia. Clin. Orthop. *212*: 89–100, 1986.
24. Phemister, D.B.: Splint grafts in the treatment of delayed and nonunion of fractures. Surg. Gynecol. Obstet. *52*:376, 1931.
25. Phemister, D.B.: Treatment of ununited fractures by onlay bone grafts without screws or tie fixation and without breaking down of the fibrous union. J. Bone Joint Surg. *29*:946, 1947.
26. Urist, M.R., Mazet, R., McLean, F.C.: The pathogenesis and treatment of delayed union and nonunion. J. Bone Joint Surg. *36A*:931, 1954.
27. Connolly, J.F.: Selection, evaluation and indications for electrical stimulation of ununited fractures. Clin. Orthop. *161*:39, 1981.
28. Day, L.: Electrical stimulation in the treatment of ununited fractures. Clin. Orthop. *161*:54, 1981.
29. Barquet, A., Silva, R., Massaferro, Cubra, A.: The AO tubular external fixator in the treatment of open fractures and infected nonunions of the shaft of the femur. Injury *19*:415, 1988.
30. Judet, R., Patel, A.: Muscle pedicle bone grafting of long bones by osteoperiosteal decortication. Clin. Orthop. *87*:74, 1972.
31. Judet, J., Judet, R.: L'ostéogénèse et les retards de consolidation et les pseudarthroses des os longs, 1960, Huitième Congrès SICOT, p. 315.
32. Jupiter, J.B., First, K., Gallico, G.G., May, J.W.: The role of external fixation in the treatment of post-traumatic osteomyelitis. J. Orthop. Trauma *2*:79–93, 1988.
33. Weber, B.C., Cech, O.: Pseudarthrosis, pathology, biomechanics, therapy, results, Berne, Switzerland, 1976, Berne, Hans Huber Medical Publisher.
34. Brav, E.A.: The use of intramedullary nailing for nonunion of the femur. Clin. Orthop *60*:69–75, 1968.
35. Kempf, I., Grosse, A., Rigaut, P.: The treatment of noninfected pseudarthrosis of the femur and tibia with locked intramedullary nailing. Clin. Orthop. *212*: 142–154, 1986.
36. Klemm, K.: Die stabilisierung infizieter pseudarthrosen mit verriegelungsnagel. Langenbecks Arch. Chir. *334*: 559–561, 1973.
37. Lhowe, D.W., Cove, J., Goodman, L.J.: The management of diaphseal nonunion of the femur. Presented at the Orthopaedic Trauma Association Annual Meeting, Los Angeles, California, September 22–24, 1994.
38. Webb, L.X., Winquist, R.A., Hansen, S.T.: Intramedullary nailing and reaming for delayed union or nonunion of the femoral shaft. A report of 105 consecutive cases. Clin. Orthop. *212*:133–141, 1986.
39. McLaren, A.C., Blokker, C.P.: Locked intramedullary fixation for metaphyseal malunion and nonunion. Clin. Orthop. *265*:253, 1981.
40. Kettelkamp, D.B., Hillberry, B.M., Murrish, D.E., Keck, D.A.: Degenerative arthritis of the knee secondary to fracture malunion. Clin. Orthop. *234*:159, 1988.
41. Johnson, E.E.: Acute lengthening of shortened lower extremities after malunion or nonunion of a fracture. J. Bone Joint Surg. *76A*:379–389, 1994.
42. Baumgaertel, F., Dahlen, C., Stiletto, R., Gotzen, L.: Technique of using the AO-Femoral distractor for femoral intramedullary nailing. J. Orthop. Trauma *8*: 315–321, 1994.
43. Chapman, M.W.: Closed intramedullary bone grafting and nailing of segmental defects of the femur. J. Bone Joint Surg. *62A*:1004–1008, 1980.
44. Klemm, K.W.: Treatment of infected pseudarthrosis of the femur and tibia with an interlocking nail. Clin. Orthop. *212*:174–181, 1986.
45. Kostuik, J.P., Harrington, I.J.: Treatment of infected ununited femoral shaft fractures. Clin. Orthop. *108*:90, 1975.
46. Patzakis, M.J., Wilkins, J., Wiss, D.A.: Infection following intramedullary nailing of long bones. Clin. Orthop. *212*:182–191, 1986.

18

Intramedullary Osteotomies

Robert A. Winquist

This chapter reviews the use of an intramedullary bone saw in femoral shortenings, derotational osteotomies, and correction of malunions. I focus on the technical details of the equipment and the surgical procedures required for using these instruments. From a historical perspective, Gerhard Küntscher, deserves credit for designing the first intramedullary bone saw in 1962.[1] This saw allowed an osteotomy of the long bone after prior intramedullary reaming.[2–4] Unfortunately, the saw was neither stable nor easily controlled. In 1973, Ray E. Pearson and the Supersonic Transport Division of the Boeing Company (Seattle, WA) were kind enough to donate their time and expertise to develop a new, more effective bone saw.[5] This saw evolved through several design stages worth brief mention. Initially, two blades were used simultaneously to make both cuts for a shortening. These blades, similar in dimension to the original Küntscher design, were thin and tended to break. Two simultaneous cuts led to excessive binding and difficulty with cutting. This intitial design was not successful and modifications were made. A bushing added to keep the saw stable in the intramedullary canal has been a tremendous help in making complete and accurately placed cuts. A measuring device, designed for simplicity, aids in accurate determination of the amount of shortening. This device fits easily over the saw and has a trochanteric rest to control depth and a lock nut to control the measurement of the second cut. Power was used to drive the original saw, but the power attachement was removed because of binding of the blade and excessive cutting with burning of the bone.

The Boeing Company turned the design over to Orthopedic Equipment Company (OEC) for manufacturing (Fig. 18–1). The various components of the saw are now interchangeable, so that only one handle with an indexing device is needed for the various bushings and blades that are available (Figs. 18–2 and 18–3).[6] After 40 surgical procedures, I decided that the range of saws should be increased. The available sizes are now 12, 13, 14, 15, 16, and 17 mm. The saws are actually 0.5 mm smaller than indicated to allow reaming to the stated size and easy placement of the saw. Blade breakage was an initial problem with the OEC saw but has been corrected through improvement of the blade attachment. Boeing had also designed a fragmenter to split and displace the central fragment.[5] The concept worked reasonably well for splitting but not for displacement. One side of the split fragment was always unstable and would move while the other side stayed in position. The fragmenter is no longer manufactured, and the internal chisel hook of Küntscher now is used to split the fragment and to move it to the side. This device is much simpler than the expansion fragmenter.

CLOSED INTRAMEDULLARY SHORTENING

Materials and Indications

Careful patient evaluation and selection are critical in intramedullary shortenings. All forms of treatment should be available to the surgeon. This procedure is not the only method of correcting leg length inequality, and the surgeon should consider the use of (1) a shoelift,

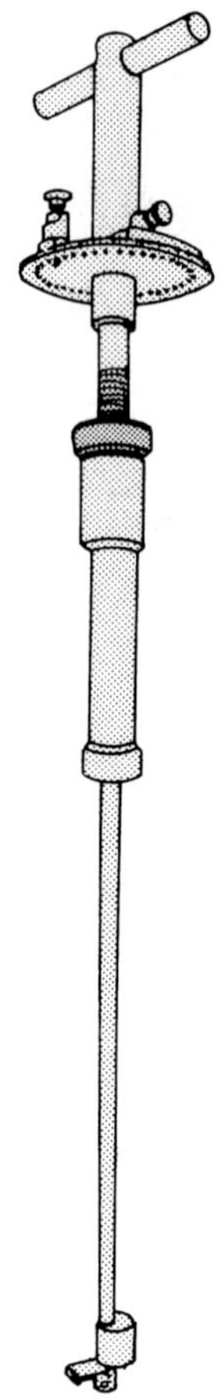

Fig. 18–1. The OEC intramedullary bone saw.

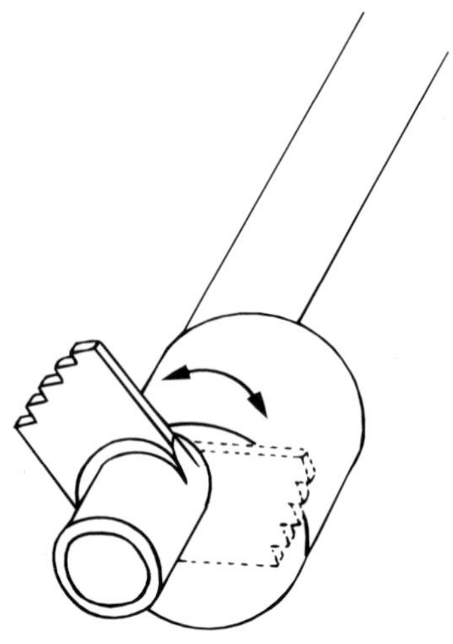

Fig. 18–3. Opening and closing of saw blade.

(2) lengthening of the tibia or femur, (3) shortening of the tibia or femur, (4) lengthening of the pelvis, (5) varus subtrochanteric osteotomies for hip dysplasia, and (6) a combination of lengthening and shortening, amputation, and epiphysiodesis. Each patient must be evaluated individually before the patient and surgeon can select the correct form of treatment. This chapter reviews only the surgical practice of closed intramedullary shortening for correction of leg length inequality.[7]

Radiographic evaluation is critical. The area of deformity should be evaluated radiographically to determine whether correction of the deformity is indicated. Scanograms or orthodiagrams are beneficial in deciding whether the discrepency is located in the pelvis, femur, tibia, or foot. Computed tomography-scan cuts can also be used to measure the reference points of the hips, knees, ankles, and feet. Standing radiographs are used to determine whether a patient with scoliosis has a fixed deformity or functional deformity. To determine the final amount of correction, the most valuable radiograph is taken with the patient standing on blocks to level the pelvis and realign the spine. This radiograph should include the lower lumbar spine, the iliac crest, and the femoral heads to help determine the correct amount of equalization.

Radiographs of the femur to be shortened are also mandatory. The variation from one patient to the next is tremendous (Figs. 18–4 through 18–8). The surgeon must carefully evaluate the size of the medullary canal and must determine the thickness of the linea and the medullary canal on both the AP and lateral radiographs. These measurements are helpful during subsequent surgical planning.

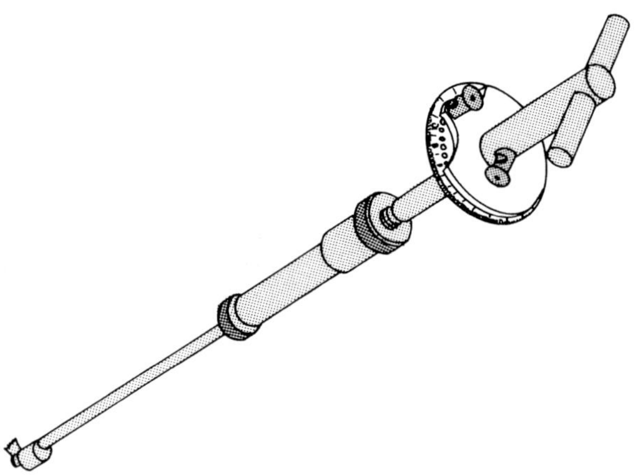

Fig. 18–2. Indexing device controls expansion of saw blade.

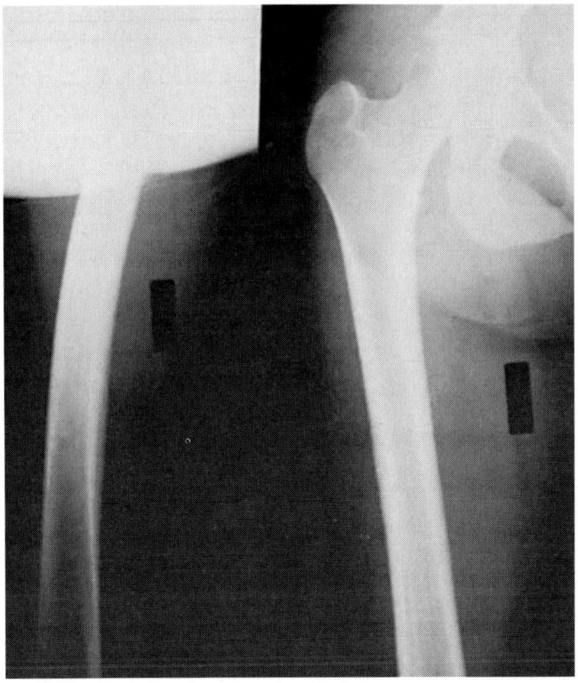

Fig. 18–4. AP and lateral views demonstrate a wide symmetrical canal, an excellent femur for shortening.

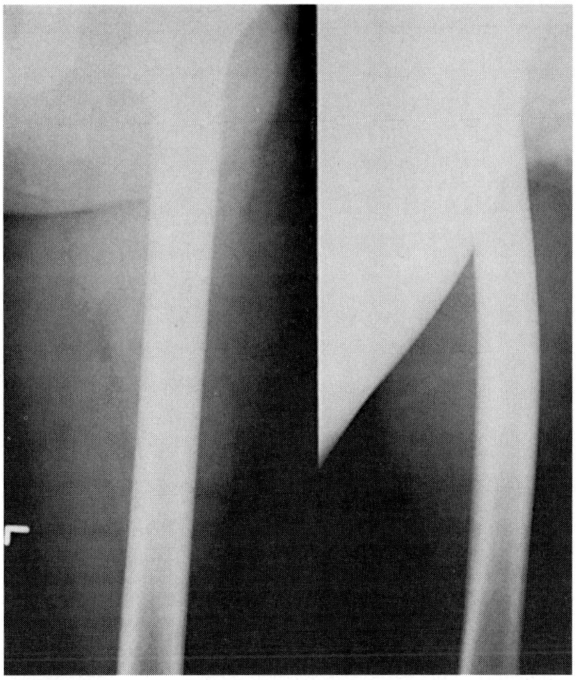

Fig. 18–5. AP and lateral views demonstrate rather thick cortices that require intramedullary reaming to allow insertion of a saw of adequate size. The cortices are symmetrical, however, and should allow good intramedullary shortening.

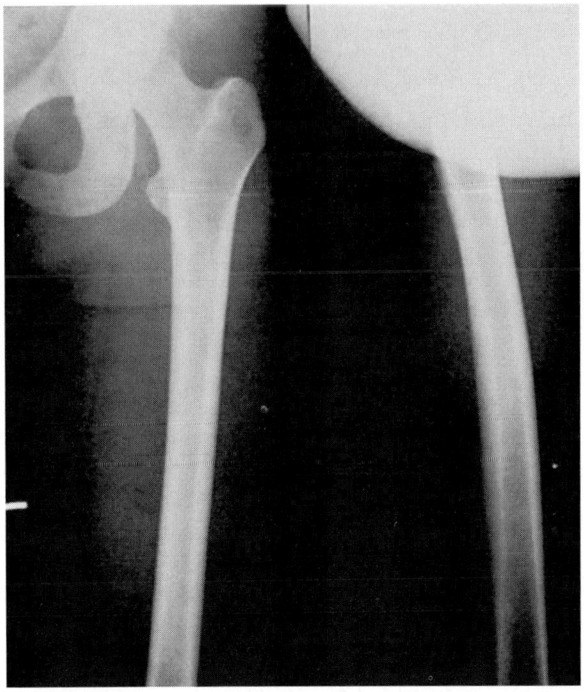

Fig. 18–6. This femoral shortening is technically more difficult. The canal is small, particularly on the AP view, and the linea is thick. Reaming is necessary but using a small saw makes it difficult to cut through the walls and linea; therefore, a percutaneous osteotome is necessary.

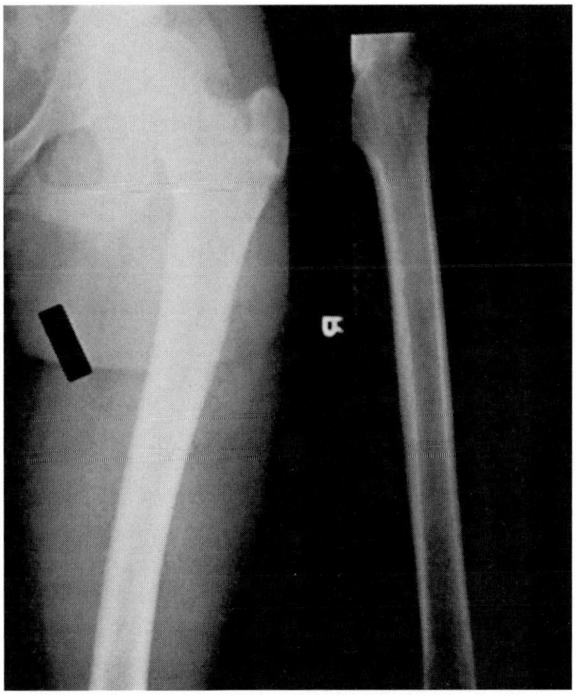

Fig. 18–7. This patient has polio. The shaft is quite straight on the lateral projection and a wide canal should make shortening easy. Unfortunately, the AP view shows a marked bowing of the femur. The tendency is to thin the lateral cortex and cause further comminution at the level of shortening.

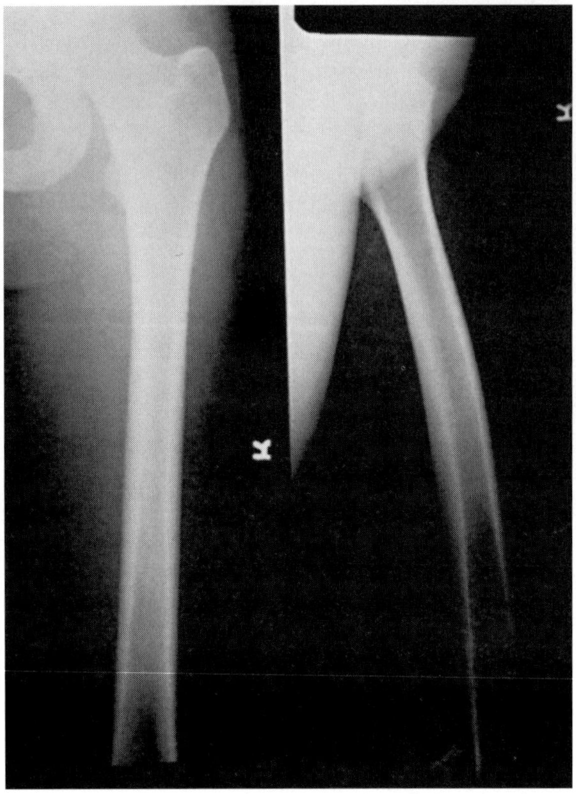

Fig. 18–8. On the lateral radiograph, the linea is thickened and a complete cut with a saw is not possible. A percutaneous osteotome is necessary.

Between 1980 and 1989, 145 patients underwent closed intramedullary shortening of the femur. Their ages ranged from 12 years to 64 years (mean = 27.7). The etiology of the inequality was varied. Femoral fractures accounted for 34% of the patients and tibial fractures for 11% of the patients. A combination of lateral-femoral and tibial fractures were seen in 9% of the patients. Idiopathic and congenital abnormalities were seen in 22% of the patients, including congenital hip disorders in 5% of the patients. Polio was the cause of leg length inequality in 5% of the patients.

The patients had the following symptoms and complaints. They are listed individually but were frequently seen in combination. Ninety patients complained of their awkward gait and limp. Back pain was seen in 87 patients, and 51 patients had scoliosis. Ankle sprains were seen in 14 patients, many of whom were wearing high lifts. The discrepency in this group of patients ranged from 2 to 10 cm. The mean discrepency was 3.8 cm. In evaluating the shape of the femur in this group of patients, it was noted that 50 patients had a thick linea and 20 patients had a narrow medullary canal. Twelve patients had an increased bow, making the shortening slightly more difficult. The amount of shortening performed was 2 to 7 cm, with a mean of 3.5 cm. The type of nail used for fixation changed during the study from a standard Küntscher nail to the routine use of a statically locked interlocking nail for all patients. The nail diameter ranged from 11 to 17 mm, with a mean of 14.3 mm. The nail length ranged from 29 to 46 cm, with a mean of 38.3 cm. Percutaneous osteotomy was required in 36% of the patients to complete the cut. Operative time averaged 98.7 minutes. The drop in hematocrit was 10.1 points, and the patients were asked to donate two units of blood prior to surgery.

Surgical Technique

Proper equipment is mandatory because of the technical nature of the procedure. This chapter explains the reasons for my personal preferences but also certainly acknowledges the alternatives. I prefer a set of OEC reamers with their deep flutes and small flexible shafts, as well as a large size range. These generate less pressure and less fat embolism than AO reamers. In addition, a long reamer (12.5 × 60 cm) is needed to clean out the medullary canal (Fig. 18–9).

I use the Chick 703 (Chick Midmark; Verailles, OH) table for this procedure. It has the advantages of a plastic peroneal post and easy access to the hip area and, therefore, allows the best visualization for intramedullary procedures. A Siemens C-arm provides the greatest mobility; rotation of the arm over 90° allows visualization of the surgical starting point. Many C-arms are larger and heavier and do not have the degree of mobility necessary to see the proximal end of the femur.

The radiographs of the femur to be shortened are analyzed carefully, and the size of the canal is measured on AP and lateral views. The degree of the bow of the femur and the thickness of the linea, as compared to the anterior cortex, must be determined. One must check for unusual bowing of the femur in the AP or lateral plane. Bowing leads to eccentric reaming and problems during the operation. The position of the cuts is determined on the AP radiographs. In most instances, the segment must be re-

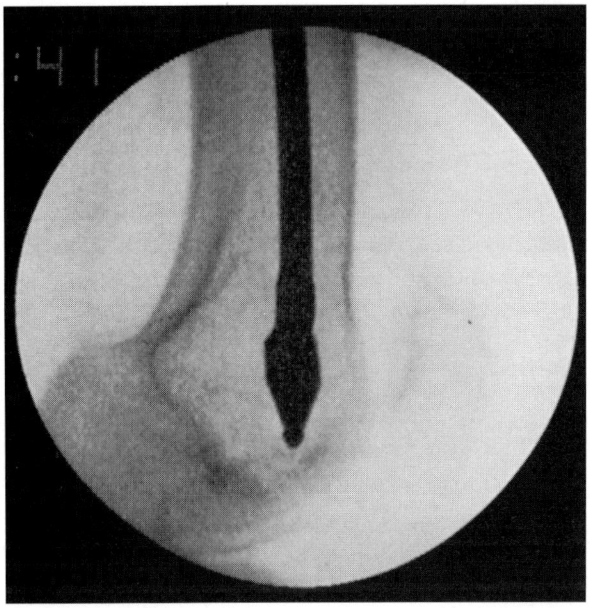

Fig. 18–9. This radiograph shows a long reamer going clear down to subchondral bone and reaming out any bone chips in the distal canal.

moved from the middle of the isthmus to allow adequate fixation on both ends. For example, if a 44-cm femur must be shortened by 4 cm, the distal femoral cut should be made 24 cm from the trochanter and the proximal cut made 20 cm from the trochanter, so that 20 cm of the femur remain in both the distal and proximal fragments. Removal of the segment from the mid-isthmus is a good rule, but the segment can be adjusted proximally and distally if the femur has an unusual shape.

Table Positioning and Reaming

The patient is placed in the lateral position on the fracture table. The C-arm is moved proximally and distally to be certain that the entire femur is well visualized. The surgical starting point in the trochanteric area must be seen on both AP and lateral fluoroscopic views.

An iodine/alcohol prep is used. The incision, which is 3 cm in length, starts 1 cm proximal to the tip of the greater trochanter and proceeds proximally in line with the femur. The fascia is split, and a finger is placed down through the muscle to palpate the free posterior edge of the greater trochanter.[9] The posterior tendinous portion of the glueus medius is palpated also. A straight T-handle reamer then is inserted in the piriformis fossa. The position is checked with both AP and lateral views on the image intensifier. The position of the straight T-handle reamer is adjusted until is is correct; this step is one of the most important in the procedure. A straight bulb-tipped guide then is inserted in this hole and is passed down to subchondral bone of the distal femoral condyle. A second bulb tip and a ruler are used for measurement. Reaming begins at 8 mm and proceeds at 1-mm increments until cortical contact is made. Reaming then proceeds at 0.5-mm increments.

Two factors must be considered during reaming. First, the largest saw possible makes the easiest cut. Second, excessive thinning of the cortex may lead to further comminution. The femur generally is reamed 1 to 2 mm larger than is normal for a fracture, and the anterior cortex must be watched on the image intensifier to prevent excessive thinning. During reaming, the bone chips frequently collect in the distal end of the femoral canal, which causes difficulty when driving the nail into the canal. When the nail hits this intramedullary bone, it tends to distract the osteotomy site. This problem is avoided by using a 12.5-mm extra-long end-cutting reamer (60 cm in length) at the conclusion of reaming to clear out the canal to the distal subchondral bone. The proximal 3 cm of femur are overreamed by 0.5 mm to allow easier insertion of the saw.

Anterotation Pins

To prevent a rotational deformity, pins are placed in the proximal and distal femur prior to the first intramedullary saw cut. One-eigth inch Steinman pins are used, as smaller pins are too flexible and bend during manipulation of the femur. The proximal pin is placed first and is the most difficult pin to place. The image intensifier is used in a lateral position. A metallic reduction rod is placed in the proximal femur to simulate the position of the nail. The guide pin goes in the trochanter anterior to the medullary canal. This is the similar position one would place a screw anterior to an intramedullary nail to fix a femoral neck fracture. The image intensifier is used to visualize this area for placement of the pin anterior to the reduction rod.

The distal pin is then placed in the shaft distal to the final position of the intramedullary nail. The image intensifier is once again used to define the distal femur, and a ⅛-inch guide pin is placed in the metaphyseal bone just above the joint. This pin is parallel to the pin in the proximal femur.

First Saw Cut

Insertion of the saw is somewhat difficult. The surgeon must palpate the hole in the trochanter and work the saw into position by turning it back and forth with an auscultating motion. The saw should be tight when going down the canal but should not be forced. Breakage at the bushing connection is possible in patients with excessive femoral bow. If the movement down this canal is too tight, the smaller saw (the next size) and bushing should be used. Once in position, the saw must be held firmly down against the trochanter. The surgeon must depend on the trochanter for subsequent measurements. The assistant surgeon holds the trochanteric rest firmly down against the trochanter during the use of the saw. The first cut is made (Fig. 18–10). The indexing device is held firmly with one hand, while the locking pin is advanced one hole at a time. The saw is turned two to three revolutions to complete the cut at each particular index setting. The blade is advanced slowly until the indexing device reaches the number 20, which indicates the maximum cutting diameter.[6] The numbers have no specific meaning, because the amount of cut varies with each saw size.

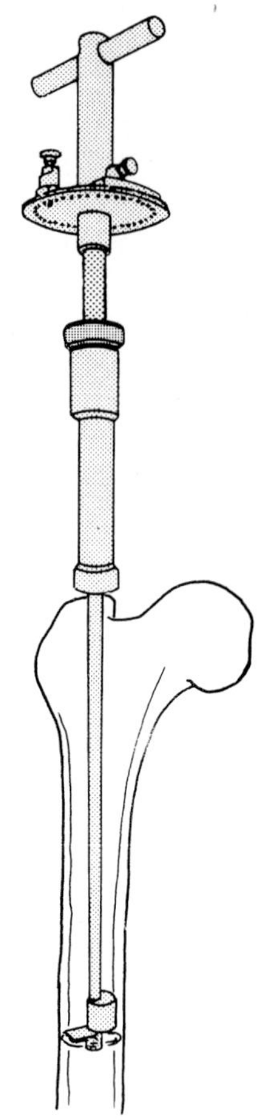

Fig. 18–10. Distal saw cut.

The saw first cuts through the anterior cortex. Some bowing in the long shaft of the saw may cause the saw to spring through the anterior cortex and bind slightly. Forcing the saw at this point may lead to breakage of the blade. If tight, the saw is backed off about five index notches and then is advanced slowly again, one notch at a time. When the indexing device reaches a maximum of 20, the cut is completed, and the blade begins to close again. The blade is then returned to a closed position at the zero mark. The saw is pulled partially out of the femur to allow advancement of the measuring device. This is accomplished holding the lock nut firmly in hand and not allowing it to move. The trochanteric rest is then advanced distally, and the gap between the trochanteric rest and the lock nut is measured until the appropriate length is achieved. The lock nut then is tightened again to prevent motion. The saw is inserted again to the maximum depth; the trochanteric rest is held carefully and firmly against the trochanter. The saw now is in position to make a second cut after manipulation of the leg, which is the next step. During manipulation, the surgeon should not hold on to the saw, because this could lead to bending of the shaft of the saw.

Osteoclasis of the Femur

Osteoclasis is generally a simple procedure. The foot is removed from traction and is held free by an assistant. The unscrubbed surgeon carefully manipulates the femur into a varus position by pressing up at the osteotomy site with one hand and pressing down on the knee with the other hand. Although the femur usually breaks quite nicely, it should not be forced. In such patients, the use of a percutaneous osteotome is much safer. A thin ¼-inch Lambotte osteotome is placed through a stab wound made by the width of a No. 10 blade. If the amount of shortening is between 2.5 and 4 cm, a single stab wound can be made directly between the two cuts. When a shortening of greater than 4 cm is anticipated, two separate stab wounds made be necessary for insertion of a percutaneous osteotome. I have been using the percutaneous osteotome more frequently, and I currently use it in approximately 36% of my patients. The osteotome is inserted carefully. The blade is parallel to the fibrous vastus lateralis. When the blade reaches the bone, it is then turned at right angles. The image intensifier is used to place the osteotome in the distal cut, which usually can be felt. The osteotome is then moved along the cut towards the posterior edge, where it is used to break through the linea. The osteotome is gripped firmly with one hand, which is held down against the skin to control over-penetration, and then it is hit briskly with the mallet to break through the linea. Although simple, this step requires great care. Again, I believe that the use of a percutaneous oteotome is a better solution than forceful breakage.

One of the most difficult and most important steps is tearing the periosteum. When the periosteum is left intact, the hook cannot be inserted to split the segment, the fragments do not move out of the way, and shortening cannot be accomplished. The periosteum is torn in the following manner: (1) the foot is removed from traction and is held by the circulating nurse; (2) the unscrubbed surgeon, who is now the most important member of the team, flexes the knee to 90° to relax the hamstrings and sciatic nerve; (3) with one hand (in a lead glove) placed on the anterior aspect of the thigh, the unscrubbed surgeon extends the fracture site approximately 70° to tear the linea; and (4) the femur is then displaced by creating a valgus force and pushing down on the lateral side. This maneuver usually allows 100% displacement of the distal shaft and, thus, allows shortening. If 100% displacement does not occur, the maneuver should be repeated as many times as necessary to achieve this goal.

Second Saw Cut

The saw is already in position. The trochanteric rest is held firmly against the trochanter by the assistant surgeon. The surgeon then completes the second saw cut in a manner similar to that of the first cut (Fig. 18–11). This step is usually quite easy. The saw is then removed. When the linea is exceptionally thick, a percutaneous osteotome is inserted again to complete the cut of the linea at the second proximal cut.

Splitting the Fragment

This step is usually not difficult. Originally, I used a fragmenter designed to expand like a Molly bolt. This fragmenter generated 65,000 lbs per square inch; it cracked the fragment but did not adequately displace it. I abandoned this device, which is not manufactured at present. Instead, I used the internal hook chisel of Küntscher to split and displace the fragments. This device is placed down the medullary canal, and its position is checked with the image intensifier (Fig. 18–12). The chisel is turned posterolaterally. A posterolateral cut is made to split the bone. If the cut is too anterior, it only

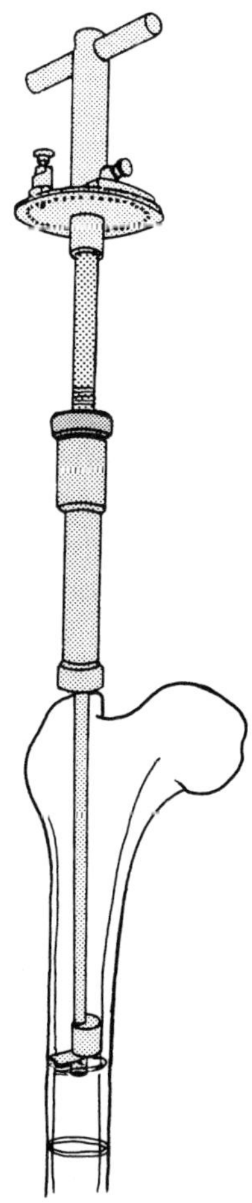

Fig. 18–11. Proximal saw cut.

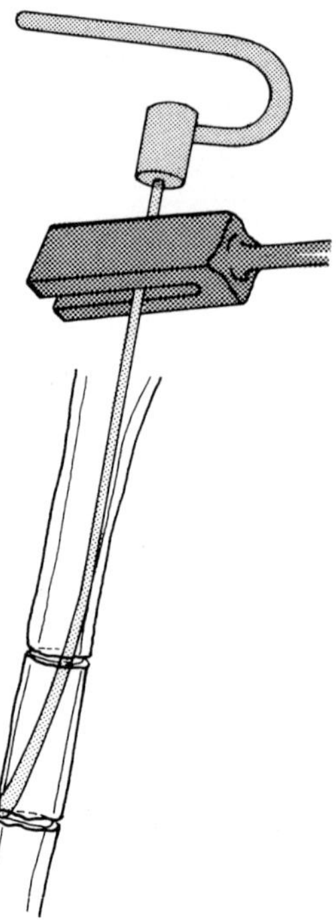

Fig. 18–12. The internal chisel hook.

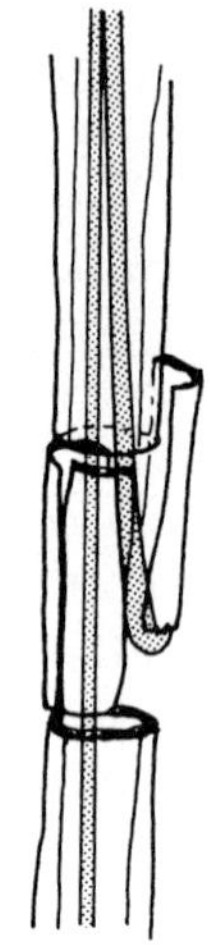

Fig. 18–13. The splitting of the fragments.

tears through the anterior cortex without splitting the segment in half. If the cut is too far posterior into the linea, it runs the risk of extending the split proximally up into the shaft when the linea is still intact. The hook, therefore, is turned towards the posterolateral part of the femur and is held down proximally to force it out against the lateral cortex. A mallet is used to pull the hook proximally and split the fragment, generally in two places (Fig. 18–13). If moved too far proximally, the hook may split up into the intact femoral shaft. Additional splits may be necessary if adequate fragmentation is not achieved.

After the bone is split, the hook is used to break through the posterior linea. The hook is kept in the split and is turned carefully in each direction. Resistance will be met, and as the hook turns further, it will crack through the linea at the proximal cut. When resistance is too great, a percutaneous osteotome should be used to help complete this split. When the hook leans against the fragment, the shaft of the hook is up against the anterolateral proximal femoral cortex and can split the cortex if the cortex is too thin or if excessive force is used. After the linea has been broken, the hook is used to try and displace the fragments as much as possible.

Shortening of the Femur and Insertion of the Intramedullary Nail

This step is the most difficult part of the procedure and should be performed by the most skilled surgeon on the team. In addition to shortening the femur, the fragments must be moved to the side, and the correct rotation must be maintained. One should not attempt to move all the fragments laterally, because they can create an uncomfortable mass. The scrub surgeon inserts a bulb-tipped guide with a slight bend. A reduction rod is inserted over the guide to allow manipulation of the proximal fragment. The osteotomy site then is impacted by using the distal shaft as a ramrod to push the pieces out of the way. The fracture then is shortened in a line. The proximal and distal antirotation pins are placed in a parallel position. This step can be extremely difficult and becomes even more so when a large segment is removed.

The position of the unscrubbed surgeon is critical. For a left femoral shortening, the lower leg is cradled in the surgeon's right arm to control rotation. The palm of the left hand pushes against the patient's knee, and the left elbow is braced against the surgeon's iliac crest (Fig. 18–14). This position is used to keep the fracture impacted during the driving of the nail. The fracture must remain impacted until the interlocking screws are placed proximally and distally. The fracture now is completely im-

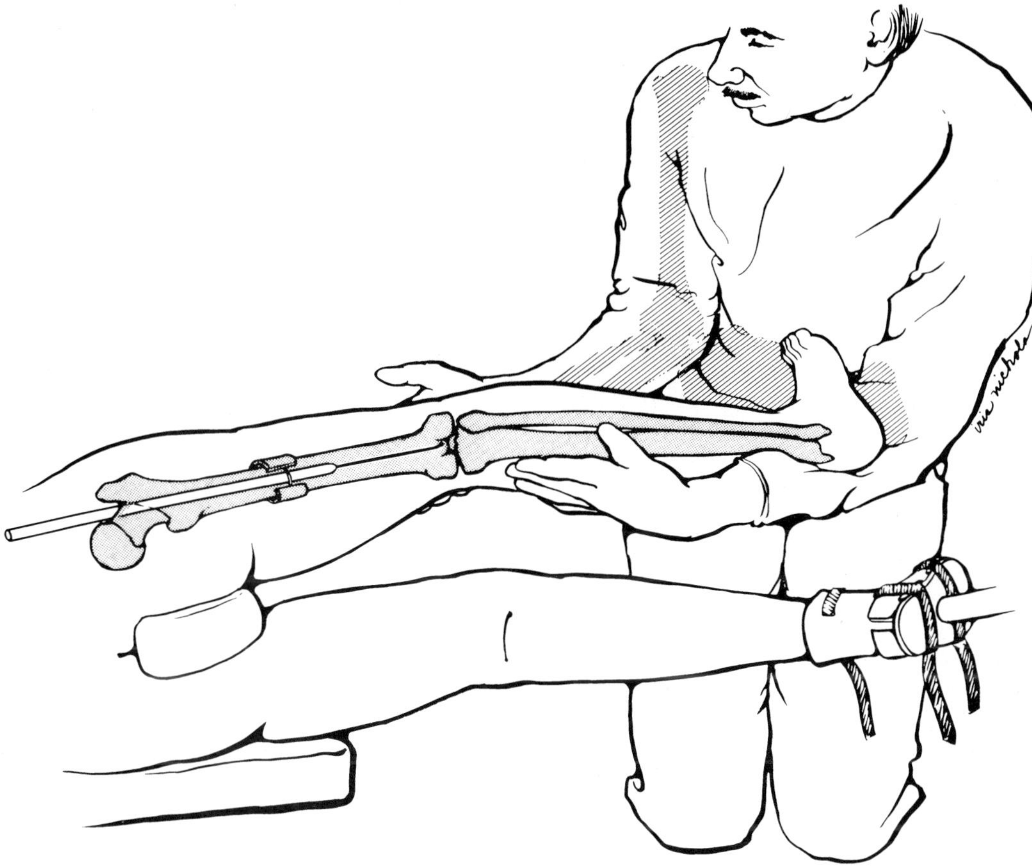

Fig. 18–14. Surgeon holds the femur with an elbow braced against iliac crest.

pacted over the bulb-tipped guide, and the distal femur is rotated slightly back and forth to improve the impaction. The proximal and distal pins should be parallel to each other. An interlocking nail is selected that is 1 mm smaller than the largest reamer which is used. The position of the nail on the AP and lateral view is checked carefully as it crosses the osteotomy site. The osteotomy site is checked repeatedly with the image intensifier during driving of the nail. The elbow of the unscrubbed surgeon is held carefully against the iliac crest to prevent distraction. The benefit of the earlier cleaning out of the distal femoral canal with a 12.5-mm extra-long cutting reamer is most evidence for this part of the procedure. The scrubbed surgeon completes the driving of the nail and checks the proximal and distal portions of the nail. A nail 2 to 3 cm shorter than the normal length for internal fixation should be selected to avoid hitting subchondral bone and distracting the osteotomy. After the nail has been fully driven, the osteotomy site is checked in two planes. If the osteotomy site has distracted during the driving of the nail, the surgeon backs up the nail, which usually impacts the fracture. It is possible to put in the distal interlocking screw and then impact the osteotomy, but care must be taken not to pull too hard on the distal screw or it may break.

Occasionally, a little spike occurs during breakage of the fragments. A spike prevents complete impaction of the fracture and must be accepted. If a fragment of bone turns on edge and is caught in the osteotomy site, the manipulation procedure must be repeated until this fragment is moved out of the way. A single interlocking screw is used proximally and distally. It is reasonable to use either of the two distal holes.

Postoperative Treatment

A prophylactic cephalosporin is administered before the surgical procedure and for 24 hours after the procedure. The day after the operation, the patient is started on quadriceps sets. Generally, the patient works on these sets for 4 to 6 weeks prior to operation to help postoperative recovery. Ice packs are used for the first 2 or 3 days. The patient is allowed to begin ambulation the morning after surgery. Range of motion of the knee has not been a problem and, consequently, does not require vigorous work by the patient. The hematocrit is repeated for the first 2 days. Interoperative blood loss is not significant, but bleeding continues internally with the lax muscles and torn periosteum. Transfusion of one to two units of auto-blood has been required by 23% of the patients.

The day following surgical intervention, the patient begins to walk with crutches bearing 30 to 50 lbs of weight. The patient uses crutches for 6 weeks following surgery. Abduction exercises are started as soon as the hip wound settles down. Radiographs are taken at 6 weeks, 3 months, and 1 year. Quadriceps rehabilitation is extremely important for knee stability and in order to avoid chondromalacia, which is a common problem. As with most major surgical procedures, rehabilitation is a long, demanding process. The patient must do most of the rehabilitation on their own. They begin with quadriceps sets and straight leg raising on their own. A physical therapy that is overly enthusiastic may exacerbate the chondromalacia. Removal of the nail and locking screws is usually performed after 1 year. Forty-seven percent of the patients had discomfort over the proximal end of the nail.

Results and Complications

The follow-up in this group of patients was 1 to 9 years with a mean of 23 months. Healing was rapid with callus formation noted between 2 and 4 weeks in 81% of the patients and between 4 and 8 weeks in 96% of the patients. Resolution of the limp, related to the leg length inequality, occurred in 100% of the patients. One of the major reasons for correction of leg length was to alleviate back pain. Eighty-seven of the patients had preoperative back pain, and following surgery and recovery, 70 of these patients had total resolution of their back pain. Seventeen patients still had back pain, with 13 of these patients showing improvement, while 3 patients still had significant pain. One patient had resolution of back pain, but it then recurred 7 years later.

Interoperative complications included two patients with a broken saw blade and two patients with broken bushings. One saw blade was retrieved by an open incision at the osteotomy site, and the other instruments were removed through the medullary canal. There was one broken reamer, which was retrieved with a bulb-tip guide. Failure of incomplete impaction at the osteotomy site occurred in 34% of the patients. This ranged from 2 mm to 12 mm This problem has decresed with the use of interlocking nails. There were no cases of clinically significant fat embolism in this series despite intramedullary reaming of a closed femoral canal. It is important to note that all patients had Küntscher reamers used with deep flutes and narrow shafts.

Rotational deformities following surgery were the most common complications. Seven patients had external rotation deformities between 10 and 25°, and 4 patients had internal rotational deformities. These all occurred prior to the use of guide pins to check rotation and interlocking nails. Because interlocking nails and guide pins have been used, there has been no rotational deformity greater than 10°. Nonunion occurred in 1 patient requiring exchange nailing. There was 1 patient with a delayed union, which healed following removal of the interlocking screws. One patient had a nonfatal pulmonary embolism requiring anticoagulation.

A common symptom was chondromalacia patellae. Avoidance of knee extension against resistance greatly decreased this symptom. Patients worked hard on quad sets and straight leg lifts to build up the quadriceps, and this then alleviated the chondromalacia. Discomfort was also noted over the displaced bone fragments in 15 patients. The symptoms were most prominent with lateral fragments, because of the lack of soft-tissue coverage and posterior fragments, which caused pressure when sitting on the edge of a chair. Only 1 patient required open removal of one of these fragments 1 year after osteotomy and at the time of nail removal.

Thirty-four patients were asked to fill out a questionnaire rating the surgery judged by patient satisfaction. The scale was 0 to 10. The mean patient satisfaction was 9.53, with a range of 7 to 10.

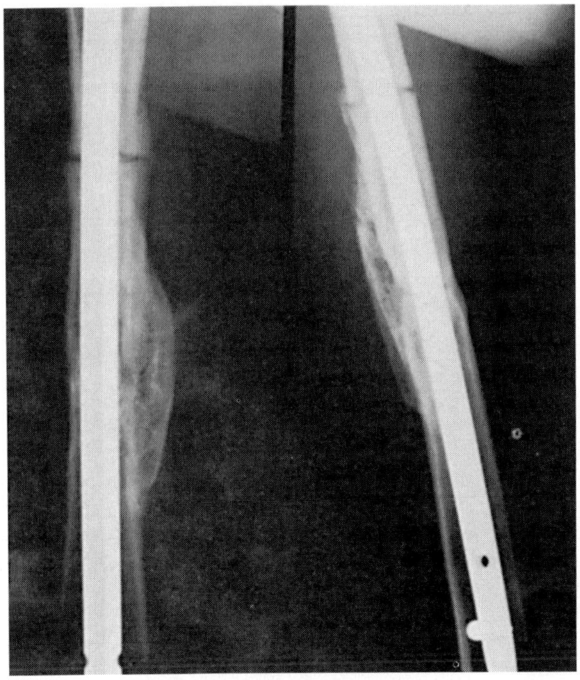

Fig. 18–15. AP and lateral postoperative radiograph demonstrate a derotation osteotomy fixed with an interlocking nail.

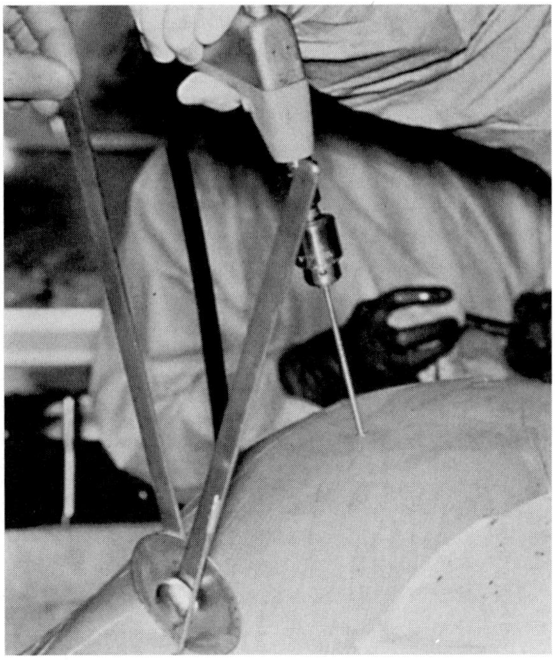

Fig. 18–17. Intramedullary osteotomy has been completed and the proximal guide pin is placed and measured with a goniometer.

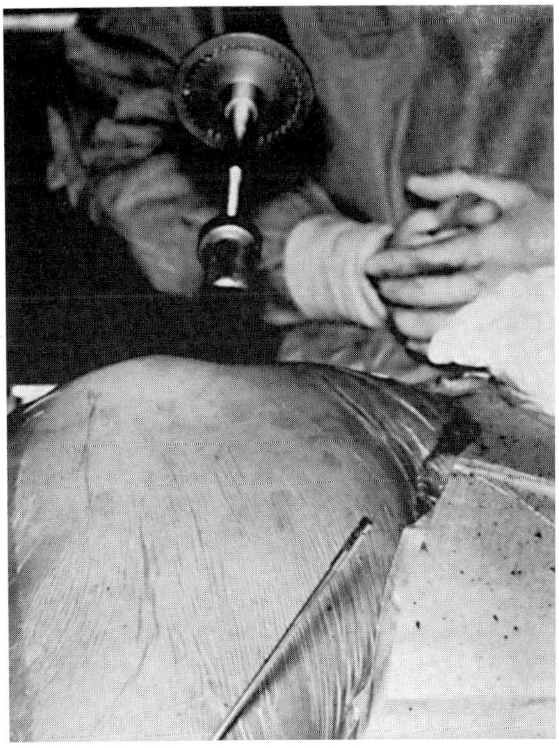

Fig. 18–16. Intramedullary saw has been inserted and distal guide pin placed.

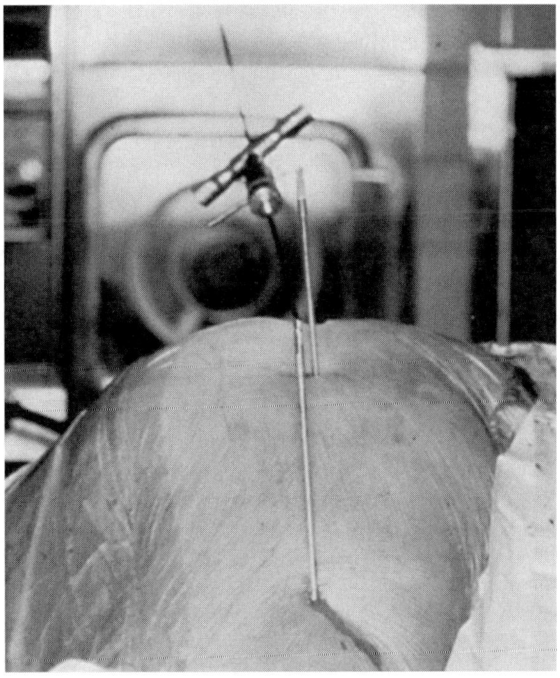

Fig. 18–18. Femur has been derotated until the guide pins are parallel.

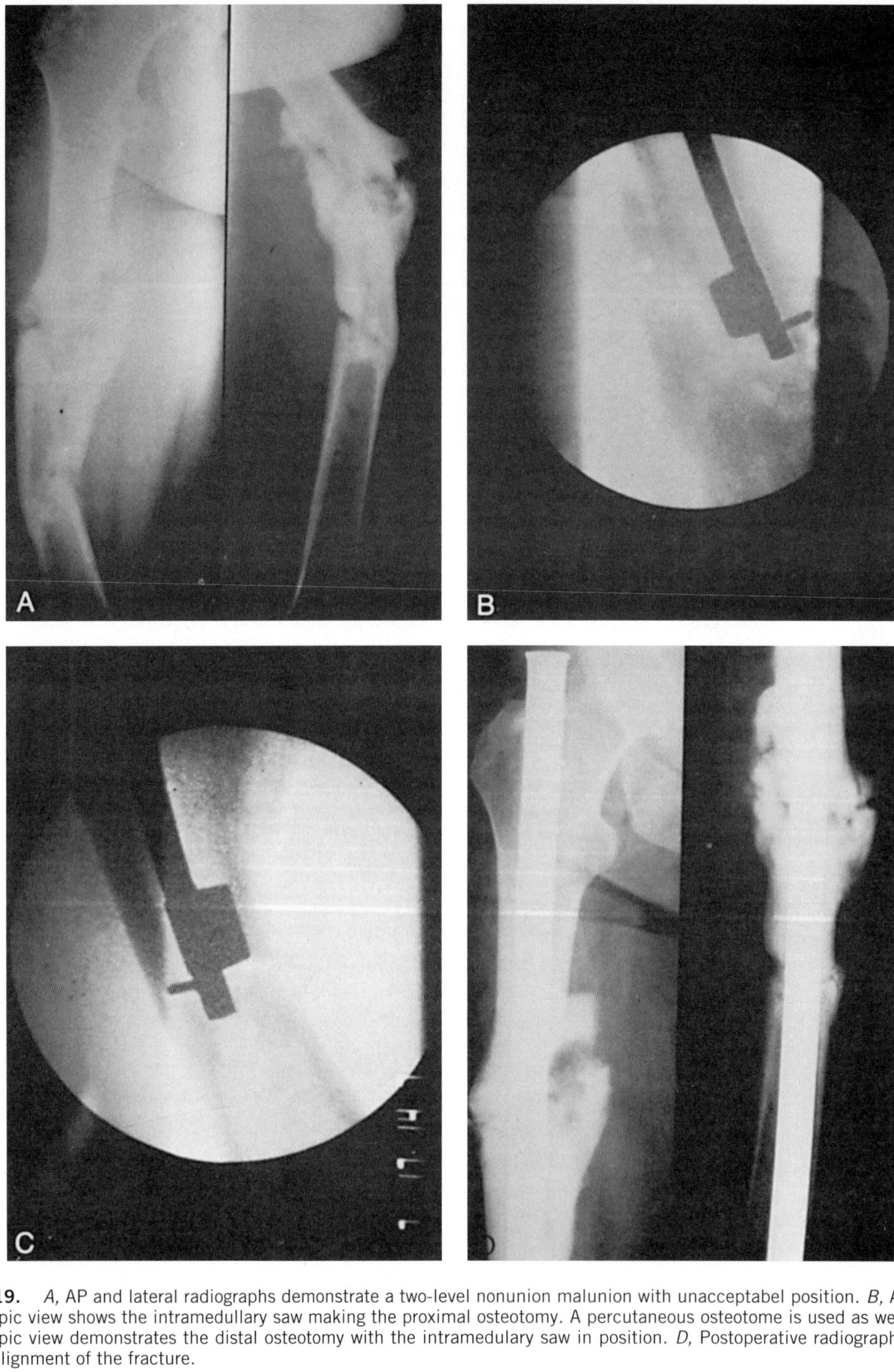

Fig. 18–19. *A,* AP and lateral radiographs demonstrate a two-level nonunion malunion with unacceptabel position. *B,* A close-up fluoroscopic view shows the intramedullary saw making the proximal osteotomy. A percutaneous osteotome is used as well. *C,* This fluoroscopic view demonstrates the distal osteotomy with the intramedulary saw in position. *D,* Postoperative radiographs demonstrate realignment of the fracture.

CLOSED INTRAMEDULLARY OSTEOTOMIES

Materials and Indications

The intramedullary saw also has been used for derotational osteotomies. Technically, this procedure is much easier than a femoral shortening. I have used this saw for 92 derotational osteotomies in 72 patients. Twenty patients had bilateral osteotomies. The etiology of the deformity was as follows: (1) post-fracture, 47 patients (4 bilateral); (2) congenital femoral anteversion, 15 patients (8 bilateral); (3) cerebral palsy, 6 patients (5 bilateral); (4) congenital retroversion, 2 patients (2 bilateral); (5) post osteotomy, 1 patient; and (6) tumor, 1 patient (1 bilateral).

The degree of deformity varied. Internal and external rotation was measured with the patient in the prone position. The leg was used to measure the arc against a perpendicular line drawn to the table. Patients with external rotational deformities had minimal internal rotation, and those with internal rotation deformities had minimal external rotation. Patients with external rotational deformities averaged fewer than 10° of internal rotation. The degree of malrotation averaged 40° in this group of patients. Patients with internal rotation deformities averaged less than 10° of external rotation. The average internal rotation was 80° in this group. The average surgical correction for both internal and external rotational deformities was 40°. In most patients, the affected leg did not have to match the normal leg, but at least 10 or 15° of internal and external rotation had to be achieved.[9]

Surgical Technique

The technique for a derotational osteotomy is much easier than that used for femoral shortening. Because many of these patients have had previous fractures of the medullary canal and the level of callus of the old fracture must be examined, the osteotomy must be done either above or below the callus to ensure its accomplishment in a simple manner (Fig. 18–15). In addition, a previous fixation device that may also distort the femoral canal may require removal. Therefore, careful evaluation of radiographs for preoperative planning is important.

The patient is placed in the lateral position on the fracture table, as in a femoral shortening. The surgical starting point is visualized carefully with AP and lateral fluoroscopy. The femur then is reamed to an appropriate size for use of an intramedullary saw. The level of the saw cut is measured with the ossimeter on the preoperative radiographs. The saw then is inserted to the correct level and is checked again with the image intensifier to be certain the cut will be above or below any previous callus.

After reaming of the intramedullary canal, a guide pin is placed in the proximal anterior trochanter, as described in the femoral shortening section. A guide pin is then placed in the distal femur using a goniometer (Fig. 18–16). The intramedullary osteotomy is completed (Fig. 18–17). The leg is then manipulated into varus to break the linea, and the femur is rotated internally or externally to correct the deformity. It is important to turn the femur beyond its planned position to make sure the periosteum is adequately torn and that springback will not occur. The guide pins are then placed parallel to each other while the nail is driven into position (Fig. 18–18). The nail is then driven across the osteotomy site and flush with the top of the trochanter. A single locking screw is placed proximally and distally.

RESULTS AND COMPLICATIONS

There were very few complications with this technique (Fig. 18–19). There were no nonunions and no infections. Callus formation was present at 6 weeks in 94% of the patients. Prior to the use of guide pins and interlocking nails, there were 4 patients who lost correction. This occurred immediately after surgery and required manipulation in all 4 patients. Two patients were placed in a spica cast. Now, all patients receive statically locked interlocking nails and loss of rotation is no longer a problem. One patient with bilateral rotational osteotomies went skiing 4 months post-surgery. She sustained a short, oblique fracture through a pin tract. This, fortunately, healed rapidly in 6 weeks and required no further treatment.

REFERENCES

1. Küntscher, G.: Die geschlossene Osteotomie der längen Röhrenknochen. Chirurg. *33*:273, 1962.
2. Fischer, S.: Geschlossene osteotomie. Chir. Praxis, *12*: 435, 1968.
3. Fischer, S.: Operativ Beinverkurzung und Beinverlangerung nach dem verfahren von Kn;autscher. der Orthopade *1*:50, 1972.

4. Küntscher, G.: Intramedullary surgical technique and its place in orthopaedic surgery. My present concept. J. Bone Joint Surg. *47A*:809, 1965.
5. Winquist, R.A., Hansen, S.T., Jr., Pearson, R.E.: Closed intramedullary shortening of the femur. Clin. Orthop. *136*:54, 1978.
6. Winquist, R.A.: Closed shortening of the femur utilizing a new type of intramedullary saw. *In* Intramedullary Nailing. Edited by Lotz, B. New York, Thieme-Stratton, 1982.
7. Morscher, E.: Atiologie und Klinik der Beinlangenunterscheide.der Orthopade *1*:1, 1972.
8. Winquist, R.A., Hansen, S.T., Jr.: Comminuted fractures of the femoral shaft treated by intramedullary nailing. Orthop. Clin. North Am., *11*:663, 1980.
9. Winquist, R.A., Hansen, S.T., Jr. Clawson, D.K.: Closed intramedullary nailing of femoral fractures. J. Bone Joint Surg., *66A*:529, 1984.

19

Intramedullary Femoral Lengthening

Kenneth J. Koval, Victor H. Frankel, and Frederick Kummer

There is a long history of femoral lengthening using external fixators both in this country and in Europe.[1–3] Although many investigators have reported successful use of external fixators for femoral lengthening, it has been demonstrated that the use of external fixation for femoral lengthening is associated with many complications.[4] The anatomic constraints of the thigh limit pin placement (particularly proximally); the thigh's muscle bulk and excursion during gait often results in pin tract problems, such as drainage and superficial and deep infection. Late sequelae of femoral lengthening using external fixators, with both small-diameter and larger-diameter pins, can include loss of hip and knee motion, knee subluxation, and femoral deformity.

Use of an intramedullary nail is an attractive alternative for femoral lengthening and appears to eliminate some of the potential complications associated with external fixators (i.e., pin tract infection). Intramedullary fracture fixation is both biologically and biomechanically superior to the use of plates and external fixators.[5–7] In addition, the osseous debris generated by reaming prior to nail placement is felt to be osteoinductive, which may accelerate regenerate consolidation as the bone is lengthened.[8,9]

Previously, intramedullary fixation for osseous lengthening has been applied primarily in children. An extensible intramedullary nail was developed by Bailey and Dubow for use in children with osteogenesis imperfecta.[10] This expanding nail is essentially a telescoping device that is locked both proximally and distally. The nail spans the child's physis and provides passive alignment. As the child's physis grows, the nail elongates with the femur and prevents bending deformities. Mixed results have been reported with use of this device; one of the most frequently reported complications is failure of the device to elongate.[10–12] A lengthening prosthesis was developed by Lewis for limb salvage in children with bone tumors.[13] This prosthesis consists of either a proximal or distal arthroplastic segment or a total osseous replacement incorporating an extensible stem. This device is inserted at the time of tumor resection; as the child grows, the device is lengthened to equalize limb lengths. However, device lengthening requires anesthesia and is accomplished by insertion of a key through the soft tissues into the device, which turns an internal worm-screw mechanism. An active intramedullary femoral lengthening nail was developed by Bliskunov.[5,14] A proximal extension arm of this nail is attached to the patient's pelvis. Femoral lengthening is achieved by externally rotating the patient's leg, which moves the arm with respect to the nail. The arm engages an internal ratchet to linearly extend the distal segment of the nail. Bliskunov has reported excellent clinical results with several hundred cases in Russia.[14,15]

More recently, intramedullary nails have been used in conjunction with external fixators during limb lengthening in order to minimize the length of time the patient spends in the external fixator. Paley et al. reported a series of 29 patients (26 femurs, 5 tibias) treated with a combination of intramedullary nails and external fixators.[16] At surgery, a dynamically locked nail was inserted in conjunction with a cortcotomy and a small wire ring external fixator. Dis-

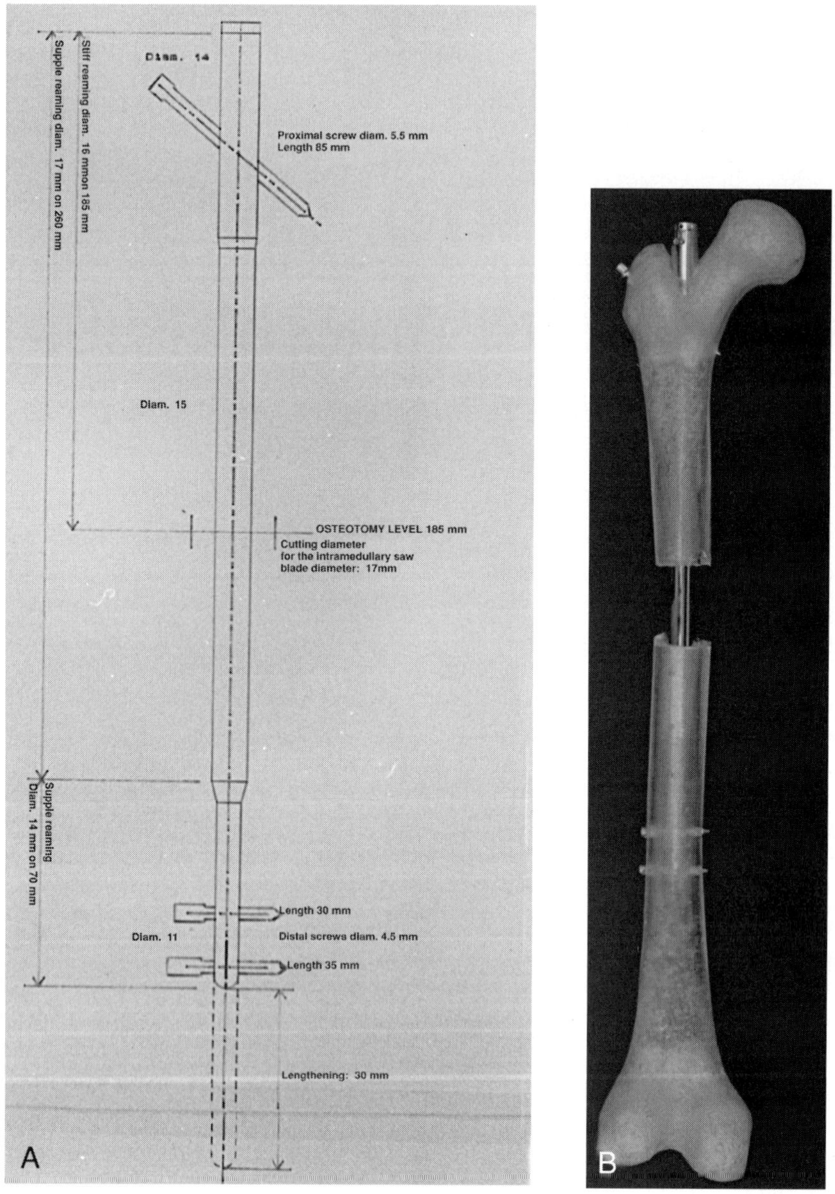

Fig. 19–1. *A,* Diagram of the gradual-lengthening nail. *B,* Photograph of the gradual lengthening nail inserted in a plastic model.

traction osteogenesis was performed using the external fixator. Once the desired length had been achieved, the external fixator was removed and the nail statically locked to prevent shortening. Sixteen femurs were treated to the point of complete osseous consolidation. Complications associated with these 16 femurs included 1 deep delayed infection of a locking screw site, 1 permanent significant loss of knee motion, and premature consolidation necessitating recorticotomy in 4 patients. However, the length of time in the external fixator averaged 0.7 months per centimeter while a matched set of patients undergoing standard Ilizarov femoral lengthening had an average time in the fixator of 1.5 months per centimeter. The investigators concluded that combining intramedullary nailing with external fixation carried a potential risk of deep sepsis but permitted earlier fixator removal.

THE FEMORAL LENGTHENING NAIL

A gradual lengthening nail has recently been designed and clinically introduced in France.[2] This telescoping device is an intramedullary femoral nail with proximal and distal locking holes and contains an internal ratchet mechanism to allow gradual, controlled distraction of the distal segment of an osteotomized femur (Fig. 19–1). This straight nail is constructed of 316L stainless steel and consists of a distal solid inner rod, which can be rotated to actuate a ratchet mechanism that distally translates this inner rod with respect to the proximal outer cylinder. Following a transverse osteotomy, fixation of the nail is accomplished through two distal 4-mm screws and a single angled 6.5-mm proximal screw. Lengthening is performed by alternately rotating the limb internally and then externally (Fig. 19–2). A lengthening of 1 mm is produced by approximately fifteen alternative rotations. Both right and left femoral nails are available with outside diameters ranging from 10 to 16 mm; there are four nail lengths which range from 120 to 240 mm. The nails lengthen between 2.5 to 4 cm, depending on nail length.

OPERATIVE PROCEDURE

The patient is placed on a fracture table or supine on a radiolucent flat table. The intramedullary canal is entered in a standard manner through the piriformis fossa. The intramedullary canal is overreamed by 1 to 2 mm using standard flexible reamers followed by straight reamers. Use of straight reamers is necessary because the nails do not have an anterior bow. An open or closed osteotomy is performed (Fig. 19–3) and the nail inserted. The nail must be inserted without force; otherwise the lengthening mechanism may not function properly. The nail is then locked proximally and distally. The proximal locking screw is inserted using a targeting device and the distal screws are inserted in a freehand manner using fluoroscopic guidance. Following nail placement with the patient anaesthetized, the nail is lengthened approximately 5 mm. This ensures that the lengthening mechanism of the device is func-

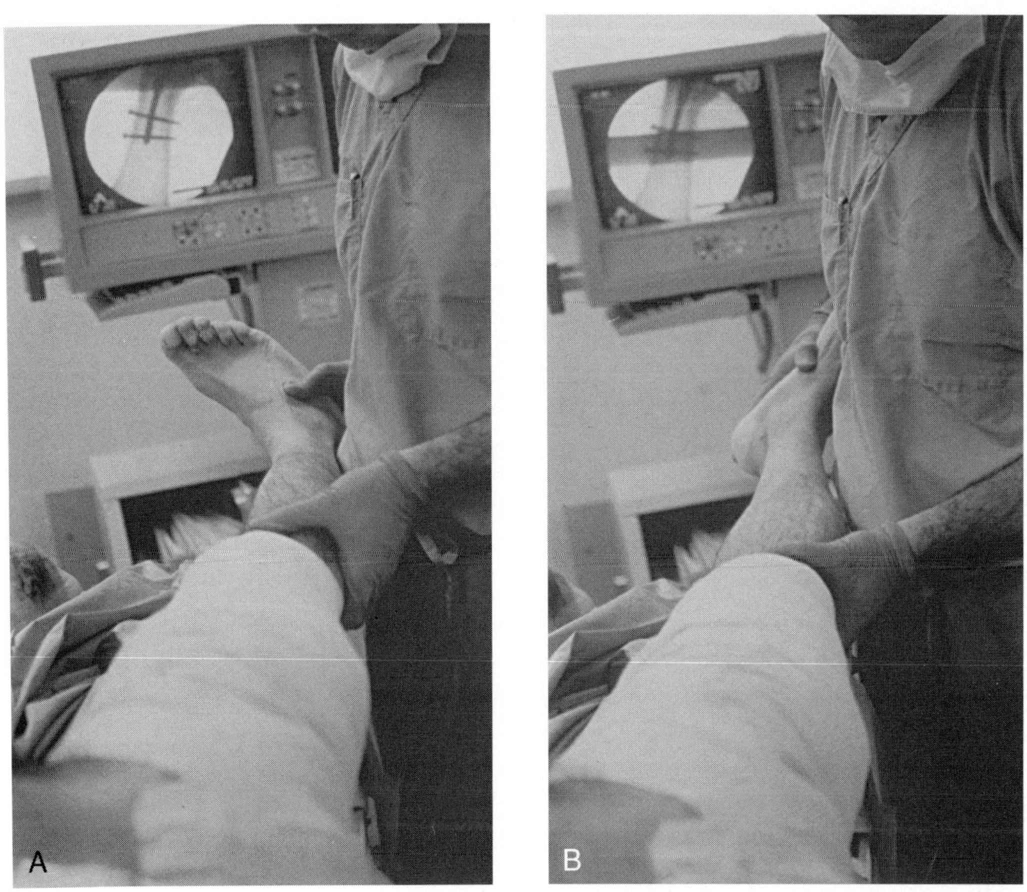

Fig. 19–2. Lengthening is performed by alternately internally (*A*) and externally (*B*) rotating the limb.

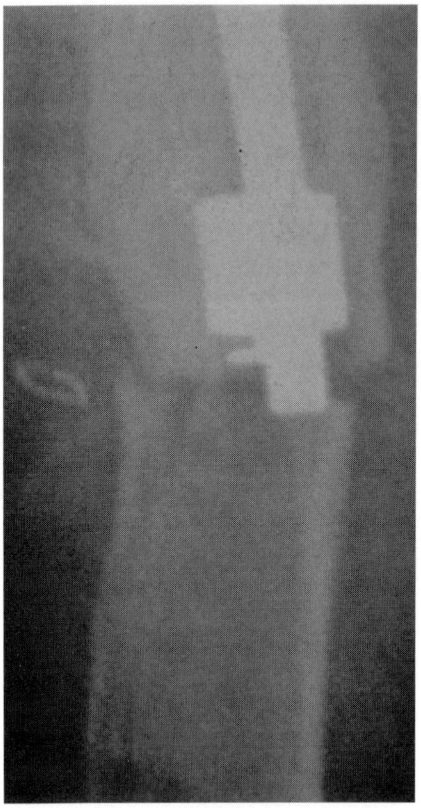

Fig. 19–3. Use of an intramedullary saw to perform a closed osteotomy prior to nail placement.

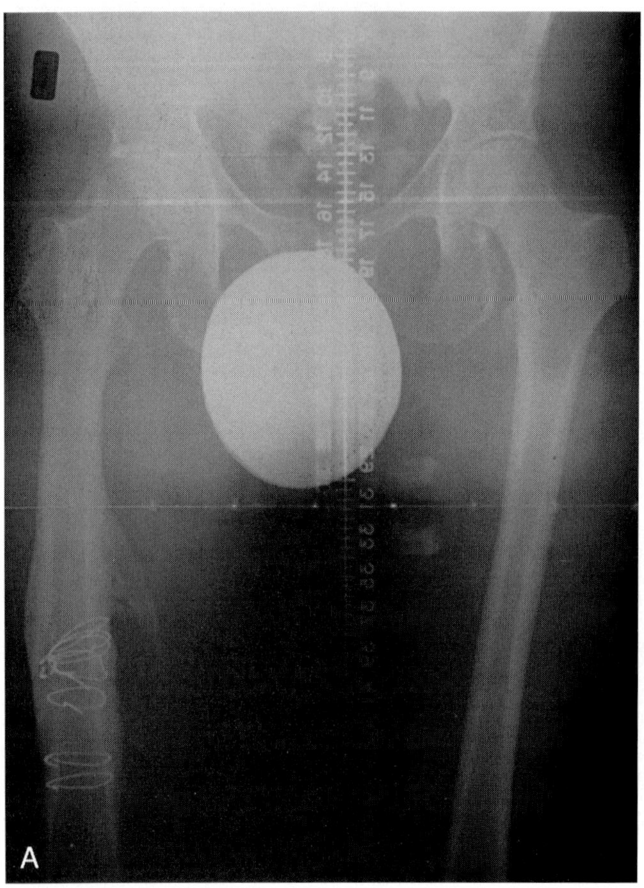

Fig. 19–4. *A,* Preoperative radiograph of a shortened right lower extremity after femur fracture. *(Figure continues)*

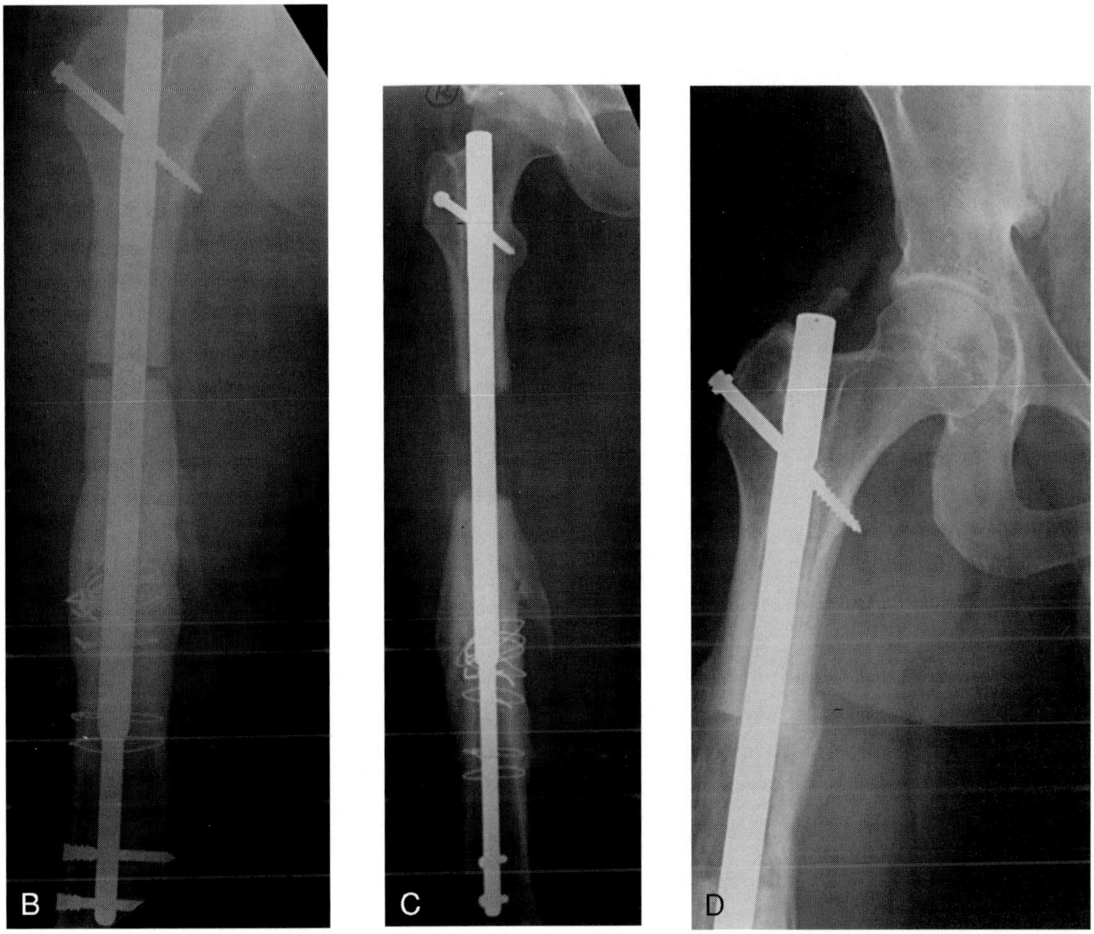

Fig. 19–4. *(continued) A,* Preoperative radiograph of a shortened right lower extremity after femur fracture. *B,* Initial postoperative radiograph after closed osteotomy and insertion of the gradual-lengthening nail. Note the initial distraction of the osteotomy fragments. *C,* AP radiograph after femoral lengthening. Note the regenerate formation laterally. *D,* AP radiograph after regenerate formation.

tioning and prevents contact of the proximal and distal fragments, which may result in patient pain during the limb rotation necessary for femoral lengthening. Postoperatively, the patient is allowed to partially bear weight. Lengthening is started on day 4 or 5 during the postoperative period. Progression of weight bearing is dependent on consolidation of the regenerate (Fig. 19–4).

BIOMECHANICAL STUDIES OF THE GRADUAL-LENGTHENING NAIL

Mechanical studies of the gradual-lengthening nail have been performed at the Hospital for Joint Diseases.[18,19] The 11-mm gradual-lengthening nail was compared to the same size Grosse-Kempf, Russell-Taylor, and Synthes nails. Four mechanical parameters were determined: bending and torsional stiffness and ultimate bending and torsional strength. Bending stiffness of the gradual-lengthening nail was examined in two positions, the initial shortened length and its maximum extended length.

For the gradual-lengthening nail, bending stiffness depended on its configuration. When the nail was shortened, the bending stiffness was approximately twice that obtained when the nail was lengthened. In both shortened and lengthened conditions, the bending stiffness of the gradual-lengthening nail was within the range obtained for the other intramedullary nails. The torsional stiffness of the lengthening nail was comparable to the torsional stiffness of the Synthes nail and the ultimate torsional strength of the gradual lengthening nail was higher. The investigators concluded that the gradual-lengthening nail had mechanical properties within the ranges of the other intramedullary nails tested.

REFERENCES

1. Cattaneo, R., Villa, A., Catagni, M.: Lengthening of the Femur. In Maiocchi, A.B. and Aronson, J. (ed): Operative Principles of Ilizarov. Baltimore, Williams & Wilkins, 1991, pp. 310–314.
2. Ilizarov, G.A., Devjatov, A.A.: Operative elongation of the leg. Ortop. Travmatol. Protez. *8*:20–25, 1971.
3. Paley, D.: Current techniques of limb lengthening. Pediatr. Orthop. *8*:73–92, 1988.
4. Paley, D.: Problems, obstacles and complications of limb lengthening. *In* Maiocchi, A.B. and Aronson, J. (ed): Operative Principles of Ilizarov. Edited by A.B. Maiocchi, J. Aronson. Baltimore, Williams & Wilkins, 1991, pp. 352–365.
5. Allen, W.C., Piotrowski, G., Burstein, A.H., Frankel, V.H.: Biomechanical principles of intramedullary fixation. Clin. Orthop. *60*:13–20, 1968.
6. Bohler, J.: Closed intramedullary nailing of the femur. Clin. Orthop. *60*:51–67, 1968.
7. Bucholz, R.W., Brumback, R.J.: Fractures of the shaft of the femur. *In* Fractures in Adults. Edited by C.A. Rockwood, Jr., R.W. Bucholz. Philadelphia, J.B. Lippincott Co., 1991, pp. 1653–1723.
8. Chapman, M.: Closed intramedullary bone grafting and nailing of segmental defects of the femur. J. Bone Joint Surg. *62A*:1004–1012, 1980.
9. Chester, S., Hallfeldt, K., Perren, S., Schweiberer, L.: The effects of reaming and intramedullary nailing on fracture healing. Clin. Orthop. *212*:18–25, 1986.
10. Bailey, R.W., Dubow, H.I.: Evolution of the concept of an extensible nail accommodating to normal longitudinal bone growth: clinical considerations and implications. Clin. Orthop. *159*:157–170, 1981.
11. Lang-Stevenson, A.I., Sharrard, W.J.W.: Intramedullary rodding with Bailey-Dubow extensible rods in osteogenesis imperfecta: An interim report of results and complications. J. Bone Joint Surg. *66B*:227–232, 1984.
12. Stockley, I., Bell, M.J., Sharrard, W.J.W.: The role of expanding intramedullary rods in osteogenesis imperfecta. J. Bone Joint Surg. *71B*:422–427, 1989.
13. Lewis, M.M.: The use of an expandable and adjustable prosthesis in the treatment of childhood malignant bone tumors of the extremity. Cancer *57*:499–502, 1986.
14. Bliskunov, A.I.: Implantable device for lengthening the femur without external drive mechanism. Meditsinskaia Tekhnika *2*:22–49, 1984.
15. Bliskunov, A.I.: Intramedullary distraction of the femur. Preliminary report. Orthop. Travmatol. Protez. *10*:59–62, 1983.
16. Paley, D., Herzenberg, J.E., Maar, D., Tetsworth, K., Goulet, J.A.: Lower extremity lengthening over intramedullary rods with external fixation. Annual meeting of the Association for the Study and Application of the Methods of Ilizarov, San Francisco, CA, February, 1993.
17. Guichet, J.M.: Doctoral dissertation, University of Aix-Marseille II, 1991.
18. Guichet, J.M., Casar, R.S., Alexander, H., Frankel, V.H.: Comparative testing of intramedullary nails stiffness and ultimate properties in bending and torsion. Annual meeting of the Orthopaedic Research Society, Washington, D.C., February, 1992.
19. Guichet, J.M., Casar, R.S., Alexander, H., Frankel, V.H.: Mechanical properties of the gradual lengthening nail. Annual meeting of the Orthopaedic Research Society, Washington, D.C., February, 1992.

20

Treatment of Infection Following Intramedullary Nailing

David Seligson and Klaus Klemm

> It was learned that a nail could be safely inserted into an infected fracture without serious consequences. It was my opinion that this method should be used as an established procedure in cases of infected fractures which had not healed as the result of usual methods of treatment.[1]

Intramedullary nailing is one of the most satisfying therapeutic measures available to patients and doctors in modern orthopedics and traumatology. In the bone-healing olympics, interlocking nailing is the high dive. One expects faultless execution and a clean entry. The patient is warned of possible infectious complications. Still, neither the patient nor the doctor really expect to hit the board. So driven are we by the need for success that the infection which surely occurs after nailing, just like it follows any other form of bone surgery, is invariably under-reported. Indeed, a search of the current literature for articles specific to the treatment of posttraumatic osteomyelitis after medullary nailing is disappointing.[2] No one wants to admit to having a series of cases. Yet, we know infection after nailing is out there, because we see and treat it in other doctors' patients. The purpose of this chapter is to provide concepts about the pathomechanics of infection following intramedullary nailing and then provide specific treatment routines for management of the various clinical situations that occur with infection after nailing. Areas for future study complete the discussion.

PATHOMECHANICS

> The first and most important step in the management of this problem is union of the fracture site. Union of the fracture site occurs only when rigid internal fixation is maintained.[3]

The placement of an intramedullary nail is an interaction between a sterile metal implant, a host with resident bioflora, and a bone that is more or less dead and more or less contaminated. The bone is greatly compromised in its blood supply by the injury and subsequently by the nailing. Dead bone is after all a sequestrum. The usual result of this procedure is the gradual colonization of the implant by bacteria,[4,5] the subsidence of inflammation, and the beginning of repair in the bone and the restoration of the integrity of the host. Both bacteria and inflammation are invariably present following nailing.[6] The transition from colonization to infection is a matter of degree. Following uncomplicated nailing, repair is the outcome, with infection, inflammation and/or tissue destruction as the result.

In our view, each patient lies somewhere on a spectrum from uncomplicated fracture healing to draining fistulous osteomyelitis. The process of union is personal and depends on the balance between host factors and organism factors.

For example, the organism most often colonizing a medullary implant is *Staphylococcus epidermidis*. In a normal host, this typically leads to a slippery coating of glycocalyx. The organism can be introduced in several ways: (1) it gets on the nail during surgery, (2) it is transferred onto the surgeon's gloves when palpating the trochanter, (3) it is rubbed off the skin as the nail is being inserted, or (4) it is transported to the nail hematogenously during an incidental bacteremia.[7] With a normal host and well-stabilized fracture, the contaminating bacteria grow sparsely on the nail and do not cause trouble. However, when a local unfavorable host factor, such as mechanical instability, or when a systemic host problem like diabetes with renal failure is added, a terrible bone-destroying infection can result (Fig. 20–1).

Local mechanical factors can be responsible for the progression to infection after nailing. Reaming, performed without generation of excessive heat, is most likely not a cause of infection after nailing. Küntscher reported an incidence of osteomyelitis of 0.3% in 1,884 nailings.[8] Unstable nails are, however, associated with the evolution of infection after nailing. These unstable situations include instability after unlocked nailing, failure of interlocking screws, and nail breakage. Particularly with flexible nailing (Rush and Ender nails) and conventional Küntscher nailing, early rotational instability can lubricate bone and the device with serum and debris. This can lead to bone resorption at the fracture site and the development of an inflammatory reaction and, subsequently, the development of overt infection. With early rotational instability, the infection spreads along the entire length of the nail. Despite good vascularity at the fracture site and attempts to heal, there is lubrication of the fractured bone ends by pus and persistence of motion and bone resorption. The infectious reaction will spread through the cortex to the outer layers of the bone. A very typical periosteal reaction is seen along the shaft (Fig. 20–2).

The pathomechanics of infection after plate osteosynthesis is entirely different. If the hallmark of infection after nailing is longitudinal contamination of the bone by spread of sepsis along the nail, infection after plate fixation is

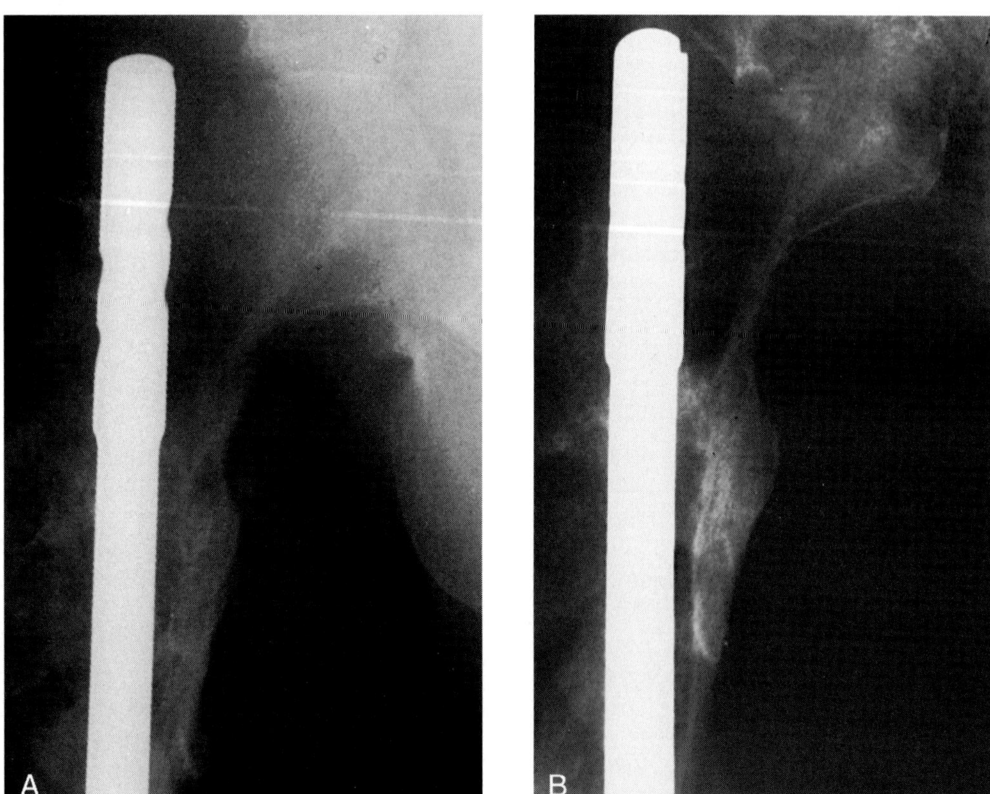

Fig. 20–1. An immuno-compromised patient underwent interlocking nailing for a subtrochanteric fracture. *A,* When the proximal locking screws became infected, they were removed. *B,* Months later there has been extensive destruction of the proximal femur without evidence of bone repair. When infection complicates a nailing, the entire device is involved.

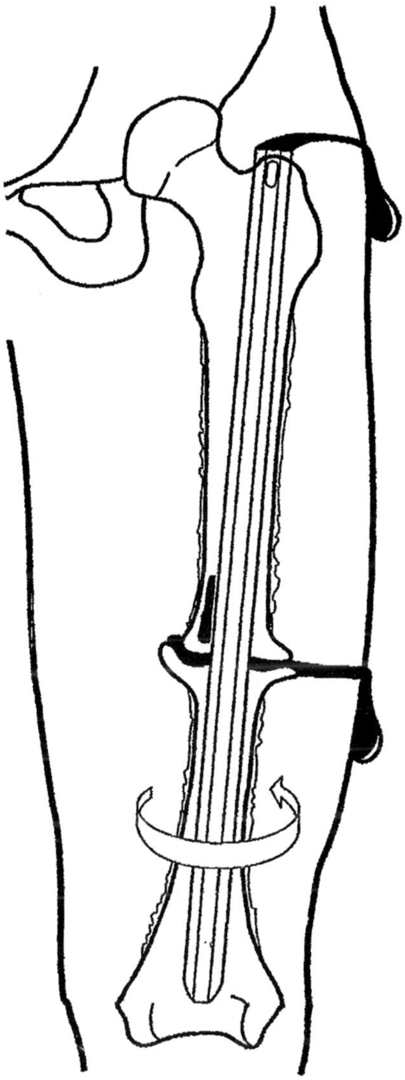

Fig. 20–2. After Küntscher nailing, infection can lead to rotational instability. Periosteal reaction is observed along the length of the nail.

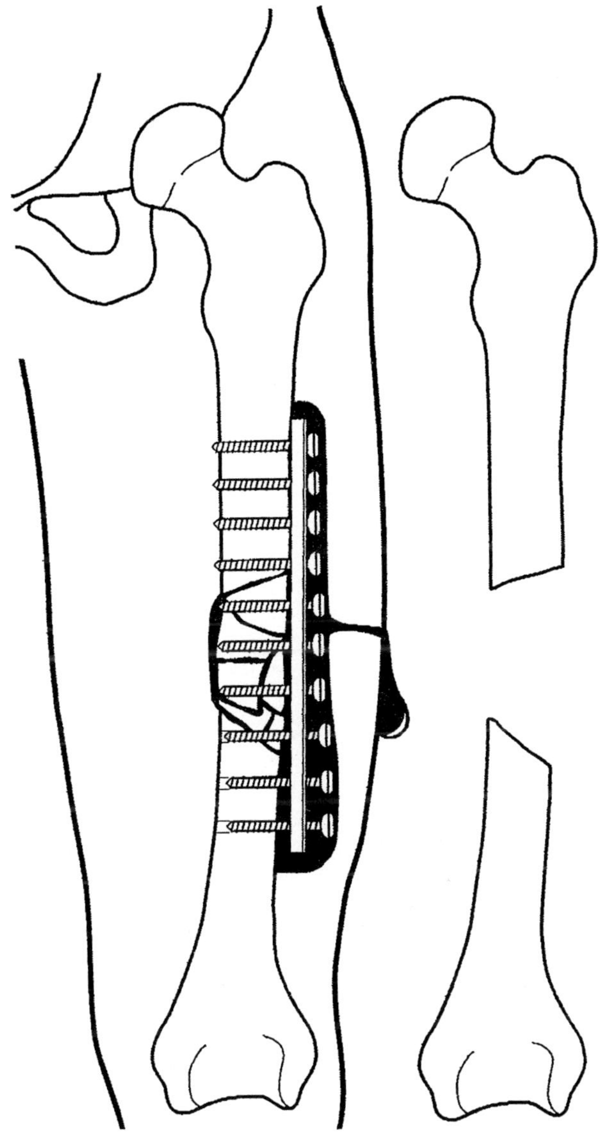

Fig. 20–3. Infection after plate osteosynthesis creates a local area of sequestrum which may need to be resected. This causes a defect.

intercalary. Here the bone is involved in the region encompassed by the plate. In the typical case, soft tissue has been dissected from the bone so that the periosteal blood supply is disturbed. Furthermore, with the initial injury at the moment of the fracture, the endosteal blood vessels are disrupted. Therefore the entire thickness of the bone and much of its circumference are avascular. The very nature of plating requires that the more complex and comminuted the fracture, the greater the devitalization needed to place a bone plate. Nor does so-called "biological" plating solve the problem, because avascular comminuted fragments may remain in the fracture locus when the plate is used as a strut across complex comminutions. When infection complicates plating, periosteal response may not occur, particularly if the devascularization has been profound. Treatment creates a defect (Fig. 20–3).[9]

The rationale for the use of interlocking nailing in the treatment of infected pseudoarthrosis is the control of instability at the fracture locus provided by the locked implant.[10] Most straightforward fractures heal with simple flexible implants, because with axial loading the fracture ends are driven together and become stable (Bigelow's rabbetting).

Biological factors at a fracture site can also contribute to the development of infection. These include nonvital bone at the fracture, contamination in compound wounds, and deficient soft tissue.[9,11] A special situation is the presence of an avascular comminution interposed at a fracture site.[12] After interlocking nailing, this avascular area may persist with only slow resorption. If the nail is dynamized or removed, there may be bone failure with collapse, instability, and infection.

Pistoning instability and angular instability are also possible. Varus-valgus instability can occur when infection loosens interlocking screws that slide in and out with stress in the plane of the screws (Fig. 20–4).

DIAGNOSIS

Fever, leucocytosis, erythema, and drainage developing after intramedullary nailing of a long bone mean infection of the entire implant and medullary canal until proven otherwise.[13–15] Acute erythema and swelling at the point

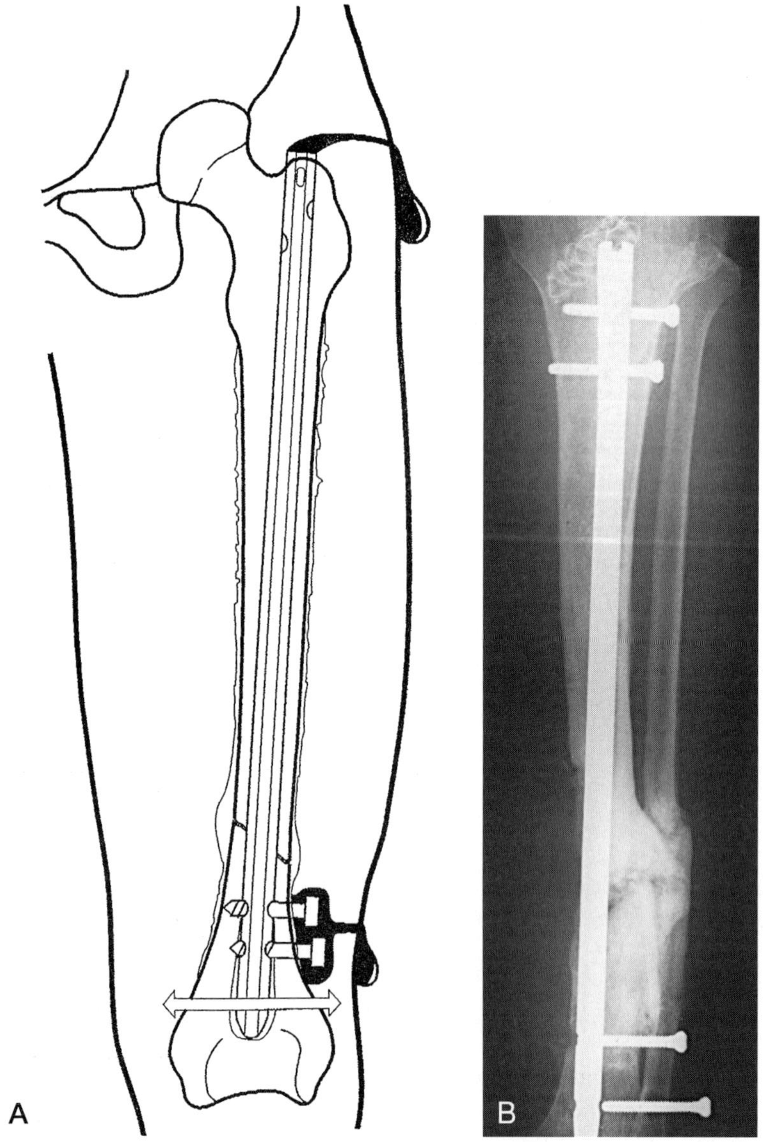

Fig. 20–4. Varus-valgus instability occurs with infection. *A,* This can cause the interlocking screws to slide in-and-out. *B,* Infection led to instability in this case where interlocking nailing was attempted after external fixation.

of insertion of the nail or where the screws for interlocking have been placed almost always mean that the entire diaphysis is involved.[16] Some surgeons persist in the concept that the infection can be localized to the point of insertion of the nail or to where the interlocking screws have been placed. In reality there is continuity throughout the length of an intramedullary nail and its screws, and the infection involves the entire implant. In the acute phase (the first 30 days after nailing), the diagnosis is made operatively. The wound is explored, drained, and operative cultures taken.[3,13,17] Here the fracture is unhealed. Delay provided by antibiotic suppression or delays for diagnostic imaging allow damage to the bone to progress, possibly complicating subsequent treatment. Baseline laboratory tests prior to surgery provide objective guides for therapy (Table 20–1). A good laboratory screen assists not only in studying the systemic response to infection but also in monitoring the possible side effects of antimicrobial agents.

The diagnosis of infection in the subacute and chronic phases after intramedullary nailing may be more difficult. Plain radiographs are essential. They answer the following important questions:

1. Is the fracture healed?
2. Is dead bone present?
3. Is the implant in or out?
4. What is the response of bone?
5. What is the response of the soft tissue?

In many respects, the assessment of osteomyelitis after intramedullary nailing is like the evaluation of a bone tumor. It is important to gauge what the infection has done to bone and what the bone is doing about the infection. Bone vascularity can be inferred from regional density differences in the plain radiographs. Dead bone still has the original density it had at the time of trauma, while bone retaining its blood supply becomes osteoporotic. Areas of bone that appear more dense, particularly in the fracture locus, may represent sequestrae. Increase in cortical width can be a measure of chronicity. Periosteal new bone formation similar to what it observed in hematogenous osteomyelitis is indicative of repair processes.[18]

The radiograph is one tool for assessing the extent of fracture healing. Persistence of the fracture line may indicate a plane of instability. Progressive resorption of bone is another sign that the fracture is not healing. Plain radiographs taken at intervals are of great assistance as they indicate trends towards repair and stability or towards resorption and failure. Radiographs can also be misleading. Slight differences in projection and technique can lead to misinterpretation of the biological phenomena under observation. An area that appears healed in one radiograph may show a wide fracture gap in a projection 10° from the first. Fluoroscopy with careful positioning and application of stress is a valuable tool toward demonstrating instability at a fracture site.

Osteomyelitis should be considered in a patient with persistent pain, weakness, fever, skin changes, or drainage long after fracture healing has taken place. This chronic infection may be present whether or not the nail has been removed.[13] Ancillary imaging techniques are available and should be used to answer specific questions raised by the physical examination and plain radiographs (Table 20–2).[3,19,20]

Each of these tests has a relative specificity and is dependent on the skill of the radiologist

Table 20–1. Laboratory survey for osteomyelitis

Hct, WBC, differential
Sedimentation rate
Prothrombin time
C-reactive protein
Antistreptolysin-O
Total protein/albumen
Bilirubin
BUN and creatine
Alkaline/phosphatase
Transaminase

Table 20–2. Supplemental diagnostic studies for osteomyelitis

Study	*Findings*
Linear tomogram	Sequestrae, fracture healing
Sinogram	Location, extent of cavity
Computerized tomogram	Extra skeletal abscesses, cortical destruction
Three-phase technetium bone scan	Osteoblastic activity
Gallium scanning	Acute inflammation
Indium-labeled WBC scan	Active osteomyelitis
Magnetic resonance scan	Fluid collection, soft-tissue changes

in selecting and manipulating images. Magnetic resonance imaging, for example, invariably overestimates the extent of fluid collections in the marrow space. It is helpful to develop a relationship with a radiologist interested in skeletal imaging and plan the sequence of examinations needed to answer specific clinical questions that are necessary to plan management.

MANAGEMENT

> On peut aussi procéder en 2 temps... Il vaut mieux, en effet, se retirer sur la pointe des pieds plutôt que de se risquer dans une difficile aventure non préparée.[21]

An infected nailing with an unhealed fracture is a difficult management problem. This problem is only made worse when treatment is undertaken without regard to biological principles.[11] The crucial consideration is not the presence of an implant but the stability of the fracture site.[3,20] Experimentally contaminated fractures heal better when they are stable.[22,23] Note that antibiotic treatment does not eliminate the infection in these cases, treatment only suppresses the infection. With interlocking nailing, when screw fixation is provided proximal and distal to a fracture (static locking) and the fixation is solid, it is rational to establish controlled drainage, suppress infection with systemic antibiotics, and allow the fracture to unite.[3,13] A final medullary cleanup can be then undertaken to reduce the possible late occurrence of an intramedullary abscess (Fig. 20–5).[16]

Many situations do not lend themselves to retention of the original nail until fracture healing. The nail itself is not the problem. The problem is unfavorable fracture site mechanics or biological factors that require removal of the implant and a multi-stage plan to first control sepsis and then restore the limb.[9,24] The initial

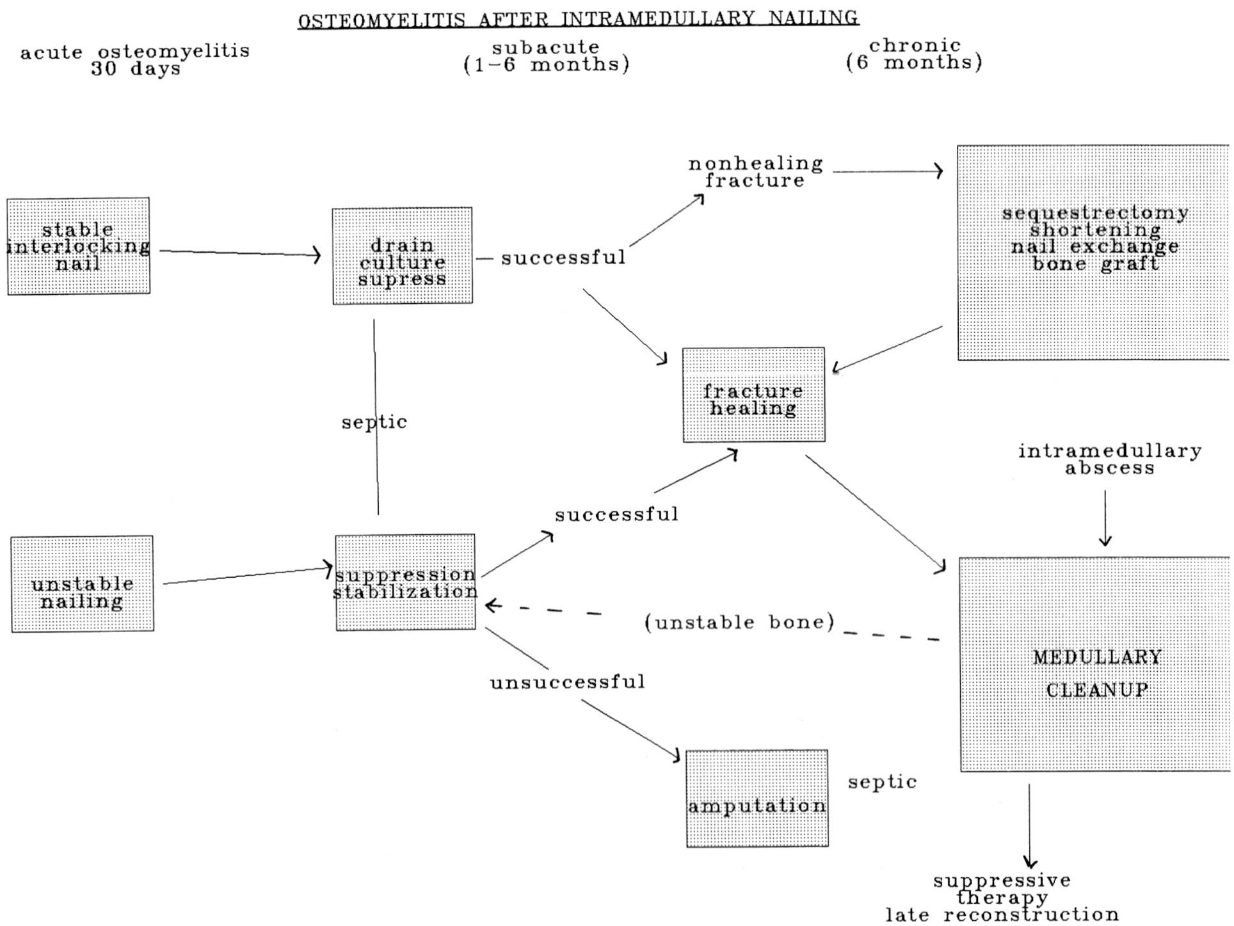

Fig. 20–5. Flow diagram for the treatment of osteomyelitis after intramedullary nailing.

step of this program is suppression followed by stabilization (Fig. 20–6). Here the medullary implant is removed to gain control of sepsis, then the limb can be restabilized to allow healing.[18] Those mechanical factors which usually require nail removal include all forms of flexible, noninterlocking nails such as Rush rods, Ender's nails, Küntscher nails, and interlocking nails that were never interlocked or in which the locking screws have failed. Except in acute cases (within the first 30 days) it is not practical to try to retain a nail that was not interlocked by placing screws through the nail. Such implants have already been cycled by loading and are fatigued. These nails may fail under the added constraints of interlocking and should be replaced. Flexible nail constructs never provide sufficient stability[25] to control infection, and they should also be removed. The therapeutic requirements are similar when infection cannot be suppressed with an interlocking nail in place. In all these situations the plan for treatment is suppression-stabilization.

The first step of suppression-stabilization is nail removal.[26] Cultures are taken from the implant and the medullary canal. In the face of active infection and instability, it is unwise to immediately introduce new implants until the infection has been drained and initial broad-spectrum antibiotic therapy has had an opportunity to control systemic and, to a lesser extent, local sepsis. A waiting period of a few days sometimes provides specific information about the bacterial spectrum of the infecting organisms.[27,28] A number of cases however will be culture-negative. Antibiotic therapy can be tailored to the specific offending organism when culture reports are available.[14,15] At least half of the time multiple organisms are recovered.[20,28] It is important for all organisms obtained from the marrow space to be identified and to obtain their antibiograms.[29] Many laboratories return reports on organisms like *Staphylococcus epidermidis* as "likely contaminant." Unless specific requests are sent to the bacteriology laboratory, important information such as methicillin resistance will be lost. During the

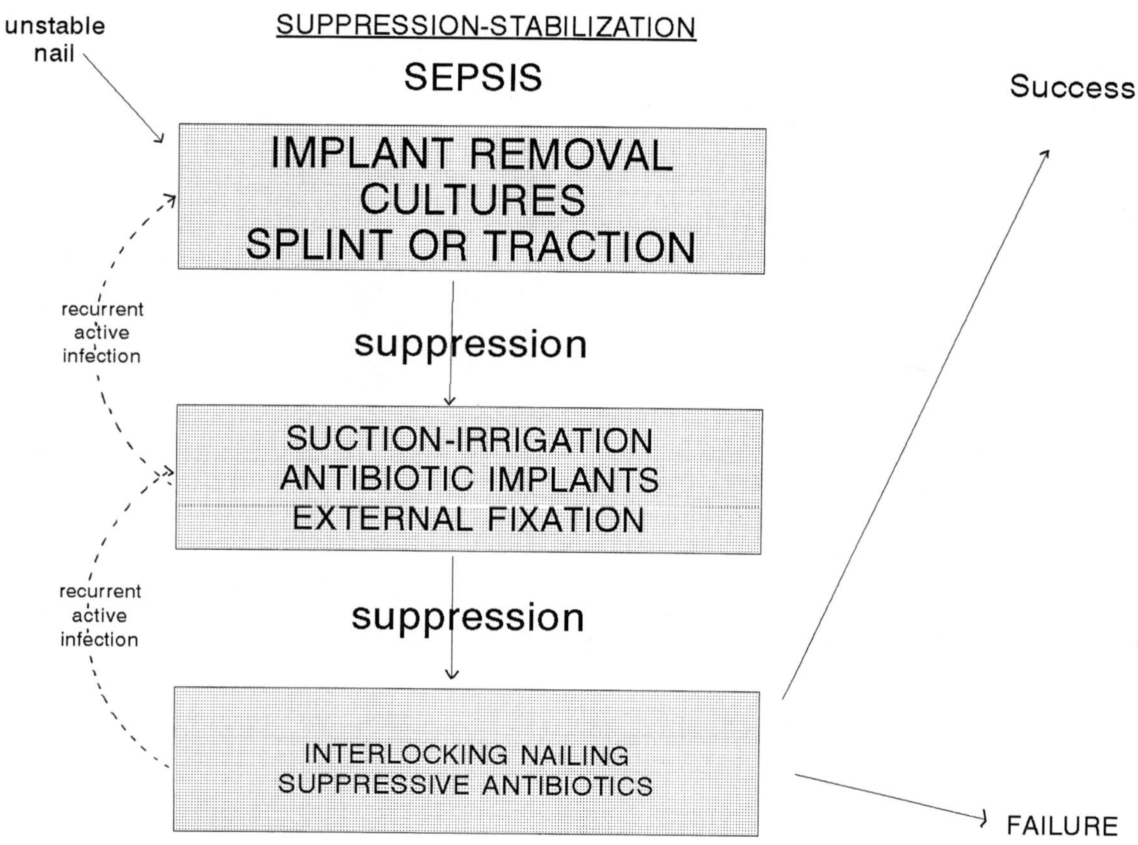

Fig. 20–6. Flow diagram for the phase of suppression-stabilization.

few days following implant removal splinting or skeletal traction controls fracture-site motion. This control is insufficient to allow the inflammatory reaction to entirely subside. Therefore when cultures are available and the patient's general condition has improved with specific therapy and general medical support, a second operation is undertaken to get better control of the infection.[30]

In the second phase of suppression-stabilization, the canal is gently debrided by reaming to remove the infected granulation tissue and lamellar sequestrae lining the inner wall, drainage is obtained and either an antibiotic-impregnated PMMA implant[31,32] (bead chains or stick) or a suction-irrigation system[33–37] is installed. PMMA bead chains can be passed using a special flexible bead chain passer which allows for placement the entire length of the medullary canal. In general the canal must be enlarged to at least 10 mm to pass the 6- to 7-mm beads successfully. A gentamicin PMMA bead stick consisting of a cylinder of antibiotic impregnated PMMA on a wire is sufficiently flexible to pass like a guide along the whole length of the canal and is much simpler to use (Fig. 20–7). Suction-irrigation is another alternative.[12,27,33,38] Here a loop drain greatly facilitates intermittent irrigation of the medullary canal (Fig. 20–8).[32] After 4 to 5 days of intermittent drainage it can be cut and both ends allowed to provide continuous drainage.

External skeletal fixation decreases patient morbidity but there is considerable risk of getting chronic pin tract drainage if it is installed prematurely. Active inflammation must sub-

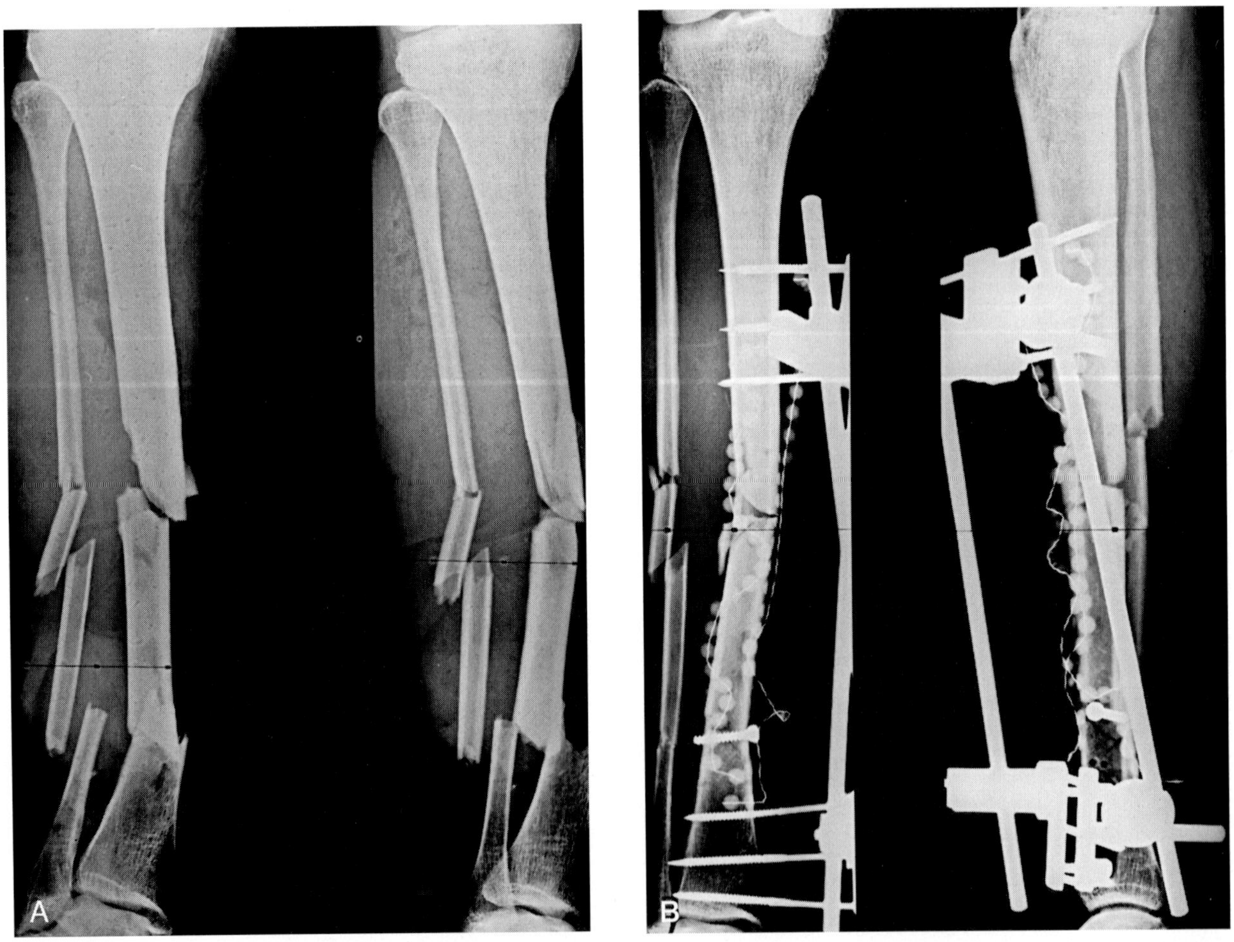

Fig. 20–7. *A,* This 31-year-old woman sustained a severe compound segmental fracture of the tibia. Her initial treatment was external fixation, implantation of gentamicin-PMMA bead chain (Septopal; Kulzer & Co. GmbH, Wehrheim, Germany), and temporary coverage with a synthetic skin substitute. Two weeks post-injury she underwent definitive coverage with a latissimus dorsi free flap *B,* After 5 months the proximal fracture had not healed. Low-grade infection was present. Therefore, a dynamic interlocking nailing was performed with insertion of a gentamicin-PMMA stick in the lumen of the nail *(Figure continues)*

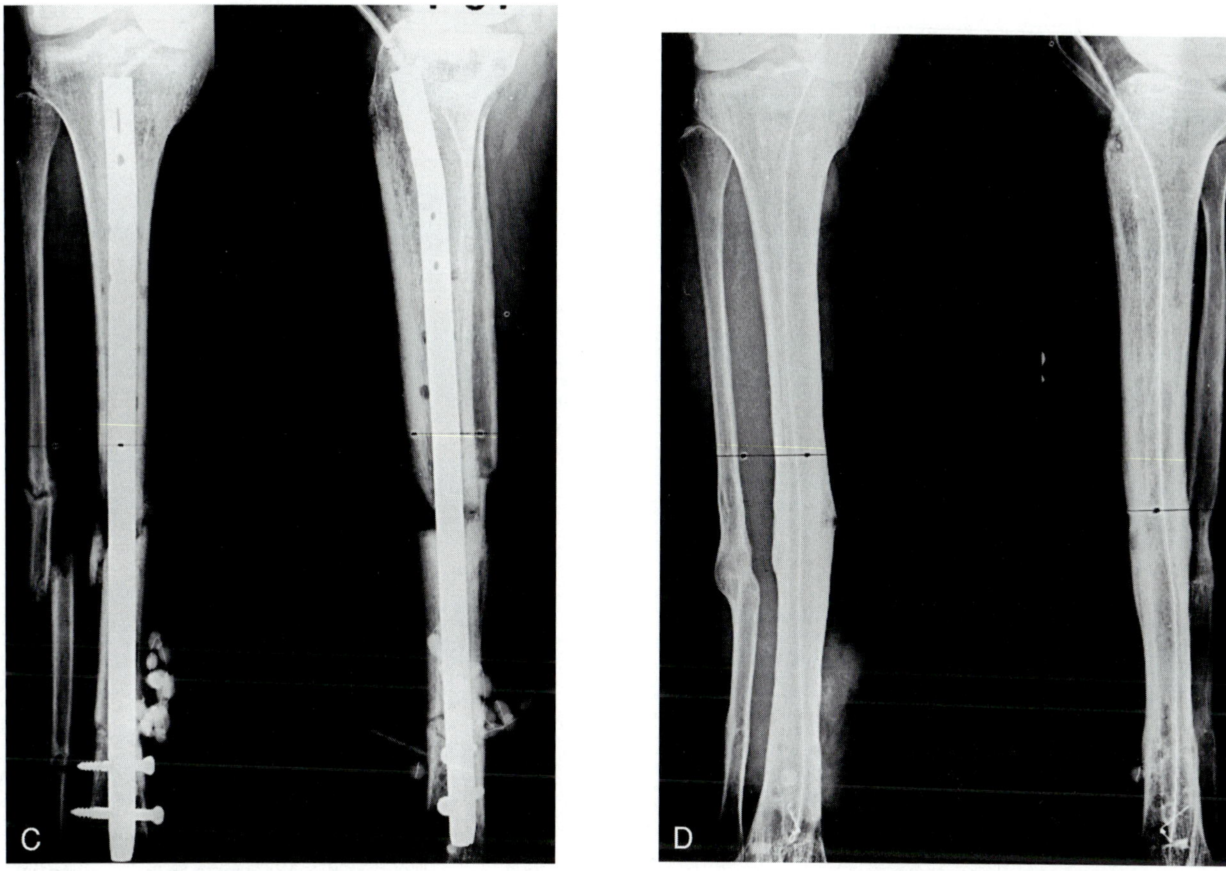

Fig. 20–7. *(continued) C,* Two years later the fractures were healed without recurrence of infection. Therefore, the nail was removed and the canal was reamed and a gentamicin-PMMA stick placed temporally to cleanup the medullary canal, *D.*

side and drainage must come under control prior to placement of a fixateur. Fixateur placement in an infected case requires attention to detail. The montage must be stable. All the pins must pass through the marrow cavity, because intracortical pins themselves are a cause of infection. The pins should be passed through drilled-pilot holes or special self-cutting pins can be used.

Antibiotic bead chains are incompatible with external fixateurs. The chains cannot be passed around pins which properly transverse the marrow space, and if the bead chains are placed first and then the pins, the bead chains cannot be removed. To solve this problem an antibiotic-impregnated PMMA stick[26] has been fabricated by extruding antibiotic-laden PMMA on a continuous monofilament wire using a process not unlike "noodle-making" (Kulzer & Co. GmbH, Wehrheim, Germany. Distributed by E. Merck, Darmstadt, Germany. Not FDA approved for U.S. sale as of January 1995). This PMMA stick passes around external fixateur pins in the medullary cavity and can be left in place longer than bead chains. Granulation tissue, while it grows around the stick, does not prevent removal as it does with the chains. Note that the greatest effect of an antibiotic-impregnated PMMA implant is in the first few days after its placement.[31,39,40] In cases where there is a persistently large quantity of drainage, the stick can be replaced in a minor procedure to maintain the highest possible level of antibiotic in the medullary canal.

Initially, we hoped that external fixation would be the method whereby fracture healing could be obtained following infection after intramedullary nailing.[41] Following placement of the frame, the fracture site was explored and debrided. Antibiotic PMMA bead chains were installed.[10,42–44] Later, the beads were removed and bone graft placed. Indeed it is possible to

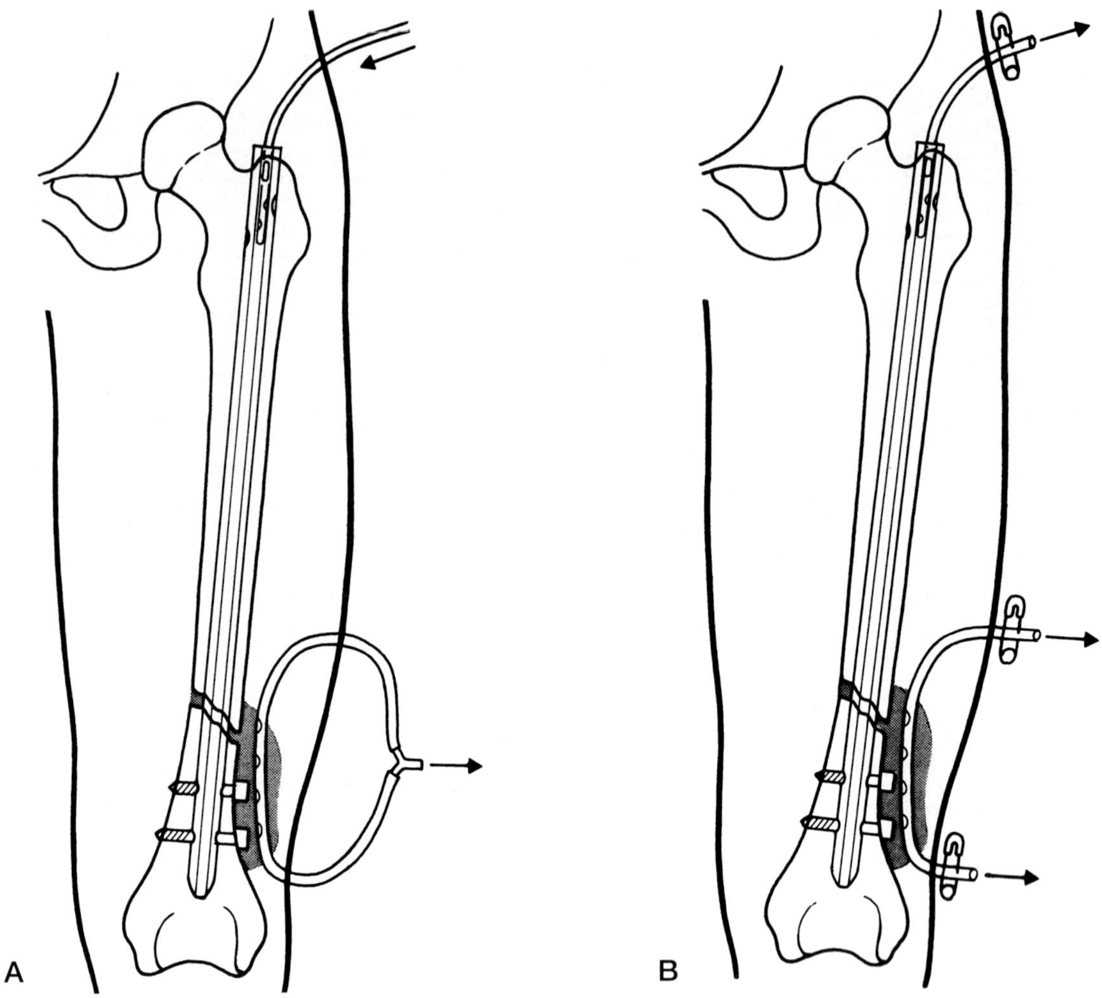

Fig. 20–8. *A,* If the interlocking nail is retained in an acute infection, a suction-irrigation system can be arranged by placing an ingress catheter in the lumen of the nail and a loop-drain at the fracture site. *B,* When the infection subsides the drains can be cut and used for chronic gravity drainage. (Reprinted from Klemm, K., Henry, S., Seligson, D.: The treatment of infection after interlocking nailing. Techniques Orthop. *3*:54–61, 1988.)

get union with this method; however, the results are not predictable and the treatment time is too long. Because the canal has been instrumented in the original nailing and subsequently became infected, external fixateur pin anchorage is not optimal. Often cumbersome frames are required, and even then the stability may be insufficient to promote union.

Therefore, the fracture site is explored and debrided only for specific indications such as the presence of a cortical sequestrum.[3,4,11] The most direct way to achieve union is to renail[1] and interlock[45] the fracture once the infection is under control. This reinstallation of an interlocking nail is called "secondary nailing" to distinguish it from "primary nailing," which is the initial placement of a nail for the treatment of an acute fracture (Fig. 20–9). Secondary nailing should be performed under perioperative antibiotic coverage. If organisms have been recovered, this therapy should be directed by their specific sensitivities.

Success after secondary nailing is observed by an improvement in the general well-being of the patient. Pulse and color return to normal and the patient has a good appetite, sleeps well, and takes less pain medication. The limb becomes less swollen. Strength and function improve. The sedimentation rate falls. The white count and differential return to normal. The patient regains an interest in his work, home, and friends. When infection does not come under

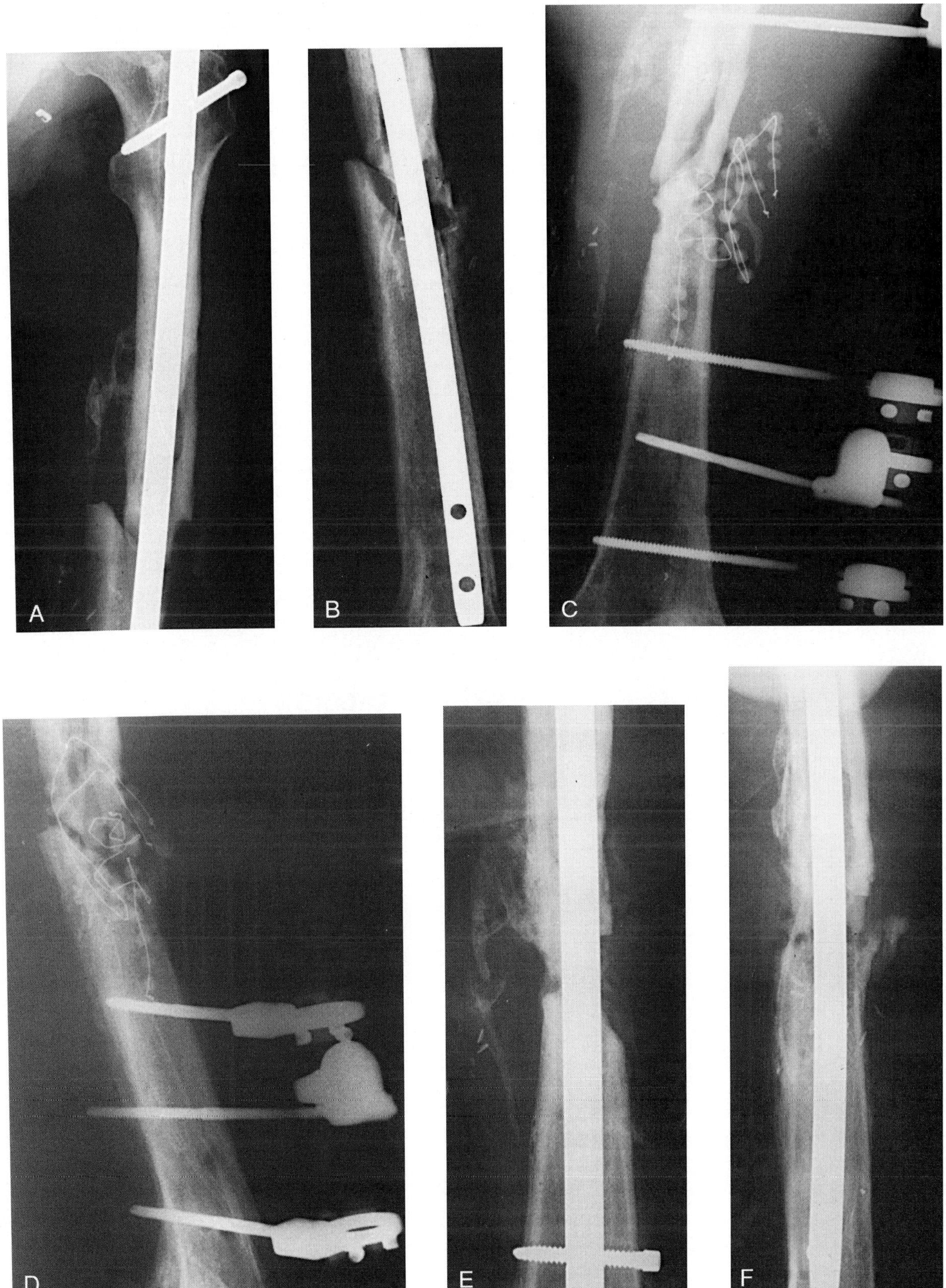

Fig. 20–9. *A,B,* Dynamization of an interlocking nailing of a femur fracture complicated by a severe soft-tissue injury and infection led to rotational instability and osteomyelitis. *C,D,* The infection came under control with nail removal, debridement, placement of antibiotic PMMA bead chains, and external fixation. *E,F,* Finally with shortening and interlocking nailing it is slowly uniting.

control and symptoms worsen, it is necessary to repeat the steps of suppression-irrigation. Sometimes two or three trials of treatment will result in success. Each treatment sequence may be characterized by a longer period of improvement. Continued failure, however, must provoke consideration of amputation in certain situations.[46] These situations involve uncontrolled systemic sepsis and persistent painful drainage, especially with highly-resistant strains of organisms such as *Proteus, Enterococcus,* and *Pseudomonas.* Insoluble problems of poor local tissue with a contracted limb and established nerve palsy, as well as insoluble systemic host problems such as collagen-vascular or immunosuppressive disorders also require bold decisions to proceed to amputation.

When treatment results in a solid bone with or without minimal drainage, the final phase of care is medullary cleanup. This treatment is also indicated for a medullary abscess which can occur years after successful nailing and implant removal.[13,47] Absolute elimination of infection, while a desirable goal, is not generally achievable with current technology. The goal is to reduce the incidence of recurrence and increase periods of low morbidity. The patient can function in society with minimum inconvenience because of good disease suppression.

Cleanup of the medullary canal is a two-step process (Fig. 20–10). First, the implant is removed and bacterial cultures are taken. These are generally negative despite the abundance of inflammatory tissue that may be present. Steps that will increase the yield of positive cultures include (1) discontinuing suppressive antibiotics for 1 week preoperatively, (2) vortexing implants (screws) to recover adherent organisms, (3) placing specimens for culture directly into medium (blood culture bottles are convenient), and (4) incubating the cultures for at least 4 days. Removing a contaminated implant

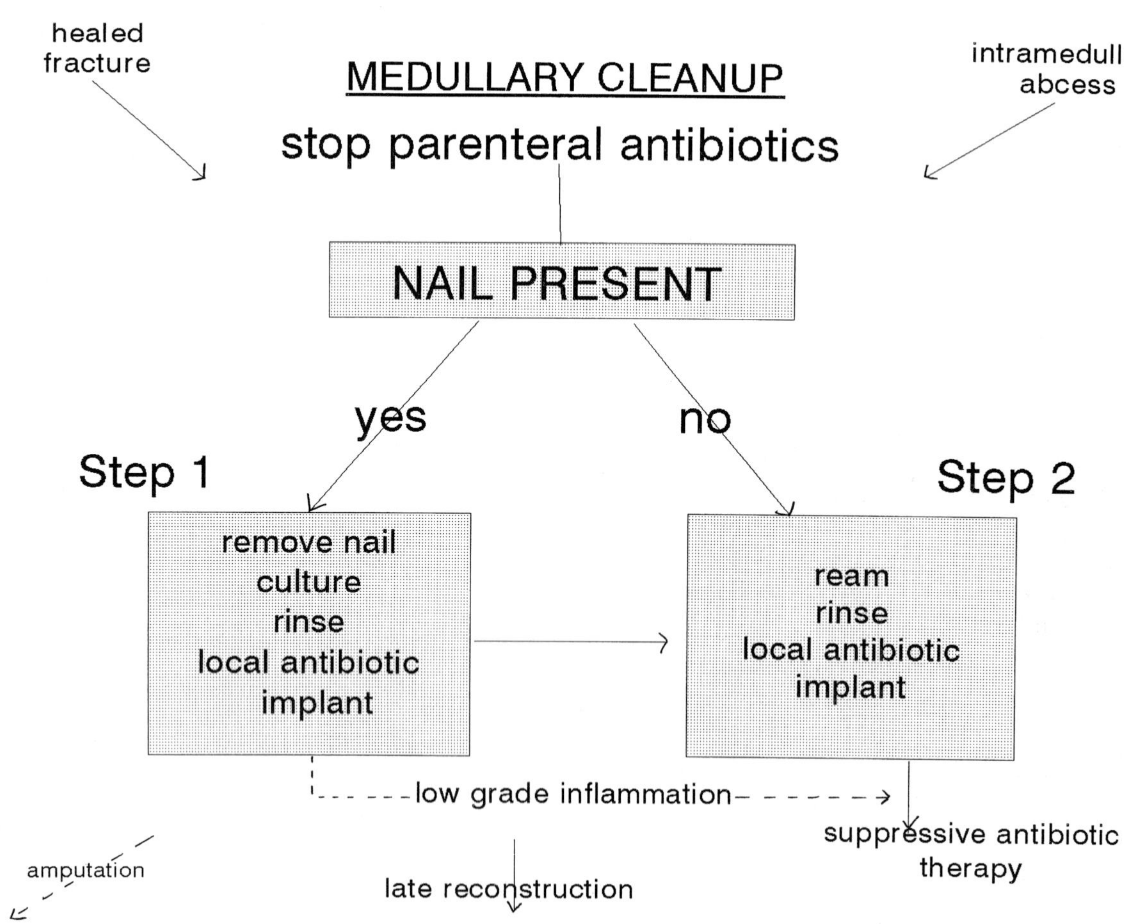

Fig. 20–10. Flow diagram for the phase of medullary cleanup.

from an intact bone is the single most important step in reducing the incidence of late morbidity.[48] Removing a stabilizing intramedullary implant from an unstable bone is the single worst step that can be taken to bring about healing. These principles are consistent but confusing. Misunderstanding can lead to a lack of productive dialogue between specialists attempting to manage an infected intramedullary nailing.

In surgery for medullary cleanup, it is helpful to gently rinse the canal. A narrow bore chest tube or red rubber catheter can be used. Mechanical brushing with a canal brush from total hip replacement surgery helps debride granulation tissue and lamellar sequestrae clinging to the endosteum. Then a chain of antibiotic PMMA beads[32] or a gentamicin PMMA stick can be placed the length of the medullary canal and the wound closed over an overflow drain. Alternatively, a suction-irrigation system can be installed and left in place for a few days.

Medullary cleanup usually requires two steps. In the second step the canal is reamed to remove endosteal sequestrae. Prior to the second operation, antibiotic therapy is initiated. This therapy is directed toward organisms that were recovered at nail removal. In the operation, antibiotic implants are first removed. The intramedullary sequestrae can be seen. They are small rice-sized islands of dead bone along the endosteal surface of the canal. Gentle reaming is carried out using flexible reamers. Generally reaming the canal 2 mm greater than the implant that was removed is sufficient. Begin reaming with the end-cutting reamer and advance in 1- or 2-mm increments until the nail size is reached. Then proceed by 0.5-mm increments. It is important to use sharp reamers and avoid the generation of heat, which can cause more damage to the endosteum. At the end of the procedure, the canal is rinsed and a chain or stick of antibiotic-impregnated PMMA can be placed temporarily or permanently in the canal. Bead chains left more than 7 to 10 days are difficult to extract, while the PMMA stick is removed quite easily. Oral suppressive antibiotic therapy slowly reduced to low doses is usually helpful for months to years following an intramedullary osteomyelitis.

In a few cases low-grade chronic infection produces thickening of the cortex and obliteration of the medullary canal. This condition is known as "sclerosing osteomyelitis of Garré."[49] Such patients are difficult to treat. In young patients consideration should be given to excising short segments and transporting bone to restore limb length. Alternatively the canal can be reestablished by reaming and an antibiotic implant placed.[50] Recurrence is the rule. Patients report painful pressure. Plain radiographs show renewed thickening of the cortex and extension of the zone of sclerosis (Fig. 20–11). Repeat debridement and suppressive systemic antibiotics seem only to slow and not to eradicate this process.[50]

THE FUTURE

Techniques of intramedullary nailing are evolving. New methods will bring new concepts that not only reduce the incidence of infection, but also will provide new approaches for the treatment of osteomyelitis. In a closed fracture, marrow nailing both initiates the infection and is the instrument for its control. Küntscher's dream of functional osteosynthesis with nailing has developed to the point of providing mechanically sound, inert metal nails that control limb length and rotation during fracture healing. The basic principles Küntscher investigated by instrumenting the marrow cavity with corrosive implants and demonstrating the formation of callus without a fracture could be applied to stimulate fracture healing.[17] Bioactive coatings applied to nails in the operating room could be customized to enhance bone formation in the zone of the fracture but not elsewhere. Nails could be coated to resist colonization by organisms and medullary implants could be designed to treat infection.

Reconstruction of shortened limbs is in its early development.[51] Interlocking nails that can be manipulated to increase length either mechanically or by miniaturized motors are coming into clinical practice. These nails will make temporary shortening an attractive option for the management of difficult infections with devitalized bone. In the future, restoration of length will probably be more predictable when performed with lengthening nails coated with bioactive peptides.

Replacement of diseased skeletal segments, as a general proposition, is a technique that requires encouragement from governmental agencies rather than microregulation. As physicians, our own lack of imagination and an unwillingness to understand the patient's per-

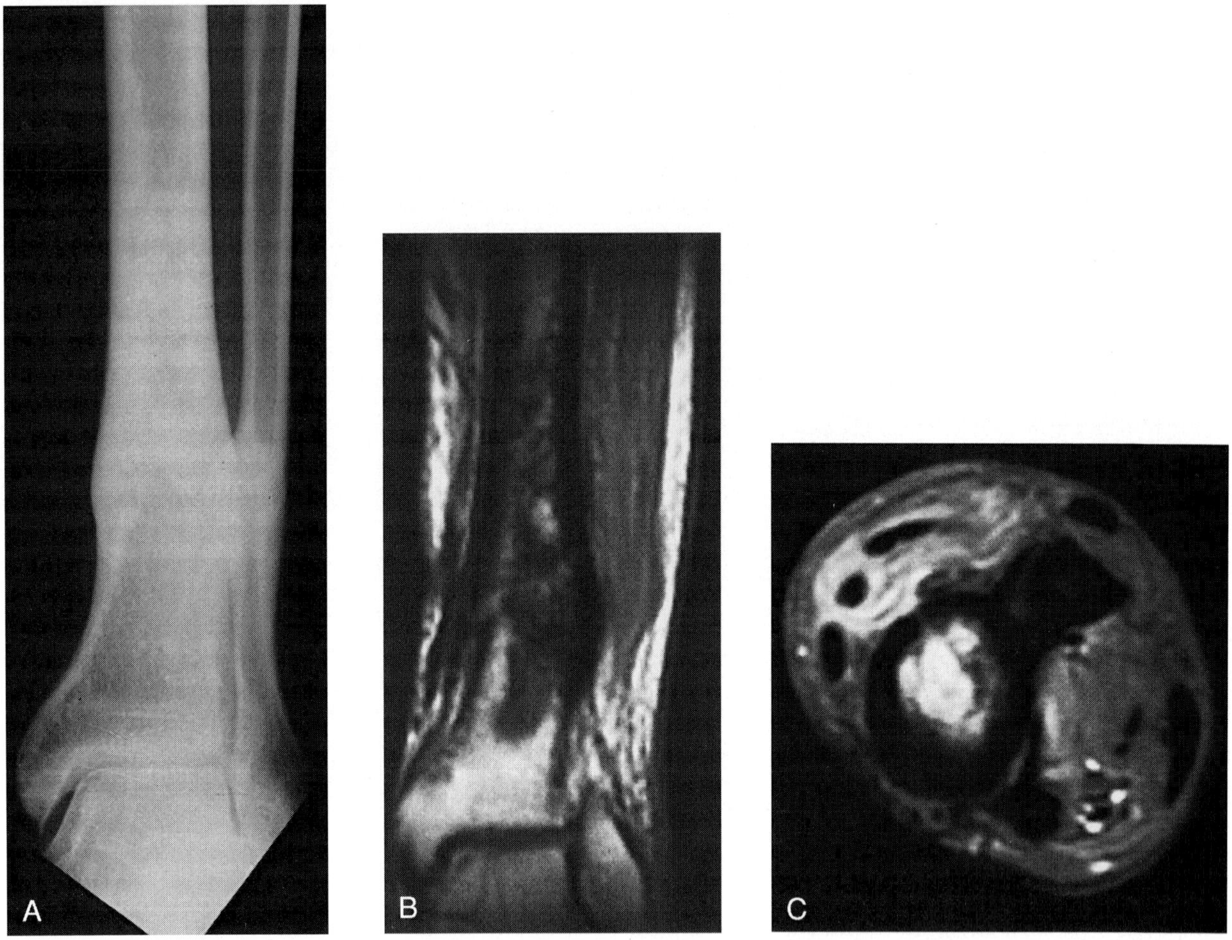

Fig. 20–11. *A,* In sclerosing osteomyelitis the cortex becomes thickened and sclerotic. *B,* The MRI shows obliteration of the marrow cavity. *C,* In cross-section an abscess is observed with extension into the anterior compartment where it surrounds the extensor tendons.

spective may equally hamper progress. Were you taught that length of the humerus was unimportant, that shoe lifts solve most lower limb discrepancies, and that amputation was more cost effective than limb reconstruction? We challenge you then to find the city where jackets with unequal arms can be purchased, where sneakers with inch lifts are sold, and where one-legged men and women function as well as their peers.

More elegant materials will ultimately be available for intramedullary fixation. Absorbable, laminated implants that guide the healing of fractures will be developed. These implants will prevent and/or treat infection and control the shape and geometry of the healed bone. They will assure restoration of cortical and medullary architecture and be of sufficient mechanical strength to allow functional use of the limb during healing.

In our professional lifetime, the treatment of femur shaft fractures, for example, has been reduced first by Küntscher nails and today with interlocking nailing from a morbid period of traction lasting 2 to 3 months followed by protected activity for a usual length of treatment of 6 months to two short hospitalizations with minimum morbidity. In advanced countries, nonoperative care is for financial reasons alone impractical. Yet, because the method of interlocking nailing has as its risk a small incidence of postoperative infection that is considered acceptable,[2,52] resources and techniques need to be released so that the few patients who suffer from an unsuccessful outcome of intramedullary osteosynthesis get the benefit of cur-

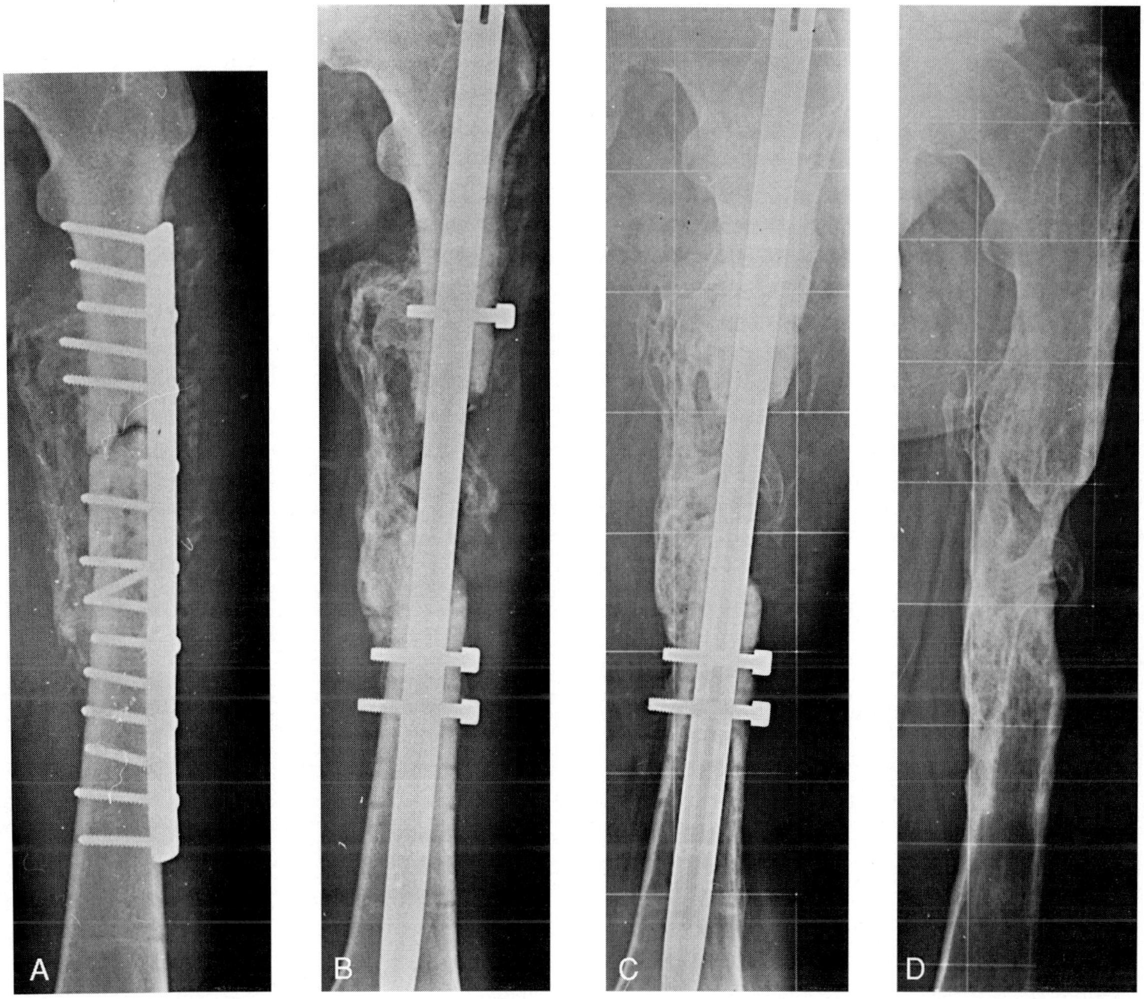

Fig. 20–12. *A,* In this historical case a 35-year-old man developed a nonunion after plate fixation of a minimally open compound femur fracture. *B,* The large sequestrum beneath the plate was excised and the femur stabilized with a prototype interlocking nail. *C,* By 14 months there was partial consolidation and the nail had been dynamized. *D,* At 3 years the fracture had healed and the nail had been removed.

rent techniques and the potential benefits of future research.

Still, today's current emphasis on outcomes analysis, cost control, and case management make it difficult to secure the resources necessary to reduce morbidity from postoperative infections. Concealing the problem, placing blame on the patient, or finding fault in the hospital are not productive ways to learn more about the treatment of infection after nailing. Challenging areas for study are improved techniques for detecting and imaging limbs at risk for medullary osteomyelitis, techniques for visualizing the endosteum intraoperatively, and development methods for determining bacterial burden in vivo. The pathophysiology of sclerosing osteomyelitis needs clarification and a method devised for its treatment. No really good methods are currently available for determining in vivo stability and quantifying fracture healing. Important epidemiologic questions need resolution. For example, what are the risks of retained implants in patients undergoing immunosuppressive treatment or in patients with immune system disorders? Do absorbable antibiotics implanted at the time of initial treatment[53] hold the promise of preventing infection after nailing altogether?

Treatment of infection after medullary nailing is difficult. However, this challenge, if met honestly, can provide a successful outcome for patient and physician (Fig. 20–12).

REFERENCES

1. Lottes, J.O.: Medullary nailing of infected fractures of the femur. Clin. Orthop. *60*:99–101, 1968.
2. Jenny, J.Y., Jenny, G., Kempf, I.: Infection after reamed intramedullary nailing. Acta Orthop. Scand. *65*:94–96, 1994.
3. MacAusland, W.R., Jr.: Treatment of sepsis after intramedullary nailing of the femur. Clin. Orthop. *60*: 87–94, 1968.
4. Gristina, A.G., Oga, M., Webb, L.X., et al.: Adherent bacterial colonization in the pathogenesis of osteomyelitis. Science *228*:990–993, 1985.
5. Oga, M., Arizono, T., Sugioka, Y.: Bacterial adherence to bioinert and bioactive materials studied in vitro. Acta Orthop. Scand. *64*:273–276, 1993.
6. Andrew, J.G., Andrew, S.M., Freemont, A.J., Marsch, D.R.: Inflammatory cells in normal human fracture healing. Acta Orthop. Scand. *65*:462–466, 1994.
7. Wilkins, J., Patzakis, M.J.: Peripheral Teflon catheters. Clin. Orthop. *254*:251–254.
8. Küntscher, G.: The incidence of infection after enlargement of the medullary cavity. Chirurg *39*:236–240, 1968.
9. Cierny, G. III, Mader, J.T.: Adult chronic osteomyelitis. Orthopedics *7*:1557–1564, 1984.
10. Klemm, K.: Die modifizierte Trummerbruchnagelung zur Stabilisierung der infizierten Pseudarthrosen am Oberschenkel. Unfallheilkunde *110*:240, 1972.
11. Nichols, E.H.: Acute, subacute and chronic infectious osteomyelitis: Its pathology and treatment. JAMA. *42*: 439–466, 1904.
12. Weber, B.G., Cĕch, O.: Pseudarthrosis. New York: Grune & Stratton, 1976.
13. Böhler, L.: Medullary Nailing of Küntscher. Baltimore, Williams & Wilkins, 1948.
14. Burri, C.: Post-Traumatic Osteomyelitis. Bern, Hans Huber, 1975.
15. Mader, J.T., Norden, C., Nelson, J.D., Calandra, G.B.: Evaluation of new anti-infective drugs for the treatment of osteomyelitis in adults. Clin. Infect. Dis. *15*(Suppl 1):S155–161, 1992.
16. Thompson, M.S.: Infections following intramedullary fixation. Clin. Orthop. *2*:60–65, 1953.
17. Küntscher, G.: Practice of Intramedullary Nailing. Springfield, IL, Charles C. Thomas, 1967.
18. Wilson, J.N.: The management of infection after Küntscher nailing of the femur. J. Bone Joint Surg. *48B*: 112–116, 1966.
19. Aliabadi, P., Nikpoor, N.: Imaging osteomyelitis. Arthritis Rheum. *37*:617–622, 1994.
20. Patzakis, M.J., Wilkins, J., Wiss, D.A.: Infection following intramedullary nailing of long bones. Clin. Orthop. *212*:182–191, 1986.
21. Litt, R., Albassir, A.: Résultats de 1' utilisation des prosthèses pour grande résection fémorale de M.E. Müller. Acta Orthop. Belg. *52*:383–389, 1986.
22. Rush, H.L., Fitts, W.T., Gibbons, J., Monroe, E.W.: Intramedullary nailing in the present of infection: An experimental study in dogs. Surg. Gynecol. Obstet. *94*: 727–732, 1952.
23. Worlock, P., Slack, R., Harvey, L., Mawhinney, R.: The prevention of infection in open fractures: An experimental study of the effect of fracture stability. Injury *25*:31–38, 1994.
24. Court-Brown, C.M., Keating, J.F., McQueen, M.M.: Infection after intramedullary nailing of the tibia. Incidence and protocol for management. J. Bone Joint Surg. *74B*:770–774, 1992.
25. Seligson, D.: Concepts in Intramedullary Nailing. Orlando, FL, Grune & Stratton, 1985.
26. Klemm, K., Henry, S., Seligson, D.: The treatment of infection after interlocking nailing. Techniques Orthop. *3*:54–61, 1988.
27. Dombrowski, E.T., Dunn, A.W.: Treatment of osteomyelitis by debridement and closed wound irrigation-suction. Clin. Orthop. *43*:215–231, 1965.
28. Patzakis, M.J., Abdollah, K., Sherman, R., Holtom, P.D., Wilkins, J.: Treatment of chronic osteomyelitis with muscle flaps. Orthop. Clin. North Am. *24*:505–509, 1993.
29. Patzakis, M.J., Wilkins, J., Kumar, J., Holtom, P., Greenbaum, B., Ressler, R.: Comparison of the results of bacterial cultures from multiple sites in chronic osteomyelitis of long bones. J. Bone Joint Surg. *76A*: 664–666, 1994.
30. Törholm, C.: Treatment of Orthopaedic Infections, thesis. University of Lund (Department of Orthopaedics), Lund, Sweden, 1984.
31. Klemm, K.K.: Antibiotic bead chains. Clin. Orthop. *295*:63–76, 1993.
32. Klemm, K.: Gentamicin-PMMA chains for the local antibiotic treatment of chronic osteomyelitis. Reconstr. Surg. Traumatol. *20*:11–35, 1988.
33. Clawson, D.K., Davis, F.J., Hansen, S.T.: Treatment of chronic osteomyelitis with emphasis on closed suction-irrigation technic. Clin. Orthop. *96*:88–97, 1973.
34. Compere, E.L., Metzger, W.I., Mitra, R.N.: The treatment of pyogenic bone and joint infections by closed irrigation (circulation) with a non-toxic detergent and one or more antibiotics. J. Bone Joint Surg. *49A*: 614–624, 1967.
35. Compere, E.L.: Treatment of osteomyelitis and infected wounds by closed irrigation with a detergent-antibiotic solution. Acta Orthop. Scand. *32*:324–333, 1962.
36. Lawyer, R.B., Eyring, E.J.: Intermittent closed suction-irrigation treatment of osteomyelitis. Clin. Orthop. *88*: 80–85, 1972.
37. Letts, R.M., Wong, E.: Treatment of acute osteomyelitis in children by closed-tube irrigation: A reassessment. Can. J. Surg. *18*:60–63, 1975.
38. Smith-Petersen, M.N., Larson, C.B., Cochran, W.: Local chemotherapy with primary closure of septic wounds by means of drainage and irrigation cannulae. J. Bone Joint Surg. *27A*:562–571, 1945.
39. Seligson, D., Klemm, K.: Antibiotic bone cement combinations. *In* Orthopedic Infections. Edited by R.D. D'Ambrosia and R.L. Marier. Thorofare, NJ, Slack, 1988.
40. Søreensen, T.S., Søreensen, A.: Bactericidal activity of gentamicin against S. aureus. Acta Orthop. Scand. *64*: 82–84, 1993.
41. Klemm, K.: Treatment of infected nonunions with gentamicin-PMMA beads and external fixation. *In* External Fixation—The Current State of the Art. Edited by A.F. Brooker and C.C. Edwards. Baltimore, Williams & Wilkins, 1979.
42. Green, S.A., Moore, T.A., Spohn, P.J.: Nonunion of the tibial shaft. Orthopedics *11*:1149–1157, 1988.
43. Klemm, K.: Infected pseudarthrosis of the femur and tibia. Clin. Orthop. *212*:174, 1986.
44. Klemm, K.: Treatment of infected fractures and pseudarthroses with external fixation and gentamicin-PMMA beads. *In* Current Concepts of External Fixation of Fractures. Edited by H.K. Uhthoff. Berlin, Springer-Verlag, 1982.
45. Klemm, K., Schellmann, W.D.: Dynamische und Statische Verriegelung des Marknagels. Mschr. Unfallheilk *75*:568, 1972.
46. D'Aubigné, R.M.: Infection in the treatment of ununited fractures. Clin. Orthop. *43*:77–82, 1965.
47. Brav, E.A., Jeffress, V.H.: Modified intramedullary nailing in recent gunshot fractures of the femoral shaft. J. Bone Joint Surg. *35A*:141–152, 1953.

48. Kovacs, A.J., Richard, L.B., Miller, J.: Infection complicating intramedullary nailing of the fractured femur. Clin. Orthop. *96*:266–270, 1973.
49. Collert, S., Isacson, J.: Chronic sclerosing osteomyelitis (Garé). Clin. Orthop. *164*:136–140, 1982.
50. Lidgren, L., Törholm, C.: Intramedullary reaming in chronic diaphyseal osteomyelitis. Clin. Orthop. *151*: 215–221, 1980.
51. Spiro, S.A., Oppenheim, W., Boss, W.K., Schneider, A.I., Hutter, A.M.: Reconstruction of the lower extremity after grade III distal tibial injuries using combined microsurgical free tissue transfer and bone transport by distraction osteosynthesis. Ann. Plast. Surg. *30*: 97–104, 1993.
52. Wickstrom, J., Corban, M.S.: Intramedullary fixation for fractures of the femoral shaft. A study of complications in 298 operations. J. Trauma *7*:551–583, 1967.
53. Jacob, E., Setterstrom, J.A., Bach, D.E., Heath, J.R. III, McNiesh, L.M., Cierny, G. III.: Evaluation of biodegradable ampicillin anhydrate microcapsules for local treatment of experimental staphylococcal osteomyelitis. Clin. Orthop. *267*:237–244, 1991.

21

The Self-Guiding Nail

Samir N. Azer and William R. Krause

Stabilization of a fractured femoral shaft has intrigued orthopaedic surgeons for over 100 years. The load-sharing construct of a nail in a cylindrical bone and the presence of an excellent soft-tissue envelope around the bone render the femur ideal for intramedullary nailing.[1] This concept was recognized as early as 1886 and 1913, when Bircher and Konig, respectively, attempted to internally splint the femur using intramedullary ivory and bone pegs. Hey Groves in 1918 reported on three cases for which he used three different nail designs resembling nails currently used today.[2] Until the popularization of intramedullary nailing by Küntscher over 55 years ago, reports of the technique remained sporadic.[3] Intramedullary nailing offers the advantages of shortening hospitalization and reducing the risk of life-threatening events such as Adult Respiratory Distress Syndrome (ARDS) and Multiple Organ System Failure in the multiple-trauma patient. While also restoring shaft alignment, and therefore allowing early functional use of the extremity and lowering the incidence of refracture, the high complication rates associated with open intramedullary nailing dampened the initial enthusiasm for the technique.[3–8] The remarkably low infection rates of 0 to 0.4%, acceleration of healing (with an average time to union of 18.4 weeks), low nonunion rates, and the preservation of the quadriceps mechanism that have been reported with closed intramedullary nailing provided the impetus for the resurgence of intramedullary nailing.[7,9–14]

In the last two decades, interest in closed intramedullary nailing has been stimulated by the successful and widely publicized experience at Harborview Medical Center in Seattle. The acquisition of radiographic image intensifiers by American hospitals has led to a dramatic increase in the method's popularity.

INTERLOCKING NAILS

With motor vehicle accidents causing the vast majority of femoral shaft fractures, comminution of the femur is a frequent finding. In the presence of comminution and in long oblique and in spiral fractures located in the supraisthmal and subisthmal regions of the femoral shaft, the noninterlocked intramedullary nail is incapable of resisting forces that result in angulation, malrotation, and shortening. This has resulted in the advent of the interlocking nail.

In 1951 Modny was the first to conceive the concept of an interlocking nail; he described an open technique using an X-beam girder with perforations throughout the entire shaft of the nail.[15] In 1967 Huckstep contributed another noncannulated nail with fenestrations for insertion of interlocking screws.[16] While Küntscher in 1968 designed the "Detensor nail" by placing transverse bolts through either end of the slotted nail, the term "interlocking nail" was not coined until Klemm and Schelmann published their report of an interlocking nail in 1972.[17] Grosse and Kempf modified the nail further to include a proximal cylindrical section that allowed attachment of instrumentation for nail and screw insertion. The wide use of interlocking intramedullary nails has been the single most important advance in the surgical treatment of long-bone fractures in the past

bifurcated tip of the SG guide rod captures and locks onto the drill bit. This establishes the distal reference point. The SG guide rod, being considerably smaller in diameter than the reamed canal, is unconstrained in the femur and, therefore, is free to be maneuvered to capture the drill bit.

The SG nail has a cross-sectional shape that is complimentary to the SG guide rod. The inside diameter of the nail is slightly larger than the outer diameter of the guide rod, which allows it to slide down over the SG guide rod without rotating. This assures correct rotational orientation of the nail within the femur and over the reference drill bit. A distal guide is then assembled onto the nail driver, forming a rigid rectangle through which the second of the two distal holes is targeted without the use of fluoroscopy.

Biomechanical Evaluation

Mechanical testing was performed on the SG nail and on four other 13-mm diameter nails, as shown in Table 21–1. The parameters determined were the bending rigidity, strength, and the torsional stiffness of all five nails.

The mechanical tests showed that the SG nail is equivalent in both bending and torsion to the other closed section nails. There was no significant difference in the bending strength or bending rigidity for the three closed-section nails and the ZMS nail. The closed-section nails had significantly greater torsional stiffness than the open section nails. The Russell-Taylor nail had a significantly greater torsional stiffness than the other four nails. The Alta nail and the SG nail were statistically equivalent. The two slotted nails had a torsional stiffness in order of magnitude lower than the closed-section nails (Fig. 21–3).[40]

Table 21–1. Intramedullary nails tested

Nail Tested	*Shape*	*Cross Section*
Russell-Taylor	circular	closed
Alta	hexagonal	closed
Self-Guiding	cloverleaf	closed
ZMS	semi-solid	slotted
AO universal	circular	slotted

Operative Procedure

Mindful attention to preoperative planning is a key element to a successful operative outcome. Subtle longitudinal fissures and nondis-

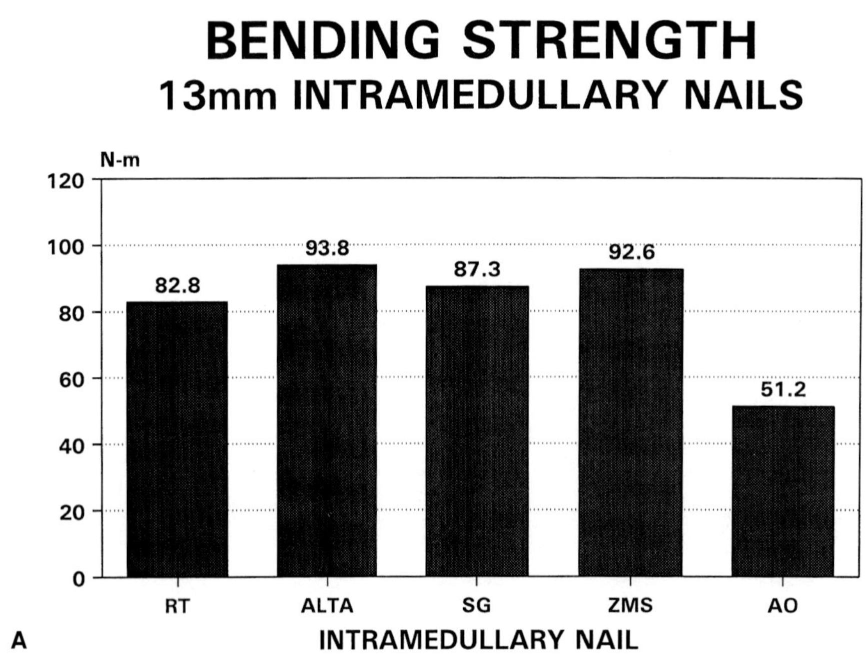

Fig. 21–3. *A*, Bending strength. *(Figure continues)*

placed comminution are best detected by careful scrutiny of the preoperative radiographs. Inadvertent lengthening or shortening of the femur can only be avoided by careful attention to detail. The contralateral femur is measured either clinically from the tip of the greater trochanter to the lateral joint line of the knee or radiographically.

Timing of Operation

Support for immediate skeletal stabilization of long-bone fractures, especially in the polytrauma patient, has been well documented in the literature.[30,41] In isolated femoral shaft fractures, immediate fixation is still preferred, although it is not critical.

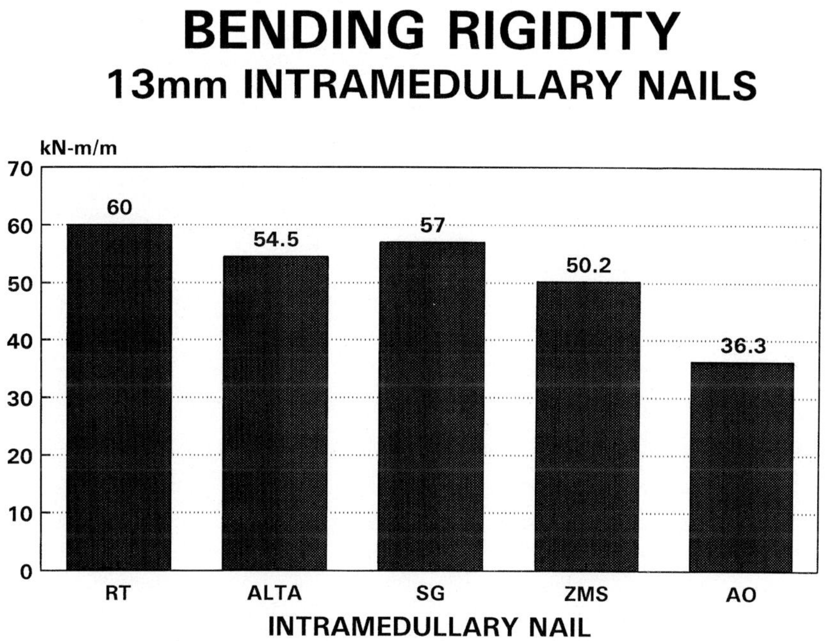

B

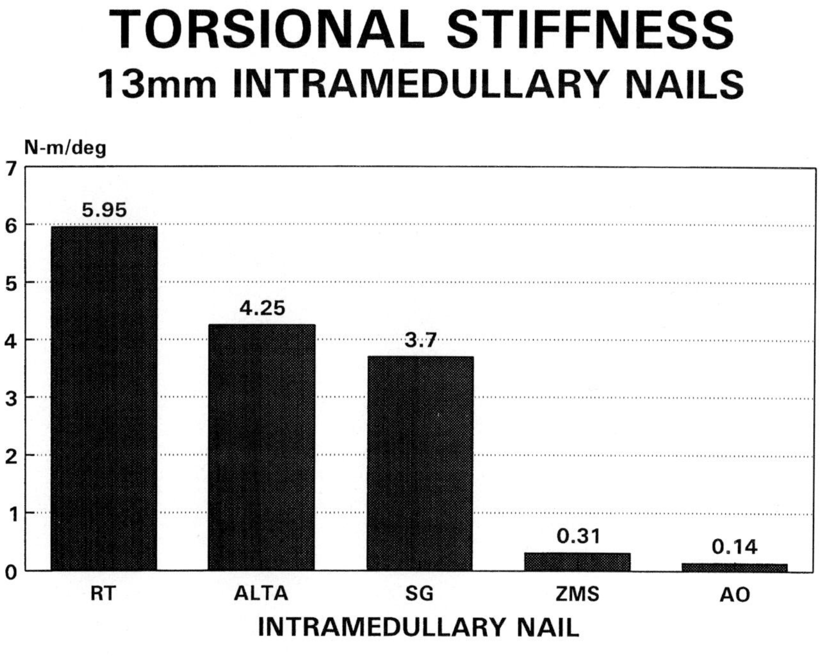

C

Fig. 21–3. *(continued) B*, Bending rigidity. *C*, Torsional stiffness.

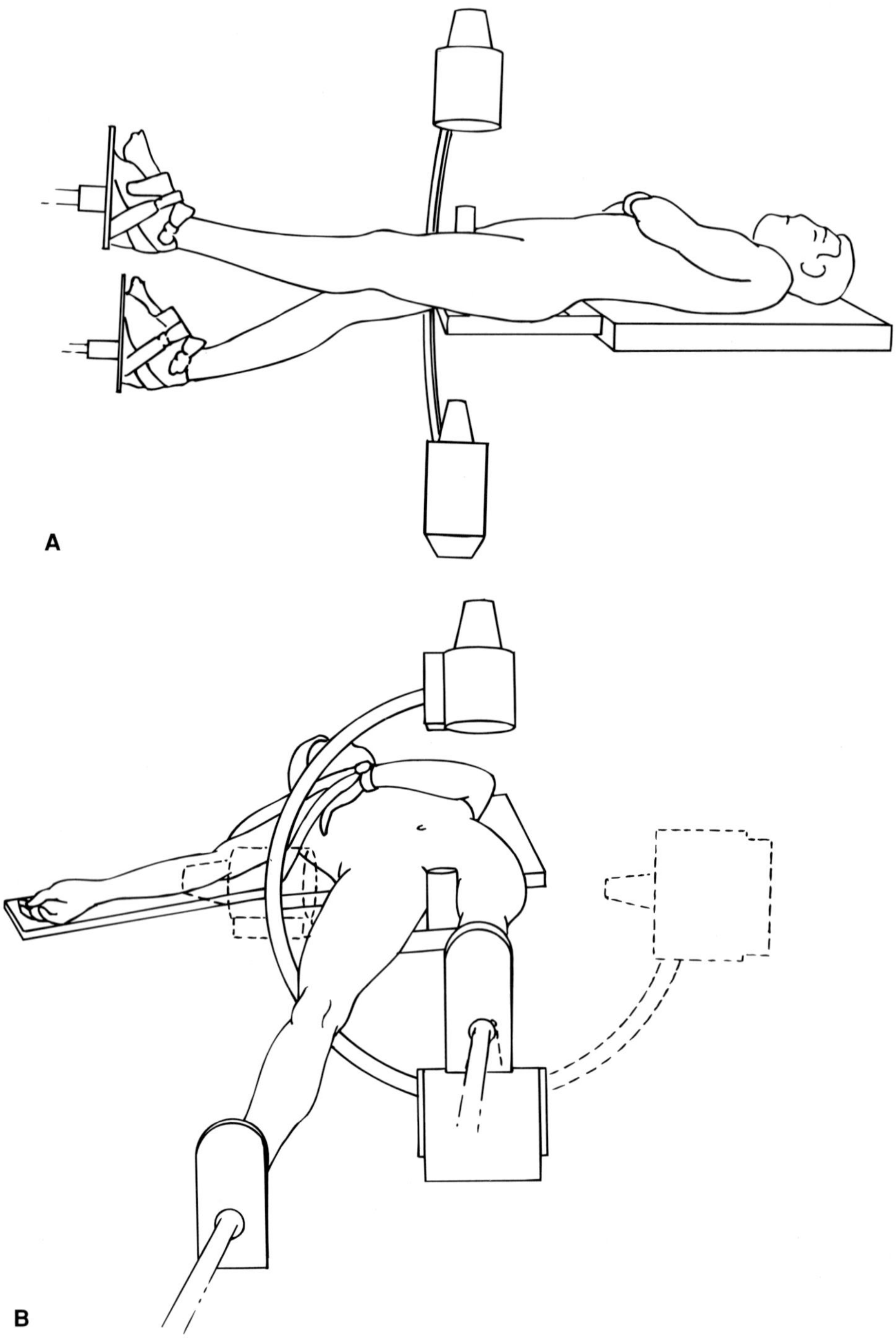

A

B

Fig. 21–4. *A*, The supine position with the legs in the scissors position, viewed from the affected side. The C-arm positioned for an AP projection. *B*, The C-arm is swung from the AP to the lateral projection and the entire femur is screened by swinging the arm cephalad and caudad.

Patient Positioning

With the extremity in tibial traction, femoral traction, or boot traction, the patient is positioned on the fracture table in either the lateral or the supine position.[42]

The Lateral Position[39]

Advantages

Easy access to the proximal femur

Disadvantages

Increased valgus deformity & rotational malalignment of the fracture
Difficult distal screw insertion
Increased pulmonary shunting

The Supine Position.[30]

The patient's torso is shifted toward the contralateral side. The affected extremity is adducted. The hip of the fractured extremity is flexed 20° to 30°.

Advantages

Easier reduction
Easier assessment of correct length and rotational alignment

Disadvantages

Difficulty in accessing the proximal femur is overcome by shifting the torso
Easier distal targeting

The well leg is placed in either exaggerated abduction with the C-arm positioned between the legs or in slight abduction with the hip slightly hyperextended. This position provides significant maneuverability for the C-arm and is our preferred position (Fig. 21–4).

Reduction

Attempts should be made to achieve reduction prior to starting the operation. Excessive intraoperative traction on the injured extremity can render the reduction more difficult and can cause sciatic nerve palsy.[43] The use of a well-padded crutch under the distal fragment is often quite helpful in reducing the fracture.[44]

Proximal one-third fractures require placing the extremity in external rotation to align the distal fragment with the externally rotated proximal fragment. Midshaft fractures are usually aligned better by placing the extremity in approximately 15° of internal rotation to offset hip anteversion. In subisthmal fractures, traction through a distal femoral pin allows flexion of the knee, which relaxes the hamstrings while still maintaining traction.[45]

Segmental fractures are dealt with by considering each segment separately and sequentially. After reaming the proximal fragment, that fragment is aligned with the middle segment using the SG guide rod. The guide wire is then advanced into the middle segment. The same process is used to align the distal segment. Shortening, especially in comminuted fractures, can be avoided by either preoperative clinical or radiographic measurement of the length of the intact femur. The adequacy of the reduction must be confirmed using the lateral radiograph, because the anteroposterior view may misrepresent the degree of distraction.

Exposure

An 8- to 10-cm incision is made starting about 2 cm distal to the tip of the greater trochanter and extended proximally in line with the fibers of the gluteus maximus. The fascia overlying the muscle is incised along the skin incision. The gluteus is split in line with its fibers, and the pyriformis fossa is palpated.

Entry

Entry Instrument. The SG awl with its double right-angled design allows direct access into the femoral canal. The awl's configuration allows alignment in the coronal and sagittal planes (Fig. 21–5).

Entry Point. The preferred entry point is posterior to the neutral point of the pyriformis fossa, because it is anatomically centered over the axis of the medullary canal (Fig. 21–6).[46] Entry through the greater trochanter leads to eccentric reaming with possible comminution and varus deformation of the proximal fragment. Splitting of the greater trochanter is also possible.[21,41,43,47] Entry through the anterior portion of the pyriformis fossa may result in nail deformation and comminution of the proximal fragment.[48] An entry point that is too far medial may lead to a fracture of the femoral neck. An inadvertent anterior entry point should be expanded to avoid comminution.[43,49]

Guide Wire Insertion

With the guide wire handle attached to control wire rotation, the bulb-tip guide wire is in-

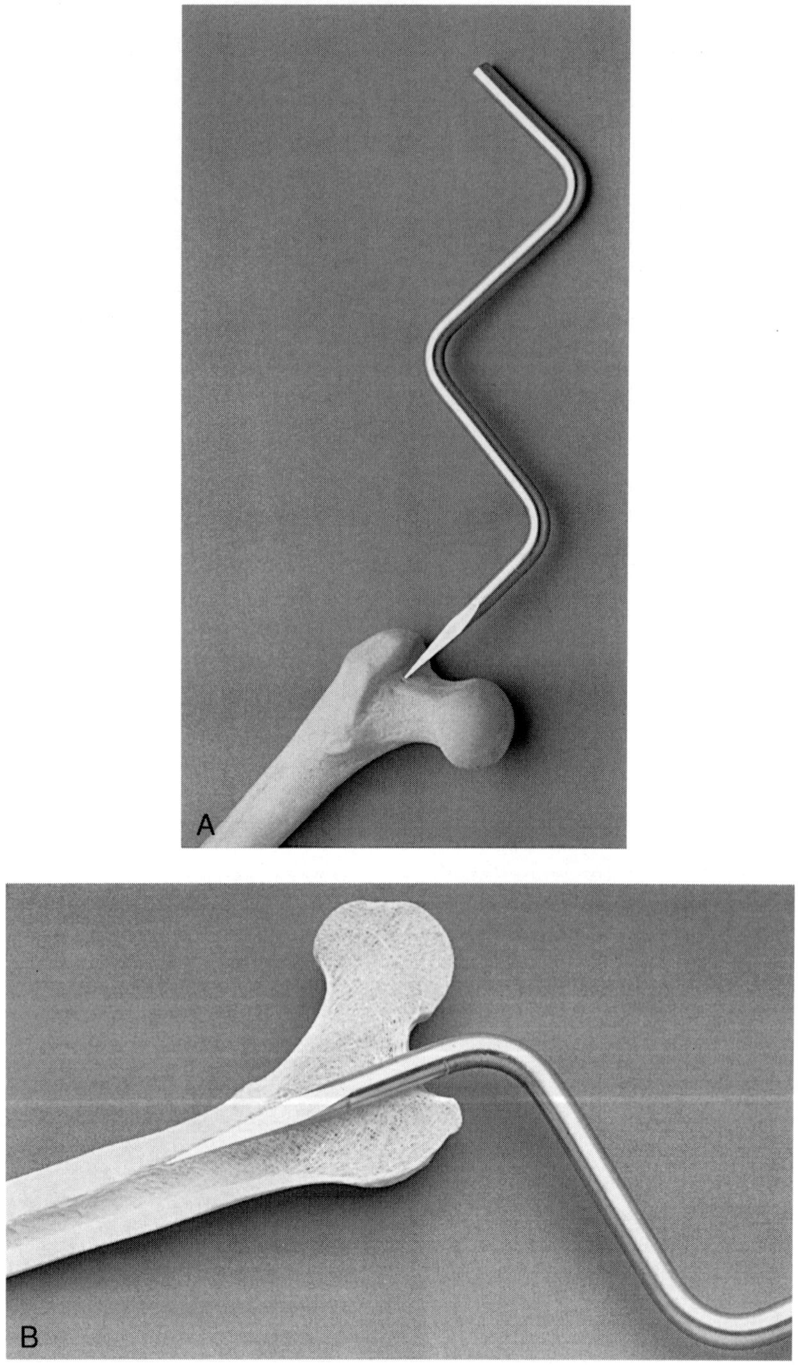

Fig. 21–5. *A*, The SG awl. The handle is away from the torso. *B*, Misdirection towards the calcar is unlikely with this design.

serted into the medullary canal past the fracture site and to the level of the intercondylar notch.

Passage of the guide wire across the fracture site and into the distal fragment is often facilitated by gently bending the guide wire into a slight curve and also bending the tip 20° to 25°.

Central placement of the guide wire is essential to prevent eccentric reaming. If the guide wire remains eccentric, its position can be controlled by introducing it through a small-diameter nail.

Reaming

Reaming is begun with the 8-mm flexible reamer placed over the guide wire. To avoid in-

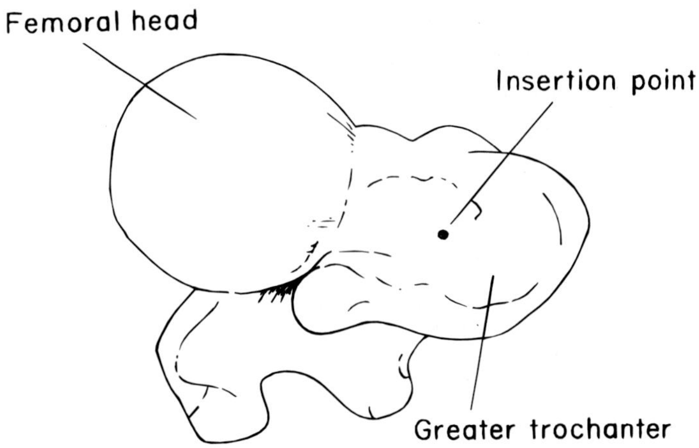

Fig. 21–6. Entry posterior to the neutral point of the pyriformis fossa.

carceration, reaming should progress in 1-mm increments until cortical contact and then in 0.5-mm increments. The canal is reamed to 1.5 mm larger than the diameter of the selected nail.[41] If the femur demonstrates an excessive amount of anterior bowing, overreaming by 2 mm may be necessary. However, reaming of more than 4 mm of cortical bone of the isthmus is not recommended.[50,51]

Careful analysis of the preoperative radiographs prevents widening or spreading apart of longitudinal fissures. Reaming at faster than the recommended speed leads to thermal necrosis of the bone.[52] When reaming across a comminuted segment, reaming should be slowed until past the area of comminution. A jammed reamer may be dislodged by either hammering back the bulb-tip guide wire or passing a smooth-tip guide wire adjacent to the reamer tip.[53]

Guide Wire Exchange and SG Guide Rod Insertion

The medullary alignment tube is introduced over the bulb-tip guide wire, which is replaced with a smooth-tip guide wire. The SG guide rod handle is then attached to the SG guide rod. The SG guide rod is introduced into the femur over the smooth-tip guide wire. Because of its smaller diameter in relationship to the reamed canal, the SG guide rod passes easily down the medullary canal while maintaining its correct rotational orientation. Passage of the SG guide rod across the fracture site is monitored on the image intensifier. In the unlikely event that the tip of the guide rod catches the cortex of the distal fragment, the guide rod is slightly withdrawn and redirected across the fracture site. This is accomplished by manipulating the guide rod by its handle. When the SG guide rod is well past the fracture site, the smooth-tip guide wire is pulled out (Fig. 21–7).

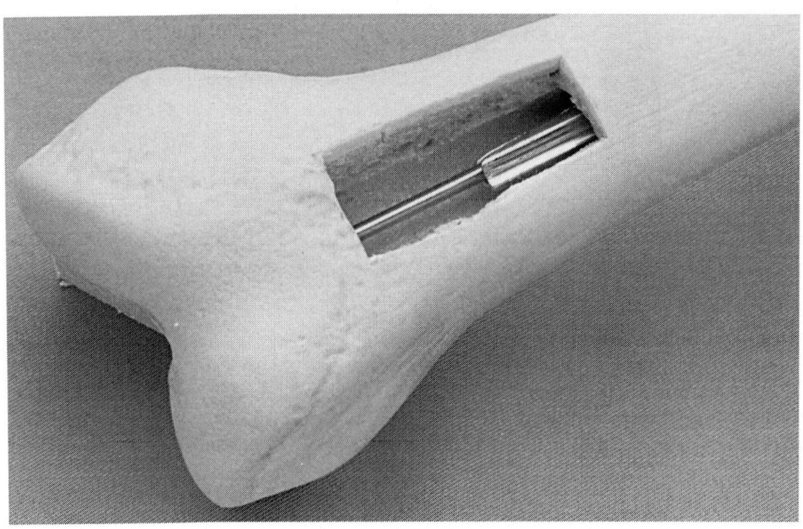

Fig. 21–7. The SG guide rod is passed over the smooth-tip guide wire.

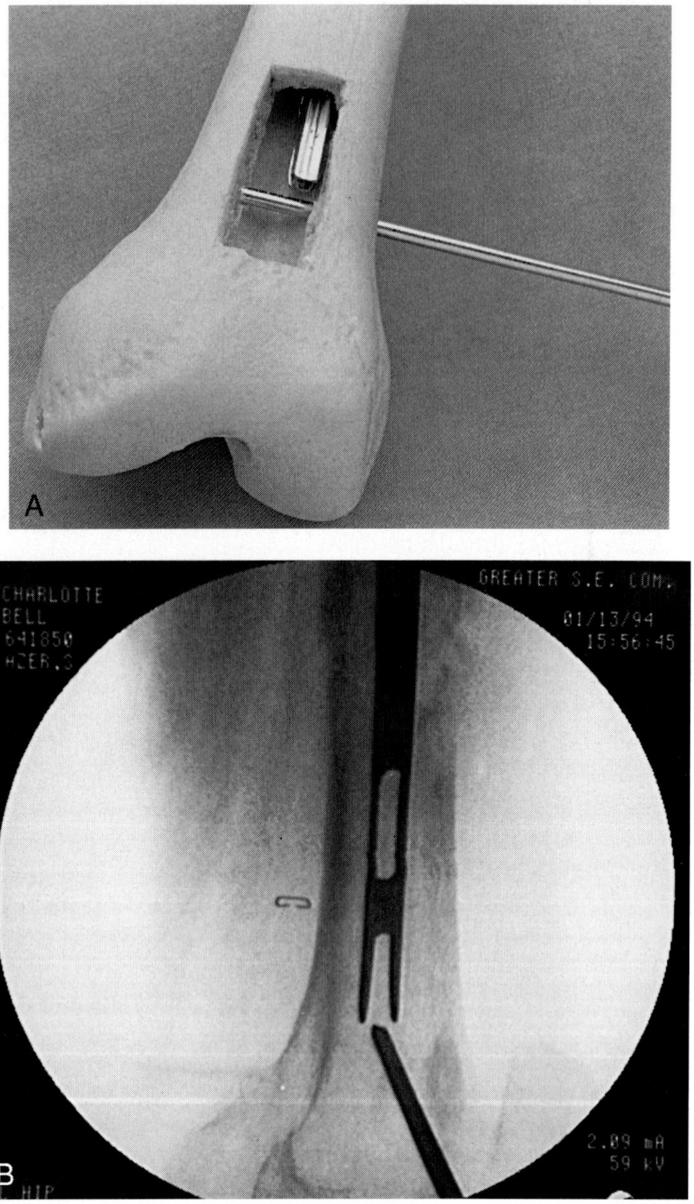

Fig. 21–8. *A*, SG guide rod near drill bit. Minor adjustments of the guide rod, by its handle, can be made to capture the drill bit. *B*, The guide rod as seen on the lateral radiograph.

The calibrations on the SG guide rod allow the surgeon to advance the rod to a precise point in the distal femur. This allows the surgeon to preselect a specific point for the most distal screw. The length of the appropriate nail is read directly off the calibrations on the guide rod.

Distal Locking

A single 5- to 6-cm lateral incision is made in the distal thigh at the site of the distal holes. The incision is carried through the fascia and down to the lateral femoral cortex. With the image intensifier viewing the lateral radiograph of the distal femur, the tip of the appropriate size drill bit is placed on the lateral femoral cortex at a point "nearing" the center of the distal bifurcation of the SG guide rod. Without the image intensifier the drill bit is drilled across the distal femur. The drill bit should be placed at right angle to the femur (Fig. 21–8).

Locking the Distal Drill Bit. Upon completion of drilling the drill bit through the medial

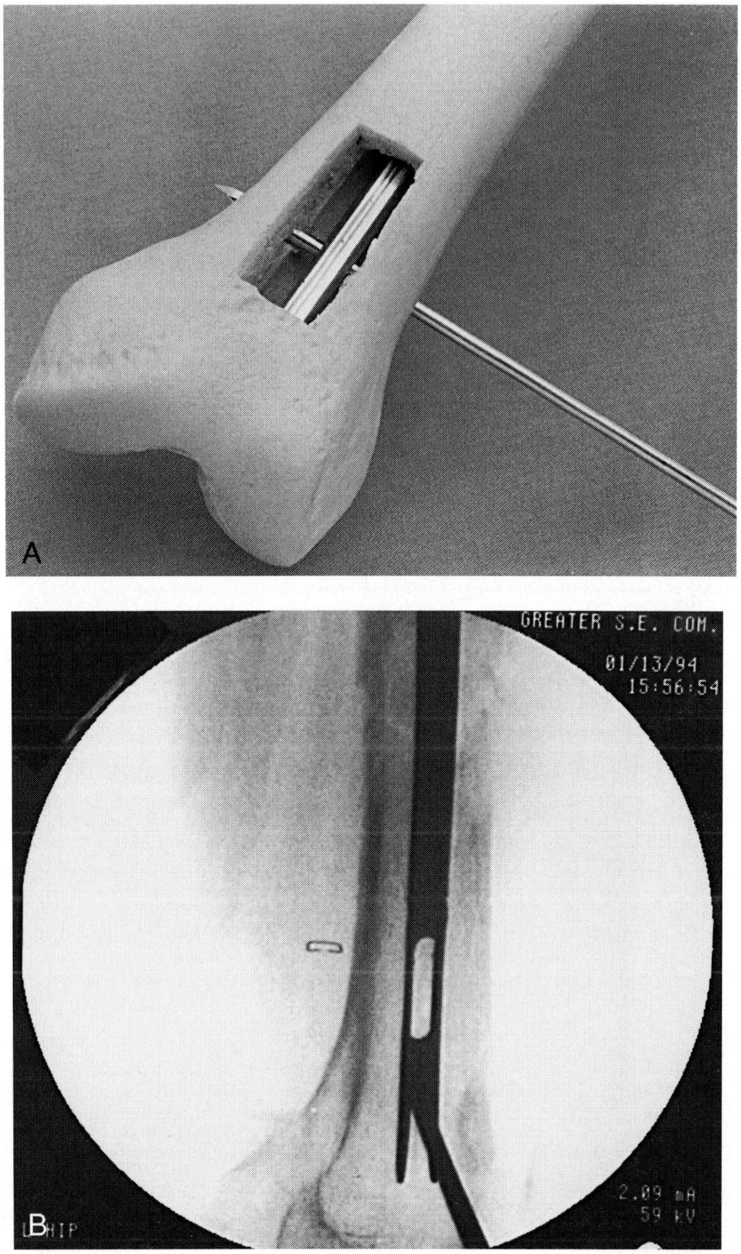

Fig. 21–9. *A*, The SG guide rod locked on the reference drill bit by a snap in its axilla. *B*, As seen on the C-arm monitor.

cortex, the SG guide rod is advanced. The bifurcation at the end of the guide rod captures the drill bit. A gentle tap on the SG guide rod handle locks the rod onto the drill bit. Locking is confirmed manually and by the image intensifier. Manual confirmation is done by pulling back on the SG guide rod. The guide rod should not withdraw (Fig. 21–9). Radiographic confirmation is done with the surgeon away from the field of radiation. The length of the appropriate nail is determined by reading the marking on the SG guide rod at the level of the tip of the greater trochanter (Fig. 21–10).

Nail Assembly and Insertion

The appropriate SG nail is selected. The locking bolt is inserted through the SG driver and screwed onto the proximal end of the nail. This locks the nail onto the driver (Fig. 21–11).

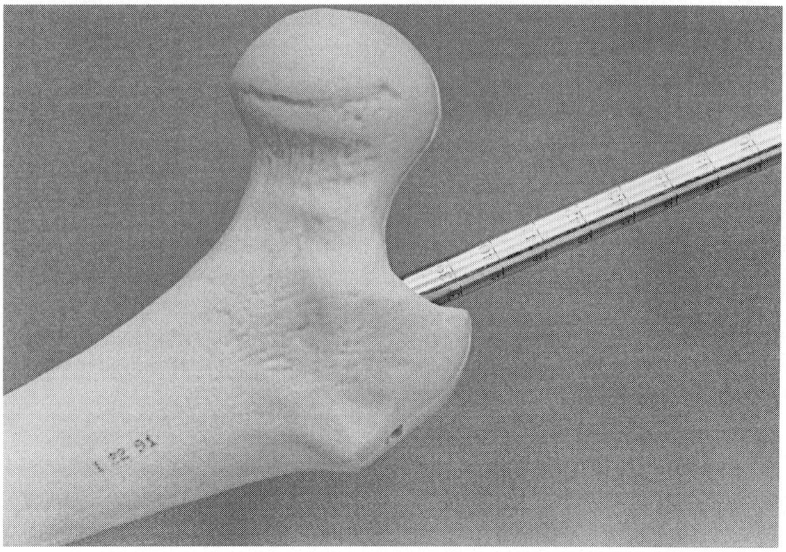

Fig. 21–10. The correct nail length is read directly off the calibration on the SG guide rod.

The SG guide rod handle is unscrewed from the rod. The SG nail is slid over the guide rod and the nail is driven down the femoral canal over the SG guide rod (Fig. 21–12). The SG nail's cross section being complimentary to that of the SG guide rod assures the nail's correct rotational orientation, while advancing in the femoral medullary canal (Fig. 21–13). The final few blows needed to advance the nail are monitored with the image intensifier (Fig. 21–14). The nail is driven down the canal until it "bottoms out," intersecting the predrilled drill bit. The nail's final position is reached when the bifurcation of the nail fully overlaps the bifurcation of the SG guide rod. Final nail position is confirmed by the surgeon with the C-arm,

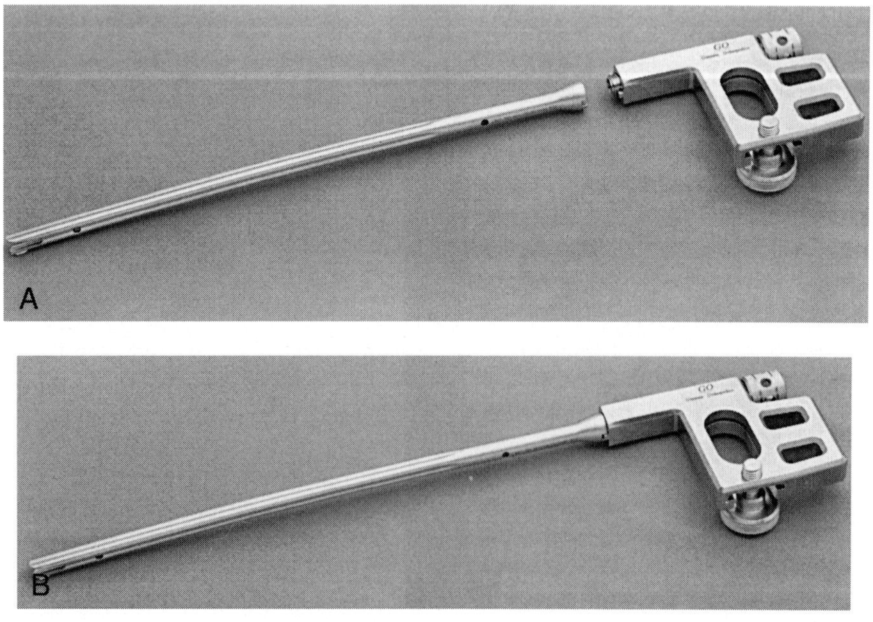

Fig. 21–11. *A*, Nail assembly. The SG nail is locked onto the nail driver by means of keyed tabs and the locking bolt. *B*, Nail assembled.

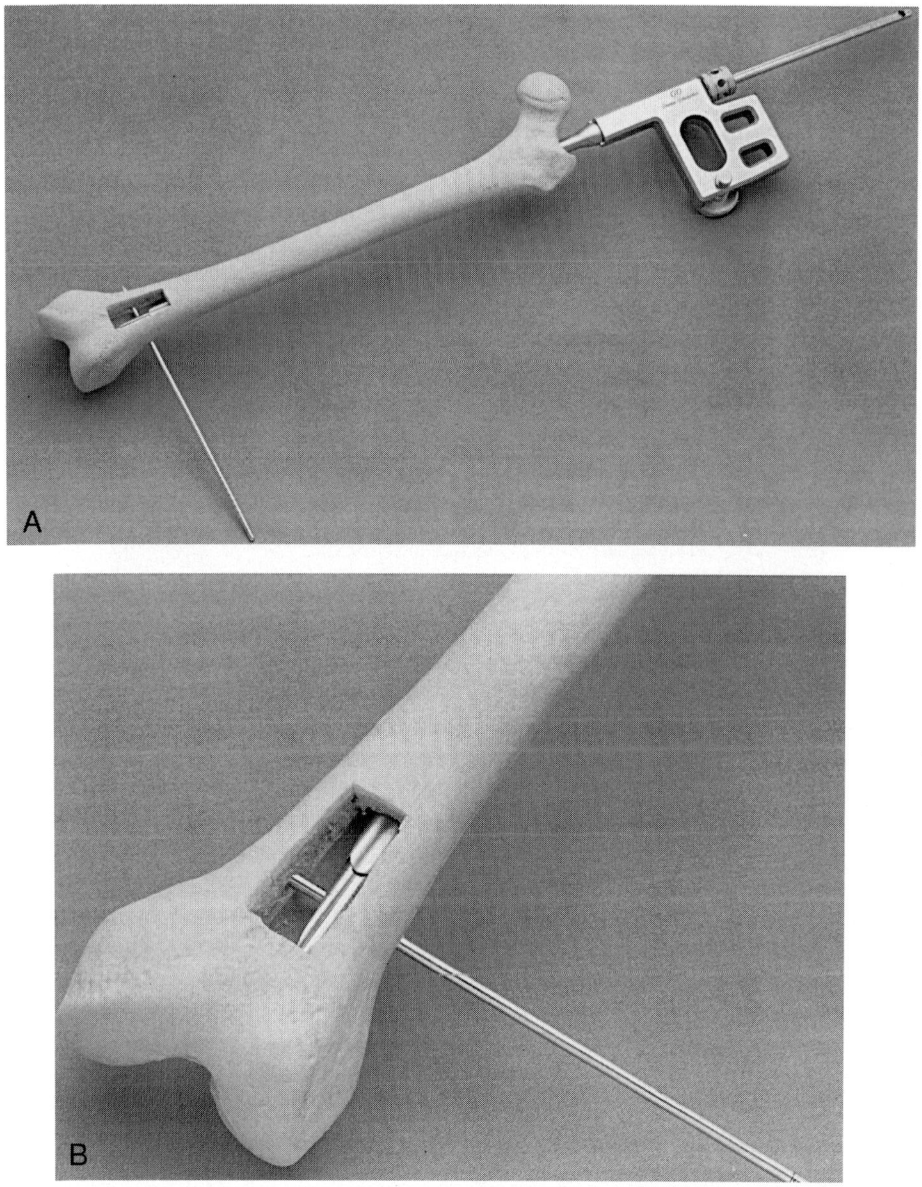

Fig. 21–12. *A*, The SG nail is driven over the guide rod. *B*, The nail approaches the reference drill bit. *(Figure continues)*

while remaining clear of the field of radiation (Fig. 21–15). The SG guide rod is then extracted with a gentle tap on the guide handle, using a mallet (Fig. 21–16).

Locating The Second Distal Hole

Distal Guide Assembly. The appropriate inner sleeves are inserted into the outer sleeves. Both sets of sleeves are then inserted through the two holes of the distal targeting box. The lateral extension rod on the distal targeting box is then slid into the proximal targeting tube. The radius of curvature of the combined lateral rod assembly corresponds to that of the nail. The assembled distal guide is then slid onto the SG driver and the predrilled drill bit (Fig. 21–17). Upon completing the assembly, the screw on the lateral extension tube is tightened to secure and lock the lateral assembly. The nut on the SG driver is then tightened to lock the entire assembly. The assembly now forms a

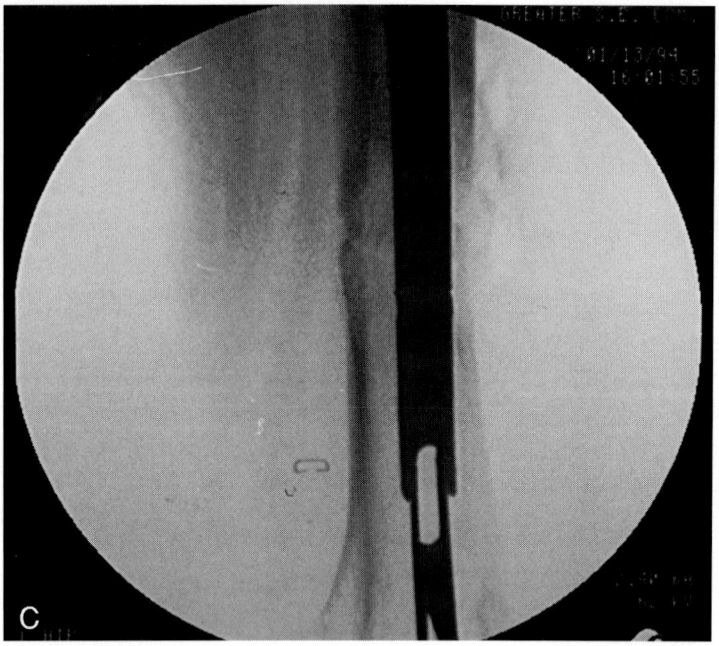

Fig. 21–12. *(continued) C,* The nail's advancement as seen on the monitor.

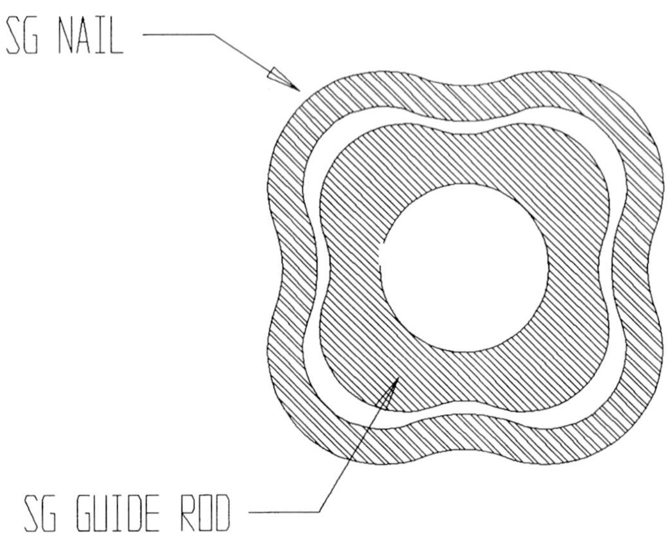

Fig. 21–13. The cross sections prevent rotation of the nail over the guide.

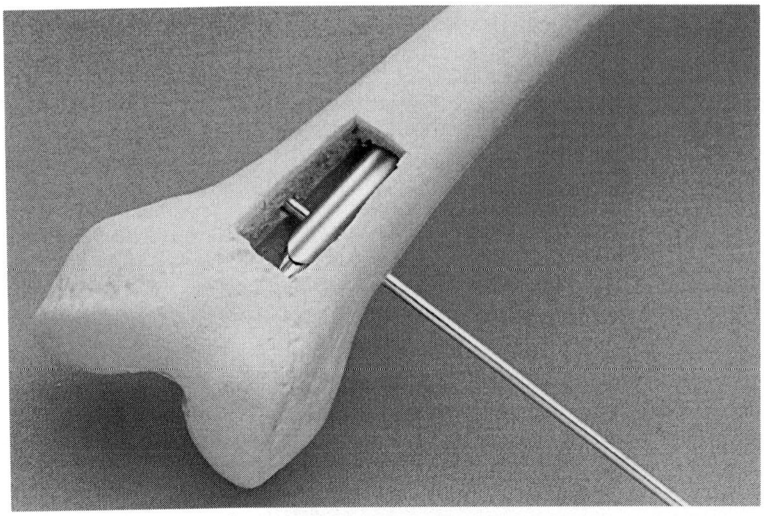

Fig. 21–14. The last two or three blows to fully seat the nail are monitored on the C-arm.

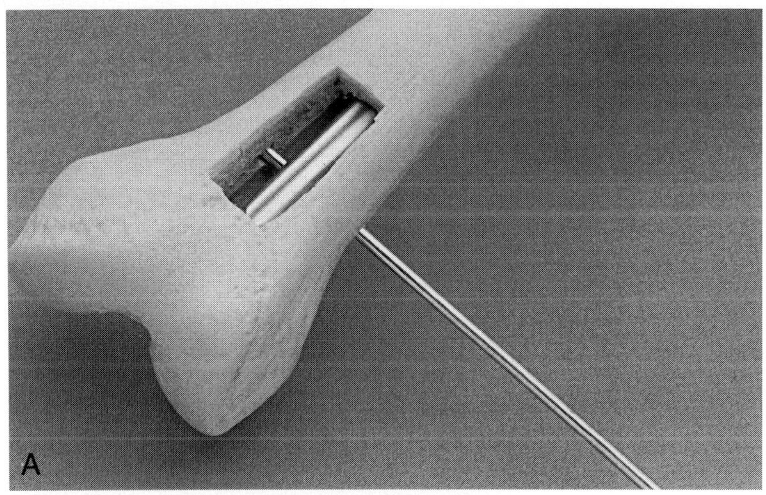

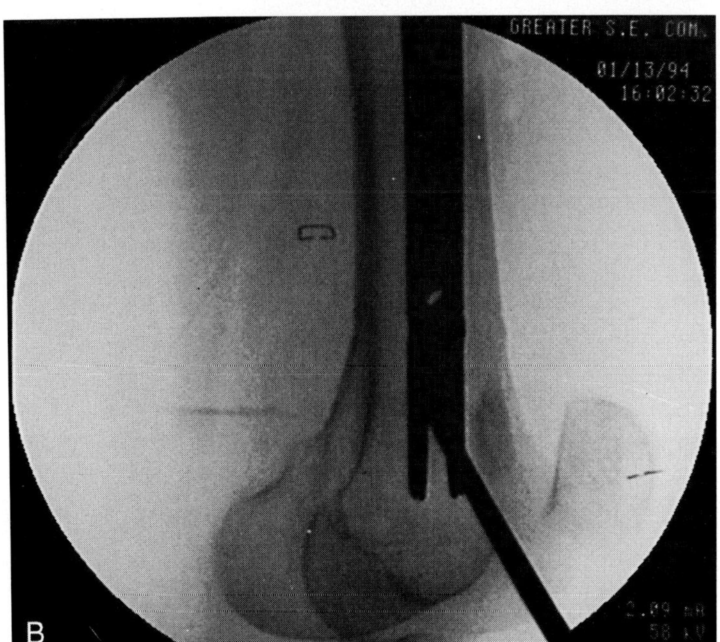

Fig. 21–15. *A*, The nail seated. *B*, The lateral radiograph is necessary for confirmation. The tips of the bifurcations on the guide rod and the nail coincide.

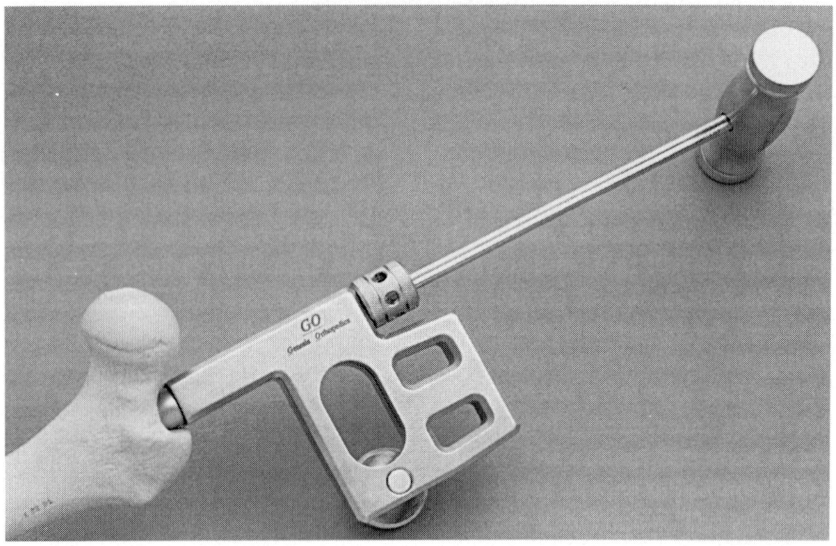

Fig. 21–16. The guide rod handle is reattached and the SG guide rod tapped out.

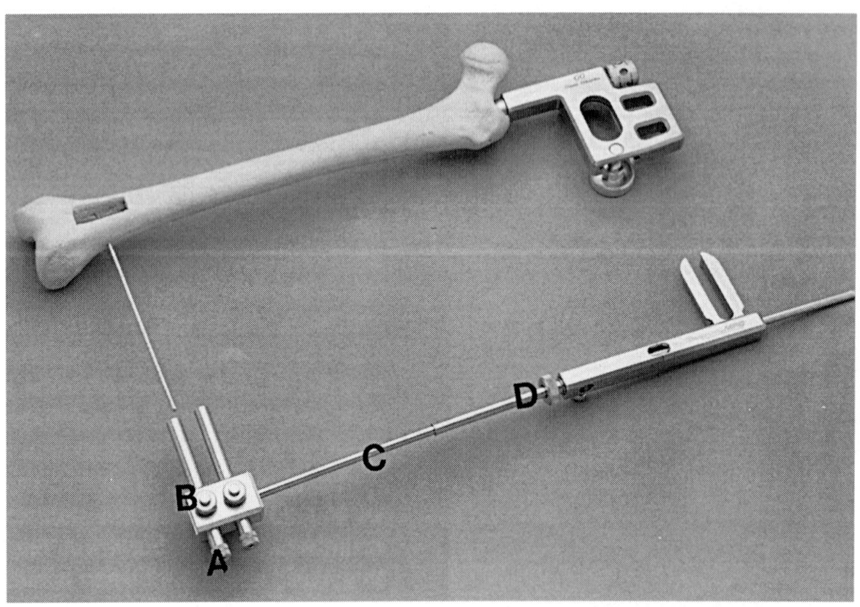

Fig. 21–17. Distal guide assembly; *A*, Inner and outer sleeves, *B*, inserted through distal targeting box; *C*, extension rod, *D*, inserted through proximal guide.

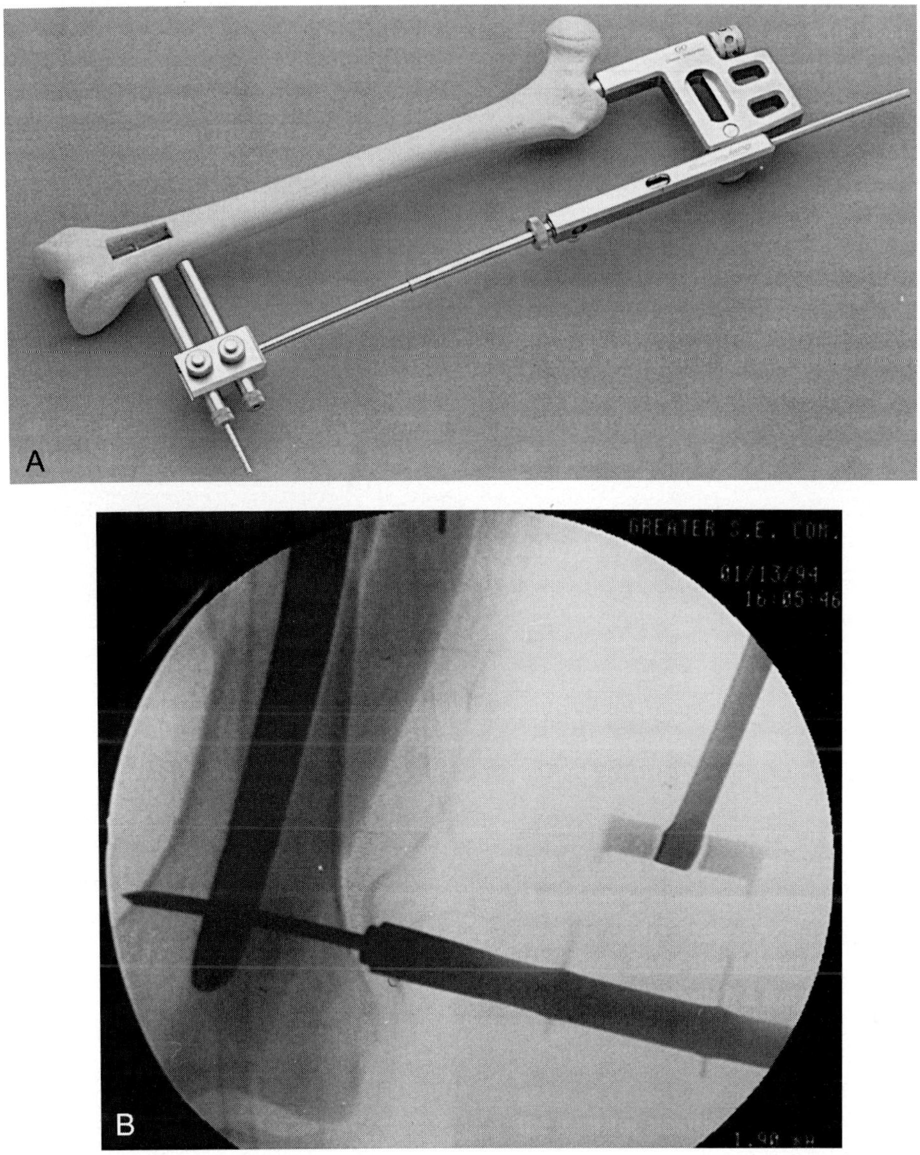

Fig. 21–18. *A*, The assembly is slid over the drill bit distally and into the SG driver proximally. *B*, The C-arm view prior to drilling the second distal hole.

rigid rectangle. The drill sleeves are then advanced to the lateral femoral cortex and secured in place by tightening the screws on the distal targeting box (Fig. 21–18). The distance between the reference drill bit and the top of the nail can be confirmed through the window in the proximal targeting tube (Fig. 21–19).

Drilling the Second Distal Hole and Inserting the Screw. The appropriate size drill bit is then inserted through the proximal of the two distal holes and drilled through the distal femur (Fig. 21–20). The inner drill sleeve of the more proximal of the two holes is removed. The drill bit is then removed and the depth gauge is used to measure the correct screw length. The appropriate screw is inserted through the outer sleeve (Fig. 21–21). The screwdriver handle is removed leaving the shaft of the screwdriver attached to the screw within the outer sleeve to maintain the alignment of the distal targeting box (Fig. 21–22). The same process is then repeated for the distal hole (Fig. 21–23).

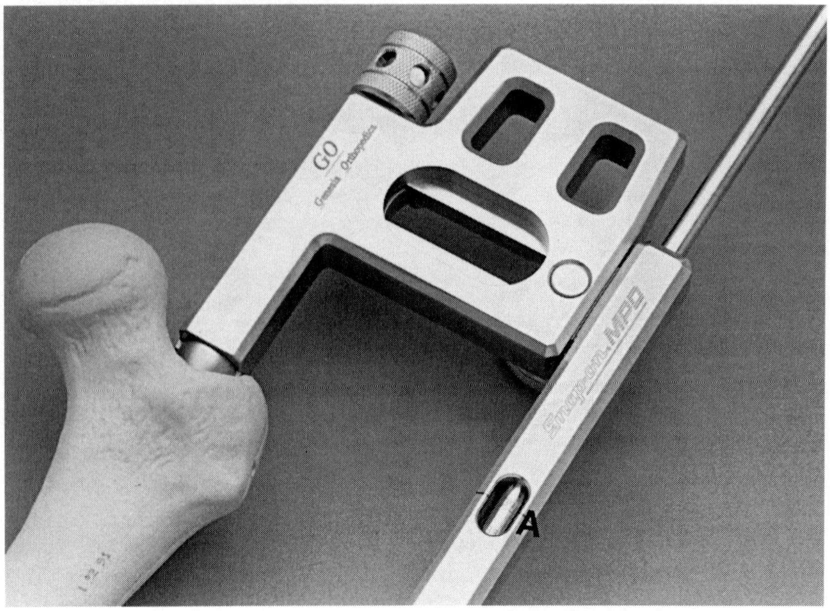

Fig. 21–19. *A*, The reading in the window (*A*) corresponds to the length of the nail.

Proximal Locking and Proximal Screw Insertion

The locking nut on the proximal targeting tube is loosened and the entire distal assembly is removed by sliding it distally. The drill sleeve assembly is then inserted through the proximal locking tube and the hole is drilled (Fig. 21–24). The inner drill sleeve is removed. The drill bit is then removed and the depth gauge is then used to measure the correct screw length. The appropriate screw is inserted through the outer sleeve.

Nail Cap Placement

At the completion of the procedure, the locking bolt is unscrewed and the nail cap is screwed onto the top of the nail using the provided screwdriver (Fig. 21–25). The wounds are then closed and dressed in the standard fashion.

Postoperative Management

With skeletal stabilization attained, the patient is allowed out of bed as soon as possible. Weight bearing, however, depends on the stability of the fracture and the rigidity of the fixation. To avoid implant or fracture failure, weight bearing is delayed in patients with fractures that are comminuted high-supraisthmal fractures and low-subisthmal fractures. Range-of-motion exercises for the knee and exercises for the quadriceps and hamstring are encouraged as soon as they can be tolerated.

CLINICAL EXPERIENCE

In a clinical study of 29 patients performed over a period of 3 years, the first 8 patients represented a pilot study, after which considerable changes were made to the system. The average age of 21 males and 8 females was 45.5 years. There were 16 fractures of the left femur and 13 fractures of the right femur. Of the fractures, 22 (73.33%) were closed. The fractures were produced by a variety of mechanisms of injury (Table 21–2). Three patients had pathological

Table 21–2. Mechanisms of injury

Mechanism of Injury	*No. of Cases*	*Percentage*
Fall	10	34
Motor vehicle accidents	7	24
Gunshot wounds	7	24
Pathological fractures	3	10
Nonunions	2	7

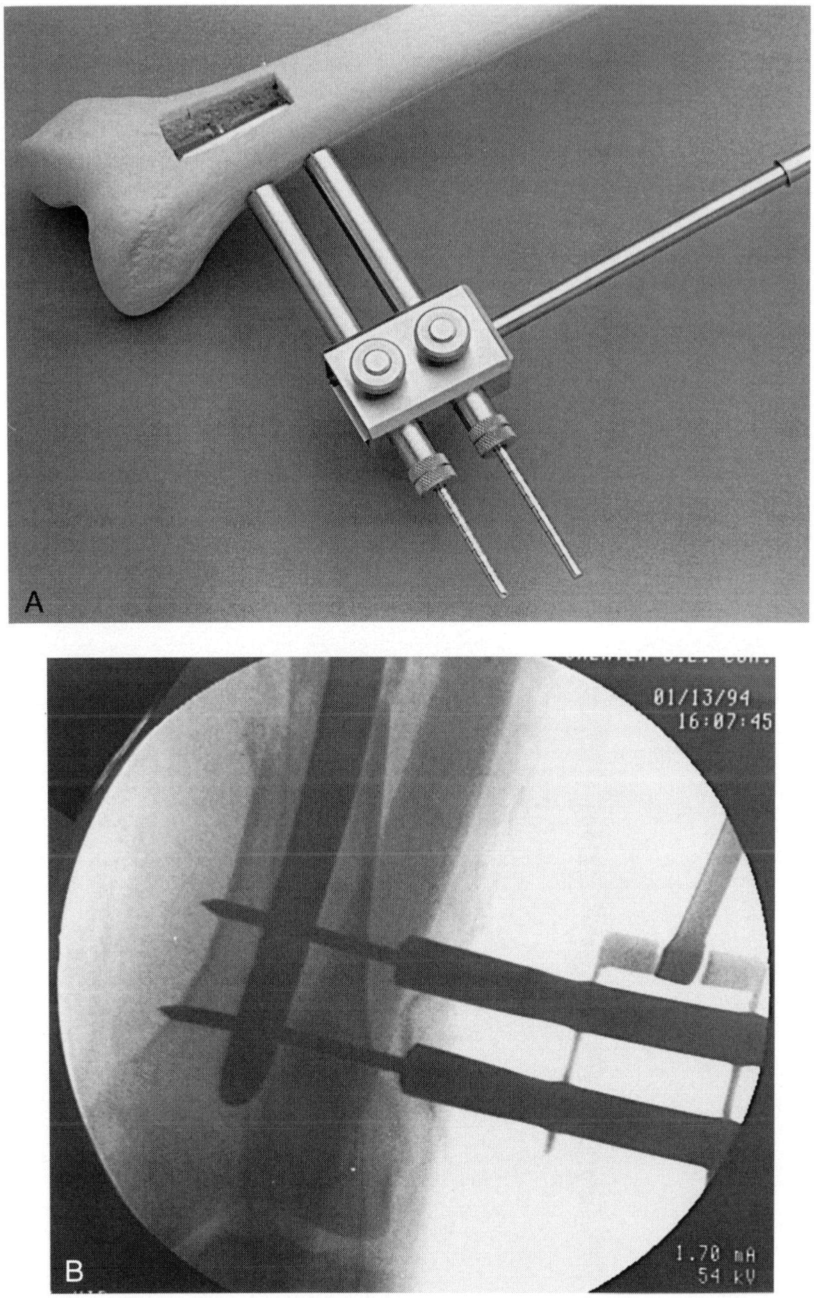

Fig. 21–20. *A*, The second drill bit is inserted through the inner sleeve. *B*, Both distal drill bits inserted and are through the medial cortex.

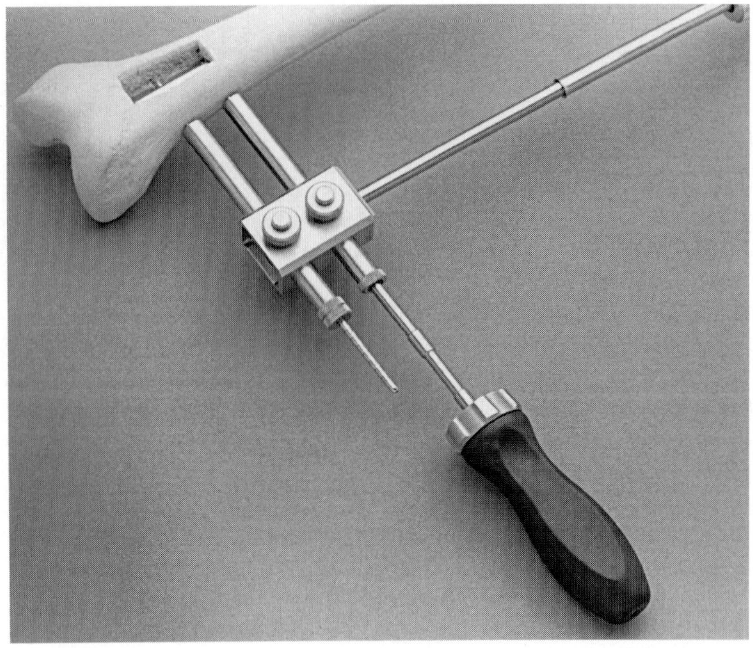

Fig. 21–21. The outer sleeve is removed and the screw is inserted.

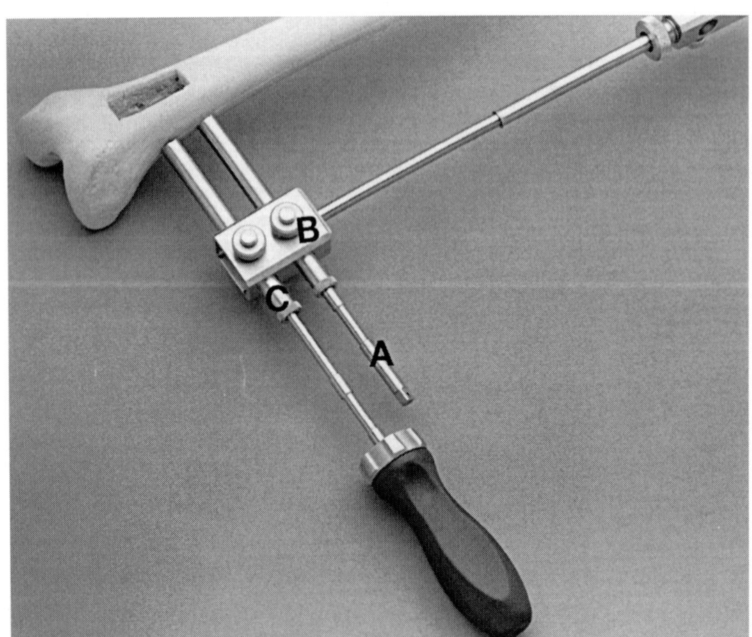

Fig. 21–22. *A*, The screw driver shaft, left in the proximal hole, (*B*) stabilizes the distal targeting box. *C*, The screw inserted in second hole.

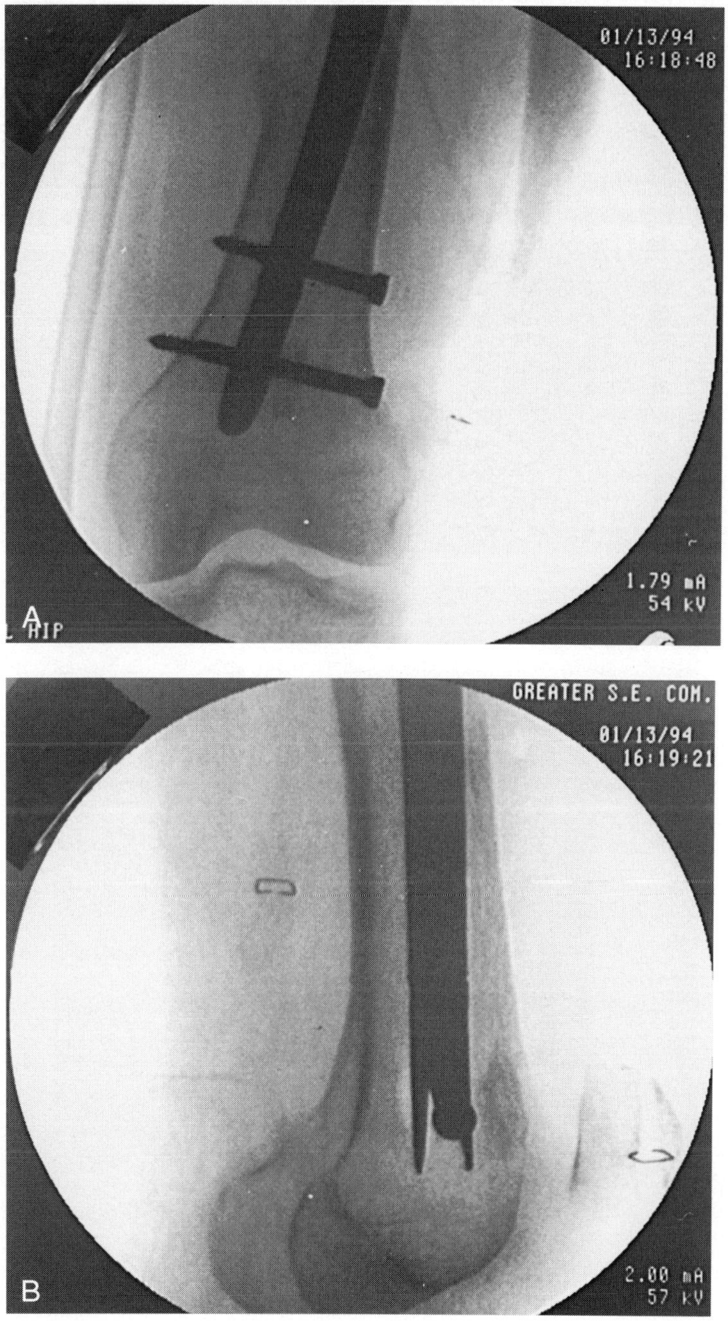

Fig. 21–23. *A*, AP radiograph. *B*, Lateral radiograph.

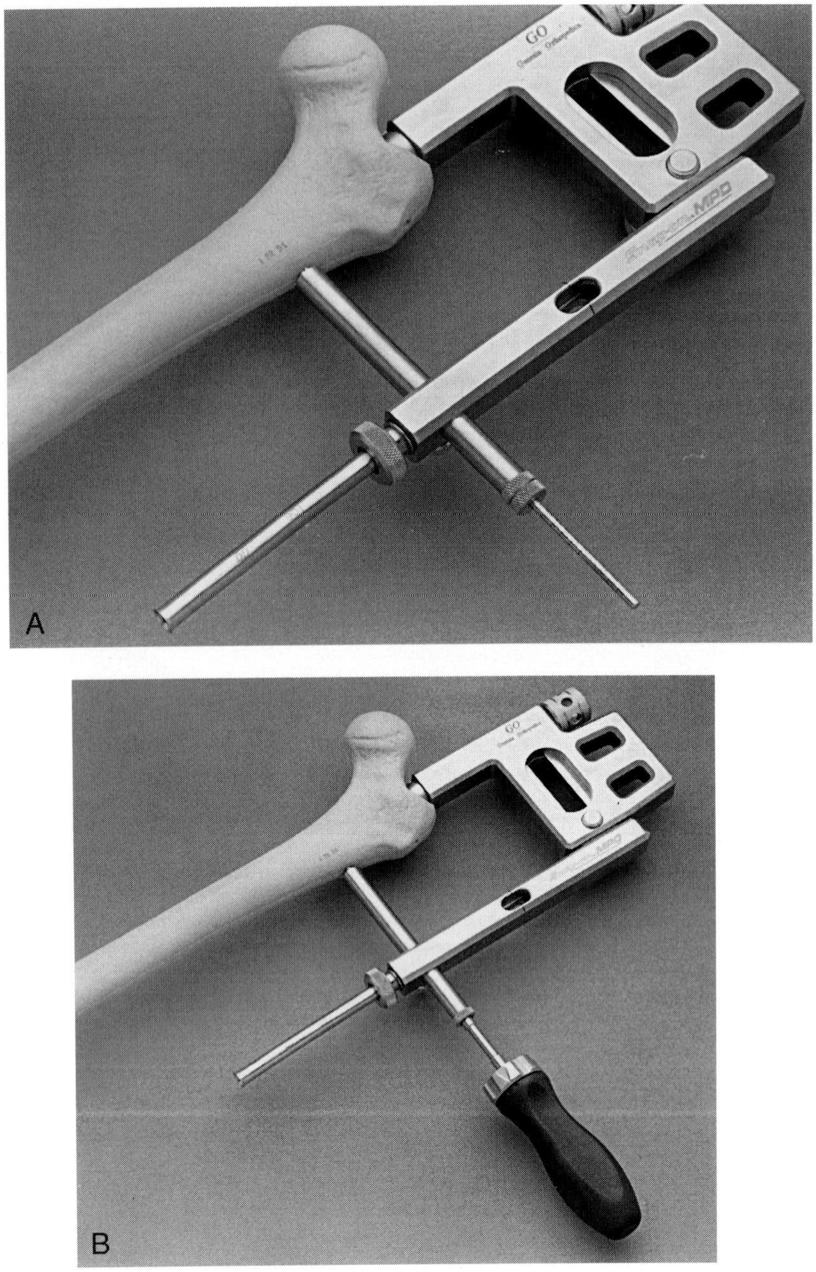

Fig. 21–24. *A*, The distal guide removed and the proximal hole drilled. *B*, Screw inserted through inner sleeve.

fractures. Two of those patients sustained fractures through metastatic lesions, and the third patient received a fracture through pagetoid bone. Two patients were treated for nonunions and both presented with broken Russell-Taylor nails. The first nonunion patient had been treated by a nail interlocked in the dynamic mode and the fracture site had been extensively opened. The second nonunion patient was treated with a nail interlocked in the static mode with the fracture distracted. Both patients were treated with closed extraction of the broken nail, reaming, bone grafting delivered through a chest tube, and insertion of SG nails. The 7 open fractures all resulted from gunshot wounds and were all comminuted. The remaining 17 fractures were either above the isthmus, below the isthmus, or were unstable

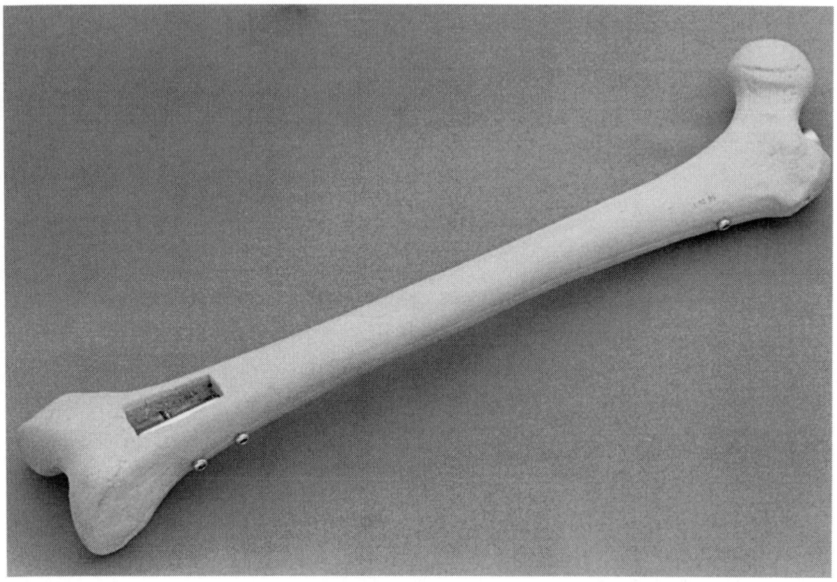

Fig. 21–25. Both ends interlocked.

through comminution or had an unstable configuration. Because the study only included fractures that were unstable, all the fractures were treated with static interlocking.

The total operative time for the first 8 patients averaged 141 minutes, of which distal targeting averaged 20 minutes. In the ensuing 21 patients, the total operative time averaged 85 minutes, of which 17 minutes were used for distal targeting. These results compare favorably to the 151 minutes of average procedure time published by Sanders (Fig. 21–26).[33]

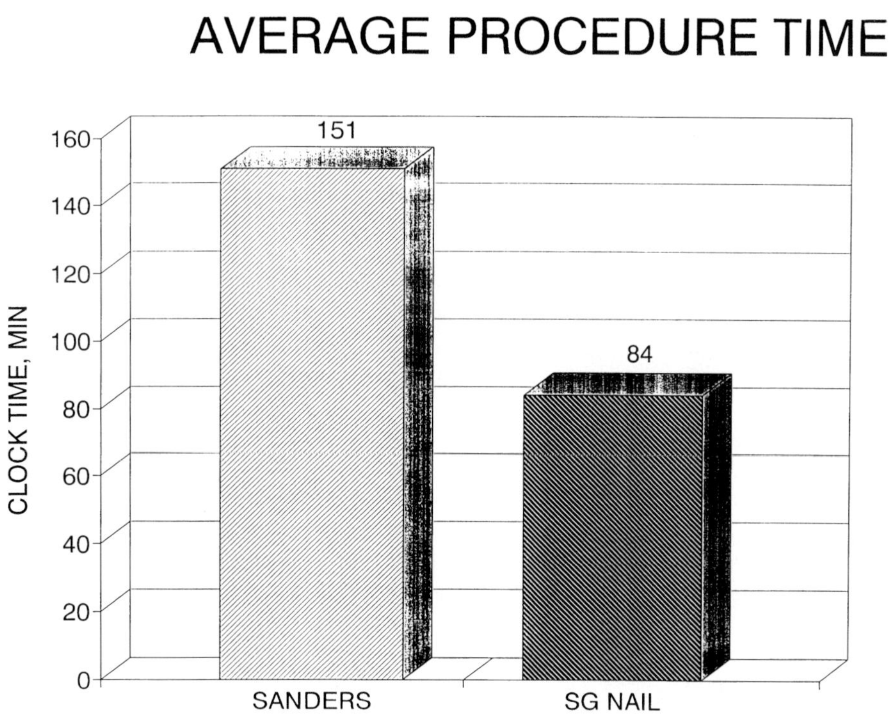

Fig. 21–26. Average procedure time.

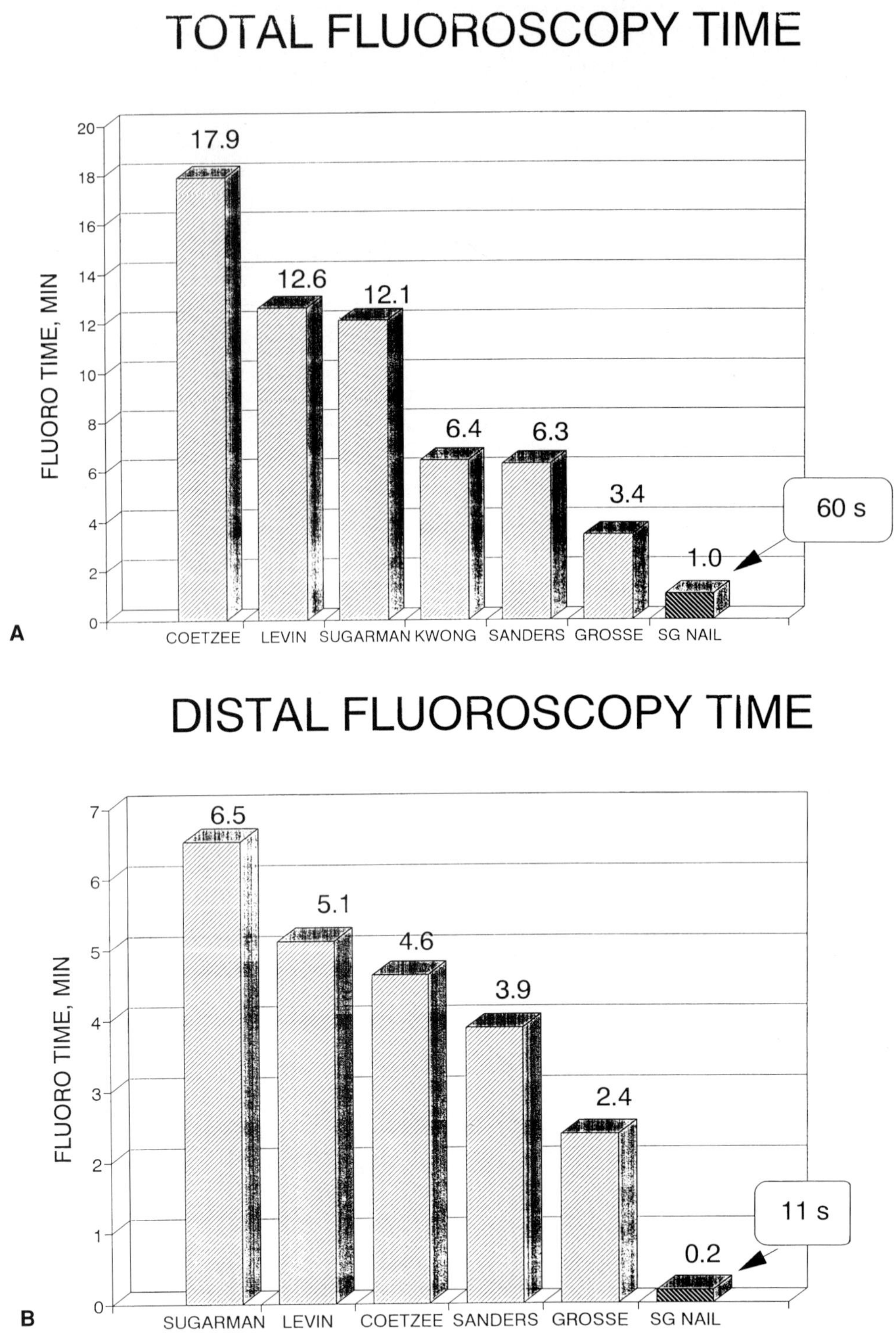

Fig. 21–27. *A*, Total fluoroscopy time. *B*, Distal fluoroscopy time.

The total fluoroscopy time for the first 8 patients was 172 seconds, while the fluoroscopy time for the remaining patients was 60 seconds. Distal targeting averaged 35 seconds for the first 8 patients and 11 seconds for the remaining 20 patients. The results obtained in this study when compared to those published by various investigators reveal a substantial diminution in both total and distal fluoroscopic times (Fig. 21–27).

Postoperative Complications

Difficulties encountered with the SG nail system have been mostly associated with the initial design. Initial targeting difficulties resulted in missed drill holes and screw placement. Additionally, two 4.5-mm screws bent with weight bearing. With the subsequent modifications made to the system, as used in the latter 21 patients, no additional targeting problems were experienced. Because a larger-diameter distal screw has been used, no other screw failures have been noted.

The complications associated with interlocking intramedullary nailing have been infrequent. Knowledge of the following general complications, applicable to all nailings and their management, is essential to the trauma surgeon.

Infection

The incidence of postoperative infection after intramedullary nailing has been reduced to less than 1% with the closed technique.[3,47,50,54,55] Clinical manifestations of infection include pyrexia, increased pain, swelling, redness, induration, or a draining sinus. Once infection is suspected, complete blood counts and sedimentation rates are obtained. Gram stains, cultures of the drainage, radiographs, and scanning studies may aid in the diagnosis.

Once the diagnosis is established, infection is managed by debridement, irrigation, sequestrectomy, and parenteral antibiotics. Implantation of antibiotic-impregnated cement beads has also been advocated.[56] Nails that continue to provide stable fixation of the fracture are not removed. Those nails not providing rigid fixation should be removed, the canal reamed, and a larger nail inserted. In cases of overwhelming infection, it may be necessary to leave the nail out and manage the fracture with external fixation.

Delayed Union and Nonunion

Investigators have generally agreed that a fractured femur that is not healed in 26 weeks is considered a delayed union. Delayed union is managed by nail dynamization in fractures that are treated by static interlocking, but only when the fracture has reached a point of consolidation so as not to risk malrotation or shortening. Dynamization is achieved by removing the locking screws farthest from the fracture.

In cases where nonunion is established, the fracture is managed by removal of the nail and reaming to a larger diameter. Morsalized bone graft is delivered to the fracture site through a chest tube and a larger nail is inserted.

Malunion

Most malunions can be avoided by careful attention to detail. Geist suggested that angulation of more than 10° and shortening of more than 10 mm should be considered malunions.[57] Closed intramedullary osteotomy and nailing are particularly useful in cases of malrotation. Angular deformities often have to be managed by open osteotomy.[58]

Implant Failure

Excessive stresses on the nail or interlocking screws with premature weight bearing, delayed union, and nonunion can result in implant failure. Metal fatigue and breakage can also be seen in fractures that are too high or too low. If a bent nail cannot be straightened by manipulation and is not easily extractable, the surgeon may have to resort to transecting the nail and removing it in two halves. Broken nails are removed by a closed technique, and the fracture is managed as in cases of nonunion.[59]

Heterotopic Ossification

Even though moderate to severe myositis ossificans and heterotopic bone formation have been reported to occur in 20% to 30% of all nailings, they are rarely symptomatic.[23,60,61]

Nerve Injuries

Sciatic nerve palsy usually results from excessive traction, while injury to the femoral and pudendal nerves is often caused by pressure from the perineal post. Injury to all three nerves occurs with a frequency of 1 to 2%.[4,23,41,62,63]

CONCLUSIONS

With careful attention to preoperative planning and close adherence to the described surgical techniques, the outcome of interlocking intramedullary nailing should be quite favorable. In this initial limited study, the SG nail system has been found to provide a reliable method for simplifying distal targeting. As demonstrated by the clinical data presented, the reduction of total operative and fluoroscopic times has been substantial. The reduction of the use of the image intensifier for distal targeting has been reproducible and seems to have addressed the need for a technique that limits radiation exposure to both the patient and the surgeon.

REFERENCES

1. Tarr, R.R., Wiss, D.: The mechanics and biology of intramedullary fixation. Clin. Orthop. *212*:10–17, 1986.
2. Street, D.M.: One hundred fractures of the femur treated by means of the diamond-shaped medullary nail. J. Bone Joint Surg. *33A*:659–669, 1954.
3. Bohler, J.: Results in medullary nailing of 95 fresh fractures of the femur. J. Bone Joint Surg. *33A*:670–678, 1951.
4. Champoux, J.A., Chandler, R.W.: Closed versus open nailing of femoral shaft fractures. Orthop. Trans. *8*:406, 1984.
5. Johnson, K.D., Johnston, D.W., Parker, B.: Comminuted femoral shaft fractures: Treatment by roller traction, cerclage wires and an intramedullary nail, or an interlocking intramedullary nail. J. Bone Joint Surg. *66A*: 1222–1235, 1984.
6. Tscherne, H., Haas, N., Krettek, C.: Intramedullary nailing combined with cerclage wiring in the treatment of fractures of the femoral shaft. Clin. Orthop. *212*:62–67, 1986.
7. Wickstrom, J., Corban, M.S.: Intramedullary fixation for fractures of the femoral shaft: A study of complications in 298 operations. J. Trauma *7*:551–581, 1967.
8. Winquist, R.A., Hansen, S.T., Jr.: Comminuted fractures of the femoral shaft treated by intramedullary nailing. Orthop. Clin. North Am. *11*:633–648, 1980.
9. Chapman, M.W.: The role of intramedullary fixation in open fractures. Clin. Orthop. *212*:26–34, 1986.
10. Chapman, M.W., Pugh, G.A., Wood, L., Day, L.J., Bovill, E.G., Jr., Blackman, R.C.: Closed intramedullary nailing of femoral shaft fractures. Orthop. Trans. *6*:326, 1982.
11. Fedders, O.: Femoral shaft fractures treated with intramedullary nailing. Acta Orthop. Scand. *50*:104, 1979.
12. Green, S.A., Larson, M.J., Moore, T.J.: Chronic sepsis following intramedullary nailing of femoral fractures. J. Trauma *27*:52–57, 1987.
13. Schneider, M.: Closed intramedullary nailing of fractures of the femoral shaft: Historical, physiological, and biomechanical aspects. Instr. Course Lect. *27*: 88–90, 1978.
14. Zdravkovic, D., Damholt, V.: Quadriceps function indirect nailing of femoral shaft fractures. Acta Orthop. Scand. *49*:73–77, 1978.
15. Modny, M.T., Lewert, A.H.: Transfixion intramedullary nail. Orthop. Rev. *15*:55–60, 1986.
16. Huckstep, R.L.: The Huckstep intramedullary compression nail: Indications, technique, and results. Clin. Orthop. *212*:48–61, 1986.
17. Smith, H.: Medullary fixation of the femur. Radiology *61*:194–199, 1953.
18. Bankston, A.B., Keating, E.M., Saha, S., Engelhardt, J.A.: Biomechanical evaluation of intramedullary rods used in distal femoral shaft fractures. Orthop. Trans. *10*:389, 1986.
19. Bray, T.J.: Indications for locked intramedullary nailing. Techniques Orthop. *3*:9–13, 1988.
20. Kyle, R.F., Schauffhausen, J.M., Bechtold, J.E.: Biomechanical characteristics of interlocking femoral nails in the treatment of complex femoral fractures. Clin. Orthop. *267*:169–173, 1991.
21. Tencer, A.F., Johnson, K.D., Serman, M.C.: Biomechanical considerations in intramedullary nailing. Techniques Orthop. *3*:1–5, 1988.
22. Beaupre, G.S., Schneider, E., Perren, S.M.: Mathematical investigation of the failures of AO/ASIF intramedullary nails. Orthop. Trans. *8*:303–304, 1984.
23. Blumberg, K.D., Foster, W.C., Blumberg, J.F., et. al: A comparison of the Brooker-Wills and Russell-Taylor nails for the treatment of patients who have fractures of the femoral shaft. J. Bone Joint Surg. *72A*:1019–1024, 1990.
24. Jenkins, N.H., Mintowt-Czyz, W.J., Draham, G.P., Jones, D.J.: New problems in old bones: Closed nailing of the shaft of the femur. Injury *18*:274–277, 1987.
25. Knudsen, K.J.M., Grobler, G.P., Close, R.E.W.: Intersecting the distal screws in a locked femoral nail. J. Bone Joint Surg. *73B*:660–661, 1991.
26. MacMillan, M., Grosse, R.H.: A simplified technique of distal screw intersection for the Grosse-Kempf interlocking nail. Clin. Orthop. *226*:252–259, 1988.
27. Pennig, D., Brug, E., Kronholz, H.L.: Operative technique: A new distal aiming device for locking nail fixation. Orthopedics *11*:1725–1727, 1988.
28. Rao, J.P., Allegra, L.P., Benevenia, J., Dauhajre, T.A.: Distal screw targeting of interlocking nails. Clin. Orthop. *238*:245–248, 1989.
29. Coetzee, J.G., Van Der Merwe, E.J.: Exposure of surgeons-in-training to radiation during intramedullary fixation of femoral shaft fractures. S. Afr. Med. J. *81*: 312–314, 1992.
30. Kempf, I., Grosse, A., Beck, G.: Closed locked intramedullary nailing. J. Bone Joint Surg. *67A*:709-720, 1985.
31. Kwong, L.M., Johanson, P.H., Zinar, D.M., et al.: Shielding of the patient's gonads during intramedullary interlocking femoral nailing. J. Bone Joint Surg. *72A*:1523–1526, 1990.
32. Levin, P.E., Schoen, R.W., Browner, B.D.: Radiational exposure to the surgeon during closed interlocking intramedullary nailing. J. Bone Joint Surg. *69A*:761–766, 1987.
33. Sanders, R., et al: Exposure of the orthopaedic surgeon to radiation. J. Bone Joint Surg. *75A*:326–330, 1993.
34. Sugarman, I.D., Adam, I., Bunker, T.D.: Radiation dosage during AO locking femoral nailing. Injury *19*: 336–338, 1988.

35. Barry, T.P.: Radiation exposure to an orthopaedic surgeon. Clin. Orthop. *182*:160–164, 1984.
36. Giachino, A.A., Cheng, M.: Irradiation of the surgeon during pinning of femoral fractures. J. Bone Joint Surg. *62B*:227–229, 1980.
37. Azer, S.N., Krause, W.R., Salman, N.N.: Self-guiding Interlocking Intramedullary Nail. Contemp. Orthop. *1*: 25–28, 1992.
38. Kinast, C., Wyder, H., Frigg, R., Perren, SM.: Biomechanical investigation of the proximal screw of interlocking nails. Orthop. Trans. *11*:295, 1987.
39. Swiontkowsky, M.F., Seiler, J.G. III: The AO/ASIF universal intramedullary nail. Techniques Orthop. *3*: 33–40, 1988.
40. Krause, W.R., Azer, S.N.: Design and evaluation of a new interlocking intramedullary nail. Paper. American Society for the study of Mechanical Engineering, Breckenridge CO, June 1993.
41. Winquist, R.A., Hansen, S.T., Jr., Clawson, D.K.: Closed intramedullary nailing of femoral fractures: A report of 520 cases. J. Bone Joint Surg. *66A*:529–538, 1984.
42. Majkowski, R.S., Baker, A.S.: Interlocking nails for femoral fractures: An initial experience. Injury *22*: 93–96, 1991.
43. Browner, B.D.: Pitfalls, errors, and complications in the use of locking Küntscher nails. Clin. Orthop. *212*: 192–208, 1986.
44. Rascher, J.J., Nahigian, S.H., Macys, J.R., Brown, J.E.: Closed nailing of femoral-shaft fractures. J. Bone Joint Surg. *54A*:534–544, 1972.
45. Stromsoe, K., Alho, A., Ekeland, A.: The Grosse-Kempf nail for distal femoral fractures. Acta Orthop. Scand. *61*:512–516, 1990.
46. Graham, G.P., Mackie, I.G.: Experience with the AO locked femoral nail. Injury *19*:249–253, 1988.
47. Hansen, S.T., Winquist, R.A.: Closed intramedullary nailing of the femur: Küntscher technique with reaming. Clin. Orthop. *138*:56–61, 1979.
48. Johnson, K.D., Tencer, A.F., Sherman, M.C.: Biomechanical factors affecting fracture stability and femoral bursting in closed intramedullary nailing of femoral shaft fractures, with illustrative case presentations. J. Orthop. Trauma *1*:1–11, 1987.
49. Brooker, A.F., Jr.: Brooker-Wills nailing of femoral shaft fractures. Techniques Orthop. *3*:41, 1988.
50. Clawson, D.K., Smith, R.F., Hansen, S.T.: Closed intramedullary nailing of the femur. J. Bone Joint Surg. *53A*:681–692, 1971.
51. Veith, R.G., Hansen, S.T., Jr.: Closed intramedullary nailing of femoral-shaft fractures following reaming: Technique and rationale. Contemp. Orthop. *4*:41–49, 1982.
52. Henry, S.L., Adcock, R.A., von Fraunhoffer, J.A., Selgison, D.: Heat of intramedullary nailing. South. Med. J. *80*:173–176, 1987.
53. Christensen, N.O.: Technique, errors and safeguards in modern Küntscher nailing. Clin. Orthop. *15*:182–188, 1976.
54. Brumback, R.J., Lakatos, R.P., Garbarino, J.L., Poka, A., Burgess, A.R.: Risks of infection with reamed intramedullary femoral fixation in multiple trauma. Orthop. Trans. *11*:490, 1987.
55. Chapman, M.W., Mahoney, M.: The role of internal fixation in the management of open fractures. Clin. Orthop. *138*:120–131, 1979.
56. Patzakis, M.J., Wilkins, J., Wiss, D.: Infection following intramedullary nailing of long bones: Diagnosis and management. Clin. Orthop. *212*:182–191, 1986.
57. Geist, R.W., Laros, G.S.: Femoral shaft fractures: Editorial comment and comparative results. Clin. Orthop. *138*:5–9, 1979.
58. Winquist, R.A.: Closed intramedullary osteotomies of the femur. Clin. Orthop. *212*:155–164, 1986.
59. Kayvanfar, J.F., Azer, S.N., Kim, D.D.: Retrieval of a broken femoral intramedullary nail using a closed technique. Contemp. Orthop. *28*:219–222, 1994.
60. Brumback, R.J., Wells, J.D., Lakatos, R., Poka, A., Bathon, G.H., Burgess, A.R.: Heterotopic ossification about the hip after intramedullary nailing for fractures of the femur. J. Bone Joint Surg. *72A*:1067–1073, 1990.
61. Marks, P.H., Paley, D.R., Kellam, J.F.: Heterotopic ossification around the hip with intramedullary nailing of the femur. J. Trauma *28*:1207–1213, 1988.
62. Seiler, J.G., Swiontkowski, M.F.: A prospective evaluation of the AO/ASIF universal femoral nail in the treatment of traumatic and reconstructive problems of the femur. J. Trauma *31*:121–126, 1991.
63. Wiss, D.A., Brien, W.W., Stenson, W.B.: Interlocking nailing for the treatment of segmental fractures of the femur. J. Bone Joint Surg. *72A*:724–728, 1990.

Index

Page numbers in *italics* indicate figures; page numbers followed by a "t" indicate tables.